Netter's
Orthopaedics

Other Netter titles include:

The Atlas of Human Anatomy

Netter's Anatomy Flash Cards

Netter's Concise Atlas of Orthopaedic Anatomy

Netter's Orthopaedics

Edited by

Walter B. Greene, MD

OrthoCarolina
Charlotte, North Carolina

Illustrations by Frank H. Netter, MD

Contributing Illustrators
Charles Boyter
John A. Craig, MD
Carlos A. G. Machado, MD
David Mascaro, MS
Mark Miller

SAUNDERS
ELSEVIER

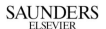

SAUNDERS
ELSEVIER

Elsevier Inc.
1600 John F. Kennedy Boulevard
Suite 1800
Philadelphia, PA 19103-2899

Netter's Orthopaedics
First Edition

ISBN-13: 978-1-929007-02-8
ISBN-10: 1-929007-02-7

NOTICE

Medicine is an ever-changing field. Standard safety precautions must be followed, but as new research and clinical experience broaden our knowledge, changes in treatment and drug therapy may become necessary or appropriate. Readers are advised to check the most current information provided by the manufacturer of each drug to be administered to verify the recommended dose, the method and duration of administration, and contraindications. It is the responsibility of the licensed health care provider, relying on experience and knowledge of the patient, to determine dosages and the best treatment for each individual patient. Neither the publisher nor the editor assumes any liability for any injury and/or damage to persons or property arising from this publication.

The Publisher

Library of Congress Catalog No.: 2001132798

Publishing Director: Linda Belfus
Executive Editor: Paul Kelly
Associate Editor: Marybeth Thiel
Art Director: Jonathan Dimes
Digital Asset Manager: Karen Oswald

Printed in China

Last digit is the print number: 10   9   8   7   6   5   4   3   2

To the many teachers, colleagues, and students who, by sharing their knowledge and enthusiasm for learning, provide ongoing stimulus for me and other practitioners to further our understanding of the amazing function and structure of the musculoskeletal system and the treatment of its disorders.

To the many highly respected medical school, residency, and fellowship teachers who kindled my ongoing love for the medical profession.

To Dr. Christian Siewers, an orthopaedic surgeon in my hometown whose patient response to my many queries and "hands-on" introduction to therapeutic procedures when I worked as an orderly in the emergency room sparked my initial interest in orthopaedic surgery.

To Dr. Charles W. Hooker, former chairman of Anatomy at the University of North Carolina, who was a great teacher and an ongoing role model in the joy of continued learning in many spheres and the correlation of structure with function and basic science with clinical medicine.

To Dr. Frank C. Wilson, chairman emeritus of Orthopaedic Surgery at the University of North Carolina and an internationally renowned orthopaedic educator, who has provided ongoing inspiration and mentoring which began when a nervous first-year medical student inquired about the possibilities of a summertime research project.

Table of Contents

Preface

Netter's Orthopaedics is an essential text on the pathophysiology, diagnosis, and treatment of musculoskeletal disorders. The need for such a book results from the commonality of these disorders, which are second only to respiratory illnesses as a reason that patients seek medical care, and their diversity, in that they comprise everything from injuries and infections to metabolic and neoplastic diseases.

Patients with conditions affecting the musculoskeletal system present in many settings, requiring that virtually all health care providers be familiar with the diagnosis and treatment of these disorders. This book, therefore, is intended for use by the many clinicians who will see these patients—students in medicine, physical therapy, and osteopathy, and residents in primary care, orthopaedics, family practice, and emergency medicine.

The first 12 chapters of *Netter's Orthopaedics* are concerned with topics related to the entire musculoskeletal system, and provide principles that can be applied to the management of many disorders. The final 7 chapters are organized by region, and offer techniques of diagnosis and treatment specific to each region. Given the widely different backgrounds of the anticipated readers of this book, we have tried throughout to make the text as accessible as possible, presenting practical information in a clear and straightforward manner.

Although the multiplicity and variety of musculoskeletal disorders may make learning this subject seem daunting, an understanding of the anatomy and basic science pertaining to the musculoskeletal system, combined with fundamental principles of evaluation and treatment, can guide most diagnostic and therapeutic interventions. Therefore, each chapter of this text begins with relevant basic science to lay the foundation for understanding the pathophysiology, diagnosis, and treatment of the clinical conditions. Because knowledge of anatomy is crucial to the evaluation and treatment of musculoskeletal conditions, this component of basic science has received particular emphasis.

All of the authors owe a great debt to Frank H. Netter, MD, the medical illustrator who created the majority of the illustrations in this book. Dr. Netter's legacy, and his importance in medical education, cannot be overstated. Through his art, Dr. Netter has been a mentor to thousands of physicians and allied health professionals. His precise and beautifully rendered depictions of the human body in health and illness communicate, as no writer can, the essential concepts of basic science and applied medicine that every student must learn. It was Dr. Netter's belief that a medical illustration is of little value if it does not provide the student with an essential point that has application in the practice of medicine. Examination of any of Dr. Netter's works in this book will demonstrate his dedication to that principle.

Although much of Dr. Netter's work is just as relevant today as it was when he created it, new techniques and procedures developed since his death in 1991 have caused us to call upon the talents of his successors, particularly John A. Craig, MD, and Carlos A. G. Machado, MD. As will be seen from their work, these artists, trained in the Netter tradition, faithfully uphold the high standards that Dr. Netter set.

The authors and illustrators hope that *Netter's Orthopaedics* will be a valuable resource for the many individuals who care for patients with these often complex and challenging conditions.

Walter B. Greene, MD

Acknowledgments

I would like to acknowledge the staff at Saunders who worked on this book and, in particular, Paul Kelly and Greg Otis who coordinated the development of this project, Jennifer Surich who managed the editorial process, Jonathan Dimes who directed the art program, and Marybeth Thiel for providing assistance and support throughout all stages of the project. I would also like to thank Mary Berry, development editor. Their extraordinary patience and skills were pivotal in this publication.

List of Contributing Authors

Walter B. Greene, MD
OrthoCarolina
Charlotte, NC

Roy K. Aaron, MD
Professor
Department of Orthopaedics
Brown University School of Medicine
Providence, RI

Jeffrey O. Anglen, MD, FACS
Professor and Chairman
Department of Orthopaedics
Indiana University
Indianapolis, IN

Judith F. Baumhauer, MD
Professor of Orthopaedics, Chief of Division
    of Foot and Ankle Surgery
Department of Orthopaedics
University of Rochester School of Medicine
    and Dentistry
Rochester, NY

Philip M. Bernini, MD
Professor of Orthopaedic Surgery
Department of Orthopaedics
Dartmouth-Hitchcock Medical Center
Lebanon, NH

Eric M. Bluman, MD, PhD
Assistant Clinical Instructor
Department of Orthopaedic Surgery
Brown University School of Medicine
Providence, RI

Susan V. Bukata, MD
Orthopaedic Research Fellow
Department of Orthopaedics
University of Rochester Medical School
Rochester, NY

Michael G. Ehrlich, MD
Vincent Zecchino Professor and Chairman
Department of Orthopaedics
Brown University School of Medicine
Providence, RI

Derrick J. Fluhme, MD
Associate Partner
South Hills Orthopaedic Surgical Associates
St. Clair Hospital
Pittsburgh, PA

Freddie H. Fu, MD
David Silver Professor and Chairman
Department of Orthopaedic Surgery
University of Pittsburgh School of Medicine
Pittsburgh, PA

Barry J. Gainor, MD
Professor
Department of Orthopaedic Surgery
University of Missouri Hospital and Clinics
Columbia, MO

Lawrence C. Hurst, MD
Professor and Chairman
Department of Orthopaedic Surgery
Stony Brook University
Stony Brook, NY

Lee D. Kaplan, MD
Assistant Professor
Department of Orthopaedics
University of Wisconsin
Madison, WI

Keith Kenter, MD
Assistant Professor and Director of Resident
    Education
Department of Orthopaedic Surgery
University of Cincinnati
Cincinnati, OH

John D. Lubahn, MD
Department Chair
Program Director
Department of Orthopaedics
Hamot Medical Center
Erie, PA

Vincent D. Pellegrini Jr., MD
James L. Kernan Professor and Chair
Department of Orthopaedics
University of Maryland School of Medicine
Baltimore, MD

Michael S. Pinzur, MD
Professor of Orthopaedic Surgery and
    Rehabilitation
Department of Orthopaedic Surgery and
    Rehabilitation
Loyola University Medical Center
Maywood, IL

David T. Rispler, MD
Assistant Professor
River Valley Orthopaedics
Michigan State University
Grand Rapids, MI

Randy N. Rosier, MD, PhD
Wehle Professor and Chair
Department of Orthopaedics
University of Rochester Medical School
Rochester, NY

Peter G. Trafton, MD, FACS
Professor and Vice Chairman
Department of Orthopaedic Surgery
Brown University School of Medicine
Providence, RI

Edward D. Wang, MD
Assistant Professor
Department of Orthopaedic Surgery
Stony Brook University Hospital and Health
    Sciences Center
Stony Brook, NY

D. Patrick Williams, DO
Clinical Professor
Orthopaedic Residency Program
Hamot Medical Center
Erie, PA

David J. Zaleske, MD
Surgical Director, Orthopaedics
Department of Orthopaedics
Children's Hospitals and Clinics
Minneapolis and St. Paul, MN

Netter's
Orthopaedics

Embryology and Formation of Bone

David J. Zaleske, MD

An understanding of embryology facilitates the study of postnatal anatomy and the treatment of patients with congenital malformations. Furthermore, as research elucidates the fascinating but complex embryologic process, it has become clear that many genes and transcription factors involved in movement from the genome to a three-dimensional organism are phylogenetically conserved. This complex and highly interactive process includes normal cytodifferentiation and morphogenesis, and it is recapitulated, at least in part, in the healing of injuries. (*Note:* Bone is the only tissue that regenerates completely after injury [fracture].) A better understanding of development should allow more precise treatment of many illnesses and, ultimately, tissue engineering with regeneration of specific organs.

CELL DIVISION AND THE MAIN EMBRYONIC PERIOD

The 9 months of prenatal human development can be divided into a period of cell division (weeks 1 and 2), a main embryonic period (weeks 3 to 8), and a fetal period (encompassing the last 7 months). Approximately 60 hours after fertilization, the *zygote* has progressed to a *morula* ("little mulberry"), a ball of cells that continues cell division as it travels through the uterine tube to the uterine cavity; it transitions to the fluid-filled *blastocyst* at approximately day 5. The blastocyst develops an inner cell mass (embryoblast) and an outer trophoblast as it adheres and then is implanted within the posterior wall of the endometrium of the uterus. By the end of week 2, the embryo is a two-layered cell disc of *endoderm* and *ectoderm* (**Figure 1-1**).

The embryonic period progresses from gastrulation to folding of the embryonic disc and eventual formation of the primordia of all organ systems. It is a very dynamic period of development and morphogenesis, in which masses of cells coalesce, migrate, and remodel (programmed cell death is included). Because this is the most active phase of differentiation, abnormalities of development that occur in the embryonic period usually result in major birth defects. The cardiovascular system is the first organ system to function at day 21/22. At that time, the embryo is too large for diffusion to satisfy the nutritional needs of the embryo.

Gastrulation is the production of mesoderm during the third week that changes the bilaminar embryonic disc into a trilaminar disc (gastrula). *Mesoderm* develops from two thickenings of ectoderm. The primitive knot (node) forms a midline cord of mesoderm, known as the *notochord*. This primitive streak gives rise to the rest of the mesoderm, including the cardiogenic mesoderm, which separates and is located in front of the oropharyngeal membrane. Gastrulation is complete when the mesoderm condenses into three, initially connected columns that flank the notochord: the *paraxial columns* (future somites), the *intermediate mesoderm*, and the *lateral plates* (**Figure 1-2**). Mesoderm that surrounds the columns becomes mesenchyme, the loose embryonic connective tissue that surrounds structures.

Shaping of the embryo involves bending of the amnion around and under the gastrula (**Figure 1-3**). Concurrently, folding of the ectoderm initiates development of the nervous system, and *somites* in the paraxial mesoderm initiate development of the axial skeleton.

The gut is formed from a tube of endoderm. The lateral plate extends and splits to form the lining of the coelomic cavities. The superior portion of the lateral plate joins with the surface ectoderm to form the ventrolateral body wall **somatopleure**, which ultimately develops into the skin, connective tissue, striated muscle, and bone in the limbs and some parts of the body wall. The inferior portion of the lateral plate joins with the endoderm to form the **splanchnopleure**, which forms the walls of visceral organs and their suspending mesenteries.

The mesodermal notochord and the paraxial columns induce ectodermal tissue to form the *neural plate*, thus beginning the process of

Figure 1-1: Cell Division: The First Two Weeks

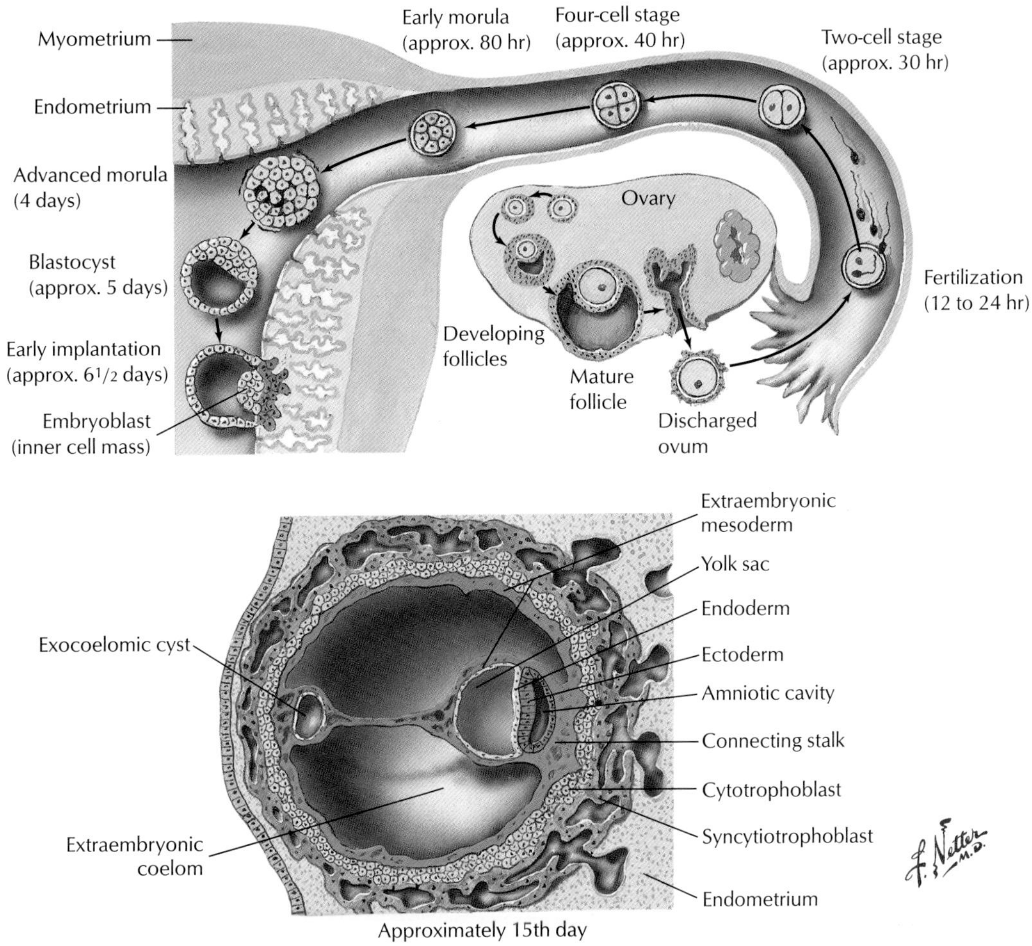

Myometrium

Endometrium

Advanced morula
(4 days)

Blastocyst
(approx. 5 days)

Early implantation
(approx. 6½ days)

Embryoblast
(inner cell mass)

Early morula
(approx. 80 hr)

Four-cell stage
(approx. 40 hr)

Two-cell stage
(approx. 30 hr)

Ovary

Developing
follicles

Mature
follicle

Discharged
ovum

Fertilization
(12 to 24 hr)

Exocoelomic cyst

Extraembryonic
coelom

Extraembryonic
mesoderm

Yolk sac

Endoderm

Ectoderm

Amniotic cavity

Connecting stalk

Cytotrophoblast

Syncytiotrophoblast

Endometrium

Approximately 15th day

neurulation; this plate then folds and invaginates to form the *neural tube*. Closure of the neural tube advances cranially and caudally. As the neural tube invaginates, ectodermal neural crest cells from each side are joined together. Later, some neural crest cells migrate to form other tissues (**Tables 1-1** and **1-2**).

HUMAN AXIAL SKELETAL EMBRYOLOGY

The axial skeleton includes the vertebrae, ribs, and sternum. Its development is initiated by paired condensations in the paraxial mesoderm—the *somites*. Each somite differentiates into a *sclerotome* and a *dermomyotome*. The sclerotomes separate and migrate around the neural tube and notochord into the somatopleure. Bone development of the axial skeleton begins with mesenchymal condensations in the sclerotome. Cells from the mesenchymal primordia differentiate into chondroblasts, which become the cartilaginous precursors of the axial skeleton and bones at the base of the cranium (**Figure 1-4**). Enchondral ossification converts these cartilage templates into various bones. Most bones of the skull and part of the clavicle develop through *intramembranous (mesenchymal) ossification* with direct formation of bone in mesenchyme derived from the neural crest.

At each level, the somites migrate ventrally to incorporate the notochord and dorsally to

Figure 1-2: Gastrulation

Formation of Intraembryonic Mesoderm from the Primitive Streak and Node (Knot)

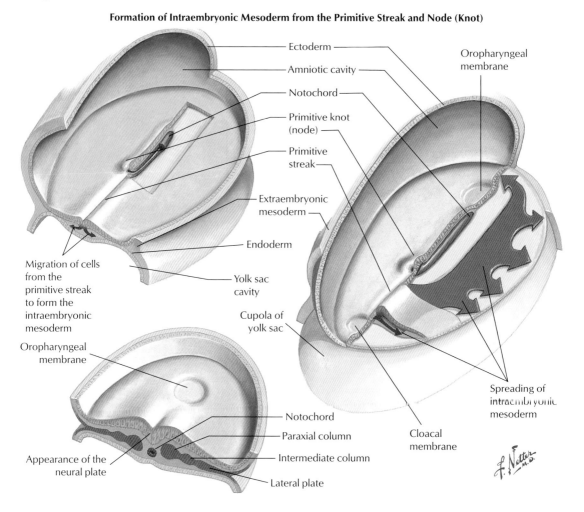

Ectoderm

Amniotic cavity

Oropharyngeal membrane

Notochord

Primitive knot (node)

Primitive streak

Extraembryonic mesoderm

Endoderm

Migration of cells from the primitive streak to form the intraembryonic mesoderm

Yolk sac cavity

Cupola of yolk sac

Oropharyngeal membrane

Spreading of intraembryonic mesoderm

Cloacal membrane

Notochord

Paraxial column

Intermediate column

Appearance of the neural plate

Lateral plate

cover the neural tube. The precursors of the axial skeleton have formed by the fourth embryonic week. Somites undergo rearrangement by division into superior and inferior halves; then, adjacent superior and inferior halves join together to form single vertebral bones (**Figure 1-5**). Thus, the vertebral arteries are relocated to the middle of the vertebral body.

Vertebral bodies, the posterior bony arch, and vertebral processes have a similar pattern of formation with various dimensions and nuances (refer to **Figures 13-2** and **13-4** in Chapter 13). Development of C1 (atlas) differs from that of C2 (axis) in that the body (cen-

trum) of the atlas fuses to the C2 body and becomes the odontoid process (dens). Parts of the somites may fail to segment, migrate, or rejoin appropriately. This failure is the basis for congenital scoliosis, which may be associated with rib fusion at single or multiple levels (see Chapter 13).

Skeletal Muscle and Peripheral Nerve Embryology

Similar to the somites, *myotomes* are paired and segmented. Each segmental myotome is innervated by a spinal nerve. The dermatomes divide into an **epimere**—the small dorsal segment—and a **hypomere**—

Figure 1-3: Folding of the Gastrula and Early Development of the Nervous System

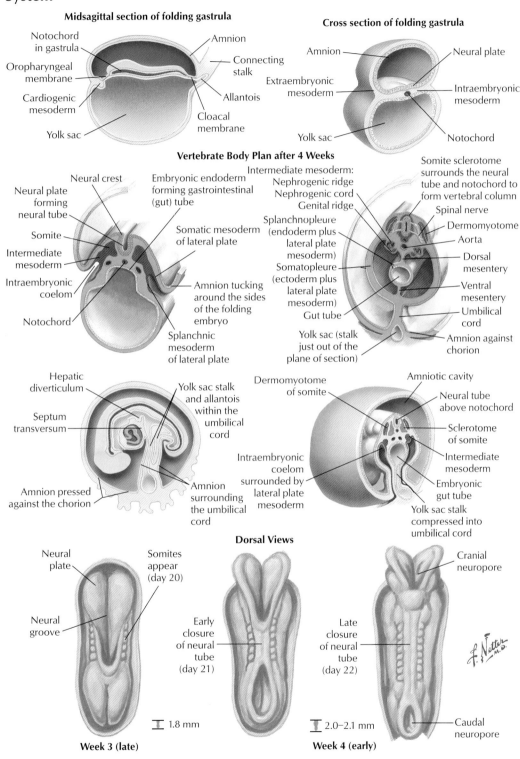

Midsagittal section of folding gastrula

Notochord in gastrula

Amnion

Oropharyngeal membrane

Connecting stalk

Cardiogenic mesoderm

Allantois

Yolk sac

Cloacal membrane

Cross section of folding gastrula

Amnion

Neural plate

Extraembryonic mesoderm

Intraembryonic mesoderm

Yolk sac

Notochord

Vertebrate Body Plan after 4 Weeks

Neural crest

Embryonic endoderm forming gastrointestinal (gut) tube

Intermediate mesoderm:
Nephrogenic ridge
Nephrogenic cord
Genital ridge

Somite sclerotome surrounds the neural tube and notochord to form vertebral column

Neural plate forming neural tube

Somite

Intermediate mesoderm

Intraembryonic coelom

Notochord

Somatic mesoderm of lateral plate

Amnion tucking around the sides of the folding embryo

Splanchnic mesoderm of lateral plate

Splanchnopleure (endoderm plus lateral plate mesoderm)

Somatopleure (ectoderm plus lateral plate mesoderm)

Gut tube

Yolk sac (stalk just out of the plane of section)

Spinal nerve

Dermomyotome

Aorta

Dorsal mesentery

Ventral mesentery

Umbilical cord

Amnion against chorion

Hepatic diverticulum

Yolk sac stalk and allantois within the umbilical cord

Septum transversum

Amnion pressed against the chorion

Amnion surrounding the umbilical cord

Dermomyotome of somite

Intraembryonic coelom surrounded by lateral plate mesoderm

Amniotic cavity

Neural tube above notochord

Sclerotome of somite

Intermediate mesoderm

Embryonic gut tube

Yolk sac stalk compressed into umbilical cord

Dorsal Views

Neural plate

Somites appear (day 20)

Cranial neuropore

Neural groove

Early closure of neural tube (day 21)

Late closure of neural tube (day 22)

Caudal neuropore

1.8 mm

2.0–2.1 mm

Week 3 (late)

Week 4 (early)

Table 1-1 **Ectodermal Derivatives**	
Primordia	**Derivatives**
Surface ectoderm	Skin epidermis
	Sweat, sebaceous, and mammary glands
	Nails and hair
	Tooth enamel
	Lacrimal glands
	Conjunctiva
	External auditory meatus
	Oral and nasal epithelium
	Anterior pituitary
	Inner ear
	Lens of eye
Neural tube	Central nervous system, including cranial nerves
	Retina/optic nerves
	Posterior pituitary
	Spinal cord, including lower motor neurons and presynaptic autonomic neurons with associated axons
Neural crest	Ganglia and sensory neurons associated with spinal dorsal root and cranial nerves
	Adrenal medulla cells
	Melanocytes
	Bone, muscle, and connective tissue in the head and neck
Amnion	Protective bag (with chorion) around the fetus

Table 1-2 **Mesodermal Derivatives**	
Primordia	**Derivatives**
Notochord	Induction of neurulation
	Intervetebral disc nucleus pulposus
Paraxial column	
Somites	Bone and cartilage
Myotome	Skeletal muscle
Dermatome	Dermis of the skin
Intermediate mesoderm	Gonads
	Kidneys and ureters
	Uterus and uterine tubes
	Upper vagina
	Ductus deferens, epididymis, and related tubules
	Seminal vesicles and ejaculatory ducts
Lateral plate mesoderm	Dermis (ventral)
	Superficial fascia and related tissues (ventral)
	Bones and connective tissues of limbs
	Pleura and mesoderm
	GI connective tissue stroma
Cardiogenic mesoderm	Heart and pericardium

the larger ventral segment. The epimere is innervated by the dorsal ramus of a spinal nerve, and the hypomere is innervated by the ventral ramus.

The epimere is the site of origin of the intrinsic back muscles (ie, splenius group, erector spinae, transversospinalis group). The hypomere gives rise to the lateral and ventral trunk wall muscles, as well as to muscles of the limbs. Myotomes fuse to form individual muscles; therefore, most muscles are innervated by more than one spinal nerve root. Back and abdominal muscles are innervated by multiple spinal nerves, whereas the brachial and lumbosacral plexuses combine multiple spinal nerves into single peripheral nerves that innervate the limb muscles. Limb muscles are divided into (1) ventral extensor compartment muscle groups innervated by anterior division branches of the ventral rami in the brachial and lumbosacral plexus, and (2) dorsal flexor compartment muscle groups innervated by posterior division branches of the ventral rami (**Figure 1-6**).

Figure 1-4: Myotomes, Dermatomes, and Sclerotomes

Differentiation of somites into myotomes, sclerotomes, and dermatomes
Cross section of human embryos

A. At 19 days

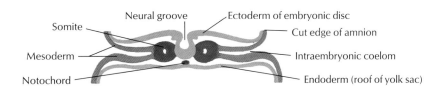

Somite — Neural groove — Ectoderm of embryonic disc
— Cut edge of amnion
Mesoderm — — Intraembryonic coelom
Notochord — — Endoderm (roof of yolk sac)

B. At 22 days

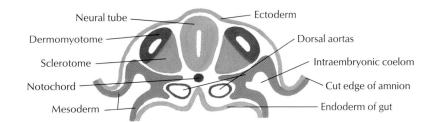

Neural tube — — Ectoderm
Dermomyotome — — Dorsal aortas
Sclerotome — — Intraembryonic coelom
Notochord — — Cut edge of amnion
Mesoderm — — Endoderm of gut

C. At 27 days

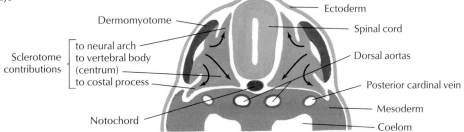

Dermomyotome — — Ectoderm
— Spinal cord
Sclerotome contributions: to neural arch / to vertebral body (centrum) / to costal process
— Dorsal aortas
— Posterior cardinal vein
— Mesoderm
Notochord — — Coelom

D. At 30 days

Note: Sections A, B, and C are at level of future vertebral body, but section D is at level between developing bodies

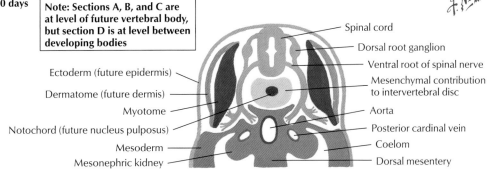

— Spinal cord
— Dorsal root ganglion
— Ventral root of spinal nerve
Ectoderm (future epidermis) — — Mesenchymal contribution to intervertebral disc
Dermatome (future dermis) —
Myotome — — Aorta
Notochord (future nucleus pulposus) — — Posterior cardinal vein
Mesoderm — — Coelom
Mesonephric kidney — — Dorsal mesentery

Figure 1-5: Muscle and Vertebral Column Segmentation

Progressive stages in formation of vertebral column, dermatomes, and myotomes

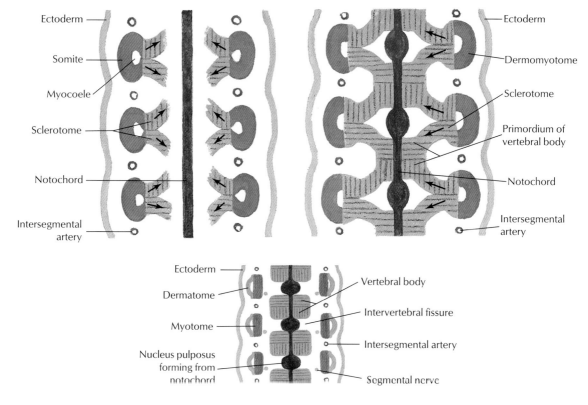

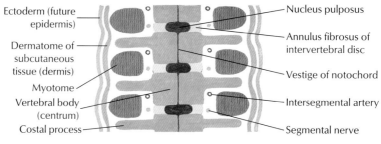

Appendicular Skeletal Embryology

Limb development begins as outpouchings (paddle-like extensions) from the **somatopleure ventrolateral body wall** that appear during the early part of the fifth embryonic week. The limb somatopleure mesenchyme is capped by the **apical ectodermal ridge**. Upper limb bud mesenchymal condensations appear 1 to 2 days before the lower limb buds appear, and morphogenesis of the upper limb continues to progress slightly ahead of lower limb development. Blood vessels develop in the limb buds early and before the development of bone or nerves. During the sixth week of gestation, the distal portion of the limb bud becomes paddle-like, with indentations and rays that ultimately develop into the digits of the hands and feet.

Mesenchymal condensations are initially continuous in the extremities. Interzonal re-

Figure 1-6: Development of Epimere and Hypomere Muscle Groups and Their Nerve Innervation

Somatic development

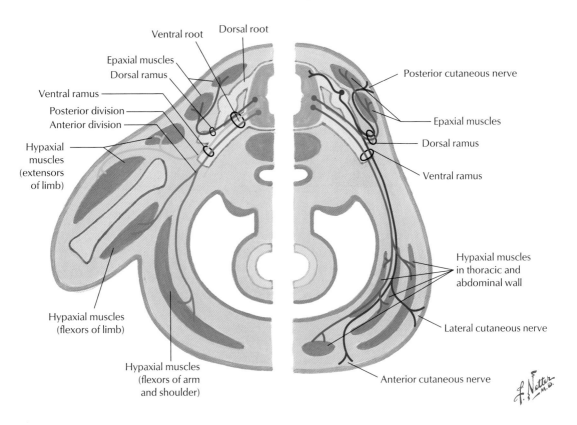

gions form between these condensations. These interzonal regions cavitate to form joints (**Figure 1-7**). Articular cartilage and intra-articular structures such as ligaments and menisci are formed from interzonal tissue.

The upper and lower limb buds rotate in opposite directions during development (**Figure 1-8**). Therefore, segmental dermatomes within the limbs also rotate and are not organized in the proximal-to-distal linear arrangement found along the trunk.

Descriptive embryology at the tissue level is increasingly elucidated at the molecular level (see **Figure 1-9**). Interaction of transcription factors, growth and inductive factors, and adhesion molecules establishes the information blueprint for bone and joint morpho-

genesis and cytodifferentiation. Specific portions of the limb bud direct this process. The *zone of polarizing activity* (ZPA), an area of mesenchymal cells located at the caudal aspect of each limb bud, directs patterning along the anteroposterior axis (anterior refers to the thumb side and posterior is the little finger) by a gradient of the gene *Sonic hedgehog* (*Shh*). Transcription molecules *Wnt7a* and *Lmx-1* are necessary for dorsoventral patterning. Proteins such as *syndecan-3, tenascin,* and *versican* mediate the formation of the mesenchymal condensations and their transformation to cartilage. *Core binding factor 1* (*Cbfa1*) and *Indian hedgehog* (*Ihh*) are involved in the cartilage maturation process leading to endochondral ossification.

Figure 1-7: Joint Development

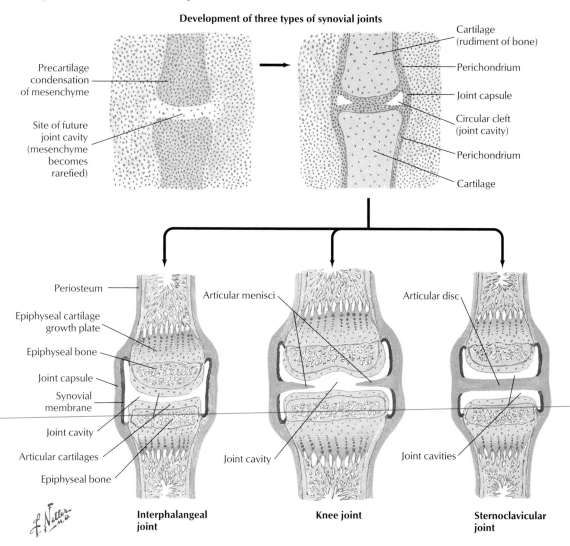

Development of three types of synovial joints

Precartilage condensation of mesenchyme

Site of future joint cavity (mesenchyme becomes rarefied)

Cartilage (rudiment of bone)

Perichondrium

Joint capsule

Circular cleft (joint cavity)

Perichondrium

Cartilage

Periosteum

Epiphyseal cartilage growth plate

Epiphyseal bone

Joint capsule

Synovial membrane

Joint cavity

Articular cartilages

Epiphyseal bone

Articular menisci

Joint cavity

Articular disc

Joint cavities

Interphalangeal joint

Knee joint

Sternoclavicular joint

Bone Formation

The term *bone* has two common meanings: (1) it may refer to osseous, or bone, tissue; or (2) it may denote an organ, such as the femoral bone.

At the end of the embryonic period and the beginning of the fetal period, the mesenchymal precursors of the skeleton begin to form osseous tissue through two methods. With *intramembranous formation*, the mesenchymal connective tissue of the neural crest condenses under the influence of specific signals.

Endothelial cells invade the condensation to form a blood supply; then, osteoblasts form new bone—a process that is followed by remodeling (**Figure 1-10**). Most bones of the calvaria, the facial bones, and, in part, the clavicle and mandible are formed through intramembranous ossification.

All other bones (ie, base of the skull, axial skeleton, appendicular skeleton with the exception of the clavicle) develop in the cartilage condensations derived from mesenchymal aggregates. Chondrocytes hyper-

Figure 1-8: Limb Rotation and Dermatomes

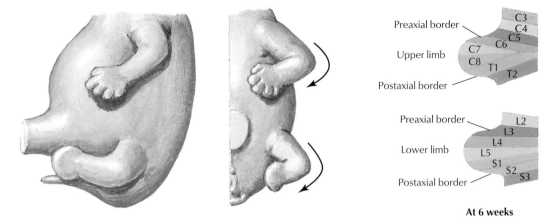

At 6 weeks. Limbs bend anteriorly, so elbows and knees point laterally, palms and soles face trunk

At 6 weeks

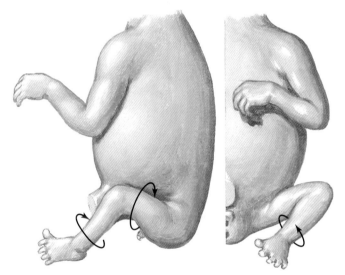

At 8 weeks. Torsion of lower limbs results in twisted or "barber pole" arrangement of their cutaneous innervation

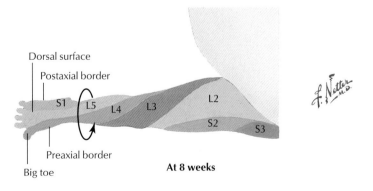

At 8 weeks

Figure 1-9: Growth Factors

Limb buds in 6-week embryo

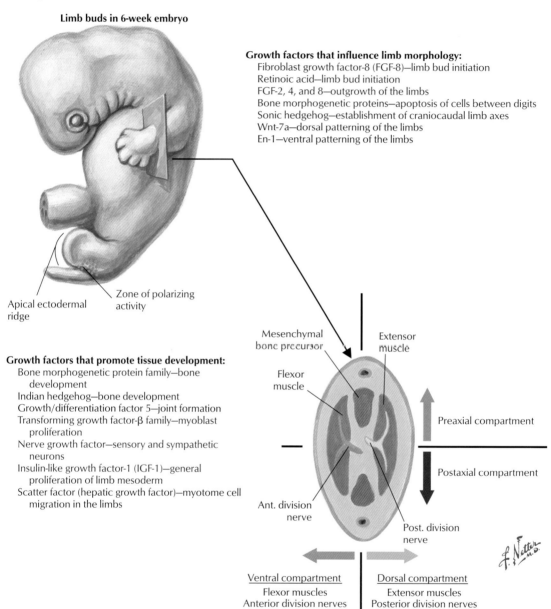

Growth factors that influence limb morphology:
Fibroblast growth factor-8 (FGF-8)—limb bud initiation
Retinoic acid—limb bud initiation
FGF-2, 4, and 8—outgrowth of the limbs
Bone morphogenetic proteins—apoptosis of cells between digits
Sonic hedgehog—establishment of craniocaudal limb axes
Wnt-7a—dorsal patterning of the limbs
En-1—ventral patterning of the limbs

Apical ectodermal ridge

Zone of polarizing activity

Growth factors that promote tissue development:
Bone morphogenetic protein family—bone
  development
Indian hedgehog—bone development
Growth/differentiation factor 5—joint formation
Transforming growth factor-β family—myoblast
  proliferation
Nerve growth factor—sensory and sympathetic
  neurons
Insulin-like growth factor-1 (IGF-1)—general
  proliferation of limb mesoderm
Scatter factor (hepatic growth factor)—myotome cell
  migration in the limbs

Mesenchymal bone precursor

Extensor muscle

Flexor muscle

Preaxial compartment

Postaxial compartment

Ant. division nerve

Post. division nerve

Ventral compartment
Flexor muscles
Anterior division nerves

Dorsal compartment
Extensor muscles
Posterior division nerves

Figure 1-10: Intramembranous (mesenchymal) Bone Formation

Initial bone formation in mesenchyme

Mesenchymal cells

Reticular fibers in extracellular
fluid of mesenchyme

Osteoblasts (from mesenchymal
cells) sending out extensions

Bundles of collagen fibers laid
down as organic osteoid matrix

Lacuna

Mineralized bone matrix
(organic osteoid and collagen
fibers impregnated with
hydroxyapatite crystals)

Osteocytes (from
osteoblasts)

Extensions of osteocytes
filling canaliculi

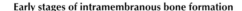

Early stages of intramembranous bone formation

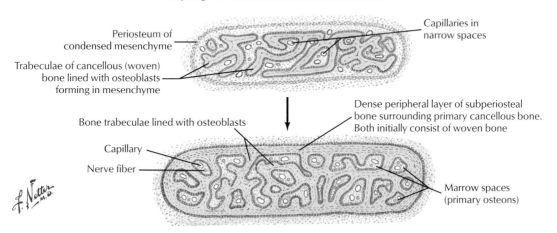

Periosteum of
condensed mesenchyme

Capillaries in
narrow spaces

Trabeculae of cancellous (woven)
bone lined with osteoblasts
forming in mesenchyme

Dense peripheral layer of subperiosteal
bone surrounding primary cancellous bone.
Both initially consist of woven bone

Bone trabeculae lined with osteoblasts

Capillary

Nerve fiber

Marrow spaces
(primary osteons)

trophy within the cartilage anlage. Capillaries invade the central region of the anlage. *Enchondral ossification* ensues, and the primary ossification center is formed (see **Figure 1-11**). Primary centers of ossification most often develop at various prenatal times that are unique to each bone. Most long-bone primary centers of ossification are present by the eighth week of gestation (**Figure 1-12**). Some small bones (eg, patella, wrist, midfoot) do not initiate ossification until early childhood.

Figure 1-11: Endochondral Ossification in a Long Bone

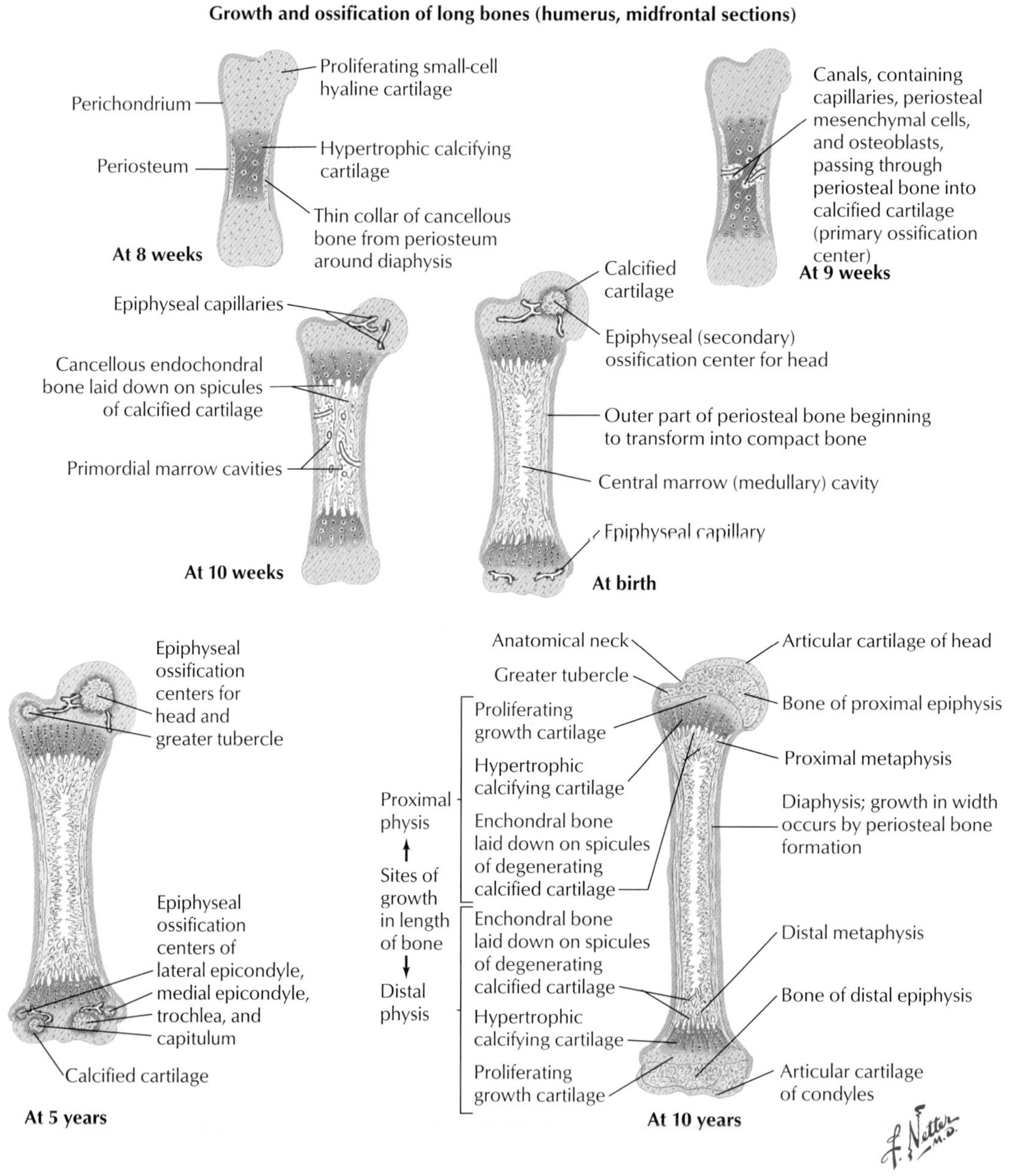

Growth and ossification of long bones (humerus, midfrontal sections)

Proliferating small-cell hyaline cartilage

Perichondrium

Periosteum

Hypertrophic calcifying cartilage

Thin collar of cancellous bone from periosteum around diaphysis

At 8 weeks

Canals, containing capillaries, periosteal mesenchymal cells, and osteoblasts, passing through periosteal bone into calcified cartilage (primary ossification center)
At 9 weeks

Epiphyseal capillaries

Cancellous endochondral bone laid down on spicules of calcified cartilage

Primordial marrow cavities

At 10 weeks

Calcified cartilage

Epiphyseal (secondary) ossification center for head

Outer part of periosteal bone beginning to transform into compact bone

Central marrow (medullary) cavity

Epiphyseal capillary

At birth

Epiphyseal ossification centers for head and greater tubercle

Epiphyseal ossification centers of lateral epicondyle, medial epicondyle, trochlea, and capitulum

Calcified cartilage

At 5 years

Proximal physis
↑
Sites of growth in length of bone
↓
Distal physis

Anatomical neck

Greater tubercle

Proliferating growth cartilage

Hypertrophic calcifying cartilage

Enchondral bone laid down on spicules of degenerating calcified cartilage

Enchondral bone laid down on spicules of degenerating calcified cartilage

Hypertrophic calcifying cartilage

Proliferating growth cartilage

Articular cartilage of head

Bone of proximal epiphysis

Proximal metaphysis

Diaphysis; growth in width occurs by periosteal bone formation

Distal metaphysis

Bone of distal epiphysis

Articular cartilage of condyles

At 10 years

Figure 1-12: Ossification Present in the Newborn

Skeleton of full-term newborn
Time of appearance of ossification centers (primary unless otherwise indicated)

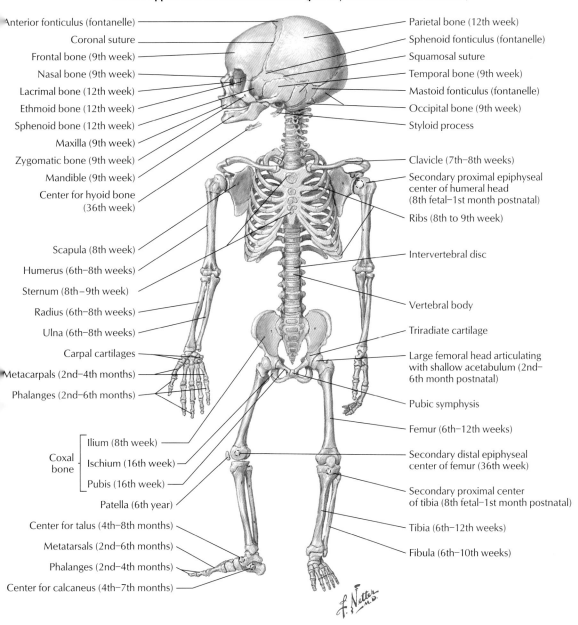

Anterior fonticulus (fontanelle)

Coronal suture

Frontal bone (9th week)

Nasal bone (9th week)

Lacrimal bone (12th week)

Ethmoid bone (12th week)

Sphenoid bone (12th week)

Maxilla (9th week)

Zygomatic bone (9th week)

Mandible (9th week)

Center for hyoid bone (36th week)

Scapula (8th week)

Humerus (6th–8th weeks)

Sternum (8th–9th week)

Radius (6th–8th weeks)

Ulna (6th–8th weeks)

Carpal cartilages

Metacarpals (2nd–4th months)

Phalanges (2nd–6th months)

Coxal bone
- Ilium (8th week)
- Ischium (16th week)
- Pubis (16th week)

Patella (6th year)

Center for talus (4th–8th months)

Metatarsals (2nd–6th months)

Phalanges (2nd–4th months)

Center for calcaneus (4th–7th months)

Parietal bone (12th week)

Sphenoid fonticulus (fontanelle)

Squamosal suture

Temporal bone (9th week)

Mastoid fonticulus (fontanelle)

Occipital bone (9th week)

Styloid process

Clavicle (7th–8th weeks)

Secondary proximal epiphyseal center of humeral head (8th fetal–1st month postnatal)

Ribs (8th to 9th week)

Intervertebral disc

Vertebral body

Triradiate cartilage

Large femoral head articulating with shallow acetabulum (2nd–6th month postnatal)

Pubic symphysis

Femur (6th–12th weeks)

Secondary distal epiphyseal center of femur (36th week)

Secondary proximal center of tibia (8th fetal–1st month postnatal)

Tibia (6th–12th weeks)

Fibula (6th–10th weeks)

The *diaphysis* is the shaft of a long bone (see **Figure 1-11**). *Metaphyses* are the adjacent flared-out regions. *Epiphyses* are the ends of a long bone. The *physis* or growth plate, which is located between the metaphysis and the epiphysis of long bones, provides longitudinal growth until the time of skeletal maturity. Growth of small bones and of the epiphysis is promoted by growth cartilage that surrounds these structures.

Bone tissue forms within the cartilaginous ends, or chondroepiphyses, of long bones, which are called *secondary centers of ossification*. In humans, the only *secondary center of ossification* that forms before birth is the one located at the distal femur, which forms at 36 weeks' gestation (see **Figure 1-12**). The appearance of various secondary centers of ossification may be used to determine the biologic or bone age of a given child.

BONE STRUCTURE AND HISTOLOGY

Bone as an organ consists of trabecular and cortical bone (**Figure 1-13**). Both types of bone contain the same cell and matrix elements, but structural and functional differences between the two are observed. *Cortical bone*, sometimes called *compact bone*, is denser (80% to 90% of the volume is calcified) and stronger than *cancellous bone*. The diaphyses of long bones primarily comprise cortical bone. Thus, shafts of long bones have a relatively small cross-sectional area that can accommodate the bulk of surrounding musculature while continuing to resist lifting and weight-bearing stresses. *Cancellous bone*, sometimes called *trabecular bone*, is a network of bony trabeculae or struts that are aligned to counteract stress and support articular cartilage. Only 15% to 25% of the medullary canal is made up of cancellous bone; the remaining volume is occupied by marrow, blood vessels, fibrous tissue, and fatty tissue. The metaphysis and the epiphysis primarily comprise cancellous bone covered by a relatively thin layer of cortical bone.

Growth of the entire human body involves a net accumulation of bone mass. Newly formed bone (during development, fracture repair, or turnover) is *woven bone*. At the microscopic level, the osteoid matrix of woven bone reveals an amorphous or patchwork pattern of osteoblasts, osteoid matrix, and randomly oriented collagen fibers. Woven bone remodels internally to *lamellar bone*. This process requires close coupling of bone formation and bone resorption. *Osteoblasts* form bone, *osteocytes* maintain bone, and *osteoclasts* (specialized macrophages) resorb bone. With successive resorption and formation, woven bone is remodeled into concentric lamellar bone, which is made up of collagen fibers, haversian systems, and interstial lamellae aligned for maximum strength per volume of bone. The cells that deposit newly formed bone, the osteoblasts, become surrounded by bone matrix and develop into mature osteocytes, which form cellular extensions for intercellular transport (**Figure 1-14**).

Bone Growth and Remodeling

Cartilaginous growth regions throughout the skeleton are programmed to add to the size of bones as organs. Absolute and relative changes in the size and shape of bones throughout the fetal and postnatal periods cause the changes in body size and proportion that result in growth of the organism. This occurs in single bones and regions. For example, the calvaria is much larger than the facial skeleton at birth (the ratio is 8:1 in a newborn compared with 2:1 in an adult). Similarly, upper limb growth is more rapid during early gestation, and it is not until birth that the length of the lower limbs is equal to that of the upper limbs.

The physis is organized to move cells along columns in a progression of cytodifferentiation (**Figure 1-15**). Cells at similar levels in adjacent columns resemble one another and constitute zones. Growth or movement occurs from the small cell phenotype on the epiphyseal side of the physis to hypertrophic cells on the metaphyseal side. The blood supply to the *reserve* and the *proliferating zones* is derived from the epiphyseal artery, whereas the *hypertrophic zone* is avascular. Metaphyseal vessels supply

Figure 1-13: Histology of Bone

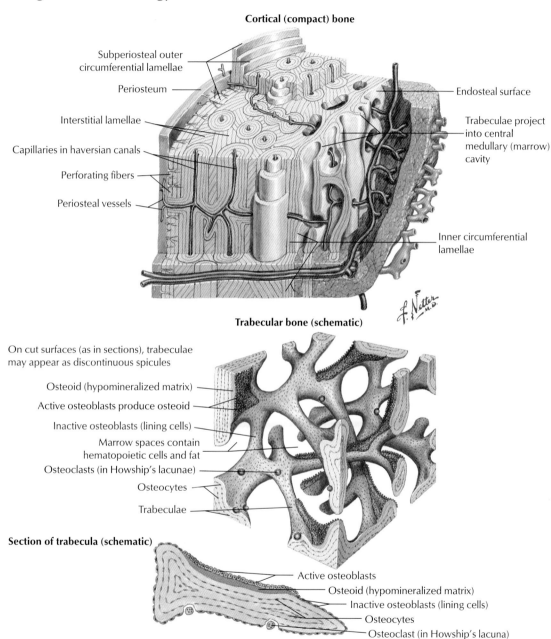

Cortical (compact) bone

Subperiosteal outer circumferential lamellae

Periosteum

Interstitial lamellae

Capillaries in haversian canals

Perforating fibers

Periosteal vessels

Endosteal surface

Trabeculae project into central medullary (marrow) cavity

Inner circumferential lamellae

Trabecular bone (schematic)

On cut surfaces (as in sections), trabeculae may appear as discontinuous spicules

Osteoid (hypomineralized matrix)

Active osteoblasts produce osteoid

Inactive osteoblasts (lining cells)

Marrow spaces contain hematopoietic cells and fat

Osteoclasts (in Howship's lacunae)

Osteocytes

Trabeculae

Section of trabecula (schematic)

Active osteoblasts

Osteoid (hypomineralized matrix)

Inactive osteoblasts (lining cells)

Osteocytes

Osteoclast (in Howship's lacuna)

Figure 1-14: Composition of Lamellar Bone

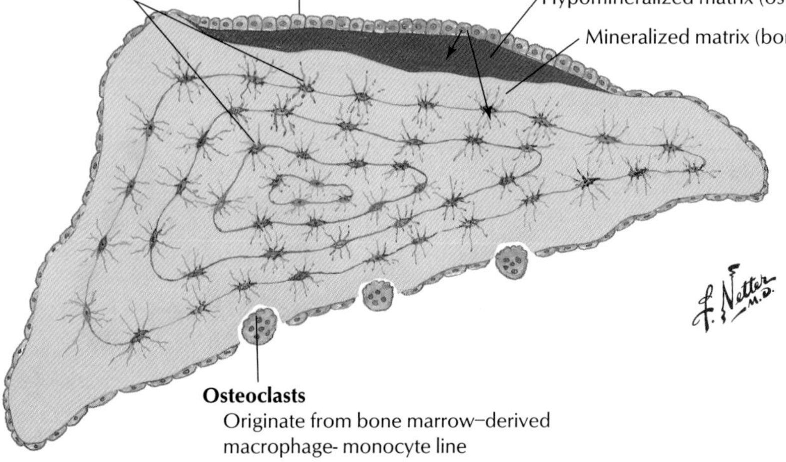

Osteocytes
Originate from osteoblasts

Osteoblasts
(Matrix-forming cells) Originate from mesenchyme

Hypomineralized matrix (osteoid)

Mineralized matrix (bone)

Osteoclasts
Originate from bone marrow–derived macrophage- monocyte line

the area of *primary spongiosa* but do not enter the physis.

Cells of the reserve zone participate in the production of matrix and the storage of metabolites that are required farther along the growth plate (see **Figure 1-15**). Stem cells for longitudinal growth reside in the upper proliferative zone. Newly formed cells progress through the proliferative zone to the hypertrophic zone, where chondrocytes enlarge and the proteoglycan matrix is degraded to disaggregated, short-chain protein polysaccharides—a process that allows the matrix to become calcified. In the upper portion of the hypertrophic zone, chondrocytes switch to anaerobic glycolysis and store calcium in the mitochondria. In the lower portion of the hypertrophic zone, the energy is depleted and calcium is discharged into the matrix, which permits *hydroxyapatite crystal formation* and provisional calcification. Progressive calcification forms longitudinal septa, on which enchondral ossification can occur. Because calcified cartilage matrix has more calcium per unit volume than does bone, the zone of provisional calcification is seen as a dense band on radiographs.

In the primary spongiosa region of the metaphysis, blood vessels bring in osteoblasts, which lay down bone on the calcified cartilage armatures. Osteoclasts immediately begin to remove the first-formed woven bone and cartilaginous septa, and osteoblasts produce more mature cancellous bone in the *secondary spongiosa*.

Remodeling is disrupted in *osteopetrosis*, a genetic disease characterized by dysfunction of the osteoclasts. In osteopetrosis, the bones appear dense or like "marble" on radiographs because the primary spongiosa with its calcified cartilage cores persists throughout the bone as an organ. Osteopetrotic bone, however, is markedly weaker than normal bone because the deficiency in internal remodeling does not permit the production of stronger lamellar bone.

The physis directs growth along the longitudinal axis. The total longitudinal growth of a bone is the height gained by a hypertrophic chondrocyte multiplied by the aggregate of all such cellular activity. Different growth plates contribute different percentages to overall longitudinal growth. For example, the distal femoral physis contributes 70% to the growth of the femur, whereas the proximal femoral physis contributes 30%.

The circumferential growth of bone occurs by *appositional intramembranous formation*.

Figure 1-15: Close-up View of Epiphysis, Physis, and Adjacent Metaphysis

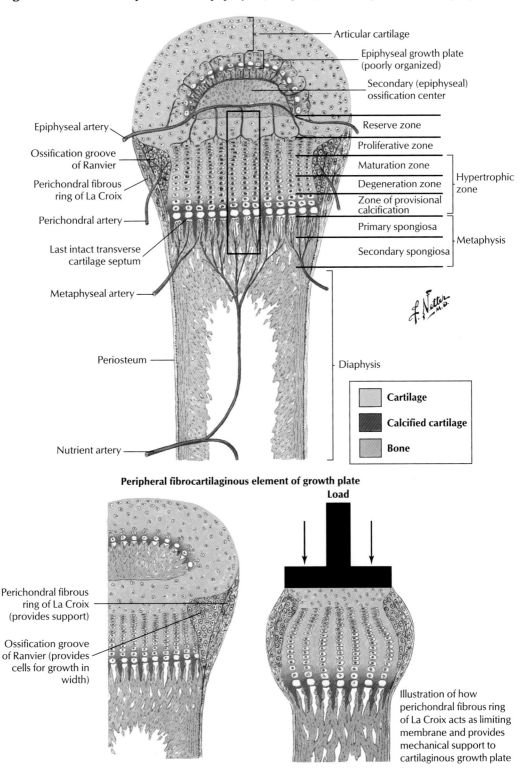

Articular cartilage

Epiphyseal growth plate (poorly organized)

Secondary (epiphyseal) ossification center

Epiphyseal artery

Reserve zone

Proliferative zone

Ossification groove of Ranvier

Maturation zone

Perichondral fibrous ring of La Croix

Degeneration zone

Hypertrophic zone

Zone of provisional calcification

Perichondral artery

Primary spongiosa

Last intact transverse cartilage septum

Secondary spongiosa

Metaphysis

Metaphyseal artery

Periosteum

Diaphysis

| Cartilage |
| Calcified cartilage |
| Bone |

Nutrient artery

Peripheral fibrocartilaginous element of growth plate

Load

Perichondral fibrous ring of La Croix (provides support)

Ossification groove of Ranvier (provides cells for growth in width)

Illustration of how perichondral fibrous ring of La Croix acts as limiting membrane and provides mechanical support to cartilaginous growth plate

Figure 1-16: Physis (Growth Plate)

Zones / Structures	Histology	Functions	Blood supply	P_{O_2}	Cell (chondrocyte) health	Cell respiration	Cell glycogen
Secondary bony epiphysis — Epiphyseal artery	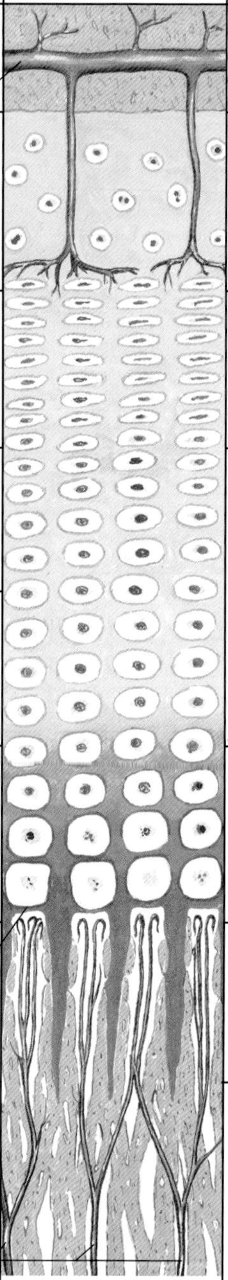						
Reserve zone		Matrix production / Storage	Vessels pass through, do not supply this zone	Poor (low)	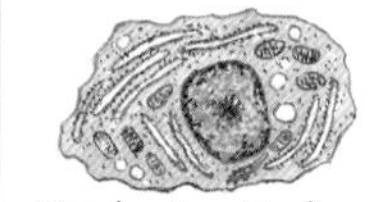 Good, active. Much endoplasmic reticulum, vacuoles, mitochondria	Anaerobic	High concentration
Proliferative zone		Matrix production / Cellular proliferation (longitudinal growth)	Excellent	Excellent / Fair	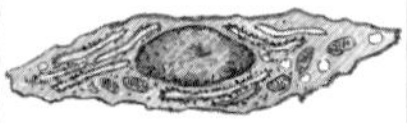 Excellent. Much endoplasmic reticulum, ribosomes, mitochondria. Intact cell membrane	Aerobic	High concentration (less than in above)
Hypertrophic zone — Maturation zone		Preparation of matrix for calcification	Progressive decrease	Poor (low) / Progressive decrease	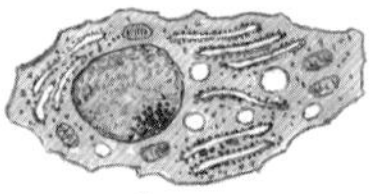 Still good	Progressive change to anaerobic	Glycogen consumed until depleted
Hypertrophic zone — Degenerative zone					Progressive deterioration	Anaerobic glycolysis	
Hypertrophic zone — Zone of provisional calcification		Calcification of matrix	Nil	Poor (very low)	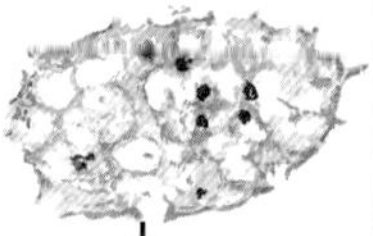 Cell death	Anaerobic glycolysis	Nil
Metaphysis — Last intact transverse septum / Primary spongiosa		Vascular invasion and resorption of transverse septa / Bone formation	Closed capillary loops / Good	Poor / Good		Progressive reversion to aerobic	?
Metaphysis — Secondary spongiosa / Branches of metaphyseal and nutrient arteries		Remodeling Internal: Removal of cartilage bars, replacement of fiber bone with lamellar bone External: Funnelization	Excellent	Excellent		Aerobic	?

20

In long bones, appositional growth results from lining of the periosteum by osteoblasts and is accompanied by concomitant osteoclastic resorption of the endosteum and widening of the medullary cavity. The broad metaphysis increases the surface area of the articular surfaces, thus decreasing the unit load on the cartilage. This funnelization of the metaphysis occurs through progressive intramembranous bone formation and subsequent osteoclastic resorption at the cutback zone. Metaphyseal cancellous bone with a thin cortex gradually transitions to typical diaphyseal compact cortical bone.

Practical Applications of Physiologic Principles

The unique regenerative capacity of bone at the tissue level in fracture repair is retained throughout life. The capacity of bone to regenerate shape at the organ level also exists throughout life but is especially notable in the immature skeleton. Displaced fractures treated by closed means typically heal with a surrounding collar of *callus* that is formed by the periosteum. This initial callus, which includes woven bone at the tissue level, is deployed broadly around the fracture site. Because woven bone is biomechanically inferior to lamellar bone the initial callus at the organ level compensates through its distribution around a larger radius, which can better resist bending and torsional moments. Internal remodeling, which continues for months, reconstitutes lamellar cortical bone, tubular proportions, and the intramedullary canal. Fracture repair and bone remodeling are discussed in greater detail in Chapter 9.

An understanding of the scientific basis of bone growth and remodeling forms the basis for provision of good clinical care. Future discoveries that will lead to control of the molecular events that mediate bone growth and remodeling will result in better clinical care.

ADDITIONAL READINGS

Cochard LR. *Netter's Atlas of Human Embryology*. Teterboro, NJ: Icon Learning Systems; 2002.

Dietz FR, Morcuende JA. Embryology and Development of the Musculoskeletal System. In: Morrisey RT, Weinstein SL, eds. *Lovell and Winter's Pediatric Orthopaedics*, 5th edition. Philadelphia, Pa: Lippincott Williams and Wilkins; 2001:1–31.

Schneider RA, Miclau T, Helms JA. Embryology of Bone. In: Fitzgerald RH, Kaufer H, Malkani AL, eds. *Orthopaedics*. Philadelphia, Pa: Mosby; 2002:143–146.

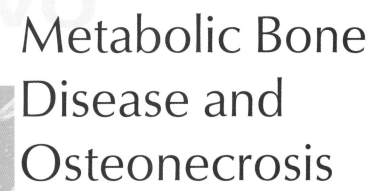

two

Metabolic Bone Disease and Osteonecrosis

**Susan V. Bukata, MD, and
Randy N. Rosier, MD, PhD**

E ach individual bone has a structure that is uniquely designed for local stability and function. Bone, that is, the skeleton, is an organ that is the major storehouse for calcium and phosphorus, and it also is a site of active hematopoietic tissue. Metabolic disease can alter normal bone deposition through conditions that alter the process of bone formation or bone resorption, or through disorders that affect both formation and resorption. Bone formation may be altered during the process of osteoblastic organic matrix (*osteoid*) formation or during the subsequent process of osteoid mineralization. Calcium and phosphate are critical in bone formation, and during the mineralization of osteoid, calcium and phosphate are transformed from the fluid phase to *hydroxyapatite crystals*.

Serum ionized calcium levels are crucial in cardiac and skeletal muscle function and neuronal activity. Therefore, despite daily fluctuations in calcium intake, ionized calcium concentrations are maintained at a remarkably constant level at between 4.5 and 5.0 mg/dL by input/output exchanges in the gut, kidney, and bone that are regulated by *parathyroid hormone (PTH)*, *1,25-dihydroxyvitamin D_3 (1,25-D_3)*, and *calcitonin* (**Figures 2-1** and **2-2**). The initial response to hypocalcemia is an increase in PTH secretion by the parathyroid gland, and the initial response to hypercalcemia is an increase in calcitonin secretion by the thyroid gland. These changes in PTH and calcitonin are augmented by changes in 1,25-D_3 levels to rapidly correct ionized calcium levels.

A seven-transmembrane, G-protein–coupled receptor found on many cell types is responsible for sensing extracellular ionized calcium. Therefore, an elevated calcium level also has a direct effect on inhibition of renal cell calcium resorption and osteoclast activity. The skeleton is the major reservoir of calcium. Calcium ions mobilized by bone resorption are replaced by bone formation. However, if bone formation does not equal bone resorption, the skeleton will be weakened (**Figure 2-3**).

Metabolic bone disease affects the entire skeleton, but because certain areas of the skeleton are under increased stress, patients with metabolic bone disease frequently have symptoms such as back pain related to compression fracture of the thoracic area and lumbar spine, as well as leg pain secondary to bowing of the femur and/or tibia and pathologic fracture of the lower limbs. Some generalized disorders of bone are influenced by the local environment; therefore, patients may develop scattered, symptomatic lesions but have normal form and function of uninvolved bones.

HYPERPARATHYROIDISM

Primary hyperparathyroidism occurs when PTH is produced in excess, even with normal or elevated serum calcium levels (**Figure 2-4**). It is generally caused by an *adenoma* of the chief cells of a single parathyroid gland. A less common cause is *hyperplasia* of all four parathyroid glands. Patients with *type I multiple endocrine neoplasia* also may have parathyroid hyperplasia. Hyperparathyroidism is caused by carcinoma in less than 0.5% of cases.

No specific genetic defect has been identified, but certain chromosomal alterations are associated with primary hyperparathyroidism. Some patients have inactivation of tumor suppressor genes on either chromosome 11 or chromosome 1. Other patients have a genetic rearrangement, with the *PRAD 1* proto-oncogene placed near the genes that control PTH production. In this situation, cell growth is stimulated when normal PTH production is stimulated, leading to adenoma formation and excessive production of PTH.

Primary hyperparathyroidism is relatively common, with an incidence of 1 in 1000. The disease can occur at all ages but is more common after 50 years. Women predominate at a 3:1 ratio. A 4- to 5-fold increase in incidence

Figure 2-1: Normal Calcium and Phosphate Metabolism

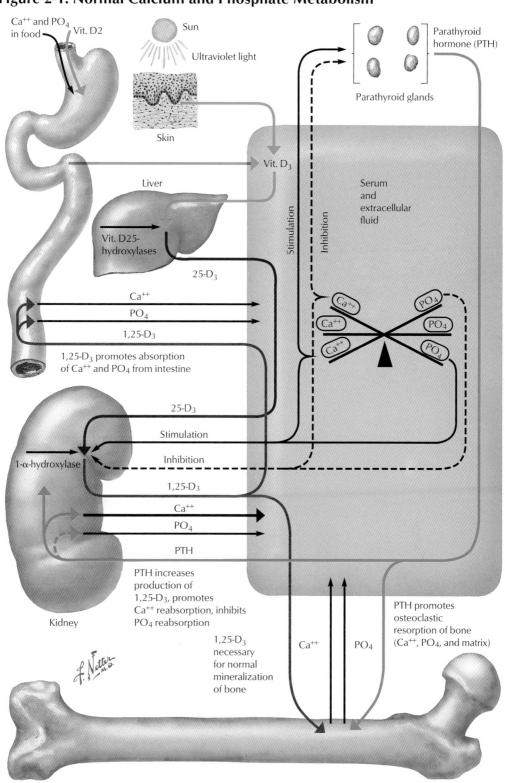

Ca^{++} and PO$_4$ in food — Vit. D2

Sun

Ultraviolet light

Skin

Parathyroid hormone (PTH)

Parathyroid glands

Vit. D$_3$

Liver

Serum and extracellular fluid

Vit. D25-hydroxylases

25-D$_3$

Stimulation

Inhibition

Ca^{++}

PO$_4$

1,25-D$_3$

1,25-D$_3$ promotes absorption of Ca^{++} and PO$_4$ from intestine

Ca^{++} PO$_4$

25-D$_3$

Stimulation

1-α-hydroxylase

Inhibition

1,25-D$_3$

Ca^{++}

PO$_4$

PTH

PTH increases production of 1,25-D$_3$, promotes Ca^{++} reabsorption, inhibits PO$_4$ reabsorption

Kidney

1,25-D$_3$ necessary for normal mineralization of bone

Ca^{++} PO$_4$

PTH promotes osteoclastic resorption of bone (Ca^{++}, PO$_4$, and matrix)

Figure 2-2: Regulation of Calcium and Phosphate Metabolism

	Parathyroid hormone (PTH) (peptide)	1,25-D$_3$ (steroid)	Calcitonin (peptide)
Hormone	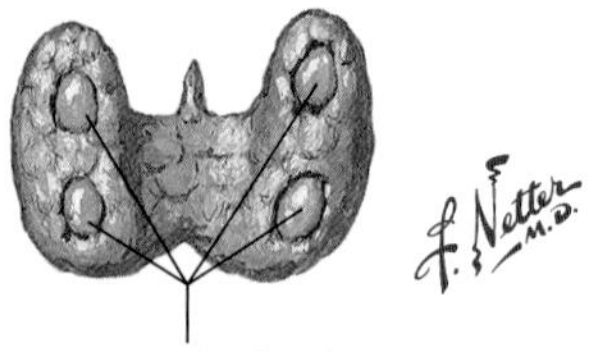 From chief cells of parathyroid glands	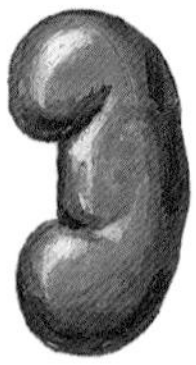 From proximal tubule of kidney	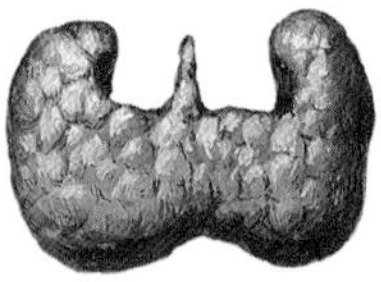 From parafollicular cells of thyroid gland
Factors stimulating production	Decreased serum Ca^{++}	Elevated PTH Decreased serum Ca^{++} Decreased serum P$_i$	Elevated serum Ca^{++}
Factors inhibiting production	Elevated serum Ca^{++} Elevated 1,25(OH)$_2$D	Decreased PTH Elevated serum Ca^{++} Elevated serum P$_i$	Decreased serum Ca^{++}
End organs for hormone action 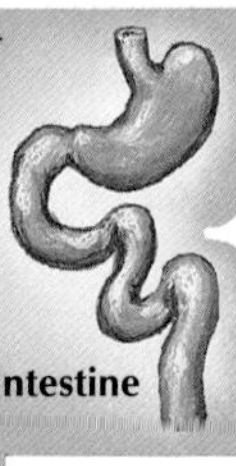 — Intestine	No direct effect Acts indirectly on bowel by stimulating production of 1,25(OH)$_2$D in kidney	Strongly stimulates intestinal absorption of Ca^{++} and P$_i$	
End organs for hormone action 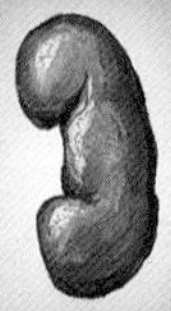 — Kidney	Stimulates 25(OH)D-1α-OH$_{ase}$ in mitochondria of proximal tubular cells to convert 25(OH)D to 1,25(OH)$_2$D Increases fractional reabsorption of filtered Ca^{++} Promotes urinary excretion of P$_i$		Increases renal calcium excretion
End organs for hormone action 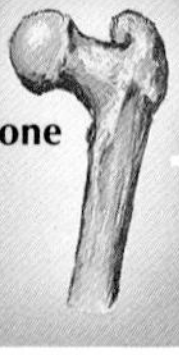 — Bone	Increases bone resorption indirectly by up-regulating osteoblast production of autocrine cytokines such as interleukin-6, which results in increased production of paracrine cytokines that stimulate osteoclast production and activity. PTH also has an anabolic effect on osteoblasts that results in overproduction of osteoid in chronic hyperparathyroidism	Stimulates bone resorption in a similar fashion to PTH and also other membrane receptors	Inhibits bone resorption by direct inhibition of osteoclast differentiation and activity
Net effect on calcium and phosphate concentrations in extracellular fluid and serum	Increased serum calcium Decreased serum phosphate	Increased serum calcium	Decreased serum calcium (transient)

Figure 2-3: Dynamics of Bone Homeostasis

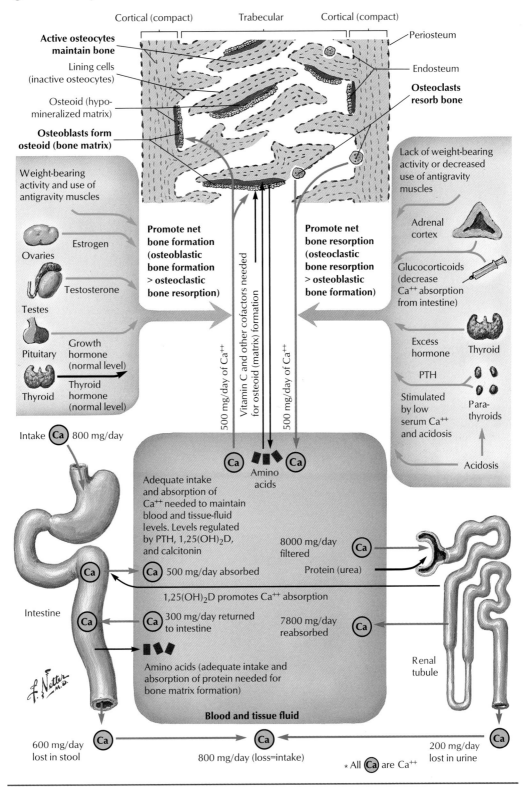

Cortical (compact) Trabecular Cortical (compact)

Active osteocytes maintain bone

Lining cells (inactive osteocytes)

Osteoid (hypo-mineralized matrix)

Osteoblasts form osteoid (bone matrix)

Periosteum

Endosteum

Osteoclasts resorb bone

Weight-bearing activity and use of antigravity muscles

Lack of weight-bearing activity or decreased use of antigravity muscles

Ovaries — Estrogen

Testes — Testosterone

Pituitary — Growth hormone (normal level)

Thyroid — Thyroid hormone (normal level)

Promote net bone formation (osteoblastic bone formation > osteoclastic bone resorption)

Vitamin C and other cofactors needed for osteoid (matrix) formation

500 mg/day of Ca^{++}

500 mg/day of Ca^{++}

Promote net bone resorption (osteoclastic bone resorption > osteoblastic bone formation)

Adrenal cortex

Glucocorticoids (decrease Ca^{++} absorption from intestine)

Excess hormone — Thyroid

PTH — Para-thyroids

Stimulated by low serum Ca^{++} and acidosis

Acidosis

Intake (Ca) 800 mg/day

(Ca) Amino acids (Ca)

Adequate intake and absorption of Ca^{++} needed to maintain blood and tissue-fluid levels. Levels regulated by PTH, $1,25(OH)_2D$, and calcitonin

8000 mg/day filtered (Ca)

Protein (urea)

(Ca) 500 mg/day absorbed

$1,25(OH)_2D$ promotes Ca^{++} absorption

Intestine

(Ca) 300 mg/day returned to intestine

7800 mg/day reabsorbed (Ca)

Amino acids (adequate intake and absorption of protein needed for bone matrix formation)

Renal tubule

Blood and tissue fluid

600 mg/day lost in stool (Ca)

(Ca)

800 mg/day (loss=intake)

200 mg/day lost in urine (Ca)

* All (Ca) are Ca^{++}

Figure 2-4: Pathologic Physiology of Primary Hyperparathyroidism

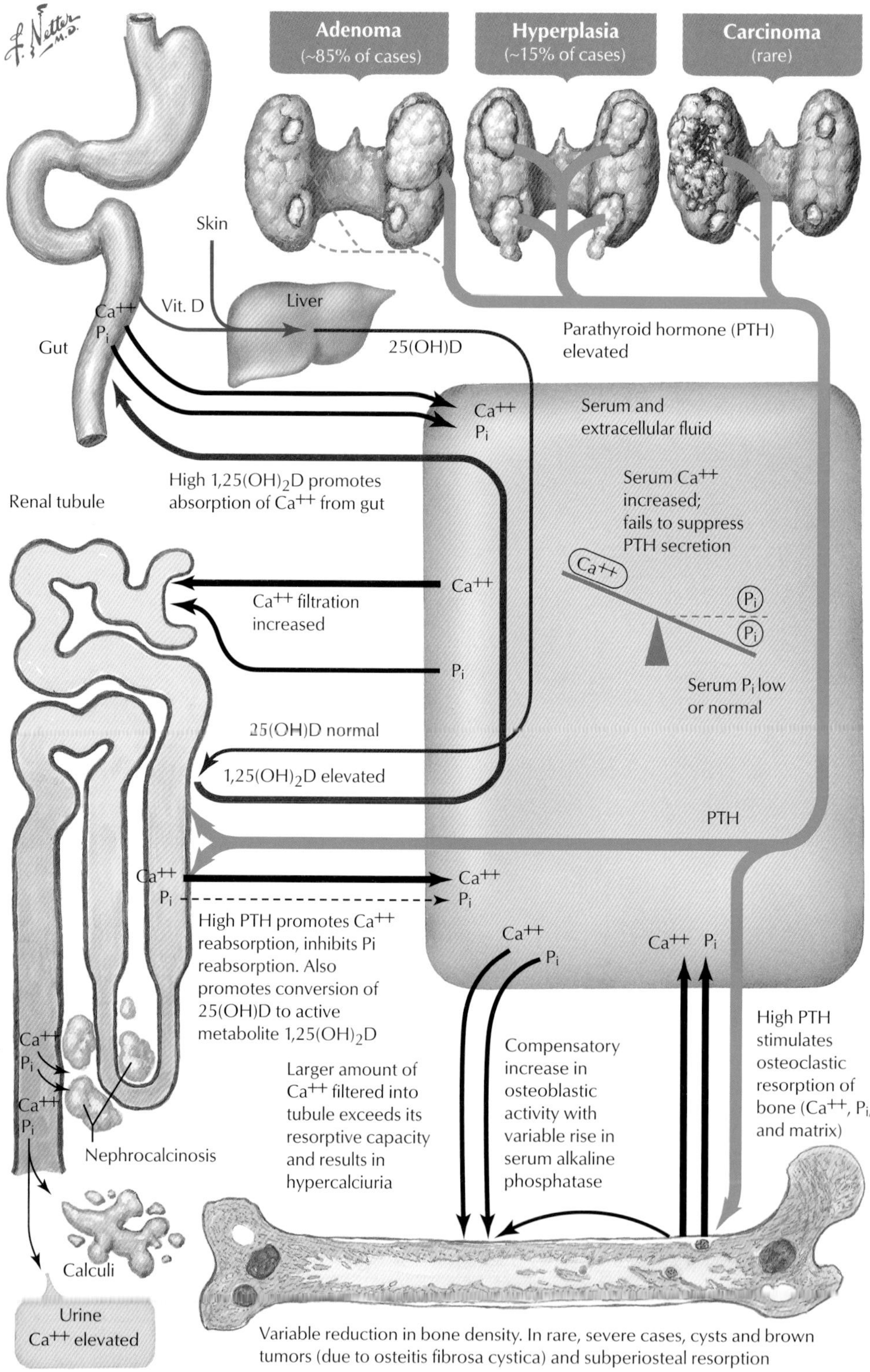

| Adenoma (~85% of cases) | Hyperplasia (~15% of cases) | Carcinoma (rare) |

Skin

Vit. D

Liver

Gut

Ca++
Pi

25(OH)D

Parathyroid hormone (PTH) elevated

Ca++
Pi

Serum and extracellular fluid

Renal tubule

High 1,25(OH)₂D promotes absorption of Ca++ from gut

Serum Ca++ increased; fails to suppress PTH secretion

Ca++

Ca++ filtration increased

Ca++

Pi

Serum Pi low or normal

25(OH)D normal

1,25(OH)₂D elevated

PTH

Ca++
Pi

Ca++
Pi

High PTH promotes Ca++ reabsorption, inhibits Pi reabsorption. Also promotes conversion of 25(OH)D to active metabolite 1,25(OH)₂D

Ca++
Pi

Ca++ Pi

High PTH stimulates osteoclastic resorption of bone (Ca++, Pi, and matrix)

Ca++
Pi

Ca++
Pi

Nephrocalcinosis

Larger amount of Ca++ filtered into tubule exceeds its resorptive capacity and results in hypercalciuria

Compensatory increase in osteoblastic activity with variable rise in serum alkaline phosphatase

Calculi

Urine
Ca++ elevated

Variable reduction in bone density. In rare, severe cases, cysts and brown tumors (due to osteitis fibrosa cystica) and subperiosteal resorption

Figure 2-5: Clinical Manifestations of Primary Hyperthyroidism

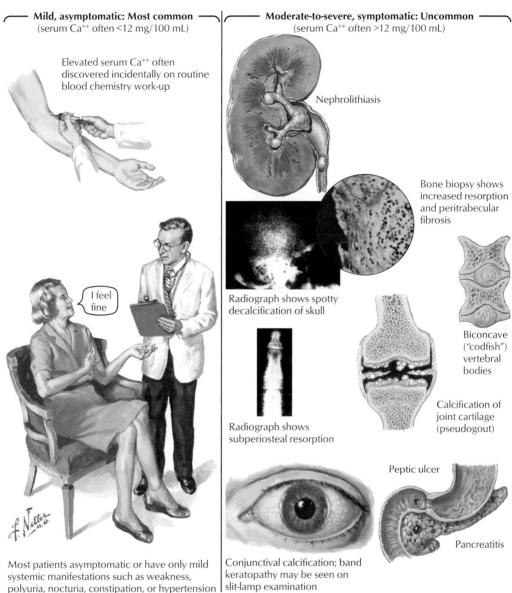

Mild, asymptomatic: Most common
(serum Ca^{++} often <12 mg/100 mL)

Moderate-to-severe, symptomatic: Uncommon
(serum Ca^{++} often >12 mg/100 mL)

Elevated serum Ca^{++} often discovered incidentally on routine blood chemistry work-up

Nephrolithiasis

Bone biopsy shows increased resorption and peritrabecular fibrosis

I feel fine

Radiograph shows spotty decalcification of skull

Biconcave ("codfish") vertebral bodies

Calcification of joint cartilage (pseudogout)

Radiograph shows subperiosteal resorption

Peptic ulcer

Pancreatitis

Most patients asymptomatic or have only mild systemic manifestations such as weakness, polyuria, nocturia, constipation, or hypertension

Conjunctival calcification; band keratopathy may be seen on slit-lamp examination

has been noted since the 1970s because of widespread use of chemistry panels. Patients are often diagnosed when elevated calcium levels are detected during routine blood tests. As a result, most patients are asymptomatic, and severe cases have dramatically decreased. Symptomatic patients complain of fatigue, weakness, and a sense of cognitive difficulty (**Figure 2-5**). Kidney stones may be the first manifestation. However, advanced bony changes caused by bone resorption, such as *brown tumors* of long bones (radiolucent lesions secondary to very high levels of PTH) and subperiosteal resorption of the distal phalanges of the hand, are now rarely seen.

The diagnosis of hyperparathyroidism is confirmed with an immunoassay for PTH. Treatment includes surgery to remove either

Figure 2-6

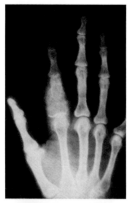

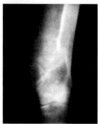

Renal Osteodystrophy and Secondary Hyperparathyroidism
Brown tumor of proximal phalanx (top) and osteitis fibrosa cystica of distal femur (bottom)

the adenoma or 3½ of the 4 hyperplastic parathyroid glands. Postoperative hypocalcemia may occur but is usually mild and does not require treatment.

Humoral *hypercalcemia of malignancy* can be a difficult problem to manage. Most cases are caused by the tumor producing *PTH-related protein*. Because PTH and PTH-related protein have similar amino acid sequences in their amino terminal domains, these two molecules bind to and activate the same receptors.

Secondary hyperparathyroidism is a secondary response to chronic dysregulation of calcium homeostasis. It usually results from renal disease (**Figure 2-6**). Renal dysfunction causes phosphate accumulation, which lowers serum ionized calcium levels; this, in turn, stimulates the parathyroid gland to a secondary hyperparathyroidism. Impaired renal function also reduces production of 1,25-D$_3$ and results in osteomalacia. In some patients, parathyroid hyperplasia may be extreme and result in overstimulation of osteoclasts and bone resorption,

called *osteitis fibrosa cystica*. Medical management includes phosphate-binding antacids and calcium carbonate. Brown tumors and severe bone pain may necessitate partial or total parathyroidectomy.

HYPOPARATHYROIDISM

Hypoparathyroidism results in hypocalcemia, hyperphosphatemia, and secondary decreased 1,25-D$_3$ levels. *Primary hypoparathyroidism* is uncommon. Isolated hypoparathyroidism results from inherited conditions that affect either PTH or the ionizing calcium–sensing receptor. Primary hypoparathyroidism may also result from more complex endocrine disorders. Clinical manifestations of chronic hypoparathyroidism include nonspecific mental symptoms such as lethargy, irritability, and depression, as well as cataracts, alopecia, and poor tooth formation. Bony changes are minimal.

Pseudohypoparathyroidism is caused by impaired response (end-organ resistance) to PTH. A variety of disorders cause pseudohypoparathyroidism, including decreased levels of G$_{s\alpha}$, the G-protein responsible for coupling the receptor in the cyclic adenosine monophosphate (cAMP) signal transduction pathway (*pseudohypoparathyroidism type 1a*); reduced expression of the PTH receptor (*type 1b*); impaired activity of adenyl cyclase, which synthesizes cAMP (*type 1c*); and other uncharacterized defects in PTH end-organ response. Individuals with pseudohypoparathyroidism type 1a and type 1c also have *Albright's hereditary osteodystrophy* (**Figure 2-7**).

OSTEOMALACIA AND RICKETS

Osteomalacia and rickets are diseases caused by altered vitamin D function or by *hypophosphatasia*, a condition in which the production of osteoid is normal but subsequent mineralization is inadequate (**Table 2-1**). Therefore, the total amount of bone is normal, but bone strength is decreased. In contrast, bone in osteoporosis is mineralized normally, but the total amount of bone is decreased. The *sine qua non* of *rickets* is inadequate mineral-

Figure 2-7

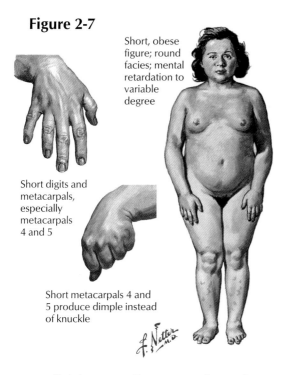

Short, obese figure; round facies; mental retardation to variable degree

Short digits and metacarpals, especially metacarpals 4 and 5

Short metacarpals 4 and 5 produce dimple instead of knuckle

Albright's Hereditary Osteodystrophy

ate. This results in a widened, disorganized maturation zone. Severe cases that cause craniotabes, rachitic rosary, and genu varum are uncommon (**Figure 2-8**).

Radiographs in adults with osteomalacia show generalized osteopenia. *Pseudofractures* result from stress fractures that heal with unmineralized bone and are seen as radiolucent lines on the compression side of bones. *Multiple pseudofractures* may be seen bilaterally, with radiolucent lines perpendicular to the axis of long bones developing from healing stress fractures. This finding is referred to as *"Milkman syndrome,"* named after the radiologist who described it; it is almost pathognomonic for osteomalacia. Because radiographs can mimic other disorders, an iliac crest biopsy showing widened unmineralized osteoid seams may be needed to confirm the diagnosis. Multiple stress fractures may result in a bowing deformity of long

ization of bone formed at the physis. Therefore, rickets occurs only in children.

The diagnosis of osteomalacia and rickets can be challenging because early in the disease process, the presenting symptoms are often vague pains in the legs and lower back, and the examination is often normal. Children with rickets may be asymptomatic, but short stature or a fracture coupled with associated risk factors may suggest the need for further evaluation. Clinical suspicion is confirmed by findings of laboratory studies and radiographs. The striking radiographic finding in rickets is widening of the physis with cupping and flaring of the metaphysis. This is particularly obvious at the more active growth plates of the distal femur, proximal tibia, distal radius, and proximal humerus. Histology of the growth plate shows a poorly defined region of provisional calcification. The cartilage cells of the maturation zone lose their orderly columnar arrangement and rapidly prolifer-

Table 2-1
Conditions That Cause Osteomalacia or Rickets

Vitamin D–deficient conditions
   Dietary lack of vitamin D
   Insufficient exposure to sunlight
   Vitamin D deficiency of prematurity
   Use of seizure medications
   Liver disease
   Intestinal disease or surgery
   Vitamin D–dependent rickets
   Renal osteodystrophy

Hypophosphatemic rachitic syndromes
   X-linked dominant hypophosphatemic rickets
   Autosomal dominant hypophosphatemic rickets
   Fanconi syndrome
   Use of aluminum-containing antacids

Impaired mineralization
   Hypophosphatasia
   Use of bisphosphonates

Figure 2-8

Childhood Rickets

Impaired growth
Craniotabes
Frontal bossing
Dental defects
Chronic cough
Pigeon breast (tunnel chest)
Kyphosis
Rachitic rosary
Harrison groove
Flaring of ribs
Enlarged ends of long bones
Enlarged abdomen
Coxa vara
Bowleg (genu varum)

Clinical findings (all or some present in variable degree)

Flaring of metaphyseal ends of tibia and femur. Growth plates thickened, irregular, cupped, and axially widened. Zones of provisional calcification fuzzy and indistinct. Bone cortices thinned and medullae rarefied

Coxa vara and slipped capital femoral epiphysis. Mottled areas of lucency and density in pelvic bones

Cartilage of epiphyseal plate in immature normal rat. Cells of middle (maturation) zone in orderly columns, with calcified cartilage between columns

After 6 weeks of vitamin D– and phosphate-deficient diet. Large increase in axial height of maturation zone, with cells closely packed and irregularly arranged

Radiograph of rachitic hand shows decreased bone density, irregular trabeculation, and thin cortices of metacarpals and proximal phalanges. Note increased axial width of epiphyseal line, especially in radius and ulna

Section of rachitic bone shows sparse, thin trabeculae surrounded by much uncalcified osteoid (osteoid seams) and cavities caused by increased resorption

Adult Osteomalacia

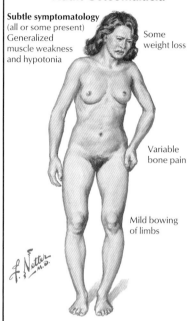

Subtle symptomatology (all or some present)
Generalized muscle weakness and hypotonia

Some weight loss

Variable bone pain

Mild bowing of limbs

f. Netter.

Radiographic findings

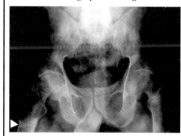

Radiograph shows variegated rarefaction of pelvic bones, coxa vara, deepened acetabula, and subtrochanteric pseudofracture of right femur

bones, and the spine may develop increased thoracic kyphosis.

Vitamin D is a steroid hormone that may be produced endogenously or via dietary sources (see **Figure 2-1**). Ultraviolet light converts *7-dehydrocholesterol* in the skin to *cholecalciferol* (*vitamin D_3*). Individuals who wear heavy garments designed to cover most of their skin may receive insufficient sun exposure for adequate vitamin D production. This condition is uncommon, however, because the sunlight exposure to the face and hands necessary to produce daily requirements is only 10 to 15 minutes in fair-skinned people. Dark-skinned persons, however, require more prolonged exposure. *Vitamin D_2* (*ergocalciferol*) may be obtained through diet. Therefore, nutritional rickets is rare in countries that supplement milk and other food products with vitamin D_2.

Vitamins D_2 and D_3 undergo hydroxylation initially at the 25-position in the liver, then in the kidneys at the 1-position, to become *1,25-D_3*, a major calcium-regulating hormone. 1,25-D_3 upregulates production of the calcium-binding proteins essential for calcium transport and absorption in the gut. This hormone also stimulates bone resorption in a manner similar to PTH.

Vitamin D–deficiency osteomalacia is seen primarily in elderly adults. Contributing factors include decreased production of 25-hydroxyvitamin D_3 with aging; reduced renal function with aging, leading to reduced levels of 1α-hydroxylase enzyme; and the greater incidence of malabsorption abnormalities that occur in the elderly.

Genetic disorders that affect the synthesis of active vitamin D also cause rickets and osteomalacia. *Type I vitamin D–dependent rickets* results from a deficiency in renal 1α-hydroxylase. *Type II vitamin D–dependent rickets* results from a defect in the vitamin D receptor, with resultant deficiency in response to 1,25-D_2. Anticonvulsant medications that activate the P-450 oxidases in the liver increase the rate of vitamin D catabolism, with resultant decreased 25-hydroxyvitamin D_3 levels and osteomalacia or rickets.

Hypophosphatemia is also associated with osteomalacia and rickets. A renal tubular defect found in *X-linked hypophosphatemic rickets* is caused by a mutation in the endopeptidase gene *PEX* (see Chapter 3). Hypophosphatemia with acidosis causes rickets in *Fanconi syndrome*. In the past, phosphate-binding antacids containing aluminum were used to treat hyperphosphatemia in patients undergoing dialysis. Unfortunately, however, aluminum from these medications is deposited in bone and disrupts normal bone mineralization.

Serum chemistries are similar in osteomalacia and rickets; patients have normal calcium levels, low vitamin D levels, elevated PTH levels, and elevated alkaline phosphatase levels. Normal calcium levels are important in distinguishing osteomalacia and rickets from primary hyperparathyroidism, in which calcium levels are elevated. Measurements of serum levels of *25-hydroxyvitamin D* and *1,25-dihydroxyvitamin D* are now routinely available, and these tests can be useful in diagnosis and in monitoring of treatment.

The treatment of patients with osteomalacia and rickets varies with the cause of the disorder. All patients should receive 1500 mg of calcium supplements daily and varying doses of vitamin D. Treatment of adult patients with vitamin D deficiencies begins with 50,000 IU of vitamin D_2 given three to five times weekly; patients are then maintained on 1000 to 2000 IU daily after the deficiency has been corrected. Patients with disorders that affect the hydroxylation of active vitamin D precursors require treatment with forms of vitamin D that are already hydroxylated. If surgical intervention for bony realignment is necessary, medical management should optimize mineralization before the operation is performed.

OSTEOPOROSIS

Osteoporosis is a bone disease that is characterized by low bone mass and microarchitectural deterioration of bone structure, leading to enhanced bone fragility and a consequent increase in fracture risk. It is the most prevalent bone disease of developed countries. Because bone loss occurs as a normal part of aging, both men and women are at risk for osteoporosis; however, because of the accelerated bone loss that begins at menopause, women are twice as likely to fracture as are men of the same age. Genetic factors are still incompletely understood but include polymorphisms in specific loci such as the vitamin D receptor and estrogen receptor genes, as well as ethnicity (whites and Asians are at greatest risk). Additional risk factors for osteoporosis include poor nutrition and low body weight (less than 85% of ideal body weight, or less than 120 pounds); limited calcium intake; chronic alcohol abuse; smoking; excessive caffeine intake; a sedentary lifestyle; and chronic exposure to certain medications, such as antiseizure medications and steroids (**Figure 2-9**).

Osteoporosis develops when the normal balance of activity between osteoblasts (the bone-forming cells) and osteoclasts (the bone-resorbing cells) is upset. *Coupling*, the normal balance between osteoblast and osteoclast activity in adults, occurs when the amount of bone formation equals the amount of bone resorption. Accelerated bone loss occurs in women after menopause because the activity of osteoclasts is enhanced. The osteoclasts make deeper and more numerous resorption lacunae, and the osteoblasts are unable to replace the resorbed bone at the same rate. This process results in net bone loss. By comparison, the bone loss that occurs with normal aging results from a decrease in osteoblast activity while osteoclasts retain normal or even slightly decreased activity.

The diagnosis of osteoporosis is based on bone density measurements at the hip and spine. *Dual-energy x-ray absorptiometry (DEXA)* is considered the standard method for obtaining bone density measurements. Radiation doses are low (1–3 mrem, compared with 25–30 mrem for a chest radiograph), and scanning times are brief (3–7 min per location). Once the density at a specific site has been determined, a *T-score* is calculated for that site. The T-score gauges the standard deviation (SD) for that specific density measurement from a standard that should be obtained when the body reaches peak bone mass (at approximately age 25 to 30 years). The World Health Organization defines *osteopenia* as mild to moderate bone deficiency with T-scores of less than 1 to 2.5 SD below peak bone mass. T-scores of more than 2.5 SD less than peak bone mass are defined as *osteoporosis* with severe bone deficiency. Although plain radiographs are useful in defining a fracture, they cannot be used in objective measurement of bone density because of variations in radiographic technique (film penetration) and, more important, because a significant amount of bone loss (at least 30%) must occur before the event can be appreciated on a plain radiograph.

Several fracture types are common with osteoporosis, including vertebral compression and fractures of the hip, femoral neck, intertrochanteric femur, distal radius, proximal humerus, distal femur, and proximal tibia. Patients who have any of these fracture types after a low-impact injury should be evaluated for osteoporosis. Patients with multiple vertebral compression fractures develop a *"dowager's hump,"* characterized by thoracic kyphosis and loss of trunk height (**Figure 2-10**).

Because osteoporosis is a dynamic disease, a single DEXA measurement cannot determine the rate of bone loss; that rate can be determined only by serial measurements over time. Serum and urine markers can be used as indicators of the relative activities of bone formation and resorption. Bone resorption activity is assessed through measurement of urinary samples of collagen byproducts of bone matrix degradation, including *N-telopeptide* and *pyridinoline*, as well as *deoxypyridinoline cross-links*. Relative bone formation activity can be assessed with the use of serum markers for *alkaline phosphatase* and *osteocalcin* (bone-specific proteins secreted by osteoblasts). Laboratory studies of bone loss activity are important in diagnosis and in monitoring the effects of treatment.

Diagnosing osteoporosis requires exclusion of osteomalacia (inadequate mineralization of bone matrix) and secondary causes of

Figure 2-9: Risk Factors for Osteoporosis

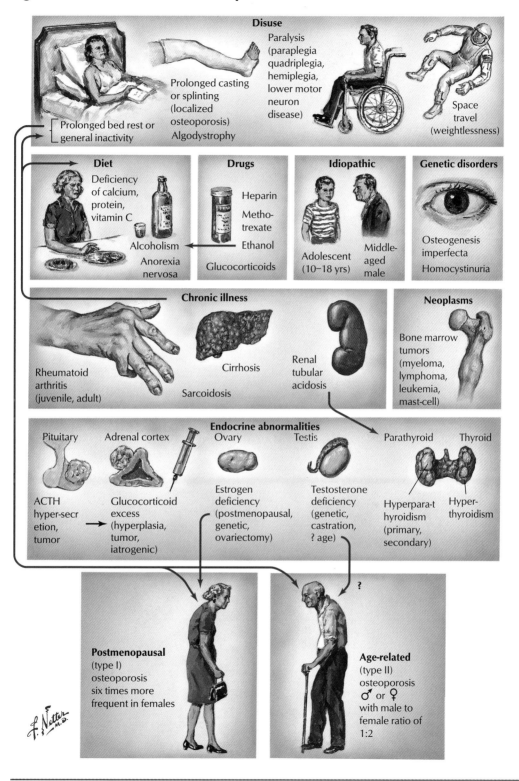

Figure 2-10: Clinical Manifestations of Osteoporosis

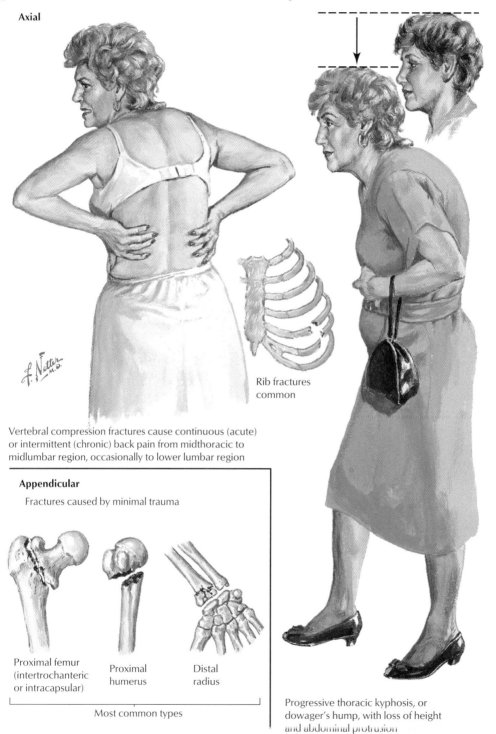

Axial

Rib fractures common

Vertebral compression fractures cause continuous (acute) or intermittent (chronic) back pain from midthoracic to midlumbar region, occasionally to lower lumbar region

Appendicular

Fractures caused by minimal trauma

Proximal femur (intertrochanteric or intracapsular)

Proximal humerus

Distal radius

Most common types

Progressive thoracic kyphosis, or dowager's hump, with loss of height and abdominal protrusion

osteopenia such as steroid use, alcoholism, eating disorders, and cancer. Abnormalities of vitamin D metabolism are the most common cause of osteomalacia. In addition to obtaining a good history, the clinician should measure serum calcium, vitamin D, phosphorus, and basic electrolyte levels, and should obtain thyroid function test results. Parathyroid hormone levels should be determined if associated alterations in calcium and phosphorus are found.

The principal goal of osteoporosis treatment is prevention. Adequate nutrition, exercise, and calcium and vitamin D intake, as well as maintenance of normal menstrual cycles, should be encouraged at all ages. The goal in children, adolescents, and young adults is to achieve a high peak bone mass. In older patients, these modalities minimize the risk of accelerated bone loss. At menopause, other therapies such as estrogen, bisphosphonates, calcitonin, and selective estrogen receptor modulators may be used to slow the rate of bone loss. Intermittent administration of PTH may stimulate osteoblastic bone formation; this treatment approach is undergoing clinical trials.

Calcium and *vitamin D supplements* decrease bone resorption, increase mineralization of osteoid, and decrease the risk of hip fracture. Although these supplements do not normalize bone resorption, they are inexpensive, relatively well tolerated, enhance the benefits of other antiresorptive agents, and are recommended for most individuals older than 50 years. The recommended daily intake of calcium is 1500 mg, an amount that most individuals do not obtain through dietary intake alone. *Calcium carbonate* or *calcium citrate* supplements are best given in divided doses of 500 mg or less to maximize absorption. Effective use of calcium carbonate requires that stomach acid be absorbed, whereas this is not the case for calcium citrate; thus, patients with *achlorhydria* (who make up a significant percentage of elderly individuals) should take calcium citrate. Vitamin D is critical to calcium absorption, and current guidelines recommend dietary supplements of 400 to 800 IU

daily. Higher doses are used to treat vitamin D deficiencies or defects in hepatic or renal vitamin D metabolism.

Estrogen receptors are found on osteoblasts and other cells. Estrogen indirectly affects calcium homeostasis by modulating intestinal calcium absorption and renal calcium excretion. Through incompletely understood mechanisms, estrogen also helps to prevent osteoclast hyperactivity. *Estrogen therapy* used to be the mainstay of osteoporosis prevention for women; however, recent reports demonstrating the detrimental effects of estrogen therapy on rates of cardiac events, uterine cancer, and breast cancer have led the US Food and Drug Administration (FDA) to recommend that the use of estrogen should be limited to females with postmenopausal symptoms or significant osteoporosis.

Selective estrogen receptor modulators (*SERMs*) take advantage of different estrogen receptors that have variable distribution and activity in different tissues. These drugs act as estrogen agonists in bone and estrogen antagonists in breast tissue. Compared with standard estrogen therapy, SERMs currently approved for use in osteoporosis reduce the risk of breast cancer by 70%, present no risk for uterine cancer, decrease the risk of spine fracture by 40%, and increase bone mass in the spine, but at a lower rate than that associated with estrogen or bisphosphonates.

Bisphosphonates are analogs of pyrophosphate that bind to the surfaces of hydroxyapatite crystals. These drugs prevent bone resorption by interfering with intracellular signaling in osteoclasts and are approved for use in men and women. Bisphosphonates are not metabolized and are excreted intact in the urine. Because they have a long half-life in bone, stopping treatment does not result in the rapid bone loss that occurs when estrogen therapy is stopped. The two most commonly used bisphosphonates, *alendronate* (10 mg daily) and *risedronate* (5 mg daily), have been shown to decrease vertebral and hip fractures. These bisphosphonates must be taken on an empty stomach with water only because calcium, food, and other beverages greatly decrease their absorption. The patient must remain upright (sitting or standing) for 30 minutes after taking the medication to minimize gastrointestinal adverse effects of esophagitis and dyspepsia that occur in approximately 10% of users.

Calcitonin is a hormone that acts directly on osteoclasts through a receptor-mediated mechanism to decrease bone resorption. This agent is available as a nasal spray and is given in doses of 200 IU daily. It has been shown to be effective in stabilizing spinal bone mass and decreasing vertebral fracture, but it appears to have no effect on hip fracture rates. Calcitonin also has a unique analgesic effect in the treatment of painful vertebral fractures.

In addition to the standard techniques for treating long-bone fractures that result from osteoporosis (ie, casting, bracing, internal fixation), a new therapy has emerged for the treatment of vertebral compression fractures. Augmentation of vertebral bodies with polymethylmethacrylate (PMMA) cement can be done through one of two techniques. *Vertebroplasty* involves the percutaneous injection of PMMA into the vertebral body, a procedure that reinforces the vertebra in its collapsed position. In *kyphoplasty*, a balloon catheter is introduced into the vertebral body and inflated, allowing for some restoration of vertebral body height. PMMA is then injected into the cavity created by the balloon catheter (**Figure 2-11**). Both therapies have demonstrated dramatic alleviation of the pain associated with vertebral fracture, allowing for earlier mobilization and return to normal activities. Complications of these procedures include infection and burns from the cement as it hardens through an exothermic reaction. The long-term effects of PMMA-supplemented vertebral bodies have not yet been determined.

PAGET DISEASE

Paget disease is a localized disorder of bone remodeling that causes dense sclerosis, enlargement, and deformity of affected bones. This disease is more prevalent in individuals of Northern European, North American, and Australian descent and is rarely seen in Asians. Affected individuals are generally older than 55 years and rarely younger than 40 years. Many patients are asymptomatic, and the disease is often discovered on radiographs taken to diagnose another problem.

The disease affects both osteoclasts and osteoblasts; however, the cause is unknown. Two studies of large kindreds have identified a gene that may increase susceptibility to the disease. Viral inclusion bodies resembling those of RNA paramyxoviruses, such as respiratory syncytial virus and measles, have been found in the osteoclasts of involved bones in some patients. The limited locations of the disease in the skeleton, the increased levels of the inflammatory cytokine interleukin-6 (IL-6) in pagetic foci, and the fact that new disease foci do not form once the disease has become established suggest that systemic factors are influenced by the local bone microenvironment to determine the establishment and extent of disease.

Three histologic phases of Paget disease have been observed. Initially, a marked increase in bone resorption is seen, with an increase in the number and size of osteoclasts. Radiographs at this phase show lucency in the affected bone. In long bones, a *wedge-* or *flame-shaped lucency* begins in the metaphysis and points toward the diaphysis. This lucency advances into the diaphysis and progresses along the length of the bone at a rate of 1 cm per year. The second phase is characterized by a rapid increase in osteoblast activity with resultant increased new bone formation and alkaline phosphatase levels. The new bone forms in a disordered pattern with widened lamellae and irregular cement lines. Woven bone, rather than normal lamellar bone, predominates, and mineralization occurs at twice the normal rate. Radiographs taken during this phase show previously lucent regions converting into radiodense regions. In the final phase, both osteoclast and osteoblast activities decrease. Radiographs show densely sclerotic deformed bones with the thickened trabecular pattern and cortices that characterize this disease.

Figure 2-11: Kyphoplasty: Pretreatment and Posttreatment Radiographs

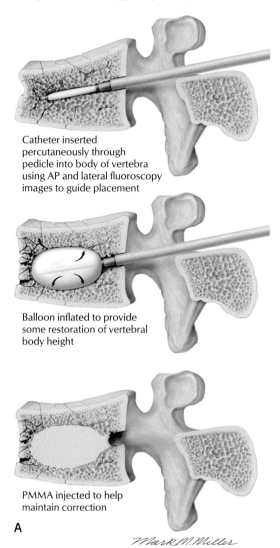

Catheter inserted percutaneously through pedicle into body of vertebra using AP and lateral fluoroscopy images to guide placement

Balloon inflated to provide some restoration of vertebral body height

PMMA injected to help maintain correction

A

Mark M. Miller

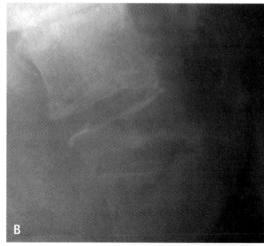

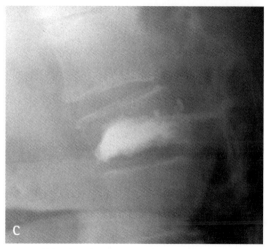

73-year-old female with acute onset of back pain after low-impact fall. Continued marked discomfort 4 weeks after injury. Lateral radiograph shows L1 compression fracture (B). Postinjection radiograph (C) shows partial restoration of vertebral height. Patient had resolution of pain and returned to prefracture function.

Most patients with Paget disease are asymptomatic. Patients with symptoms report bone, joint, or low back pain (**Figure 2-12**). A bone scan will be positive during the early phases of the disease and may help demonstrate foci before they become evident on plain radiographs. Paget disease of the spine commonly affects the lumbar vertebrae, resulting in a "picture frame" appearance of these vertebrae with their thickened end plates and thickened subcortical bone. Enlargement of the vertebrae can cause nerve root compression with associated pain, weakness, and numbness in the region innervated by the affected nerve. Lesions located adjacent to joints may cause osteoarthritis. Fractures are more common and frequently occur on the convex (tension) side of affected bones, resulting in a bowing or angular deformity. Paget disease also can precipitate high-output cardiac failure due to increased vascularity of the affected bones and the subsequent demand on the cardiovascular system.

Patients with suspected Paget disease should have plain radiographs taken of the affected areas. Biochemical markers of bone turnover, such as serum alkaline phosphatase and urinary collagen breakdown markers, should be measured during the initial evaluation and followed during treatment. Symptomatic patients should receive bisphosphonates. Oral therapy with alendronate, risedronate, and tiludronate prevents the mineralization defects associated with prolonged etidronate treatment. Calcitonin, administered as a nasal spray, is an alternative for individuals who cannot tolerate bisphosphonates; however, its effectiveness is variable.

Patients with severe osteoarthritis may be helped by joint replacement procedures, but the high vascularity of their bone often increases intraoperative bleeding. Hypercalcemia also may occur after major orthopaedic procedures in patients with active disease.

An unusual complication that occurs in approximately 1% of patients is the development of a high-grade sarcoma within a pagetic lesion. These tumors most commonly are osteosarcomas, but fibrosarcomas and chondrosarcomas also may be seen. Furthermore, carcinomas occasionally metastasize to pagetic foci because of the increased vascularity of these regions. This emphasizes the need for periodic radiographs and biopsy of lesions that appear to be evolving.

OSTEONECROSIS

Osteonecrosis, also known as *avascular necrosis*, occurs when circulation of blood is impaired in a region of bone, with resultant death of osteocytes and other cells in the involved area. Osteonecrosis may occur in any bone, although it is most commonly seen in the femoral head, the humeral head, the femoral condyles, the hand (lunate and scaphoid bones), and the foot (navicular or talar bones). Bone infarction also may occur in the medullary canals of long bones such as the femur, the tibia, and the humerus.

Disruption of the circulation may result from trauma, such as a fracture or dislocation causing tearing and/or compression of vulnerable blood vessels (**Figure 2-13**). Fractures of the femoral neck, the scaphoid, and the talus are associated with an increased risk that osteonecrosis will develop.

Bone infarction also may occur without trauma. Patients with conditions that disrupt the flow of blood in the small arterioles and venules, with resultant vascular stasis, have an increased incidence of osteonecrosis. Examples of these conditions include sickle cell anemia; decompression sickness (dysbarism); Gaucher disease; hypercoagulable disorders caused by decreased protein C, protein S, factor V Leiden mutant, or antithrombin III; and hypofibrinolysis resulting from increased levels of plasminogen activator inhibitor-1, pregnancy, or malignancy. Alcohol abuse and steroid use are both associated with osteonecrosis. The exact mechanism of their effect on bone circulation is not known, although the effect is thought to result from alterations in lipid metabolism, with resultant fat emboli and abnormal circulating lipids becoming trapped in end arterioles.

Death of the osteocytes and bone marrow cells occurs within hours after disruption of blood circulation in a bone. Biopsy of bone at this early stage demonstrates empty osteocyte lacunae and necrosis of adjacent marrow fat and hematopoietic cells. Repair of the necrotic bone is attempted, beginning at the boundary of viable bone and extending into the area of infarction. The early repair process in cancellous bone is characterized by the laying down of new bone (woven bone) on the dead trabeculae. This repair process is slower in cortical bone because cones of necrotic cortical bone must be resorbed by osteoclasts before new bone can be formed. Because the necrotic bone is removed more quickly than new bone is formed, normal mechanical stresses may cause the region of

Figure 2-12: Paget Disease

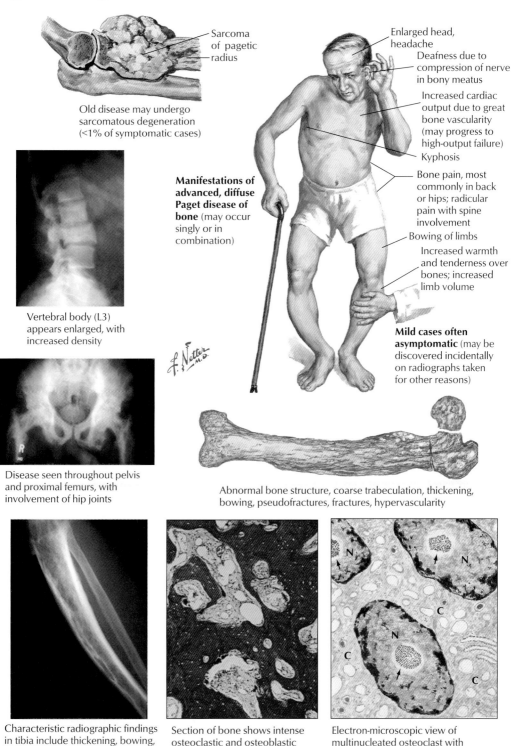

Sarcoma of pagetic radius

Old disease may undergo sarcomatous degeneration (<1% of symptomatic cases)

Enlarged head, headache

Deafness due to compression of nerve in bony meatus

Increased cardiac output due to great bone vascularity (may progress to high-output failure)

Kyphosis

Bone pain, most commonly in back or hips; radicular pain with spine involvement

Bowing of limbs

Increased warmth and tenderness over bones; increased limb volume

Manifestations of advanced, diffuse Paget disease of bone (may occur singly or in combination)

Vertebral body (L3) appears enlarged, with increased density

Mild cases often asymptomatic (may be discovered incidentally on radiographs taken for other reasons)

Disease seen throughout pelvis and proximal femurs, with involvement of hip joints

Abnormal bone structure, coarse trabeculation, thickening, bowing, pseudofractures, fractures, hypervascularity

Characteristic radiographic findings in tibia include thickening, bowing, and coarse trabeculation, with advancing radiolucent wedge

Section of bone shows intense osteoclastic and osteoblastic activity and mosaic of lamellar bone

Electron-microscopic view of multinucleated osteoclast with nuclear inclusions that may be viruses (arrows). N = nuclei; C = cytoplasm

Figure 2-13: Osteonecrosis After Fracture

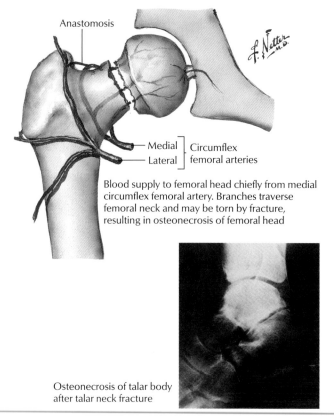

Blood supply to femoral head chiefly from medial circumflex femoral artery. Branches traverse femoral neck and may be torn by fracture, resulting in osteonecrosis of femoral head

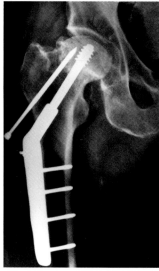

Osteonecrosis after fracture of the femoral neck. Note collapse and sclerosis of femoral head

Osteonecrosis of talar body after talar neck fracture

bone undergoing repair to collapse. When this occurs in subchondral bone, collapse and disruption of the underlying articular surfaces may be seen. Buckling of the articular surface typically begins several months after the initial insult and is the event that precipitates symptoms. The resultant joint incongruity, coupled with further collapse of osteonecrotic bone, initiates the process of secondary arthritis that may eventually (over several years) cause a debilitating arthritis.

Patients with osteonecrosis typically present with gradually increasing pain that is further increased by activity. Some patients develop sudden sharp pain that is thought to be secondary to the acute collapse (fracture) of a relatively large area of subchondral bone and subsequent joint incongruity. At initial presentation, most patients show mild limita-

tion of motion. With progression of arthritic changes, joint motion is further restricted, and gait becomes more antalgic.

At the onset of osteonecrosis, no changes are seen on plain radiographs. Three months after the initial insult, radiographs sometimes show very subtle osteopenia. When the subchondral bone begins to collapse, a radiolucency, called a *crescent sign,* is sometimes seen. With progression of the arthropathy, joint incongruity with flattening and narrowing of the articular surface is observed. Medullary infarctions, as they are repaired, show *ringed regions of radiodensity* on plain radiographs that often resemble smoke rising from a chimney. This radiographic pattern results from saponification of marrow fat and its calcification. Because many medullary infarctions are asymptomatic, these lesions

Figure 2-14: Stages of Osteonecrosis of the Femoral Head

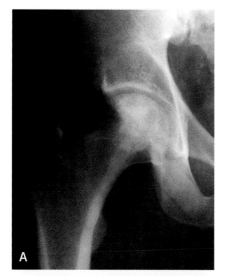

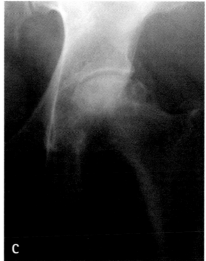

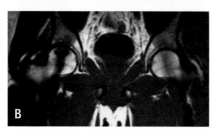

52-year-old male with 2 month history of activity-related anterior thigh pain. AP radiograph (A) shows sclerosis but no evidence of crescent sign or subchondral collapse. MRI (B) shows anterior-middle third signal changes consistent with osteonecrosis but no evidence of subchondral disruption.

AP radiograph (C) of left hip in a 52-year-old male with 1.5 year history of progressive bilateral hip pain. Radiograph of left hip shows step-off in contour of bone and decreased cartilage thickness consistent with advanced stage osteonecrosis.

are often incidental radiographic findings (**Figure 2-14**).

Magnetic resonance imaging (MRI) is 95% sensitive and specific for diagnosing osteonecrosis and is used both in defining the extent of the osteonecrosis and in early detection. Signal changes on MRI are observed within a few days after the insult occurs, even though the patient is asymptomatic. Because 60% of individuals with osteonecrosis of the femoral head have bilateral disease, it is important that an MRI of the asymptomatic hip be obtained in these individuals so that osteonecrosis can be detected in its earliest stages.

Treatment of osteonecrosis is based on the location of the infarct, its size, and the stage at which it is diagnosed. Medullary infarctions

are generally treated symptomatically and observed for healing.

Osteonecrosis of the femoral head frequently requires intervention because approximately 80% of these cases progress to a significant arthropathy. Restricted weight bearing does not appear to prevent progression of associated hip arthropathy. In the early stages of osteonecrosis, decompression of the femoral head with removal of a core of cancellous bone up to the subchondral margin can decrease the intraosseous pressure surrounding the infarction and provide a route for vascular ingrowth and bone repair. Patients often experience immediate relief of pain, but they must remain on crutches with limited weight bearing on the treated limb until enough bone healing has occurred to prevent articular surface collapse. These cored-out tunnels are sometimes packed with bone graft in an attempt to stimulate new bone formation. Up to two thirds of patients treated with *core decompression* before articular surface incongruity develops will have a satisfactory result, compared with only one quarter of patients who do not undergo surgical intervention. Some studies have reported that similar success may be attained in patients with more advanced stages of osteonecrosis by supplementation of the *core decompression with a vascularized fibular bone graft*. However, this procedure is technically demanding and has a 20% complication rate. After subchondral bone and articular surfaces have collapsed and flattened, patients in the later stages of osteonecrosis are treated symptomatically for their arthritis until joint replacement is required.

Osteonecrosis in other locations is treated symptomatically. The humerus is not a weight-bearing bone, and pain, even from a collapsed articular surface, often may be treated nonoperatively. If pain is severe and shoulder function becomes greatly limited, the patient may undergo shoulder hemiarthroplasty. Osteonecrosis of the talus (which generally results from talar neck fracture) or of the navicular (which can occur spontaneously) is treated initially with limited weight bearing. Fusion of the ankle or midfoot may be performed when significant disability persists. Both osteonecro-sis of the scaphoid due to fracture and spontaneous osteonecrosis of the lunate (Kienböck disease) are treated with casting or bracing until pain improves. If pain persists, operative alternatives include vascular pedicle transplantation, joint leveling by a radial shortening or ulnar-lengthening osteotomy, proximal row carpectomy, limited intercarpal arthrodesis, and wrist arthrodesis. Osteonecrosis of the knee is treated similarly to osteonecrosis of the femoral head, except that the initial treatment of limited weight bearing is more acceptable in the knee because of more rapid healing at this site and the reduced tendency for articular collapse. Persistent pain may be relieved by core decompression. Arthritis caused by articular surface collapse is treated symptomatically; however, severe pain or functional limitations may require that knee arthroplasty be performed.

ADDITIONAL READINGS

Favus MJ, ed. *Primer on the Metabolic Bone Diseases and Disorders of Mineral Metabolism*, 5th edition. Washington, DC: American Society for Bone and Mineral Research; 2003.

Flynn WF, Lane JM, Cornell CN. Metabolic bone disease. In Chapman MW, ed. *Chapman's Orthopaedic Surgery*, 3rd edition. Philadelphia: Lippincott Williams and Wilkins; 2001:3483–3503.

Hernigou P, Poignard A, Nogier A, Manicom O. Fate of very small asymptomatic stage-I osteonecrotic lesions of the hip. *J Bone Joint Surg Am*. 2004;86:2589–2593.

http://www.osteo.org/ (NIH Osteoporosis and Related Bone Disease-National Resource Center).

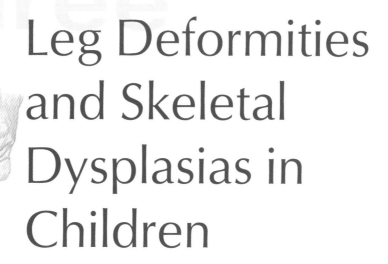

three

Leg Deformities and Skeletal Dysplasias in Children

Walter B. Greene, MD

The oft-quoted statement, "Children are not just small adults," is particularly germane to the diagnosis and treatment of pediatric disorders of the musculoskeletal system. Growth and its associated remodeling potential may be a tremendous ally in the treatment of some pediatric disorders. For example, in a newborn with a dysplastic dislocated hip, simple splinting often results in a normal joint that provides normal function for a lifetime. Growth, however, may exacerbate some conditions. Excessive pressure on a growth plate, particularly one that has some dysfunction, causes further inhibition of growth and progressive angulation of the limb. Examples include progressive genu varum observed in infantile tibia vara, rickets and other skeletal dysplasias, and progressive curvature of the spine as observed in some pediatric spinal disorders.

Erosion of articular cartilage caused by skeletal malalignment takes time to develop. As a result, severe pain from skeletal deformities often is absent during childhood. An understanding of the natural history of these conditions is critical for knowing whether observation, bracing, or surgical treatment is needed. Furthermore, the lower extremity undergoes changes in alignment during growth. An understanding of these physiologic changes is necessary before it can be determined whether a child is normal for age or needs further evaluation.

This chapter reviews the angular and rotational changes that occur during growth, as well as genetic diseases that affect skeletal growth and function. Juvenile rheumatoid arthritis, pediatric and neuromuscular disorders, infectious disease, tumors and childhood disorders localized to a specific site are described in other chapters.

IN-TOEING AND OUT-TOEING

Intrauterine packaging influences the position and alignment of the extremities, particularly the lower limbs. Neonates have moderate hip flexion, abduction, and external rotation contractures; mild knee flexion contractures; and excessive ankle dorsiflexion. With more room to move, the infant typically stretches out the knee and ankle in a few weeks; however, hip external rotation capsular tightness does not resolve fully until the child begins to walk.

In-toeing and out-toeing are common parental concerns after a child begins to walk. In-toeing, the more common concern, may be secondary to increased internal femoral torsion (*femoral anteversion*), increased *internal tibial torsion*, foot deformities, or some combination of the three conditions. Out-toeing may be secondary to external femoral torsion (*femoral retroversion*), increased *external tibial torsion*, foot deformities, or some combination of the three conditions. An understanding of normal development is critical because in-toeing and out-toeing are frequent variations of normal development.

Femoral torsion (anteversion) is greatest at birth (approximately 40°) and gradually declines to adult values (10° to 15°) by age 8 years (**Figure 3-1**). Although it does not provide an absolute measurement, the easiest way to assess femoral anteversion is through measurement of hip rotation with the child prone and the hips extended. However, it is important to realize that clinical measurement of hip rotation does not profile the degree of femoral torsion until the neonatal hip external rotation contracture fully resolves, which usually occurs by 1 year of age; however, it may take longer.

In children, the total arc of hip rotation is typically 80° to 100°, and the average range of rotation for a child older than 2 years is approximately 50° internal rotation and 40° external rotation. Increased internal rotation coupled with decreased external rotation indicates *increased femoral anteversion*. Likewise, increased external rotation coupled with decreased internal rotation indicates reduced femoral torsion (*femoral retroversion*). Femoral torsion is within normal limits unless internal or external rotation is less than 20°.

Tibial torsion, measured by the relationship

Figure 3-1: Internal Femoral Torsion (In-Toeing)

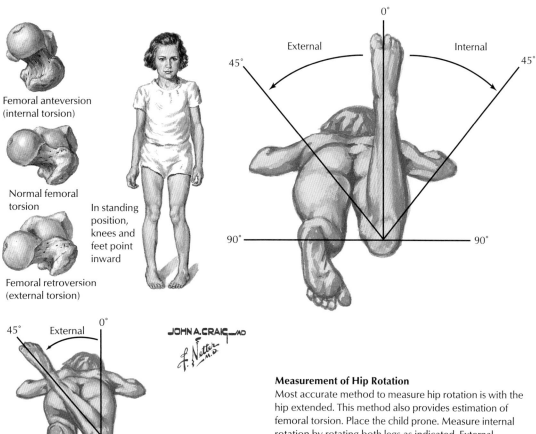

Femoral anteversion
(internal torsion)

Normal femoral
torsion

In standing
position,
knees and
feet point
inward

Femoral retroversion
(external torsion)

JOHN A. CRAIG—MD

F. Netter
M.D.

Measurement of Hip Rotation
Most accurate method to measure hip rotation is with the hip extended. This method also provides estimation of femoral torsion. Place the child prone. Measure internal rotation by rotating both legs as indicated. External rotation can only be measured by assessing one extremity at a time. Place one hand on the buttocks and with the other hand move the hip into external rotation as depicted. Maximum external rotation is noted when the pelvis starts to tilt. In children 2 years of age or older, the average internal and external rotation is equal at 45° to 50° each and the total arc of hip rotation is 90° to 100°. Patients who have greater internal rotation and less external rotation have more femoral anteversion. Patients with greater external rotation and less internal rotation have less torsion of the femur.

of the transmalleolar axis to the coronal axis of the proximal tibia, is typically neutral, or 0°, at birth and gradually increases to approximately 20° by age 10 years (range, 0° to 40°). Tibial torsion is often asymmetric, with the left side commonly less externally rotated. Although it is not a direct measurement, tibial torsion also may be assessed through measurement of the thigh-foot angle (**Figure 3-2**).

This angle is easier to measure and parallels the transmalleolar axis, but average values are typically 5° greater internally.

Parents often seek medical attention for their children because of concern about how they are walking. Children with severe in-toeing may stumble or trip more frequently as they catch their toes on the back of the trailing leg. Neuromuscular disorders also cause in-toeing or out-

Figure 3-2

Internal tibial torsion
Child seated with knees flexed 90°. Patellae point directly forward, indicating that femurs are in neutral position, but feet point inward, suggesting tibial torsion. Measure tibial torsion by positioning the thigh in neutral rotation, then placing the thumb of one hand over the tibial tuberosity and with the other hand placing the thumb over the prominence of the medial malleolus and the long finger over the prominence of the lateral malleolus. The degree of tibial torsion is the estimate of the angle made by the transmalleolar axis and the axis of the coronal plane of the proximal tibia.

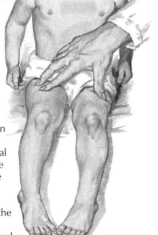
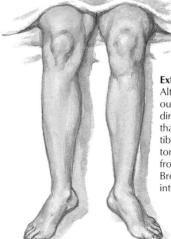

External tibial torsion
Although feet are turned outward, knees point directly forward, showing that toeing out is due to tibial, not femoral, external torsion. This case resulted from overuse of Denis Browne splint to correct internal femoral torsion.

Thigh-Foot Angle

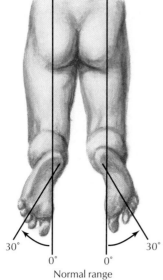
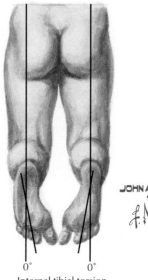

30° 30°
0° 0°
Normal range

0° 0°
Internal tibial torsion

toeing, and children with these conditions—most often mild cerebral palsy—may be brought to the physician for evaluation of their "abnormal walking" before the underlying neuromuscular disorder has been diagnosed. Therefore, children undergoing evaluation for in-toeing and out-toeing should be screened for development of appropriate motor milestones (**Table 3-1**) and examined for spasticity, muscle contractures, and a stiff or unbalanced gait.

Physical examination should include the following steps:

+ Measurement of foot progression angle (the angle that the foot makes relative to the line of progression as the child walks)

+ Measurement of hip rotation (femoral torsion)

Table 3-1 Gross Motor Developmental Screening During Early Childhood	
Age	**Activity**
2 years	Climbs up and down stairs, one step at a time
2.5 years	Jumps
3 years	Climbs stairs, alternating feet
4 years	Hops on one foot
5 years	Skips

+ Measurement of tibial torsion (thigh-foot and ankle)
+ Inspection of the foot
+ Evaluation for possible neuromuscular disorders

The foot progression angle does not indicate the site of the problem, but it quantifies the severity of the problem and distinguishes it as either in-toeing or out-toeing. By age 2 years, children typically walk like adults in that the foot is turned out relative to the line of progression. A normal foot progression angle is 10° (range, 0° to 20°).

Metatarsus adductus and *clubfoot* are foot conditions that may cause or contribute to in-toeing (see Chapter 19). Increased heel valgus, typically associated with pes planovalgus, may contribute to out-toeing.

External rotation contracture of the hip during infancy may persist to a degree that causes concern when the child is between the ages of 6 and 12 months—a time when limb alignment is more obvious because children are in walkers or are starting to pull to a stand (**Figure 3-3**). Associated factors include male gender and black race. Examination typically reveals 60° to 70° of external rotation and only 20° to 30° of internal rotation. Hip rotation is usually symmetric, but out-toeing is greater on the right because tibial torsion is usually more external on that side.

Most children who exhibit in-toeing after 2 years of age have increased femoral anteversion. Regardless of the source of the in-toeing or out-toeing, however, most children with these conditions do not require treatment. Shoe modifications, braces, and exercises do not alter the development of femoral or tibial torsion. Casting occasionally is necessary in metatarsus adductus. In normal children, enough correction or compensation for increased femoral and tib-

Figure 3-3: External Rotation of Hips

Rotational Deformities of Lower Limb: Toeing Out

In external rotation of hips, when feet are turned maximally inward, knees are in neutral position or, at most, in slight internal rotation

Knees and feet point laterally, indicating femoral origin of toeing-out deformity. Common in newborns but usually corrects spontaneously when child begins to walk.

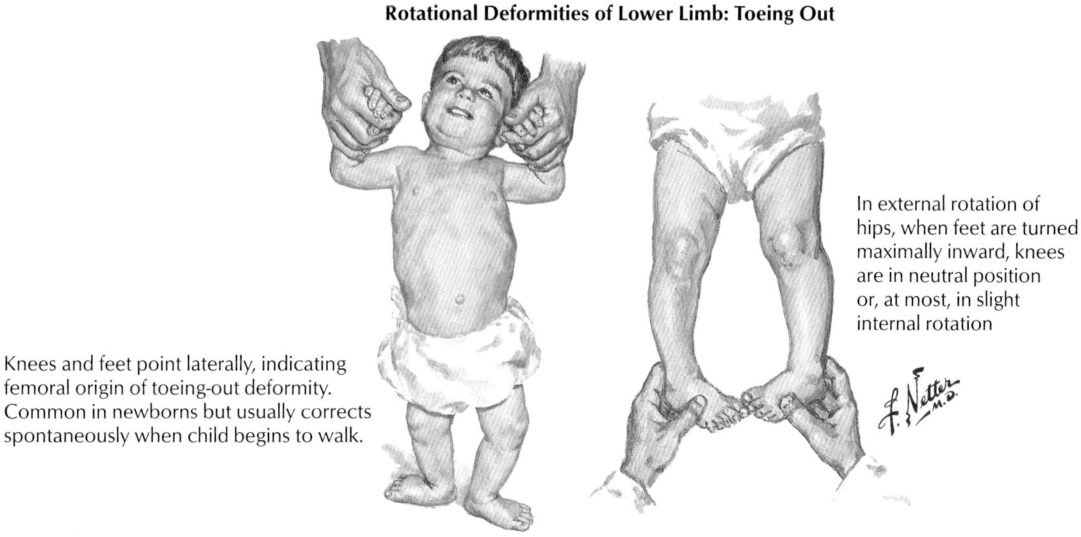

Figure 3-4: Malalignment Syndrome

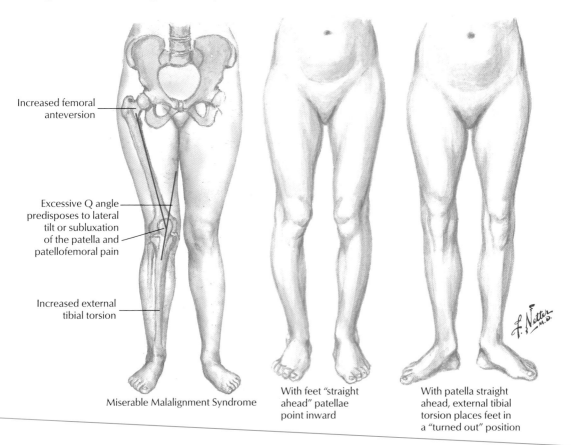

Increased femoral anteversion

Excessive Q angle predisposes to lateral tilt or subluxation of the patella and patellofemoral pain

Increased external tibial torsion

Miserable Malalignment Syndrome

With feet "straight ahead" patellae point inward

With patella straight ahead, external tibial torsion places feet in a "turned out" position

ial torsion occurs so that walking and running are not adversely affected. Although uncommon, if the child is 8 to 10 years of age and the in-toeing remains severe, then a rotational osteotomy of the femur may be indicated. Patellofemoral tracking problems occasionally result from increased femoral anteversion and concomitant external tibial torsion. With persistent knee pain, this so-called *miserable malalignment syndrome* requires corrective osteotomies of the femur and tibia (**Figure 3-4**). In children with cerebral palsy or other neuromuscular disorders, abnormal femoral and tibial torsion is more likely to persist to a degree that requires surgical correction.

GENU VARUM AND GENU VALGUM

At birth, bowleg (genu varum) of 10° to 15° is normal. The limbs gradually straighten

to a neutral tibiofemoral angle by the age of 12 to 20 months. Continued growth then results in progressive valgus, with genu valgum reaching maximum values at age 3 to 4 years. Genu valgum at this age is typically 10° to 15°, but it should be noted that young children have a fairly wide range of normal knee alignment (2 SD is ±10°). With further growth, the tibiofemoral angle gradually straightens, so that by age 7 years, normal adult genu valgum of approximately 5° is typically achieved (**Figure 3-5**).

Parents of an otherwise apparently healthy child typically become concerned about genu varum when bowleg is still present at 14 to 24 months. Several conditions should be considered when these children are evaluated (**Table 3-2**). The most common cause of genu varum at this age is physiologic genu

Figure 3-5: Bowleg

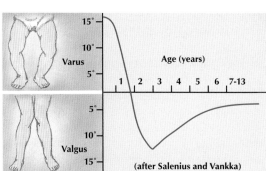

Graph depicts normal developmental changes in tibio-femoral angle. Substantial deviation suggests pathologic cause such as rickets, Blount's disease, or other disorders requiring specific treatment.

Two brothers, younger (left) with bowleg, older (right) with knock-knee. In both children, limbs eventually became normally aligned without corrective treatment

varum, sometimes called physiologic bowlegs, a condition that is a normal variation of growth and resolves without treatment.

Examination involves measuring height and plotting it on a height nomogram. Children with short stature need further evaluation.

Table 3-2
Differential Diagnosis of Genu Varum at Age 1 to 2 Years (no previous diagnosis)

+ Physiologic genu varum (variant of normal development)
+ Infantile tibia vara (depressed growth of the medial aspect of the proximal tibial physis; more common in African Americans, obese children, and early walkers)
+ Hypophosphatemic rickets (short stature, widening of the physis, low serum phosphorus level)
+ Metaphyseal dysplasia (short stature, widening of the physis, normal serum phosphorus level)
+ Fibrocartilaginous dysplasia (bowing proximal tibia, increased density in the medial aspect of the proximal tibial metaphysis)

One can quantify the genu varum by using a goniometer to measure the angulation, or measure the intercondylar (IC) width (distance between the medial femoral condyles when the lower extremities are positioned with the ankles touching). The IC distance is easier to measure in small children and can be compared in follow-up visits but has the disadvantage of being a relative, rather than an absolute, measurement.

Radiographs are appropriate when the child is at less than the 25th percentile for height, the varus is relatively severe for the child's age, excessive internal tibial torsion is observed, the varus is progressively increasing after age 16 months, or significant asymmetry of the two limbs is noted. Assess the tibiofemoral angle, the width of the growth plate, and the slope of the proximal tibia (the medial aspect is depressed in infantile tibia vara). It may be difficult to differentiate infantile tibia vara and physiologic genu varum at this age, but a tibial metaphyseal-diaphyseal angle greater than 14° to 16° is highly suggestive of infantile tibia vara.

Genu valgum typically becomes a parental concern when the child is $2\frac{1}{2}$ to $3\frac{1}{2}$ years of age. Most of these children have physiologic genu valgum, but other disorders should be considered (**Table 3-3**). An indirect measurement of genu valgum is the intermalleolar width (distance between the medial malleoli with the medial femoral condyle touching). Radiographs usually are not necessary but should be considered when the genu valgum is greater than 15° to 20°, the genu valgum is significantly asymmetric, or the child has short stature. For an otherwise normal 3- to 4-year-old child, observation is the treatment of choice. With subsequent growth, increased genu valgum spontaneously corrects more than 99% of the time. Furthermore, shoe modifications are ineffective. If abnormal genu valgum persists, a hemiepiphysiodesis can be performed at age 10 to 13 years.

SKELETAL DYSPLASIAS

Skeletal dysplasias result from genetic disorders that alter the proteins making up bone, articular cartilage, or growth plate tissue. Our understanding of skeletal dysplasias is progressing at a rapid pace. Classification of these disorders also is in a period of transition. Previously, the cause of skeletal dysplasia was so poorly understood that most dysplasias were grouped according to descriptive radiographic features. A clearer understanding of skeletal dysplasias not only will result in better treatment for these disorders but also will enhance our understanding and classification of the pathologic processes involved.

Achondroplasia—Fibroblast Growth Factor Receptor 3 Disorders

Achondroplasia is the most common cause of dwarfism (disproportionate shortening) and demonstrates greater genetic homogeneity than any other autosomal dominant disorder. Most cases result from new mutations that almost always cause a single amino acid change (arginine to glycine) in the membrane portion of the gene that codes *fibroblast growth factor receptor 3 (FGFR3)*.

FGFR3 is expressed in all growth plates and apparently regulates progression of chondrocyte maturation. The mutation in achondroplasia causes disorganization and inhibition of chondrocyte proliferation in the physis. Intramembranous bone formation, however, is normal. Therefore, these patients have a normal, but relatively large, skull with frontal bossing but hypoplasia of the midface that develops from endochondral ossification (**Figure 3-6**).

Trunk length is relatively normal, but the extremities have rhizomelic shortening, with the humeri and femora being the more foreshortened portions of the extremities. Upper extremity abnormalities include mild flexion contractures of the elbows and the "trident hand" caused by extra space between the third and fourth fingers. Disproportionate shortening of the upper extremities causes mild difficulties with personal hygiene, but otherwise, upper extremity function is not affected. Some degree of hip flexion contracture is universal. Genu varum or genu valgum may develop. Distal tibia vara is common and may require corrective osteotomy.

Kyphosis of the thoracolumbar junction is common during infancy, but this condition usually improves with age. The interpedicular distance progressively narrows in the lumbar spine, which is opposite the normal pattern. As a result, spinal stenosis is a frequent problem, and patients may develop neurogenic

---

Table 3–3

Differential Diagnosis of Genu Valgum at Age 2½ to 3½ Years (no previous diagnosis)

+ Physiologic genu valgum (variant of normal development)

+ Hypophosphatemic rickets (short stature, widening of the physis, low serum phosphorus level)

+ Multiple epiphyseal dysplasia (short stature, decreased height of epiphysis, delayed carpal ossification)

+ Pseudoachondroplasia (short stature, possibly windswept knees)

+ Growth stimulation after proximal tibial metaphyseal fracture

Figure 3-6: Achondroplasia

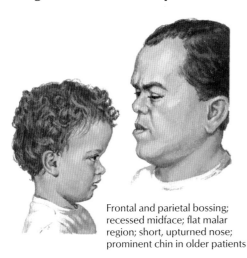

Frontal and parietal bossing; recessed midface; flat malar region; short, upturned nose; prominent chin in older patients

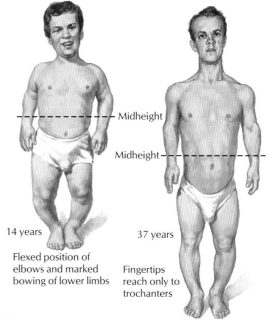

Midheight

Midheight

14 years

37 years

Flexed position of elbows and marked bowing of lower limbs

Fingertips reach only to trochanters

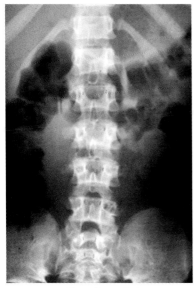

Trident hands with short fingers (held in three groups)

Infant with severe thoracolumbar kyphosis that usually reverses to characteristic lordosis at weight-bearing age. If it does not, true gibbus with cord compression may result. Neurologic signs and vertebral wedging are indications for surgery

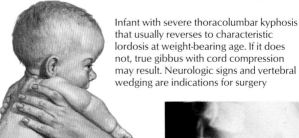

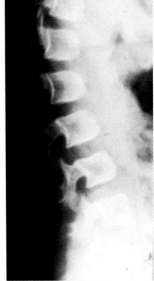

Lateral radiograph shows scalloped posterior borders of lumbar vertebrae and short pedicles, causing sagittal spinal stenosis

Anteroposterior radiograph shows progressive decrease in interpedicular distance (in caudad direction) in lumbar region, with resultant transverse narrowing of vertebral canal

claudication in the third or fourth decade that requires laminectomy and decompression of the spinal cord.

The clinical and radiographic features of achondroplasia are unique, and the diagnosis is typically straightforward. The differential diagnosis is usually *hypochondroplasia*, a less severe condition that is secondary to mutation of the tyrosine kinase portion of *FGFR3*.

Osteogenesis Imperfecta—Type I Collagen Disorder

Osteogenesis imperfecta (OI) is the most common genetic disorder that causes increased fracture susceptibility in children. The mutation affects *type I collagen*, which, in addition to its function as a "fiber-strengthening" material in bone, is found in ligaments, tendons, skin, sclera, and dentin. Autosomal dominant inheritance accounts for most cases. Fractures, bony deformities, joint laxity, hernias, mild cardiac abnormalities, blue sclera, premature deafness, and dentinogenesis imperfecta may occur. Clinical heterogeneity in OI is considerable. The Sillence classification (**Table 3-4**) is commonly used, but because very few families have the same

mutation, many cases do not fit easily into one of the categories.

Type I disease, the mildest form of OI, usually is caused by mutations that produce normal but reduced amounts of type I collagen. In type IA, clinical variability is noted, even within the same family, in the color of the sclera and in the number of fractures; some patients experience numerous fractures after the onset of walking, and others have only one or two fractures during late childhood (**Figure 3-7**).

In types II, III, and IV, most cases result from point mutations that cause substitutions in the repeated glycine amino acids. As a result, either the proα1(I) protein chain or the pro-α 2(I) protein chain is structurally abnormal. These patients may have fractures at birth or may develop fractures in the first year of life. Radiographic features include osteopenia and cortical thinning. Patients with type III OI routinely develop excessive bowing and deformity of the limbs, shortening of the limbs from bony deformity and disruption of the physis, and vertebral body compression fractures with shortening of the trunk and scoliosis (**Figure 3-8**).

Patients with severe forms of OI present with fractures at birth or soon after birth. The condition is easy to diagnose in these patients. In other cases, the diagnosis may be more problematic. Child abuse, metabolic bone disorders, other genetic conditions that weaken bone, and juvenile osteoporosis should be considered.

Bisphosphonate therapy can increase bone mass in patients with OI. This increase has been documented with the use of cyclic intravenous pamidronate in children with severe OI. Randomized trials of patients with other types of OI and with other types of bisphosphonate therapy are ongoing. Bone marrow transplantation also is being investigated.

Severe bowing of the long bones requires osteotomies, frequently at more than one level of the shaft, as well as internal fixation, preferably with an expanding type of intramedullary device (**Figure 3-9**). Progressive

---

Table 3-4

Sillence Classification of Osteogenesis Imperfecta

Type	Associated Features
I	Mild OI with blue sclera, possibly with premature deafness; autosomal dominant
II	Perinatally lethal
III	Severe, multiple fractures; progressively deforming; autosomal recessive
IV	Mild to moderate OI; white sclera

Types I and IV are subdivided into group A or B based on (A) absence or (B) presence of dentinogenesis imperfecta.

Source: Modified from Sillence DO, Senn A, Danks DM. Genetic heterogeneity in osteogenesis imperfecta. *J Med Genet* 1979;16:101–116.

Figure 3-7: Type I Osteogenesis Imperfecta

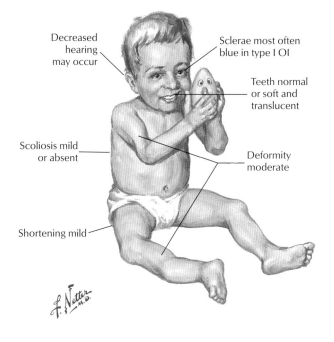

Decreased hearing may occur

Sclerae most often blue in type I OI

Teeth normal or soft and translucent

Scoliosis mild or absent

Deformity moderate

Shortening mild

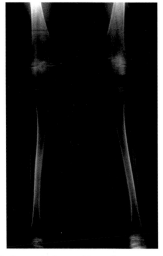

Radiograph shows thin and osteoporotic bones (variable). Fracture rate moderate; deformity mild, often amenable to intramedullary fixation

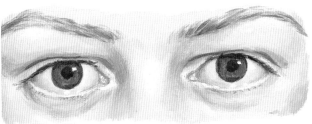

Sclerae usually blue

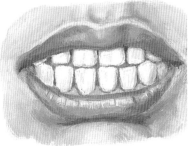

Teeth normal or soft and translucent

scoliosis necessitates a spinal fusion, a procedure that is difficult to perform in patients with OI because of marked bone fragility and severe spinal curvatures.

Type II Collagen Disorders

Type II collagen is the major structural component of articular cartilage (discussed in Chapter 4). Defects in the gene that codes for type II collagen result in disorders ranging from the perinatally lethal achondrogenesis to relatively mild disorders characterized by early osteoarthropathy. Because our understanding of type II collagen disorders is in-

complete, patients are still most often classified according to syndromes that were identified when knowledge of the condition was limited to radiographic and clinical features. As a result, clinical heterogeneity is common, and some syndromes include mutations in more than one gene.

Spondyloepiphyseal dysplasia congenita (SED congenita) is a heterogenous group that is evident at birth and is distinguished by disproportionate short-trunk dwarfing. The severe phenotype is secondary to abnormal αl(II) chains that result in structurally deficient type II collagen (triple helix fibrils retained).

Figure 3-8: Types III and IV Osteogenesis Imperfecta

Severe involvement; present with fractures at birth or within first 1-2 years of life

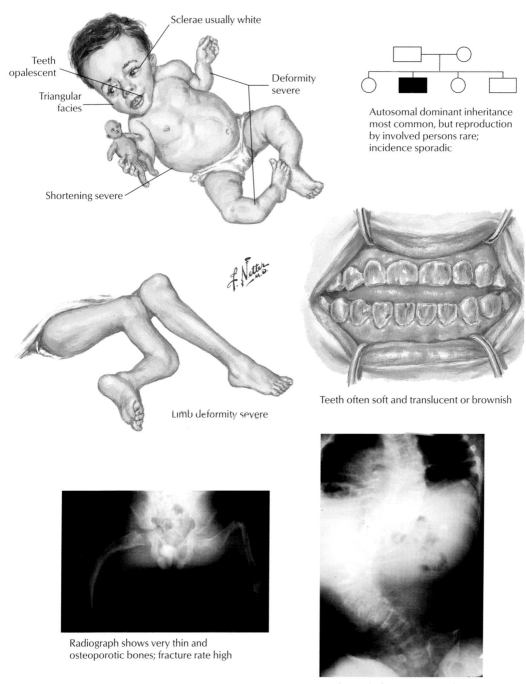

Sclerae usually white

Teeth opalescent

Triangular facies

Shortening severe

Deformity severe

Autosomal dominant inheritance most common, but reproduction by involved persons rare; incidence sporadic

Limb deformity severe

Teeth often soft and translucent or brownish

Radiograph shows very thin and osteoporotic bones; fracture rate high

Radiograph shows severe scoliosis and chest deformity

Figure 3-9: Treatment of Osteogenesis Imperfecta by Intramedullary Fixation

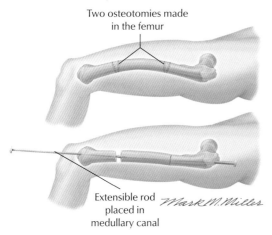

Two osteotomies made in the femur

Extensible rod placed in medullary canal

Mark M. Miller

Most cases result from new mutations of an autosomal dominant gene.

Flattening of the midface is seen in patients with SED congenita. The neck is short, as is the trunk. The chest is barrel-shaped, with thoracolumbar kyphosis and increased lumbar lordosis. Rhizomelic shortening of the extremities is observed, particularly in the lower extremities. The hips show coxa vara and a markedly irregular articular contour. The knees may develop genu varum, genu valgum, or windswept knee deformities (genu varum on one side and genu valgum on the other). The hands and feet appear relatively normal (**Figure 3-10**).

Radiographs are characterized by delayed ossification, fragmentation of the epiphyseal portion of long bones, and marked flattening of the vertebrae (platyspondyly). Patients often develop scoliosis. Odontoid hypoplasia is very common, and approximately one third of patients with SED congenita develop symptomatic C1-C2 instability that requires occiput-to-C2 fusion. Degenerative joint disease develops early, particularly in the hips. Lower extremity deformities may require osteotomies, but because of progressive degeneration of the articular cartilage, the results are somewhat unpredictable. Before anesthesia is given, flexion-extension views of the cervical spine should be obtained in all patients.

Kniest-type SED is characterized by a prominent forehead, flat nasal bridge, cleft palate, hearing loss, short stature, disproportionately short trunk, flat and irregular epiphysis, and broad metaphysis. A distinguishing feature is stiff joints that appear to be enlarged because of the broad metaphysis. Retinal detachment and glaucoma may cause blindness. Most mutations are noted to occur between exons 12 and 24 of the *COL2A1* gene. Orthopaedic treatment is similar to that provided to children with SED congenita.

Spondyloepiphyseal dysplasia tarda is distinguished from SED congenita by milder features and later patient age at diagnosis (**Figure 3-11**). Different types of genetic inheritance have been reported, but the most common is an X-linked disorder, with males more commonly and more severely affected. The diagnosis tends to be made after age 4 or 5 years. Patients commonly present with hip or back pain, and SED tarda initially may be misdiagnosed as bilateral Legg-Perthes disease. Osteotomies of the hips or knees or early total joint replacement may be required.

Stickler syndrome (hereditary arthroophthalmopathy) is an autosomal dominant disorder characterized by myopia, predisposition to retinal detachment, and premature osteoarthritis, particularly of the hips. Mutations that affect *COL2A1*, *COL11A1*, and *COL11A2* are associated with Stickler syndrome, with most cases being secondary to *COL2A1*. Other potential problems include midfacial underdevelopment, cleft palate, hearing loss, and mild spondyloepiphyseal dysplasia.

Familial precocious osteoarthritis may be associated with a mutation in the gene that codes for type II collagen. Patients typically develop early arthritis of the hips. Undoubtedly, future studies will result in a better understanding of the association of minor abnormalities in particular cartilage components that are predisposed to early degenerative changes.

Cartilage Oligomeric Matrix Protein Disorders

Cartilage oligomeric matrix protein (COMP) is a large glycoprotein that is found in the extra-

Figure 3-10: Spondyloepiphyseal Dysplasia Congenita

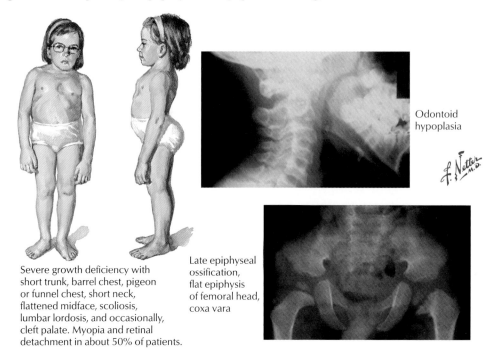

Odontoid hypoplasia

Severe growth deficiency with short trunk, barrel chest, pigeon or funnel chest, short neck, flattened midface, scoliosis, lumbar lordosis, and occasionally, cleft palate. Myopia and retinal detachment in about 50% of patients.

Late epiphyseal ossification, flat epiphysis of femoral head, coxa vara

Figure 3-11: Spondyloepiphyseal Dysplasia Tarda

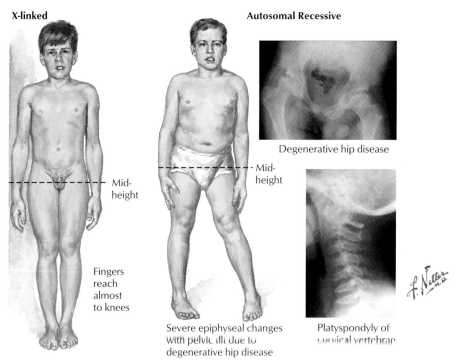

X-linked

Autosomal Recessive

Mid-height

Fingers reach almost to knees

Mid-height

Degenerative hip disease

Severe epiphyseal changes with pelvic tilt due to degenerative hip disease

Platyspondyly of cervical vertebrae

cellular matrix surrounding chondrocytes, as well as the extracellular matrix of ligaments and tendons. Pseudoachondroplasia and some forms of multiple epiphyseal dysplasia are secondary to defects in COMP.

Pseudoachondroplasia

In patients with pseudoachondroplasia, an abnormal form of COMP accumulates in the rough endoplasmic reticulum of chondrocytes, tendons, and ligaments. The matrix progressively loses its ability to support and maintain the shape and function of cells. Therefore, pseudoachondroplasia is not apparent at birth on clinical examination, but platyspondyly may be evident on radiographs. Short stature, however, becomes apparent at between 1 and 3 years of age. Other presenting signs include genu varum, genu valgum, and windswept knee deformities. Head size and face are normal.

Radiographs may show mild odontoid hypoplasia, but clinically significant cervical instability occurs in only a small percentage of patients with pseudoachondroplasia. The spine has platyspondyly that is not as severe as that observed in SED congenita. The extremities show delayed ossification of the epiphysis, irregular epiphysis, and joint incongruity, particularly at the hips and knees. The metaphyses are broad and irregular.

Consistent with the progressive accumulation of COMP, limb shortness and disproportionate dwarfism increase with growth (**Figure 3-12**). Marked joint incongruity with associated flexion contractures and recurvatum leads to early osteoarthritis of the hips and knees. Abnormalities in the hands and feet are mild. Thoracic kyphosis and lumbar lordosis often increase. Mild scoliosis develops, but most patients do not require surgical stabilization.

The cervical and thoracic spine should be monitored for potential instability and scoliosis. Realignment osteotomies may be required for hip dysplasia or severe angular deformities at the knee. However, because of progressive abnormalities in growth (physeal cartilage) and in joint surface congruity

(articular cartilage), the risk of recurrence is high.

Multiple Epiphyseal Dysplasia

Multiple epiphyseal dysplasia (MED) is a group of disorders characterized by flattening of the epiphysis of the long bones (particularly at the hip and knee), delay in ossification of the carpal bones, and normal spine or only mild spinal involvement. Clinical problems associated with MED include short stature, coxa vara, Legg-Perthes changes in the hips, and early degenerative joint disease of the shoulder, hips, knees, and ankles. In the past, MED was frequently separated into Fairbanks dysplasia (more severe type) and Ribbing dysplasia (milder involvement) (**Figure 3-13**). It is now understood that MED may be secondary to a mutation in the *COMP* gene or may be caused by a mutation in the gene for the $\alpha_2 2$ fibrils of collagen type IX (*COL9A2*). Obviously, the *COMP* mutation in MED causes a less severe alteration in COMP than occurs in patients with pseudoachondroplasia. Collagen type IX is located on the surfaces of collagen type II fibrils. It is hypothesized that collagen type IX helps to maintain the long-term integrity of articular cartilage.

Diastrophic Dysplasia Transporter Disorders

Diastrophic dysplasia (DD) is a skeletal dysplasia that is characterized by numerous severe and disparate skeletal abnormalities. Clinical features include short stature, rhizomelic shortening of the limbs, kyphoscoliosis, limitations of finger flexion, hitchhiker thumbs, foot deformities ranging from metatarsus adductus to severe clubfoot, and painful osteoarthritis that manifests by 20 to 40 years of age, particularly in the hips and knees (**Figure 3-14**).

DD is an autosomal recessive disorder that is caused by mutations in the gene that codes for sulfate transporter protein. Normal cartilage requires proper sulfation of proteoglycans if it is to be sufficiently negatively charged to function properly. A defect in the *DD* gene results in undersulfation of proteo-

Figure 3-12: Pseudoachondroplasia

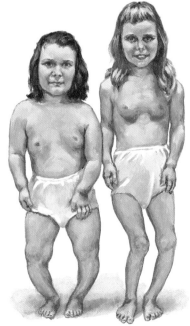

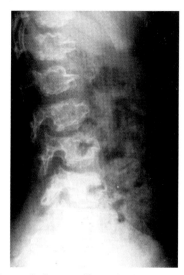

Squared-off, tonguelike projections on anterior borders of lumbar vertebrae due to defects in growth plates. This radiographic sign often disappears as growth plates mature

Sisters with short upper and lower limbs. Girl on left has bilateral bowing of lower limbs; girl on right shows genu valgum on one side and genu varum on the other side, causing pelvic obliquity that may lead to scoliosis.

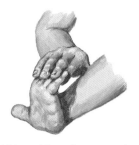

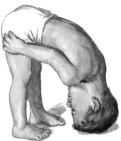

Wrist and finger hyperextension due to ligamentous laxity. Because of body disproportion, head can touch floor easily.

glycans and progressive degeneration of articular cartilage, as well as abnormalities in physeal and epiphyseal cartilage.

Metaphyseal Chondrodysplasias

The metaphyseal chondrodysplasias are a group of disorders characterized by irregularity in the metaphysis; however, the name is a misnomer because the primary defect causes abnormal ossification of the cartilaginous columns in the physis. As a result, the physis is widened and shortening of the bones is noted, particularly of the weight-bearing long bones (femur and tibia). The many different types of metaphyseal chondrodysplasia are secondary to mutations in several genes that code for different proteins. The differential diagnosis for a metaphyseal chondrodysplasia includes various types of rickets and hypophosphatasia.

The most common metaphyseal chondrodysplasia is the Schmid type, which is an

Figure 3-13: Multiple Epiphyseal Dysplasia

Fairbanks type

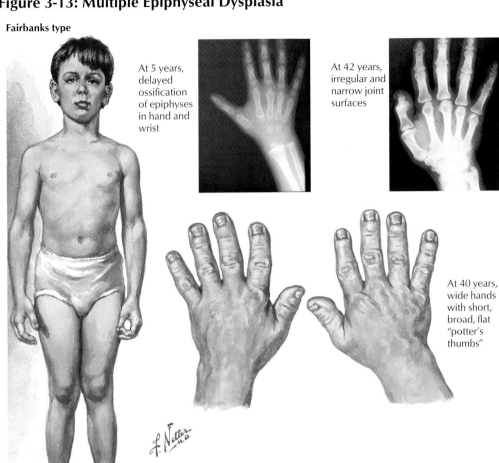

At 5 years, delayed ossification of epiphyses in hand and wrist

At 42 years, irregular and narrow joint surfaces

At 40 years, wide hands with short, broad, flat "potter's thumbs"

Relatively normal habitus, body proportions, and facies; mildly short stature. Joint stiffness may lead to progressive incapacitation.

Slanted distal articular surfaces of tibias; usually evident after epiphyseal fusion at puberty

Figure 3-14: Diastrophic Dysplasia

Diastrophic Dwarfism

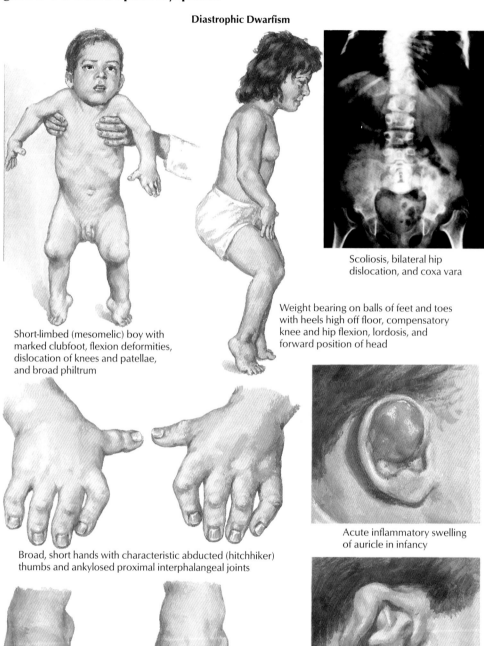

Scoliosis, bilateral hip dislocation, and coxa vara

Weight bearing on balls of feet and toes with heels high off floor, compensatory knee and hip flexion, lordosis, and forward position of head

Short-limbed (mesomelic) boy with marked clubfoot, flexion deformities, dislocation of knees and patellae, and broad philtrum

Broad, short hands with characteristic abducted (hitchhiker) thumbs and ankylosed proximal interphalangeal joints

Acute inflammatory swelling of auricle in infancy

Marked clubfoot resistant to correction

Progression to typical cauliflower deformity

autosomal dominant disorder caused by a mutation in the gene that codes for the α_1 chain of type X collagen. Type X collagen is a short-chain homotrimer (consisting of three identical chains linked together) that is synthesized only by hypertrophic chondrocytes. Absence of or abnormalities in type X collagen in the extracellular matrix of the physis affect enchondral ossification with resultant mild disorganization of mineralization and trabecular bone formation. Weight-bearing stresses exacerbate the growth abnormalities; therefore, the upper extremities have radiographic abnormalities but no clinical dysfunction. Patients appear normal at birth but typically present between 1 and 5 years of age with short stature, genu varum, coxa vara, and a waddling gait. If severe bowlegs develop, realignment osteotomies are required (**Figure 3-15**).

Other relatively common metaphyseal chondrodysplasias include the *McKusick type* (also known as *cartilage hair hypoplasia*; **Figure 3-16**), Jansen metaphyseal dysplasia (caused by a defect in the receptor for parathyroid hormone–parathyroid hormone–related peptide receptor [PTH-PTHrP]), and the *Kozlowski type* (spondylometaphyseal dysplasia with mild platyspondyly).

Hypophosphatemic Rickets

Hypophosphatemic (vitamin D–resistant) rickets is most often due to an X-linked dominant disorder characterized by short stature, bowleg deformities, and hypophosphatemia. Similar to Schmid-type metaphyseal chondrodysplasia, this disorder is not clinically evident at birth. Unless there is a positive family history, children with this condition typically are brought to medical attention when they are between 1 and 4 years of age because of progressive short stature and bowed legs. An occasional patient has excessive genu valgum. Radiographs show widening of the physis and bowing of the extremities. The bowlegs and short stature are caused by defective mineralization in the zone of provisional calcification plus the inhibition of growth by weight-bearing forces. Similar to Schmid-type metaphyseal chondrodysplasia, the degree of mineralization in hypophosphatemic rickets is adequate enough that upper extremity alignment, range of motion, and function are normal.

Hypophosphatemic rickets causes decreased proximal tubular reabsorption of phosphate with resultant hypophosphatemia. Previous theories proposed that this condition may occur secondary to an intrinsic defect in the kidney; however, recent studies suggest

Figure 3-15: Metaphyseal Chondrodysplasia, Schmid Type

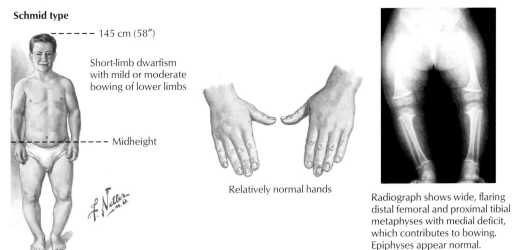

Schmid type

145 cm (58")

Short-limb dwarfism with mild or moderate bowing of lower limbs

Midheight

Relatively normal hands

Radiograph shows wide, flaring distal femoral and proximal tibial metaphyses with medial deficit, which contributes to bowing. Epiphyses appear normal.

Figure 3-16: Metaphyseal Chondrodysplasia, McKusick Type

McKusick type

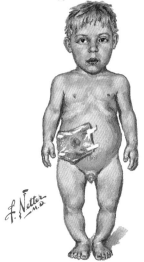

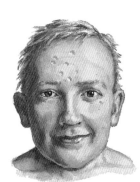

Greatly magnified hairs from six siblings. A, B, D, and F from normal siblings; C and E from siblings with metaphyseal chondrodysplasia.

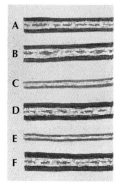

19-year-old patient with sparse, fine hair, normal face; scars from severe chickenpox

4¹/₂-year-old boy with short-limb dwarfism, sparse, fine hair, and Harrison grooves on chest. Colostomy for megacolon.

Section of costochondral junction shows paucity of chondrocytes and failure to form columns for calcification and bone formation

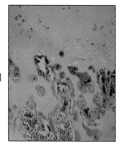

that patients produce a humeral factor that induces phosphate wasting. Some families have mutations in the *PEX* gene on the *X* chromosome (phosphate-regulating gene with homologies to endopeptidases). Further delineation of the pathogenesis of this condition will result in the development of specific therapies to correct phosphate wasting.

Current treatment requires large doses of oral phosphate and 1,25-dihydroxyvitamin D₃. This therapy, however, only partially corrects the defective mineralization. Therefore, early identification of these patients is important. If the disorder can be diagnosed before walking and subsequent inhibition of growth by weight-bearing forces commence, then many of these patients will have only mild genu varum that does not require surgical intervention. For significant genu varum, realignment osteotomies at the femur and tibia are required.

Individuals with a positive family history of hypophosphatemic rickets should undergo early testing of serum phosphorus levels. With an affected father, all female offspring will have the condition, but none of the males will be affected. If the mother is affected, then each child, whether male or female, has a 50/50 chance of having the disorder.

Marfan Syndrome

Marfan syndrome is an autosomal dominant disorder caused by a mutation in the gene that codes for fibrillin 1 (*FBN1*). Fibrillin, a large glycoprotein present in many tissues, is a structural component of microfibrils, which have important functions in the formation and homeostasis of the elastic matrix and matrix cell attachments. Defects in *FBN1* usually result in decreased amounts of fibrillin and a structurally weakened elastin; this combination causes ocular, cardiovascular, and skeletal manifestations. Patients demonstrate considerable heterogenous expression that is most dependent on the exact mutation; however, variable manifestations also occur within families. A typical patient with Marfan syndrome is tall and thin with arachnodactyly and ligamentous laxity. The mean adult height is greater than the 95th percentile, but the final adult height is less than that predicted in childhood, because the peak height velocity occurs at an earlier age in children with Marfan syndrome, averaging $7^{1}/_{2}$ years in girls and $10^{1}/_{2}$ years in boys. Musculoskeletal problems include scoliosis, pes planovalgus, and protrusio acetabuli. Other features include ectopia lentis, myopia, retinal detachment, crowding of the teeth, striae of the skin, and cardiovascular problems such as aortic or mitral valve regurgitation, dilatation of the ascending aorta, and aortic dissection (**Figure 3-17**).

The diagnosis of Marfan syndrome is based on family history and clinical findings. An abnormal arm span to height ratio (>1.05:1) with an abnormal Walker-Murdoch wrist sign suggests the need for further evaluation. In the absence of family history or a documented mutation in *FBN1*, a diagnosis of Marfan syndrome requires two major criteria in different systems, plus involvement of a third system (**Table 3-5**).

Cardiac complications are frequent, and the possibility of their occurrence should be evaluated before any elective surgery is performed. β-Blockers and reconstructive cardiac surgery often are needed. Scoliosis is the most common reason for orthopaedic reconstructive surgery. Bracing does not work well in Marfan syndrome, and curves of greater than 40° should be stabilized. Dural ectasia and meningoceles may be present. Compared with idiopathic scoliosis, spinal surgery in these patients involves increased blood loss and increased risk of infection and cerebrospinal leak.

Congenital Contractural Arachnodactyly

Congenital contractural arachnodactyly is an autosomal dominant disorder caused by a mutation in the gene that codes for fibrillin 2 (*FBN2*). Children with this condition have the same skeletal features as children with Marfan syndrome, but they develop contractures of the joints instead of ligamentous laxity.

Hereditary Multiple Exostosis

Hereditary multiple exostosis is an autosomal dominant condition caused by a defect in one of two genes: *EXT1* or *EXT2*. The more severe phenotypic involvement is usually noted in *EXT1* cases. *EXT1* and *EXT2* are ubiquitously expressed genes that were previously theorized to act as tumor suppressor genes but probably act to regulate bone growth.

Patients with hereditary multiple exostosis experience *multiple osteochondromas* (bony exostosis covered with a cartilaginous cap) (see Chapter 8). Involvement at the metaphyseal region of long bones is most common, but an exostosis may occur at other locations, such as the pelvis, scapula, ribs, or fingers. The exostosis continues to enlarge until growth is complete. Clinical problems include irritation of surrounding muscles and nerves, bony malalignment, limb-length inequality, and occasional malignant degeneration. Bony malalignment is more frequent in the forearm and legs. Typically, the smaller of the two bones (ulna and fibula) demonstrates inhibited growth. As a result, valgus can develop at the wrist, knee, and ankle. Malignant transformation, fortunately, is uncommon (occurs in approximately 1% of patients) and usually is a chondrosarcoma that develops after maturity.

Radiographs are diagnostic. The exostosis can be *sessile* or *pedunculated* and is continuous with the main part of the bone. If a patient develops significant discomfort or malalignment, the exostosis should be removed. In an adult, enlargement of the exostosis or the development of pain necessitates investigation into possible malignant transformation.

HEMATOPOIETIC CONDITIONS

Hematopoietic tissue is a component of bone. Several hematopoietic disorders affect skeletal growth and development. The more common of these disorders are described in the following sections.

Sickle Cell Disease

Approximately 1 of every 300 African Americans has sickle cell disease. The three common genotypes are:

Figure 3-17: Marfan Syndrome

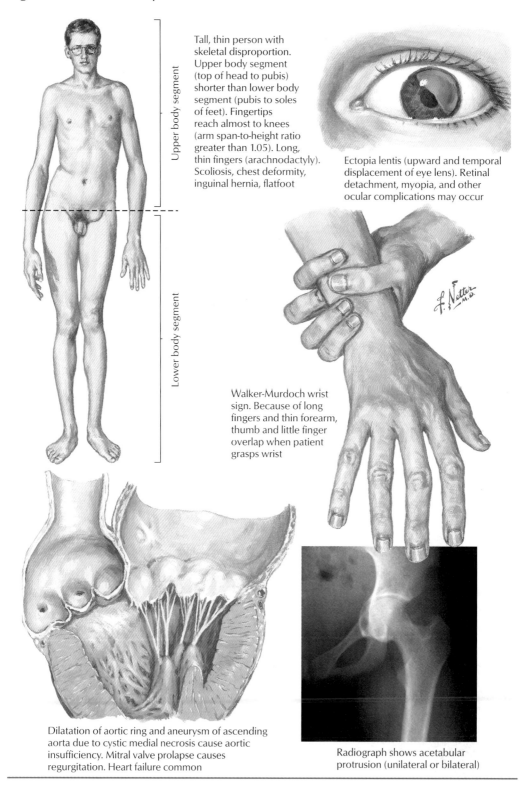

Tall, thin person with skeletal disproportion. Upper body segment (top of head to pubis) shorter than lower body segment (pubis to soles of feet). Fingertips reach almost to knees (arm span-to-height ratio greater than 1.05). Long, thin fingers (arachnodactyly). Scoliosis, chest deformity, inguinal hernia, flatfoot

Ectopia lentis (upward and temporal displacement of eye lens). Retinal detachment, myopia, and other ocular complications may occur

Walker-Murdoch wrist sign. Because of long fingers and thin forearm, thumb and little finger overlap when patient grasps wrist

Dilatation of aortic ring and aneurysm of ascending aorta due to cystic medial necrosis cause aortic insufficiency. Mitral valve prolapse causes regurgitation. Heart failure common

Radiograph shows acetabular protrusion (unilateral or bilateral)

Table 3-5
Diagnosis of Marfan Syndrome

Major Criteria

+ Dilatation of ascending aorta
+ Dissection of ascending aorta
+ Ectopia lentis
+ Dural ectasia
+ >4 skeletal findings
+ Affected relative
+ Proven mutation

Skeletal Features (Need >4)

+ Pectus carinatum
+ Pectus excavatum requiring surgery
+ Arm span/height > 1.05
+ Wrist and thumb signs
+ Scoliosis > 20°
+ Spondylolisthesis
+ Elbow flexion contractures
+ Pes planovalgus
+ Acetabular protrusio

Source: Pyeritz RE. The Marfan syndrome. In: Royce PM, Steinmann B, eds. *Connective Tissue and Its Heritable Disorders: Molecular, Genetic, and Medical Aspects.* New York, NY: Wiley-Liss; 1993:437–468.

+ SS disease, which is homozygous for hemoglobin S
+ SC disease, which is heterozygous for hemoglobin S and hemoglobin C
+ Sβ disease, which is heterozygous for hemoglobin S and hemoglobin β-thalassemia

Vasoocclusion and *hemolysis* are the basic pathologic events involved in sickle cell disease. When hemoglobin S is deoxygenated, it polymerizes and changes to a gel of intertwined fibers. As a result, erythrocytes become distorted and fragile and are rapidly destroyed. The paradox is that sickle cells not only are more fragile but also are relatively rigid and more viscous. Therefore, in addition to increasing hemolysis, these erythrocytes clog small blood vessels and infarct tissues. Bone and joint problems in sickle cell disease include sickle cell

crisis, dactylitis, osteonecrosis, osteomyelitis, septic arthritis, reactive arthritis, and leg ulcers.

A sickle cell crisis results from a localized area of infarction. Extremity pain occurs secondary to bone marrow infarction, whereas abdominal pain is most likely secondary to infarction in the intestines. Supportive measures are the mainstay of therapy.

Dactylitis, or hand-foot syndrome, occurs secondary to infarction of bone marrow in the hand or foot; frequently, it is the first clinical manifestation after hemoglobin F has been replaced by hemoglobin S. Problems with dactylitis cease with the disappearance of hematopoietic marrow in the hands and feet, and the syndrome has not been reported in patients older than 6 years.

Osteonecrosis is common in sickle cell disease; patients older than 45 years have an incidence of femoral head osteonecrosis higher than 30% and an incidence of humeral head osteonecrosis higher than 20%. If osteonecrosis develops before 10 years of age, the prognosis is relatively good, but progressive disability and pain are common in adolescents and young adults with the condition.

Disorders of the Monocyte-Macrophage System

Functions of the monocyte-macrophage system include macrophage "cleanup" of normal tissue breakdown and remodeling. Storage diseases of the reticuloendothelial system, also called *lysosomal storage diseases,* have profound effects on the phagocytic system. The common pathogenesis involves deficiency of a catabolic enzyme normally found in lysosomal particles of the cell cytoplasm. As a result, products of cellular metabolism accumulate that would normally be degraded and excreted, the lysosomes are overloaded and the cell becomes dysfunctional. Abnormal accumulation of macrophages and subsequent organ dysfunction occur.

Gaucher disease, the most common lysosomal storage disease, is an autosomal recessive disorder caused by a mutation in the gene that codes for *glucocerebrosidase,* a lysosomal enzyme that hydrolyzes glucocere-

Figure 3-18: Gaucher Disease

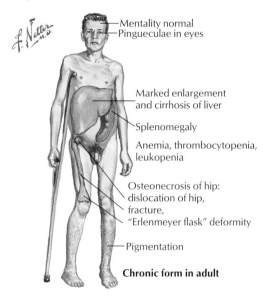

Mentality normal
Pingueculae in eyes

Marked enlargement and cirrhosis of liver

Splenomegaly

Anemia, thrombocytopenia, leukopenia

Osteonecrosis of hip: dislocation of hip, fracture, "Erlenmeyer flask" deformity

Pigmentation

Chronic form in adult

broside, an important component of cell wall membranes. In patients with Gaucher disease, necrosis of cells, especially leukocytes, causes gradual accumulation of glucocerebroside in the macrophages. Resultant Gaucher cells are large, lipid-laden cells found mostly in the spleen, liver, and bone marrow. Clinical manifestations are attributable to accumulation of these abnormal macrophages or are a secondary consequence of the resultant organ dysfunction. For example, thrombocytopenia and clotting deficiency resulting from hepatosplenomegaly may precipitate severe leg or back pain, referred to as Gaucher crisis.

Three types of Gaucher disease are recognized, with type I being the most common. Clinical heterogeneity depends on the site of mutation. Common findings include splenomegaly and hepatomegaly with resultant anemia and thrombocytopenia. Skeletal manifestations include abnormal widening of the metaphysis (Erlenmeyer flask deformity), osteopenia, Gaucher crisis, osteomyelitis, pathologic fracture, avascular necrosis, and early arthritis (**Figure 3-18**). Enzyme replacement therapy markedly diminishes clinical problems, but it is expensive.

Hemophilia

Any of the coagulation factors may be deficient, but musculoskeletal problems are found primarily in patients with factor VIII or factor IX hemophilia. The pathophysiology and treatment of hemophilic arthropathy are discussed in Chapter 4.

ADDITIONAL READINGS

Herring JA, ed. *Tachdjian's Pediatric Orthopaedics*, 3rd edition. Philadelphia, Pa: WB Saunders; 2002.

Morrisey RT, Weinstein SL, eds. *Lovell and Winter's Pediatric Orthopaedics*, 5th edition. Philadelphia, Pa: Lippincott Williams and Wilkins; 2001.

Staheli LT. *Fundamentals of Pediatric Orthopaedics*, 3rd edition. Philadelphia, Pa: Lippincott Williams and Wilkins; 2003.

Arthritic Disorders

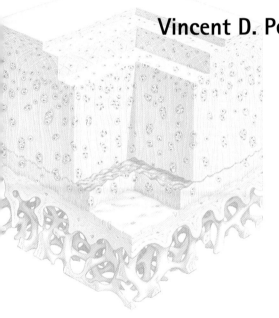

Vincent D. Pelligrini, Jr., MD

Arthritis literally means "inflammation of a joint." Arthritic disorders range from osteoarthritis (OA), which includes limited synovitis, to the other end of the spectrum epitomized by rheumatoid arthritis, with its marked inflammatory changes involving multiple joints and frequent systemic manifestations. Arthritis is common and is a major cause of pain, disability, and loss of work time. In one report, patients with rheumatoid disease and osteoarthritis averaged 7 days of restricted activity, 2.5 days out of work each month, and nearly one third were retired or unemployed because of arthritic disease. The 1998 National (USA) Ambulatory Medical Care Survey recorded almost 14 million physician visits for arthritis, of which 63% were for osteoarthritis, 20% for rheumatoid and other inflammatory arthritides, and 17% for other and unspecified arthropathies.

ANATOMY AND PHYSIOLOGY OF THE JOINT

A synovial (diarthrodial) joint includes the articular cartilage of adjacent bones; an inner synovial membrane (synovium); an outer ligamentous capsule; and, in the normal situation, a small amount of synovial fluid (<2 mL, even in large joints) (**Figure 4-1**). The joint capsule and associated ligaments are composed primarily of type I collagen. Their functions are to contain the adjacent bones in a defined relationship to one another, and to constrain abnormal motion. Synovium inserts at the cartilage-bone junction; however, folds of synovial tissue extend beyond this site.

Articular cartilage is a highly effective tissue that provides pain-free movement with load bearing. The very smooth, almost frictionless motion of normal joints is put in perspective by comparison of the significantly lower coefficient of friction of normal articular cartilage (range, 0.003−0.006) with that of ice (0.1 at 0°C). Articular cartilage is avascular and receives its nutrition by diffusion from synovial fluid. Because articular cartilage is not innervated, arthritic pain is secondary to activation of stress receptors in the capsule and other periarticular structures.

Normal hyaline cartilage is a matrix of proteoglycan aggregates, type II collagen, and

Figure 4-1: Synovial Joint

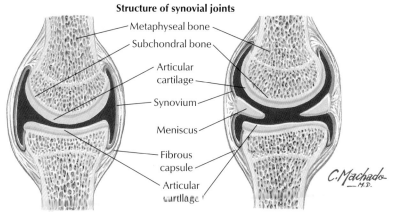

Structure of synovial joints

Metaphyseal bone
Subchondral bone
Articular cartilage
Synovium
Meniscus
Fibrous capsule
Articular cartilage

Typical synovial joints exhibit congruent articular cartilage surfaces supported by subchondral and metaphyseal bone and stabilized by joint capsule and ligaments. Inner surfaces, except for articular cartilage, covered by synovial membrane (synovium)

interspersed chondrocytes. Similar to other soft tissues, cartilage comprises mostly water (80% of wet weight); however, in contrast to other soft tissues, cartilage is a turgid gel and is remarkably firm. The large proteoglycan aggregates consist of proteoglycan aggrecan molecules bound by link protein to hyaluronate, an unsulfated glycosaminoglycan. The aggrecan molecules include a central protein core and radiating glycosaminoglycan chains of chondroitin-4-sulfate, chondroitin-6-sulfate, and keratan sulfate. The proteoglycan aggregates, buttressed by collagen bundles, are responsible for the compressive strength and load-absorbing properties of cartilage. The hydrophilic nature and high density of negative charges on the glycosaminoglycan chains are key to articular cartilage resilience when tissue pressures may be as great as 3 atmospheres (**Figure 4-2**).

Loss of proteoglycans characterizes the early stages of a number of arthritic diseases. As this happens, the cartilage loses its resilience, and the resultant softening promotes further degeneration of the proteoglycan aggregate, as well as changes in the subchondral bone.

Type II collagen is found only in hyaline cartilage, and its characteristic triple-helix formation of three identical peptide chains provides tensile strength to the cartilage surface. Tensile properties of the collagen fibers provide a counterbalancing force that neutralizes and contains the expansile tendency of the proteoglycan aggregates and resulting oncotic pressure. The minor collagens that are found in articular cartilage (types V, VI, IX, X, and XI) contribute to matrix assembly, and their dysfunction likely plays a role in osteoarthritic disease.

The *superficial zone* of articular cartilage is the thinnest layer, and it consists of very fine, tangentially oriented collagenous and non-collagenous proteins with a low proteoglycan content and a few flattened chondrocytes (**Figure 4-3**). The *middle zone* includes larger, somewhat randomly oriented collagen fibrils and spherical chondrocytes surrounded by a generous quantity of proteoglycans. The *deep layer* demonstrates a more orderly alignment of spherical chondrocytes, radially oriented collagen bundles, the highest concentration of proteoglycans, and the lowest water content. On hematoxylin and eosin stains, the *tidemark* is a wavy bluish line that separates the deep and calcified zones. The *calcified zone* secures the articular cartilage surface to the underlying bone with collagen fibrils that pass from the radial deep zone of the cartilage through the tidemark to the underlying subchondral bone.

Synovial fluid is essentially a transudate of serum. Its purpose is joint lubrication and nourishment of articular cartilage. The superficial synovial capillaries constitute an extensive fenestrated network that facilitates rapid exchange of small solutes and water. To nourish articular cartilage, molecules leaving the synovial capillaries traverse the loosely meshed synovial tissue, the synovial fluid, and the layers of cartilage matrix. Intermittent cartilage compression and release provides for imbibition of synovial fluid into the cartilage interstitial fluid. Synovial fluid is the lubricant for *fluid film lubrication*, which is the primary means of joint lubrication. However, under high loads or with long duration of contact, *boundary lubrication* adds a monolayer of lubricating glycoproteins to augment fluid film mechanics (see **Figure 4-2**).

Usually, large molecules such as immunoglobulin M (IgM) or fibrinogen are largely excluded from normal joint fluid, but in diseases that cause synovitis, the barrier to diffusion of large molecules into the joint is lowered. Therefore, in conditions such as septic arthritis, rheumatoid arthritis, and gout, the synovial fluid resembles an exudate with considerable cellular content, as well as depletion of glucose and an accumulation of lactic acid, carbon dioxide, and large protein molecules. In an inflammatory arthritis, synovial fluid cell counts typically exceed $50,000/mm^3$, with more than 90% of cells being polymorphonuclear leukocytes. Inflammatory synovial fluid is less translucent, is less viscous, and has

Figure 4-2: Composition of Articular Cartilage

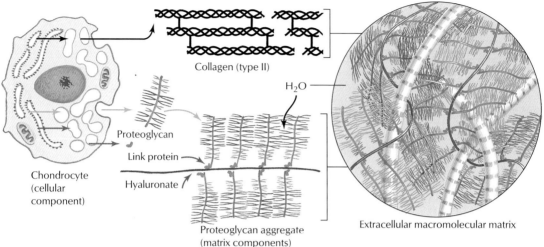

Collagen (type II)

H_2O

Chondrocyte
(cellular
component)

Proteoglycan

Link protein

Hyaluronate

Proteoglycan aggregate
(matrix components)

Extracellular macromolecular matrix

Chondrocytes synthesize collagen (structural framework) and hydrophilic proteoglycans,
which interact with collagen fibrils to form hydrated macromolecular matrix of articular cartilage

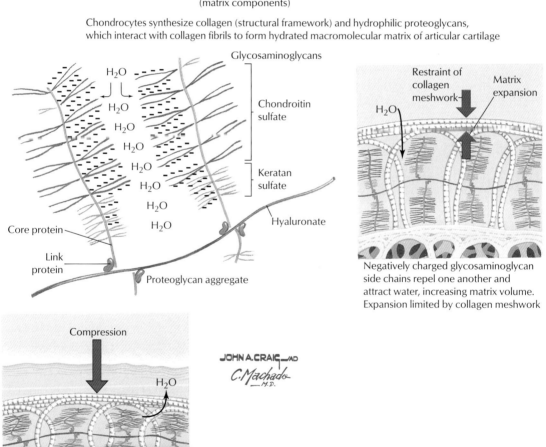

Glycosaminoglycans

H_2O

H_2O

Chondroitin
sulfate

H_2O

H_2O

H_2O

Keratan
sulfate

H_2O

H_2O

Hyaluronate

H_2O

Core protein

Link
protein

Proteoglycan aggregate

Restraint of
collagen
meshwork

Matrix
expansion

H_2O

Negatively charged glycosaminoglycan
side chains repel one another and
attract water, increasing matrix volume.
Expansion limited by collagen meshwork

Compression

H_2O

JOHN A. CRAIG__AD
C. Machado
M.D.

Compression of matrix pushes glycosaminoglycan side chains together, releasing
water and decreasing matrix volume. Decompression allows reexpansion of molecule
and matrix volume

Figure 4-3: Structure of Articular Cartilage

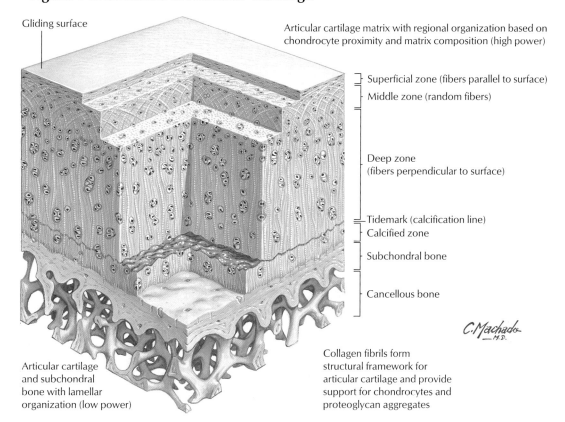

Gliding surface

Articular cartilage matrix with regional organization based on chondrocyte proximity and matrix composition (high power)

Superficial zone (fibers parallel to surface)

Middle zone (random fibers)

Deep zone
(fibers perpendicular to surface)

Tidemark (calcification line)

Calcified zone

Subchondral bone

Cancellous bone

Articular cartilage and subchondral bone with lamellar organization (low power)

Collagen fibrils form structural framework for articular cartilage and provide support for chondrocytes and proteoglycan aggregates

C.Machado
—M.D.

decreased lubricating properties compared with normal synovial fluid (**Figure 4-4**).

A greater volume of synovial fluid is found in arthritic joints. Synovial effusion is particularly increased in the early stages of an inflammatory arthritis, and in superficial joints, the resultant joint swelling is readily apparent. The effusion distends the joint, and the resultant pain causes the patient to limit movement of the joint and to hold the joint in a position that minimizes stretch of the pericapsular structures. However, with longstanding arthritis, the capsular structures become thickened and fibrotic, and at this stage, the resultant joint contracture is a primary cause of decreased joint motion.

In normal articular cartilage, chondrocytes synthesize and replace matrix components at a continuous, albeit relatively slow, turnover rate. Chondrocytes also elaborate degradative enzymes that facilitate normal catabolism

and accelerate pathologic turnover of the matrix elements. Cytokines, such as *interleukin-1* and *tumor necrosis factor (TNF)*, are elaborated by macrophages in the synovial membrane during disease states, and can adversely affect matrix degradation and cartilage function. Likewise, anabolic growth factors such as *tumor growth factor-β* and *insulin growth factor-I* stimulate proteoglycan synthesis. Even though metabolic activity is increased in OA, the hyperactive machinery is also producing abnormal components or normal components that aggregate abnormally. The resulting repair material does not function as normal articular cartilage does, and progressive erosions result in end-stage arthritis.

OSTEOARTHRITIS

Although all degenerative conditions of diarthrodial joints are frequently labeled as *osteoarthritis* (OA), this term should be reserved

Figure 4-4: Synovial Fluid Examination

Gross appearance
A. Normal. Clear to pale yellow, transparent
B. Osteoarthritis. Slightly deeper yellow, transparent
C. Inflammatory. Darker yellow, cloudy, translucent (type blurred or obscured)
D. Septic. Purulent, dense, opaque
E. Hemarthrosis. Red, opaque. Must be differentiated from traumatic tap

The clarity of the fluid is assessed by expressing a small amount of fluid out of the plastic syringe into a glass tube. Printed words viewed through normal and noninflammatory joint fluid can be read easily

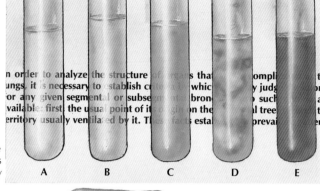

A   B   C   D   E

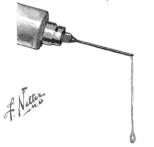

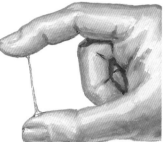

Viscosity. Drop of normal or noninflammatory fluid expressed from needle will string out 1 in or more, indicative of high viscosity. Inflammatory fluid evidences little or no stringing. Viscosity may also be tested between *gloved* thumb and forefinger

for conditions caused by primary degeneration of articular cartilage. The associated synovitis in OA is relatively mild and is secondary to an inflammatory response from synovial macrophages that respond to breakdown products of cartilage erosion.

Primary idiopathic osteoarthritis describes the condition in patients when no obvious underlying cause can be discerned. *Secondary osteoarthritis* is degenerative joint disease that is secondary to specific conditions that cause accelerated erosion of articular cartilage. For example, a child with developmental dysplasia of the hip and a resultant incongruent joint may develop secondary OA. Because pressure equals force divided by area, angular skeletal deformities that asymmetrically load articular cartilage also may cause secondary OA. *Traumatic arthropathy* is a type of secondary OA that is usually secondary to intra-articular fractures and resultant joint incongruity.

Primary OA is increasingly prevalent with advancing age. Some arthritic changes are part of the normal aging process, as evidenced by the decreased range of motion of virtually all joints, even in people who are asymptomatic. However, after the age of 75 years, more than 80% of persons are symptomatic and are limited to some degree by OA in one or more joints. Common sites of OA include the distal and proximal interphalangeal joints of the fingers, the carpometacarpal joint of the thumb, the cervical and lumbar spine, the hip, the knee, and the the metatarsophalangeal joint of the great toe. Premature primary OA is seen as severe degenerative changes in one or more joints by 50 to 60 years of age, without apparent predisposing events. No doubt our understanding and treatment of OA will progress as knowledge expands concerning mutations and resultant dysfunction of the various proteins that are part of the cartilage matrix.

In the early stages of OA, articular cartilage loses its pearly white appearance. Progressive changes include softening, fissuring, and flaking of the cartilage surface (**Figure 4-5**). When full-thickness loss of cartilage occurs, the subchondral bone becomes eburnated. Radiographic findings include narrowing of the joint space secondary to thinning of articular cartilage, subchondral sclerosis representing new bone formation and response to healing microfractures, osteophytes at the joint margin, and subchondral cysts that typically communicate with the joint space. As the disease progresses, the joint space may become completely obliterated, and subchondral cysts and proliferative osteophytes may markedly distort normal joint congruity.

The early pathologic process of OA is both degradative and hypermetabolic, with early proteoglycan loss and subsequent increased proteoglycan synthesis characterized by relatively increased amounts of chondroitin sulfate and relative insufficiency of link protein. Collagen is relatively preserved in the early stages of OA. Catabolic enzymes such as interleukin-1, neutral proteases, and metalloproteinases are increased and are a factor in progressive OA. Histologically, these changes manifest as loss of basophilic staining, appearance of chondrocyte clones, and fibrillation of the superficial cartilage. The increased synthesis of functionally impaired building blocks ultimately fails to rescue and restore the diseased matrix. The altered and weakened hyaline cartilage is susceptible to further erosion under load-bearing conditions and becomes ineffective in buffering the subchondral trabeculae against impact loading and microfracture. Eventually, full-thickness loss of hyaline cartilage occurs from the combined effect of biochemical breakdown of the matrix and abnormal biomechanical forces.

Patients with OA present with local signs and symptoms that are specific to the affected joint. Of note, symptoms expressed by patients with arthritic disease are generally independent of etiology and generally focus toward pain, limitation of motion, and impaired function. Pain is initially provoked by load-bearing activity, is relieved by rest, and then is aggravated on resumption of activity after rest. As symptoms progress, the pain may become constant, being present even at rest and awakening the patient at night. Examination shows variable functional limitations and loss of joint motion (**Figure 4-6**).

Although OA as manifested by decreased motion is found as often in males as in females, symptomatic OA is more common among females, particularly the primary generalized osteoarthritis (GOA) that is characterized by visible osteophytes at the distal interphalangeal joints of the fingers (Heberden nodes) and other arthritic joints, specifically, the proximal interphalangeal joints of the fingers and the carpometacarpal joint of the thumb (**Figure 4-7**). Involvement of the weight-bearing joints of lower extremities is less common but causes greater functional disability. Knee arthritis is associated with GOA and hand arthritis; hip arthritis has only a weak association with GOA.

Compared with OA at other joints, OA of the knee is most likely to cause functional impairment. The reported incidence of OA of the knee is 30% or greater after the age of 65 years. Associated factors in knee OA include female gender and obesity. In contrast, OA of the hip is less common than that of the knee and exhibits neither a female predilection nor meaningful association with obesity.

The nonoperative management of OA depends on which joint is involved, but the principles of treatment include activity modification, intermittent rest and splints, nonforceful strengthening exercises, external aids to reduce load-bearing stress, and nonaddictive pain medication. Nonsteroidal antiinflammatory drugs (NSAIDs) do not alter the natural course of OA, and in some patients, they may be no more effective than acetaminophen; however, they offer the theoretical advantages of reduced pain and alleviated synovitis. Selection of a particular NSAID is determined by cost, convenience of dosing interval, and individual tolerance of gastrointestinal, renal, and cardiac adverse effects.

Figure 4-5: Histopathology of Osteoarthritis

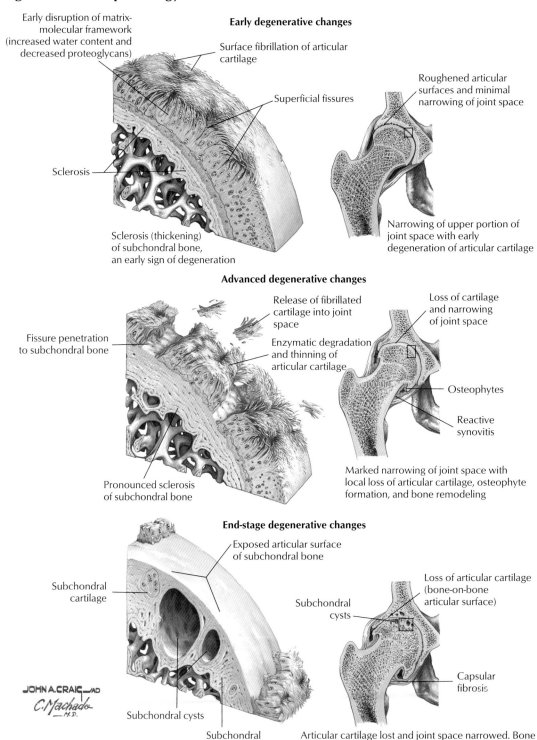

Early degenerative changes

Early disruption of matrix-molecular framework (increased water content and decreased proteoglycans)

Surface fibrillation of articular cartilage

Superficial fissures

Roughened articular surfaces and minimal narrowing of joint space

Sclerosis

Sclerosis (thickening) of subchondral bone, an early sign of degeneration

Narrowing of upper portion of joint space with early degeneration of articular cartilage

Advanced degenerative changes

Release of fibrillated cartilage into joint space

Enzymatic degradation and thinning of articular cartilage

Loss of cartilage and narrowing of joint space

Fissure penetration to subchondral bone

Osteophytes

Reactive synovitis

Pronounced sclerosis of subchondral bone

Marked narrowing of joint space with local loss of articular cartilage, osteophyte formation, and bone remodeling

End-stage degenerative changes

Exposed articular surface of subchondral bone

Subchondral cartilage

Subchondral cysts

Loss of articular cartilage (bone-on-bone articular surface)

Subchondral cysts

Capsular fibrosis

JOHN A. CRAIG—MD
C. Machado
—M.D.

Subchondral cysts

Subchondral sclerosis

Articular cartilage lost and joint space narrowed. Bone shows remodeling osteophyte and subchondral cysts

Figure 4-6: Clinical Findings in OA

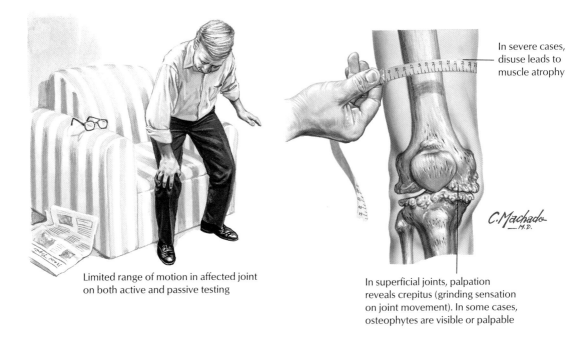

Limited range of motion in affected joint on both active and passive testing

In severe cases, disuse leads to muscle atrophy

In superficial joints, palpation reveals crepitus (grinding sensation on joint movement). In some cases, osteophytes are visible or palpable

Figure 4-7: Hand in OA

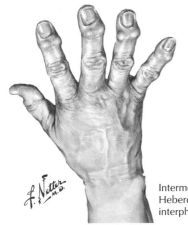

Intermediate-stage Heberden nodes at distal interphalangeal joints

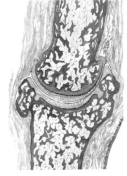

Section through distal interphalangeal joint shows irregular, hyperplastic bony nodules (Heberden nodes) at articular margins of distal phalanx. Cartilage eroded and joint space narrowed.

Figure 4-8: Surgical Alternatives for Osteoarthritis

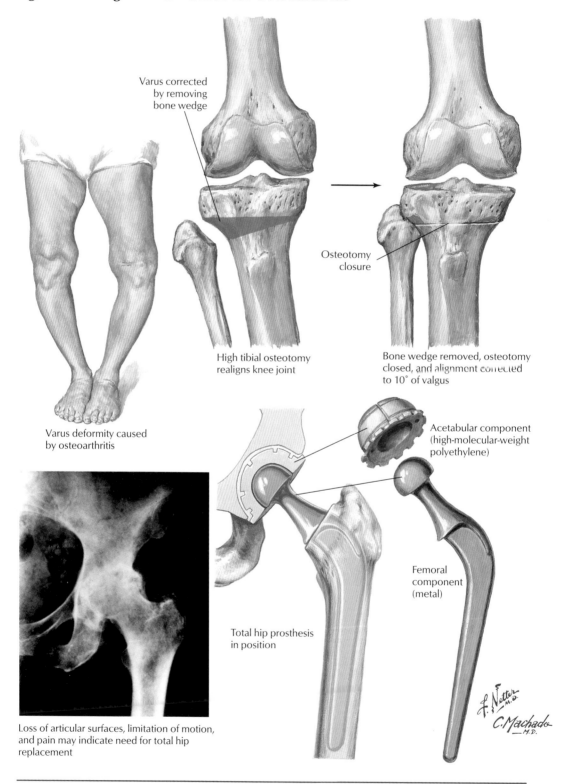

Varus corrected by removing bone wedge

Osteotomy closure

High tibial osteotomy realigns knee joint

Bone wedge removed, osteotomy closed, and alignment corrected to 10° of valgus

Varus deformity caused by osteoarthritis

Acetabular component (high-molecular-weight polyethylene)

Femoral component (metal)

Total hip prosthesis in position

Loss of articular surfaces, limitation of motion, and pain may indicate need for total hip replacement

The surgical treatment of OA varies according to the anatomy of the joint, the severity of the disease, and the demands of the patient. The goals of OA reconstructive procedures are to relieve or decrease pain, to correct deformity, and to improve function. The procedures usually fit into one of four categories: *osteotomy*, to realign joint surfaces so as to redistribute load to a relatively preserved portion of the joint, thus reducing pain and forestalling prosthetic replacement; *resection arthroplasty*, with or without release of contracture and/or interposition of a biologic spacer (used more commonly in the upper extremity to buy time or as a definitive procedure); *arthrodesis*, to fuse the end-stage joint and thus alleviate pain when anatomic considerations do not permit effective joint replacement, or in a young patient who has functional demands in excess of those reasonably expected of a prosthetic arthroplasty; and *prosthetic arthroplasty (total joint replacement)* for end-stage disease in an older patient or one with moderate functional demands (**Figure 4-8**).

RHEUMATOID ARTHRITIS

Rheumatoid arthritis (RA) is a systemic autoimmune disease of unknown cause characterized by an inflammatory synovitis that is destructive to articular cartilage. The incidence of RA increases with advancing age, with peak onset during the fourth and fifth decades. The female-to-male ratio is 2.5:1. Female hormones appear to influence the development of RA because there is a decreased incidence with the use of oral contraceptives, an increased risk in nulliparous women, remission of symptoms during pregnancy, and increased onset of the disease around the time of menopause. Genetic factors also have a role, as suggested by family association and increased prevalence of class II human leukocyte antigen HLA-DR1 and HLA-DR4 (**Figure 4-9**).

RA is probably triggered by an altered response in the interaction between T cells and antigen-presenting cells. The primary pathologic event in RA takes place in the synovium, suggesting that the offending agent

Figure 4-9: Immunogenetics of Rheumatoid Arthritis

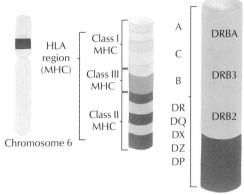

HLA genes located on short arm of chromosome 6. Locus divided into three classes, which are subdivided into smaller regions that encode amino acid sequence of class II MHC receptor. RA-susceptible persons share alleles with common sequence (or with minor substitutions) between positions 66 and 74 (shared epitope). In nonsusceptible persons, more substitutions in these regions

JOHN A.CRAIG—AD

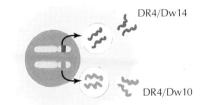

Each person receives one copy of class II MHC allele from both mother and father and therefore produces two forms of class II molecules

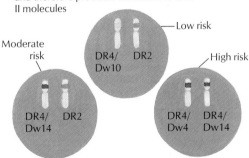

Persons with no RA-associated alleles are at low risk. Presence of single RA-associated allele increases susceptibility to and severity of disease. Heterozygosity (two RA-associated alleles) increases by 50% both disease severity and risk of aggressive disease

is carried to the joint via the bloodstream (**Figure 4-10**). The subsequent activation of cytokines, B cells, and other inflammatory mediators causes a marked synovitis, with polymorphonuclear leukocytes proliferating in the superficial lining of the synovium and joint fluid, while T cells, B cells, fibroblasts, and plasma cells congregate around small blood vessels in the deeper layer of the synovium. The synovium hypertrophies, develops villous formation, and also can produce a *pannus*, an invasive granulation tissue that invades and erodes adjacent subchondral bone and cartilage. Catabolic enzymes produced by the inflamed synovium initiate proteoglycan and collagen destruction. Additional stress to the articular cartilage is caused by associated joint effusion, which stretches the capsule and causes ligamentous instability.

The onset of RA is characterized by the insidious development of symptoms over a period of several weeks to months. The arthritis is typically symmetric, with early involvement more common in the hands, wrists, feet, and ankles (**Figure 4-11**). The inflammatory nature of the patient's arthritis is suggested by morning stiffness and stiffness with inactivity (gel phenomenon). Generalized malaise and fatigue also are noted at disease onset. Accepted criteria for the diagnosis of RA are the presence of at least four of seven findings that continue for at least 6 weeks (**Table 4-1**). No laboratory study is diagnostic of RA, but approximately 80% of patients with RA have abnormal levels of *rheumatoid factors* (IgM or IgG antibodies that bind to the Fc portion of IgG to form immune complexes). High levels of rheumatoid factor are associated with severe disease and greater extra-articular involvement. Occasionally, a patient may present with acute monoarticular arthritis, but this finding is more consistent with an underlying septic arthritis.

RA is a systemic disease, and most patients have extra-articular manifestations. Subcutaneous *rheumatoid nodules* composed of T lymphocytes clustered in focal aggregates and surrounded by collections of plasma cells typically form over pressure points such as

the olecranon and heel. *Tenosynovitis*, particularly around the hands and feet, is common and can progress to dysfunction or rupture of the tendon (**Figure 4-12**). *Localized vasculitis* is common and is manifested by conditions such as palpable purpura, nailfold infarct (subungual and splinter hemorrhages), and leg ulcer. Systemic vasculitis is uncommon. The most common ocular manifestation in RA is *keratoconjunctivitis sicca*, which may cause only dry eye or may include burning, foreign body sensation, and mucoid discharge. Episcleritis, scleritis, and scleromalacia may also occur.

Interstitial lung disease is found to be present by histologic review at autopsy in most patients with RA, but clinical symptoms are much less prevalent, perhaps because multiple-joint arthritis imposes limited

Table 4-1
American Rheumatism Association 1987 Revised Criteria for the Diagnosis of Rheumatoid Arthritis
Morning stiffness of at least 1 hour*
Arthritis in at least three joint areas[†] with swelling or fluid*
Arthritis of hand joints (at least one wrist, MCP, or PIP joint swollen)*
Symmetric joint swelling and involvement*
Subcutaneous nodules
Radiographic changes typical of rheumatoid arthritis
Positive rheumatoid factor

*Specified criteria that must be present for at least 6 weeks.

[†]Right or left proximal interphalangeal (PIP), metacarpophalangeal (MCP), wrist, elbow, knee, ankle, and metatarsophalangeal (MTP) joints.

Source: Arnett FC, Edworthy SM, Bloch DA, et al. The American Rheumatism Association 1987 revised criteria for the classification of rheumatoid arthritis. *Arthritis Rheum.* 1988;31:315–324.

Figure 4-10: Immunopathogenesis of Rheumatoid Arthritis

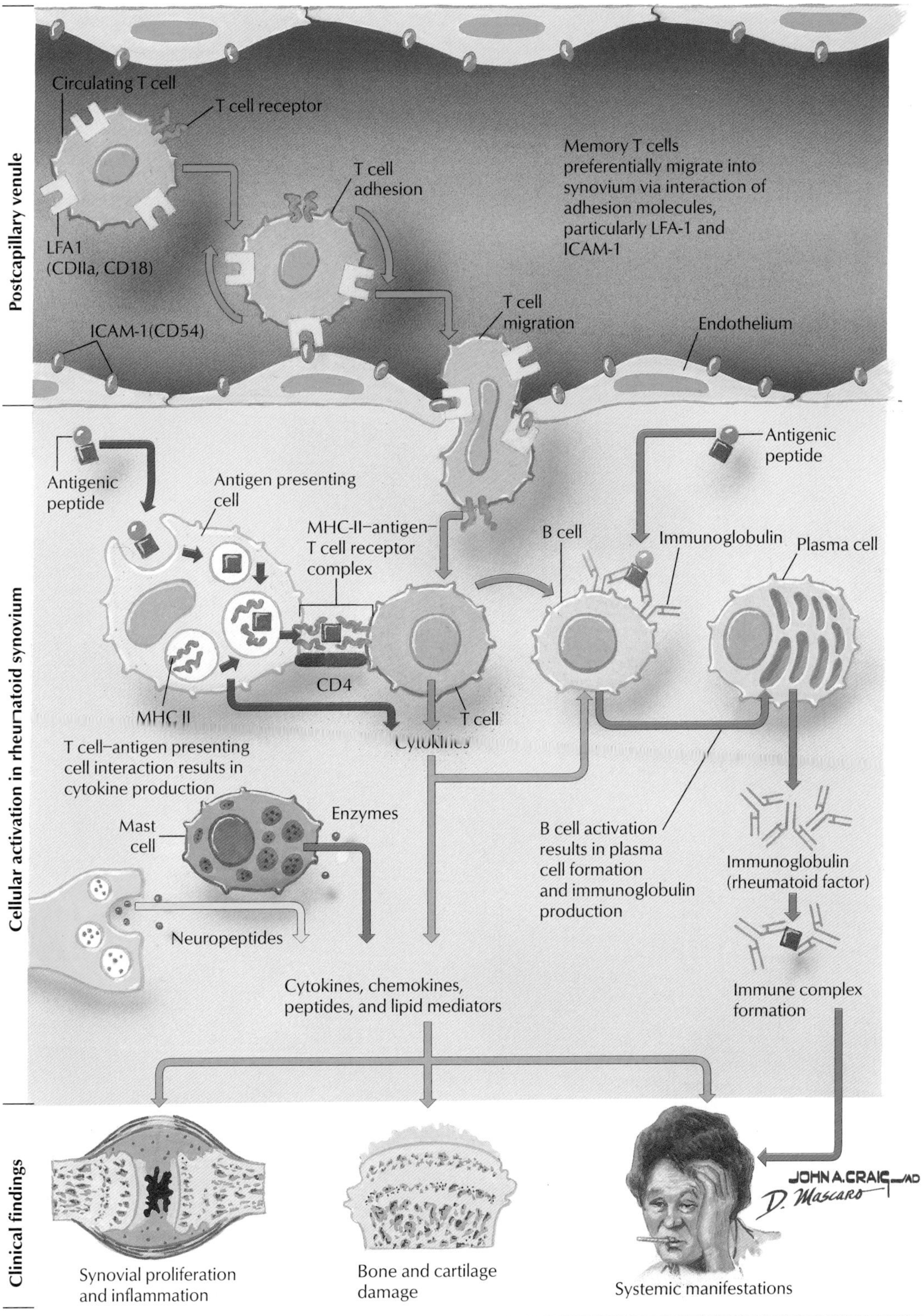

Postcapillary venule

Circulating T cell

T cell receptor

T cell adhesion

LFA1 (CDIIa, CD18)

ICAM-1(CD54)

Memory T cells preferentially migrate into synovium via interaction of adhesion molecules, particularly LFA-1 and ICAM-1

T cell migration

Endothelium

Cellular activation in rheumatoid synovium

Antigenic peptide

Antigen presenting cell

MHC-II–antigen– T cell receptor complex

B cell

Antigenic peptide

Immunoglobulin

Plasma cell

CD4

MHC II

T cell

T cell–antigen presenting cell interaction results in cytokine production

Cytokines

Mast cell

Enzymes

Neuropeptides

B cell activation results in plasma cell formation and immunoglobulin production

Immunoglobulin (rheumatoid factor)

Cytokines, chemokines, peptides, and lipid mediators

Immune complex formation

Clinical findings

Synovial proliferation and inflammation

Bone and cartilage damage

Systemic manifestations

JOHN A. CRAIG—MD
D. Mascaro

Figure 4-11: Clinical Presentation of Rheumatoid Arthritis

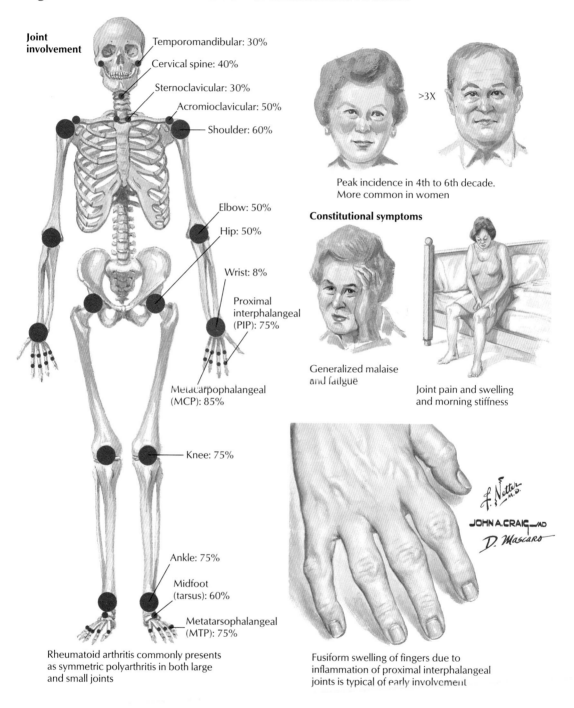

Joint involvement

Temporomandibular: 30%

Cervical spine: 40%

Sternoclavicular: 30%

Acromioclavicular: 50%

Shoulder: 60%

Elbow: 50%

Hip: 50%

Wrist: 8%

Proximal interphalangeal (PIP): 75%

Metacarpophalangeal (MCP): 85%

Knee: 75%

Ankle: 75%

Midfoot (tarsus): 60%

Metatarsophalangeal (MTP): 75%

>3X

Peak incidence in 4th to 6th decade. More common in women

Constitutional symptoms

Generalized malaise and fatigue

Joint pain and swelling and morning stiffness

Rheumatoid arthritis commonly presents as symmetric polyarthritis in both large and small joints

Fusiform swelling of fingers due to inflammation of proximal interphalangeal joints is typical of early involvement

Figure 4-12: Extra-articular Manifestations of RA

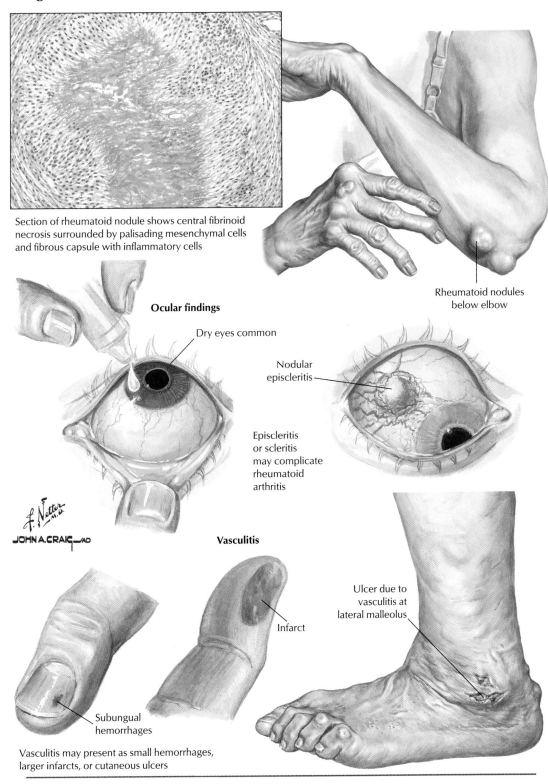

Section of rheumatoid nodule shows central fibrinoid necrosis surrounded by palisading mesenchymal cells and fibrous capsule with inflammatory cells

Rheumatoid nodules below elbow

Ocular findings

Dry eyes common

Nodular episcleritis

Episcleritis or scleritis may complicate rheumatoid arthritis

J. Netter M.D.
JOHN A. CRAIG—MD

Vasculitis

Infarct

Ulcer due to vasculitis at lateral malleolus

Subungual hemorrhages

Vasculitis may present as small hemorrhages, larger infarcts, or cutaneous ulcers

walking activity. Pulmonary nodules tend to be observed in peripheral locations, measure 1 to 6 cm in diameter, and may cavitate and cause pleural effusions. Likewise, *pericarditis* is observed electrocardiographically and at autopsy in approximately 50% of patients with RA. A similar percentage of patients with RA undergoing echocardiography demonstrate cardiac effusion; however, most remain asymptomatic.

At disease onset, the involved joints have a boggy synovitis, effusion, and limitation of motion. With continued synovitis, the ligaments are stretched and are unable to provide adequate support. With chronic synovitis, the joints develop contractures, limitations in motion, and characteristic rheumatoid deformities. Particularly common are radial deviation of the wrist, ulnar deviation of the metacarpophalangeal joints, and swan-neck and boutonnière deformities of the fingers.

The cervical spine may be involved in RA. Chronic synovitis of the diarthrodial facet joints causes progressive instability of the upper and/or lower cervical vertebrae. Subluxation of C1 on C2 or cranial settling of C1 into the foramen magnum of the occiput can occur and may result in cervical myelopathy. Complaints of occipital headache warrant evaluation with flexion and extension cervical spine radiographs. These radiographic studies should be included as preoperative evaluation before intubation for a general anesthetic.

Radiographic characteristics of RA include osteopenia, subchondral erosion, and uniform narrowing of the joint space (**Figure 4-13**). These features may be contrasted with the sclerosis and asymmetric joint erosion that typify OA.

Initial treatment of RA includes education of the patient regarding the disease, protective splinting of the small joints of the hand, appropriate orthotics for foot involvement, and low-impact strengthening exercises. Anti-inflammatory medications are particularly important in treating RA. Initial treatment begins with NSAIDs, but many patients require disease-modifying agents such as methotrexate.

Figure 4-13: Radiographic Changes in RA

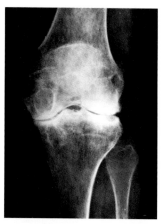

Radiograph shows thinning of cartilage in both compartments of knee joint

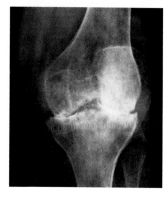

Same patient 4 years later. Progression of bone erosion and marked osteoporosis

Recently, the introduction of *anti-Tumor Necrosis Factor (TNF)* medications has greatly enhanced the medical management of RA. Clinical response to anti-TNF agents has been more dramatic than to any other drugs to date, but whether long-term use of these drugs will be well tolerated remains to be determined. Corticosteroids provide symptomatic relief but do not stop progression of the disease. Their adverse effects are multiple; therefore, these agents are used most often for life-threatening vasculitis that complicates RA.

If the disease progresses despite optimal medical management, then surgical intervention may be beneficial. Tenosynovectomy or synovectomy for uncontrolled inflammation of a tendon sheath or joint may improve function and prevent the complication of tendon rupture. Pain and disability associated with marked joint erosions involving the shoulder, elbow, hips, knees, or finger metacarpophalangeal joints usually necessitate prosthetic joint replacement. Because multiple joints are involved in these patients, arthrodesis is used less frequently in RA. However, arthrodesis may be the best alternative for the wrist, ankle, finger proximal interphalangeal joint (PIP), and great toe joints.

Juvenile Rheumatoid Arthritis

The four criteria listed by the American Rheumatism Association for diagnosing juvenile rheumatoid arthritis (JRA) are (1) chronic synovial inflammation of unknown cause, (2) onset in children younger than 16 years, (3) objective evidence of arthritis in one or more joints for 6 consecutive weeks, and (4) exclusion of other diseases. The three categories of JRA include pauciarticular, polyarticular, and systemic. *Pauciarticular JRA* involves four or fewer joints after 6 months of symptoms, whereas *polyarticular JRA* involves five or more joints. *Systemic JRA* is characterized by an illness that begins with high, spiking fevers and is likely to be complicated by pericarditis, pleural effusions, and enlargement of the liver, spleen, and lymph nodes.

Pauciarticular JRA is the most common pattern and is characterized by onset before 4 years of age and a female-to-male ratio of 4:1. Pain, swelling, and stiffness are strikingly less severe at disease onset in pauciarticular JRA compared with adult RA. Parents typically note some morning stiffness and reluctance of the child to actively play. The disease commonly begins in a single joint, most frequently the knee, ankle, wrist, or finger joints.

Polyarticular JRA is characterized by symmetric involvement of the knees, wrists, fingers, and ankles, and it is more common in girls. The onset of seronegative polyarticular JRA occurs typically between the ages of 1 and 3 years. The seropositive form usually begins in adolescence and is virtually indistinguishable from adult RA.

Systemic JRA accounts for approximately 10% of all cases. Onset commonly is noted between 4 and 9 years of age. At onset, patients appear systemically ill and have daily, or even twice-daily, spiking fevers that are often accompanied by a characteristic salmon-pink evanescent rash (**Figure 4-14**).

Iridocyclitis (inflammation of the anterior uveal tract) is most likely to develop in pauciarticular JRA, occurring in 75% of those patients who also have a positive antinuclear

Figure 4-14: Systemic Juvenile Rheumatoid Arthritis

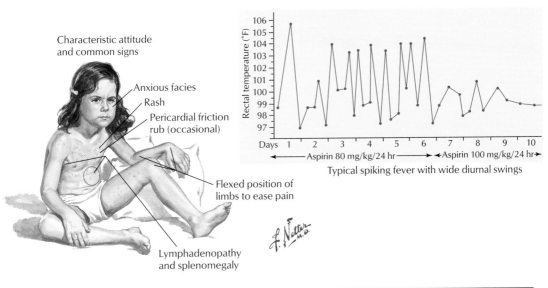

antibody (ANA) test. Most commonly, iridocyclitis begins shortly after joint involvement, but it may develop before joint involvement or as late as 10 years after the onset of joint symptoms. The condition is usually chronic and insidious, and it may result in serious damage to the eye, including synechiae with resultant irregular pupil, band keratopathy with obstructed vision, and secondary cataracts (**Figure 4-15**). Because these children rarely complain of symptoms, early detection is dependent on timely and ongoing slit lamp examinations by ophthalmologists.

The diagnosis of JRA is one of exclusion. No diagnostic tests are available, and even the erythrocyte sedimentation rate is often normal in children with pauciarticular and polyarticular JRA. The differential diagnosis includes leukemia, osteomyelitis, and septic arthritis. Leukemia is associated with night pain and with pain that is associated more with the bone than the joint. Osteomyelitis presents with fever and more severe pain. Septic arthritis is characterized by single-joint involvement, severe pain, and fever.

Spontaneous remission is common, but end-stage arthritis may occur, particularly in patients with systemic and late-onset polyarticular disease. Treatment begins with NSAIDs. Other medications, such as methotrexate, are used if synovitis is persistent. Surgical intervention is used primarily to treat end-stage destructive arthritis.

SERONEGATIVE SPONDYLOARTHROPATHIES

The *seronegative spondyloarthropathies*, which include ankylosing spondylitis, psoriatic arthritis, reactive arthritis, and arthritis associated with inflammatory bowel disease,

Figure 4-15: Ocular Manifestations in Juvenile Rheumatoid Arthritis

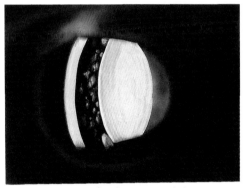

Deposits in anterior chamber seen on slit lamp examination

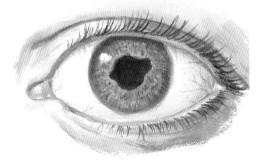

Irregular pupil due to synechiae

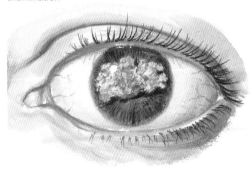

Band keratopathy

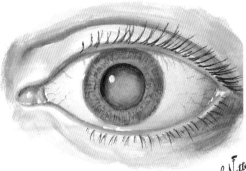

Cataract

are a group of multisystem inflammatory disorders characterized by enthesitis (destructive inflammation at sites of tendon and ligament insertion into bone), involvement of the spine and sacroiliac joints, oligoarticular peripheral joint arthritis, and associated unique skin, eye, and intestinal manifestations. *Seronegative* refers to the absence of rheumatoid factor. A genetic component to these disorders is suggested because many patients are positive for the *HLA-B27 antigen.*

Ankylosing Spondylitis

Ankylosing spondylitis (AS) particularly involves the spine and sacroiliac joints. Peripheral joint arthritis in AS correlates with the severity of the disease but typically is milder than that observed in the other seronegative spondyloarthropathies. In the past, AS was thought to predominantly affect men; however, it is now understood that the sex distribution is more equivalent, but with milder disease observed in women.

Approximately 90% of patients with AS are positive for HLA-B27, and nearly 100% of patients with aortitis or uveitis carry this gene. The *HLA-B27* gene is known to have a role in the binding of antigenic peptides and their presentation to killer T cells. However, because the likelihood that AS develops in an identical twin is only 60%, other "environmental" factors are involved in the expression of this disease.

Patients with early-stage AS typically describe insidious onset of low back pain that has a striking component of morning stiffness. Occasionally, patients, particularly those who have disease onset in the second decade, present with a peripheral joint arthritis or a painful enthesitis such as plantar fasciitis or Achilles tendinitis.

Spondylitis and marked limitation of lumbar spine motion are common in AS and are most easily detected by the skin distraction test (**Figure 4-16**). With the patient standing, one measures a 15-cm span from the posterior iliac spine (dimples of Venus) to the upper lumbar region. Then, the patient is instructed to flex forward as much as possible. The distance between the two points should normally increase by 5 to 7 cm, but in patients with AS and spondylitis, the skin distraction is markedly decreased. Patients with sacroiliitis will have buttock pain on the FABER test (flexion, abduction, and external rotation of the hip, causing stress across the sacroiliac joint).

Subchondral inflammatory disease at the site of ligament insertion is gradually replaced by fibrocartilage repair tissue that ultimately undergoes mineralization and ossification. Radiographs taken early in AS commonly demonstrate squaring of the superior and anterior margins of the vertebral bodies from inflammation and subsequent ossification at the insertion of the outer fibers of the annulus fibrosus. As the disease progresses, bridging syndesmophytes create a "bamboo spine." Sacroiliitis progresses to obliteration and fusion of the sacroiliac joints.

With progression of AS, the thoracic and cervical spine may become involved. Lumbar lordosis is decreased, thoracic kyphosis is increased, and the cervical spine may become virtually immobile. Paradoxically, a spine that is stiffened by bridging syndesmophytes is limited in flexibility and in load-bearing capacity and becomes osteopenic. Any acute increase in neck or back pain should raise the question of a fracture. These injuries may be difficult to identify through an ankylosed, osteopenic spine on routine radiographs.

End-stage arthritis may develop in the hip joints but is uncommonly severe at other sites. Uveitis is common but is typically controllable with topical steroid therapy. Aortic insufficiency and conduction defects may occur.

Psoriatic Arthritis

Inflammatory arthritis affects approximately 10% of patients with psoriasis. The sex ratio is approximately equal. Skin disease usually, but not always, precedes joint symptoms by several months to years. However, approximately 15% of patients with psoriatic arthritis (PA) develop dactylitis or arthritis before they develop skin manifestations. The *HLA-Cw6* and *HLA-B27* genes are associated with PA, but the HLA-B27 association is much

Figure 4-16: Ankylosing Spondylitis

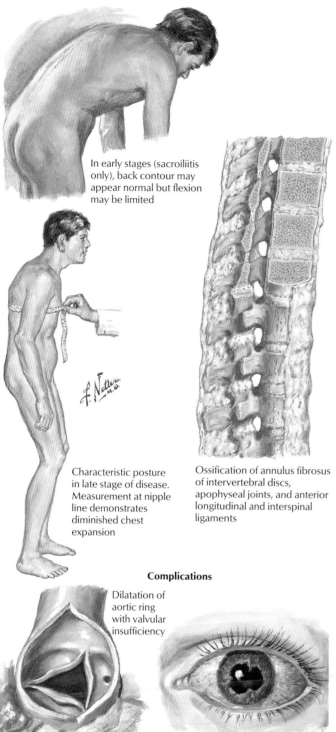

In early stages (sacroiliitis only), back contour may appear normal but flexion may be limited

Characteristic posture in late stage of disease. Measurement at nipple line demonstrates diminished chest expansion

Ossification of annulus fibrosus of intervertebral discs, apophyseal joints, and anterior longitudinal and interspinal ligaments

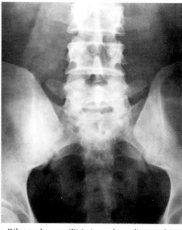

Bilateral sacroiliitis is early radiographic sign. Thinning of cartilage and bone condensation on both sides of sacroiliac joints

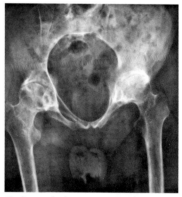

Radiograph shows complete bony ankylosis of both sacroiliac joints in late stage of disease

Complications

Dilatation of aortic ring with valvular insufficiency

Iridocyclitis with irregular pupil due to synechiae

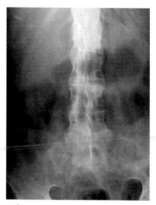

"Bamboo spine." Bony ankylosis of joints of lumbar spine. Ossification exaggerates bulges of intervertebral discs.

weaker than that observed in AS or arthritis of inflammatory bowel disease. The clinical similarities of PA to reactive arthritis and the identification of cross-reactivity between streptococcal antigens and skin keratin suggest a postinfectious relationship.

The pattern of joint involvement varies, but most patients with PA have *asymmetric oligoarticular peripheral joint arthritis*, with only 25% to 30% manifesting spinal involvement. *Dactylitis* is relatively common in PA; results from periosteal inflammation and enthesopathy of the finger or toe joints; and causes a markedly swollen, "sausage" digit with periarticular erosions and thickening of the phalanges from new bone formation (**Figure 4-17**). Hand and foot involvement in PA may include aggressive bone destruction, with characteristic whittling of the proximal side of

the interphalangeal joints, resulting in a "pencil point-in-cup" appearance and asymmetric distal interphalangeal involvement. *Arthritis mutilans* is a particularly aggressive variant of PA with severe osteolysis of the phalanges, metacarpals, and metatarsals and severe deformity and dysfunction of the digits.

Nail disorders may assist in the identification of patients likely to develop PA. Pitting, ridging, and onycholysis of the nails occur in 80% of psoriatic patients with associated joint disease and in only 20% of those without joint involvement. Conjunctivitis and iritis develop in approximately 30% of patients with PA.

Laboratory abnormalities are generally nonspecific and include elevation of the erythrocyte sedimentation rate; normocytic, normochromic anemia; and synovial fluid white cell counts ranging up to 50,000/mm^3.

Figure 4-17: Psoriatic Arthritis

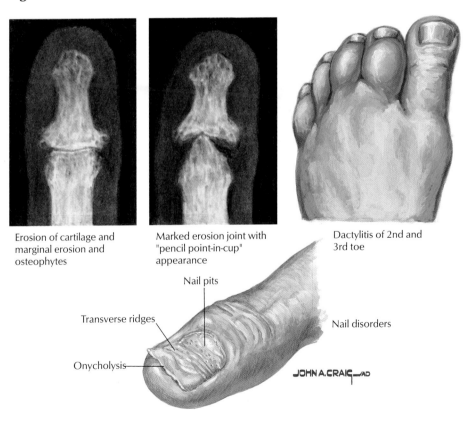

Erosion of cartilage and marginal erosion and osteophytes

Marked erosion joint with "pencil point-in-cup" appearance

Dactylitis of 2nd and 3rd toe

Nail pits

Transverse ridges

Nail disorders

Onycholysis

JOHN A. CRAIG—AD

Reactive Arthritis

Reactive arthritis is typically an asymmetric oligoarthritis of the lower extremities that starts 2 to 8 weeks after an infection. Reactive arthritis is also known as *Reiter syndrome* because a 1916 report by H. Reiter described a patient with a triad of arthritis, urethritis, and conjunctivitis. Sequence homology of some bacterial cell wall components with the human HLA-B27 antigen may account for the cross-reactivity of human antigen-antibody complexes with the infectious agent that triggers the disease process. The pathogens known to cause reactive arthritis include *Chlamydia trachomatis* (nongonococcal urethritis) and *Salmonella, Shigella, Campylobacter,* and *Yersinia* organisms (infectious diarrhea).

Musculoskeletal manifestations of reactive arthritis include *enthesitis* of the Achilles tendon or plantar fascia, dactylitis, and sacroiliitis (**Figure 4-18**). *Conjunctivitis* is common, occurring in approximately half of patients, and it is typically mild and transient. *Acute uveitis* with anterior inflammation (iritis) may occur. Urethritis is more common in men. *Balanitis circinata* may be present and is characterized by small, shallow, painless ulcers on the glans penis and urethral meatus. *Keratoderma blennorrhagicum*, a hyperkeratotic skin rash that occurs most frequently on the soles of the feet, also may appear on the palms and toes and is very similar to pustular psoriasis. Cardiac involvement is infrequent, occurs in patients with more severe joint disease, and includes conduction abnormalities and aortic insufficiency.

Radiographic features are similar to findings in other seronegative spondyloarthropathies. Laboratory findings include elevated erythrocyte sedimentation rate and synovial fluid counts ranging up to 50,000/mm^3.

Arthritis Associated With Inflammatory Bowel Disease

Reactive arthritis associated with inflammatory bowel disease occurs primarily in patients with ulcerative colitis or Crohn disease. The incidence of arthritis is 10% to 20%; it is more common among patients with Crohn

Figure 4-18: Reactive Arthritis

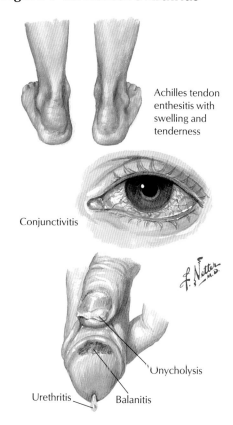

Achilles tendon enthesitis with swelling and tenderness

Conjunctivitis

Onycholysis

Urethritis

Balanitis

disease. In patients who develop arthritis, the HLA-B27 antigen incidence is 50% to 70%.

Arthritic manifestations include sacroiliitis, spondylitis, and peripheral arthritis that involves the lower extremities. The peripheral arthritis usually parallels the course of the bowel disease, but the severity of the spondylitis does not correlate with the severity of the bowel disease. Peripheral arthritis is typically pauciarticular, asymmetric, and, most commonly, transient and migratory. Both large and small joints may be involved. The arthritis is most often nondestructive. Enthesitis with resultant plantar fasciitis and Achilles tendinitis may occur, as well as dactylitis. Bowel surgery influences the course of peripheral arthritis only in ulcerative colitis.

Therapy

Treatment for the seronegative spondyloarthropathies varies depending on the severity of the disease. Education of the patient, NSAIDs, and regular exercise (particularly in AS) are the first lines of treatment. Sleeping flat without a pillow, maintaining good posture, and performing back extension exercises are particularly important in AS to minimize progressive spinal deformities. Indomethacin may be the most effective NSAID, particularly in AS. Sulfasalazine may benefit patients with AS who have peripheral arthritis and short duration of disease. Methotrexate therapy has been helpful in psoriatic and reactive arthritis. The use of TNF inhibitors, although relatively new in AS and PA, has resulted in decreased disease activity and reduced symptoms in both disorders.

Reconstructive surgery can be helpful for patients with end-stage arthritis. Total joint arthroplasty is most often used for hip disease in AS. Patients should receive postoperative irradiation to prevent heterotopic ossification. Patients with AS who have severe kyphosis of the thoracolumbar spine may benefit from spinal osteotomy.

Aortitis in AS may cause aortic insufficiency and conduction defects. Pacemakers and valvular replacement may be required. Uveitis is usually self-limited in patients with AS, but corticosteroid therapy may be required to prevent progressive visual impairment.

CRYSTALLINE ARTHROPATHY

Crystalline arthropathies are secondary to deposits of crystals in the synovium and other tissues with subsequent reactive synovitis. These disorders are characterized by episodes of severe pain in a single joint. Over time, more than one joint may be involved, and joint destruction may occur. Gout is better known, but calcium pyrophosphate dihydrate crystal deposition disease (CPPD) and other calcium phosphate–related conditions occur with greater collective frequency.

Gout

Gout, caused by deposition of *uric acid crystals*, is a relatively common disease that occurs in approximately 2% of the general population. Men are twice as commonly afflicted as women because circulating estrogen in the menstruating female promotes renal excretion of uric acid. Disease incidence increases with age (peak incidence in the fifth decade) and with increasing serum uric acid concentrations. Hyperuricemia by itself is not synonymous with gouty arthritis or renal disease, but the duration and severity (>10 mg/dL) of hyperuricemia are important in the development of symptomatic arthritis or urolithiasis.

Uric acid is the normal breakdown product of purine metabolism. An abrupt increase in production or ingestion of purine-containing compounds can overwhelm the renal excretory mechanism, resulting in increased uric acid levels in serum and related body fluid spaces. Predisposing factors include an inherited deficiency aggravated by male gender and dietary indulgences in meat and red wine (**Figure 4-19**).

Typically, monosodium urate crystals precipitate in supersaturated solutions. Lower temperatures decrease the solubility of uric acid, explaining the propensity of toe and finger joint involvement. Repetitive microtrauma, such as occurs in the first metatarsophalangeal joint of the great toe and the distal interphalangeal joints of the hand, explains greater involvement of these joints.

The typical onset of symptomatic gout is an acute and dramatically painful arthritis that begins at night in a single joint, most commonly the metatarsophalangeal joint of the great toe. In a small segment of patients, joint symptoms are preceded by nephrolithiasis. Associated fever, chills, swelling, and periarticular erythema may be confused with cellulitis or septic arthritis. As the inflammation subsides, desquamation of the skin overlying the affected joint may be noted.

Initial attacks subside spontaneously over 3 to 10 days, even without specific therapy. Patients are asymptomatic until the next episode, even though monosodium urate crystals may be aspirated from the involved joints or even from joints that have not been affected. Over time, attacks occur more frequently, involve more joints, persist for longer periods, and may result in end-stage arthritis.

Figure 4-19: Gouty Arthritis

Natural History

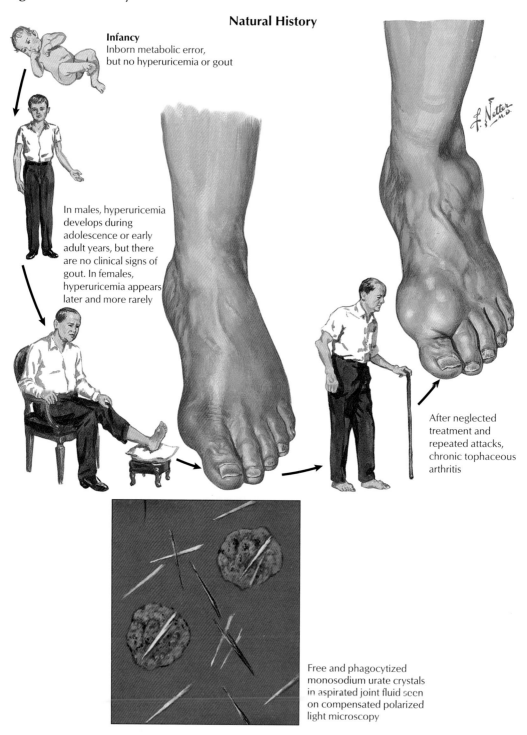

Infancy
Inborn metabolic error, but no hyperuricemia or gout

In males, hyperuricemia develops during adolescence or early adult years, but there are no clinical signs of gout. In females, hyperuricemia appears later and more rarely

After neglected treatment and repeated attacks, chronic tophaceous arthritis

Free and phagocytized monosodium urate crystals in aspirated joint fluid seen on compensated polarized light microscopy

Chronic recurrent attacks of gouty arthritis and persistent hyperuricemia may result in the deposition of uric acid crystals in the synovium, subcutaneous tissue, bursae, subchondral bone, and helix of the ear. Resultant *tophi* (uric acid deposits with surrounding histiocytic reactions) typically appear an average of 10 years after the initial gouty attack. Tophaceous material is characteristically chalky white and exhibits uric acid crystal morphology on examination under polarized light microscopy. Occasionally, tophi spontaneously extrude through the skin from superficial locations.

Kidney stones of uric acid are 10 times more common among patients with symptomatic gouty arthritis than among normouricemic individuals. Related renal dysfunction, proteinuria, and hypertension may be seen in patients with gout, but these are usually mild.

Radiographs during early acute attacks are normal except for associated soft tissue swelling. Advanced destruction in joints affected by gout is characterized by subchondral erosions with a sclerotic margin; these are round or oval, suggesting pressure-related erosion of adjacent bone. The joint space is relatively well preserved until late in the disease.

The diagnosis of gout is confirmed by demonstration of *intracellular, negatively birefringent monosodium urate crystals*. These needle-shaped crystals appear yellow under polarized light microscopy. Synovial fluid white counts may be normal or in the range of 100,000/mm^3. If high white cell counts are present, the gouty effusion may be mistaken for septic arthritis until crystals are identified and joint cultures are found to be negative. Serum uric acid levels are important in the long-term management of gout but are of limited use in the diagnosis of acute gout because these levels may be normal at the time of an acute gouty attack.

Treatment approaches include medications to diminish the inflammatory response of an acute attack and reduction of serum uric acid to minimize the risk of recurrent attacks and progressive joint destruction. *Colchicine* interferes with leukocyte migration and function, and 90% of patients with acute gout have decreased pain and swelling when colchicine is initiated within a few hours of disease onset. Although quite effective, oral colchicine is associated with gastrointestinal adverse effects, and approximately 80% of patients treated with colchicine experience cramping diarrhea and/or nausea and vomiting. Therefore, in patients who do not have severe pain, NSAIDs are the most common medications used in treatment of an acute gout attack. Chronic gout and hyperuricemia are managed by first determining whether the patient is a perpetual overproducer or underexcreter of uric acid. Overproducers are treated with *xanthine oxidase inhibitors*, such as allopurinol, and underexcreters are managed with a *uricosuric agent*, most commonly probenecid.

Calcium Pyrophosphate Dihydrate Crystal Deposition Disease

Calcium pyrophosphate dihydrate crystal formation occurs primarily in cartilage. Predisposing factors to crystal formation include aging, familial predisposition, metabolic diseases (hypophosphatasia, hyperparathyroidism, hemochromatosis, Wilson disease, and hypomagnesemia), and osteoarthritis. Crystals may be shed into the joint, causing calcium pyrophosphate dihydrate deposition disease (CPPD). Chondrocalcinosis, pseudogout, and chronic pyrophosphate arthropathy are the three clinical manifestations of CPPD.

Chondrocalcinosis is calcification of fibrocartilage or hyaline cartilage. The incidence of chondrocalcinosis increases with advancing age, and by the ninth decade of life, nearly half of all persons manifest radiographic evidence of joint cartilage calcification; nearly 5% have gross evidence of CPPD at the time of autopsy. Females are affected two to seven times as frequently as males. Fortunately, patients with chondrocalcinosis are frequently asymptomatic.

Pseudogout is the most common cause of acute monoarthritis in the elderly. The acute attack mimics, but is less severe than, gout, with rapid onset of severe joint pain, swelling, and erythema. The knee is involved in more than half of episodes. The wrist is also a common site of involvement, but any joint, including the first metatarsophalangeal joint, may be involved. Acute pseudogout may occur spontaneously or may be associated with an intercurrent illness, trauma, surgery (particularly parathyroidectomy), or thyroxine replacement.

Chronic pyrophosphate arthropathy is more common in females. The knees, wrists, shoulders, elbows, hips, and hands are frequently affected. Symptoms include early morning stiffness, and multiple joints are often involved. Affected joints show swelling and limited motion. Synovitis is typically more severe than with OA but less severe than with RA.

The diagnosis of CPPD can be confirmed by demonstration of the weakly positive, birefringent, rhomboid-shaped calcium pyrophosphate crystals associated with typical symptoms. The synovial fluid white count is usually around 20,000/mm^3 (**Figure 4-20**).

Acute episodes of pseudogout may be relieved by joint aspiration alone. NSAIDs may also help relieve the acute attack. NSAIDs combined with activity modification, weight reduction, low-impact exercise, and use of canes may be indicated for patients with chronic CPPD symptoms. Most patients do not require surgical reconstructive procedures.

Hemophilia

Any of the 14 coagulation factors may be deficient in patients with hemophilia, but musculoskeletal problems are found primarily

Figure 4-20: Calcium Pyrophosphate Dihydrate Crystal Deposition Disease

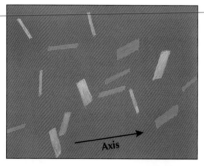

Calcium pyrophosphate dihydrate (CPPD) crystals, indicative of pseudogout, appear as rhomboids or rods, blue when parallel to axis, yellow when perpendicular to it (positive elongation)

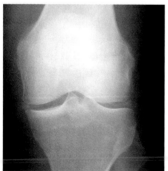

Anteroposterior radiograph of knee reveals densities due to calcific deposits in menisci

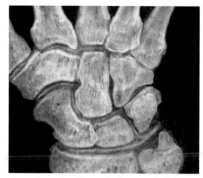

Drawing of radiograph shows calcific deposits in articular cartilages of carpus as fine lines between carpal bones and in radiocarpal joint

in patients with deficits of factor VIII or factor IX. The other inherited coagulation disorders are uncommon and, more important, are characterized by mucosal hemorrhage; they rarely demonstrate hemorrhage into a joint.

Hemophilic arthropathy begins with a *hemarthrosis*, particularly when two or three bleeding episodes occur in a joint within a short period. As blood inside the joint is catabolized, breakdown products must be absorbed by the synovium. Iron is the most damaging element. Synovial cells can absorb only a limited amount of iron; when that quantity is exceeded, the cell disintegrates and releases lysozymes that not only destroy articular cartilage but also inflame the synovial tissue. The result is a hypertrophic and hypervascular synovium that, in a person with a clotting deficiency, is fragile and tends to bleed easily. Thus begins the vicious cycle of recurrent hemarthrosis followed by more synovitis and joint destruction.

Chondrocytes take up iron as well, and with excessive amounts of iron in the joint, the chondrocytes also disintegrate and release lysosomes that destroy the cartilage matrix. Furthermore, the factory (the chondrocyte) also is destroyed. This combination of synovitis and primary articular cartilage erosion explains the rapid and severe arthropathy seen in hemophilic patients who do not have access to adequate replacement therapy.

Radiographic changes in the early stages of hemophilic arthropathy are similar to those observed in rheumatoid arthritis. Erosions at the joint margin, subchondral cysts, subchondral irregularity, widening of the intercondylar notch of the femur, and enlargement of the radial head are characteristic changes as the arthropathy progresses. With end-stage arthropathy, narrowing of the articular cartilage is obvious, but the subchondral bone is more sclerotic in hemophiliacs than in patients with rheumatoid arthritis (**Figure 4-21**).

Transfusion to replace the missing clotting factor is most critical in the management of any hemarthrosis. Major joint bleeding should be followed by a period of prophylactic transfusion therapy. Aspiration of the joint can remove the bulk of blood and may reduce the amount of iron that must be absorbed. If hypertrophic synovitis develops, the patient may be treated with radiation synovectomy, arthroscopic synovectomy, or open synovectomy. The enlarged and incongruent radial head is most often also excised at the time of an elbow synovectomy. Total joint arthroplasty can be helpful with end-stage arthritis.

Ochronosis

Ochronosis, or alkaptonuria, is an uncommon autosomal recessive condition that occurs secondary to complete deficiency of *homogentisic acid oxidase*. As a result, the metabolism of phenylalanine and tyrosine results in excessive retention of homogentisic acid, a pigmented polymer that is subsequently deposited in cartilage, skin, and the sclera. In articular cartilage, it is bound to collagen in the deeper layers, resulting in a more brittle articular surface that is easily fibrillated and eroded. Diseased cartilage is prone to

Figure 4-21: Hemophilic Arthritis

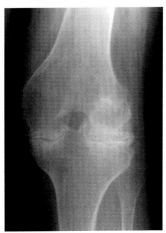

Severe arthritis in young male with hemophilia and history of recurrent hemathrosis and hypertrophic synovitis. Note widening of intercondylar notch, marked joint incongruity, and subchondral sclerosis.

Figure 4-22: Ochronosis

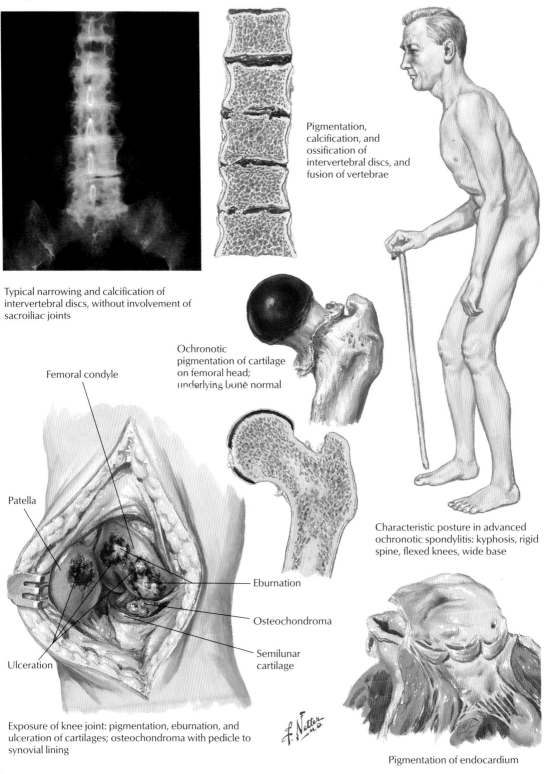

Typical narrowing and calcification of intervertebral discs, without involvement of sacroiliac joints

Pigmentation, calcification, and ossification of intervertebral discs, and fusion of vertebrae

Ochronotic pigmentation of cartilage on femoral head; underlying bone normal

Femoral condyle

Patella

Ulceration

Eburnation

Osteochondroma

Semilunar cartilage

Characteristic posture in advanced ochronotic spondylitis: kyphosis, rigid spine, flexed knees, wide base

Exposure of knee joint: pigmentation, eburnation, and ulceration of cartilages; osteochondroma with pedicle to synovial lining

Pigmentation of endocardium

fragment and develop osteochondral loose bodies. In addition, homogentisic acid has a propensity for deposition in the nucleus pulposus, resulting in a brittle and stiffened disc space (**Figure 4-22**).

Onset of symptoms occurs typically in the fourth decade of life. Patients with ochronotic spondylosis may present with acute back pain. Progression of the spondylosis results in a stiffened lumbar spine and loss of normal lordosis. Peripheral arthropathy typically involves the large joints and is characterized by prominent osteochondral loose body formation, chronic effusions, and secondary chondrocalcinosis.

Radiographs demonstrate multiple disc vacuum signs with eventual ossification of the discs and intervertebral ligaments. In contrast to ankylosing spondylitis, the sacroiliac and apophyseal joints are spared. The peripheral joints are characterized by loose bodies and osteoarthritic changes, with involvement of the shoulder, hip, and knee, and sparing of the smaller joints. The diagnosis is suggested by a history of the patient's passing black urine and is confirmed upon observation of freshly passed urine that turns black upon exposure to air. Synovial fluid is characteristically clear and yellow because it does not darken with alkalinization. Symptomatic treatment is similar to that for other osteoarthritic conditions. Arthroscopic removal of osteochondral loose bodies is indicated for mechanical symptoms of locking or instability. Total joint arthroplasty is the treatment for end-stage arthritis.

ADDITIONAL READINGS

Cassidy JT, Petty RE. *Textbook of Pediatric Rheumatology*, 5th edition. Philadelphia, Pa: WB Saunders; 2006.

Pirsch JD. Care of the transplant patient. *Clinical Symposia*. 1998;Vol. 51, No. 1.

Harris ED Jr., Budd RC, Firestein GS, Genovese MC, Sergent JS, Ruddy S, Sledge CB. *Kelley's Textbook of Rheumatology*, 7th edition. Philadelphia, Pa: WB Saunders; 2005.

Moskowitz RW, Howell DS, Altman RD, Buckwalter JA, Goldberg VM. *Osteoarthritis*. Philadelphia, Pa: WB Saunders; 2001.

Rott KT, Agudelo CA. Gout. *JAMA*. 2003;2857–2860.

five

Disorders of Muscles, Tendons, and Ligaments

David T. Rispler, MD

The more than 400 skeletal muscles in the body provide movement and account for 40% to 45% of total body weight. Furthermore, muscle strains are the most common diagnosis associated with visits to physicians' offices, and even when an injury is a fracture or sprain, the rehabilitation program is devoted primarily to muscle strengthening.

ANATOMY AND PHYSIOLOGY OF MUSCLE

Individual muscles vary greatly in size and shape. Their intrinsic framework, however, is similar. The primary structural element is the muscle fiber, or *myofiber*, which is a multinucleated syncytium formed from multiple *myoblasts* that have fused together to extend from the bone of origin across one or more joints to insert into a tendon that then inserts into bone. Endomysium, perimysium, and epimysium are the various connective tissue membranes that provide protective coverage but are loose enough to allow for functional changes in muscle length (**Figure 5-1**).

In an immature myoblast, the nucleus is located centrally; with maturity, the nucleus shifts to an eccentric position and lies just under the sarcolemma (the plasma membrane that surrounds each myofiber). The sarcolemma supports and protects the *sarcoplasm* (the myoblast cytoplasm) and interacts with the *basement membrane*, a three-part connective tissue layer that surrounds the sarcolemma. *Satellite cells* are stem cells located between the basement membrane and the sarcolemma. These cells proliferate after muscle injury and form new myoblasts and myofibers.

In muscles that require fine motor control, a single motor axon typically sends branches to relatively few myofibers (eg, 6 to 10 myofibers in ocular muscles); however, in power muscles such as the gastrocnemius, a single axon innervates more than 1000 myofibers. Each muscle fiber, however, is connected to only one nerve branch at the motor end plate. An electrical impulse from the nerve triggers chemical transmission of acetylcholine across the synapse of the motor end plate, with subsequent depolarization and spread of an action potential through the full length of the muscle membrane. This electrical impulse reaches the interior of the myofiber via an intricate *sarcoplasmic reticulum system* (**Figure 5-2**). In response to the electrical impulse, calcium is released from the reticular channels into the sarcoplasm. The increased concentration of calcium activates contractile proteins in the sarcoplasm.

Skeletal muscle derives its striated appearance and function from the contractile proteins. The *sarcomere*, the contractile unit, is composed of *thin filaments* (mostly actin, but also tropomyosin and troponin molecules) and *thick filaments* (myosin molecules). A sarcomere extends from one Z line to the next Z line (see **Figure 5-1**). The bands and zones in a sarcomere differ, depending on whether thin, thick, or interdigitating thick and thin filaments are present (**Figure 5-3**).

When a myofiber is in a relaxed state, *tropomyosin* blocks the binding sites on actin. When the influxing calcium binds to *troponin*, a structural reconfiguration induces tropomyosin to move into a groove on the actin, thus exposing actin binding sites and allowing cross-linking between the thick and thin filaments; this cross-linking results from bridging of the paired, paddle-like heads of the *myosin* molecules to the *actin* molecules.

Muscle contraction and sliding of the thick and thin filaments occur with cross-bridging; however, each cross-bridge results in only a small amount of shortening, and the process of binding and release must be repeated multiple times before functional contraction of the myofiber is achieved. The energy for each cross-bridge comes from the hydrolysis of adenosine triphosphate (ATP).

Muscle relaxation occurs through the active transport of calcium back into the tubules of the sarcoplasmic reticulum. With dissociation of calcium from troponin, tropomyosin

Figure 5-1: Organization of Skeletal Muscle

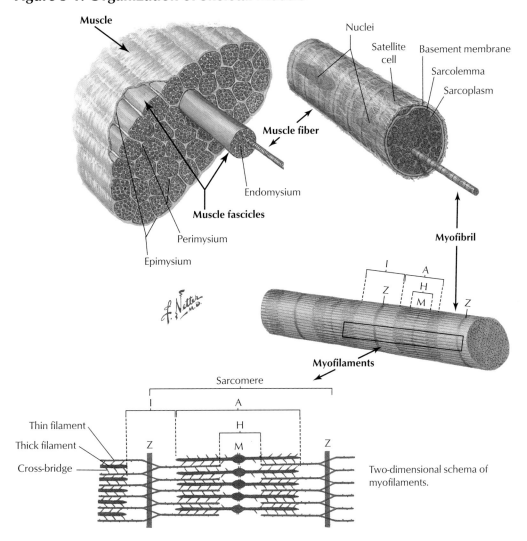

Two-dimensional schema of myofilaments.

reverts back to the state in which it blocks actin and myosin bridging.

Muscle activity typically is described as *contraction* or shortening of the muscle-tendon unit. Muscles, however, also function with activation of actin and myosin bonds in *isometric* and *eccentric* modes. In an isometric "contraction," force is generated, but the muscle length stays the same and the joint does not move. In an eccentric action, actin and myosin bonds form as the muscle lengthens. Eccentric activity provides controlled joint motion as objects are moved, for example, active function of the biceps muscle allows controlled extension of the elbow while a heavy object is lowered.

For a single muscle fiber, the strength or tension of activation depends primarily on length-tension relationships. Maximum force is exerted when the length of the sarcomere permits activation of all possible actin and myosin cross-bridges. This situation occurs when the myofiber is at resting length. If the muscle fiber is in a shortened or lengthened position, less cross-bridging occurs, and less muscle tension (power) is produced (**Figure 5-4**).

Figure 5-2: Sarcoplasmic Reticulum and Initiation of Muscle Contraction

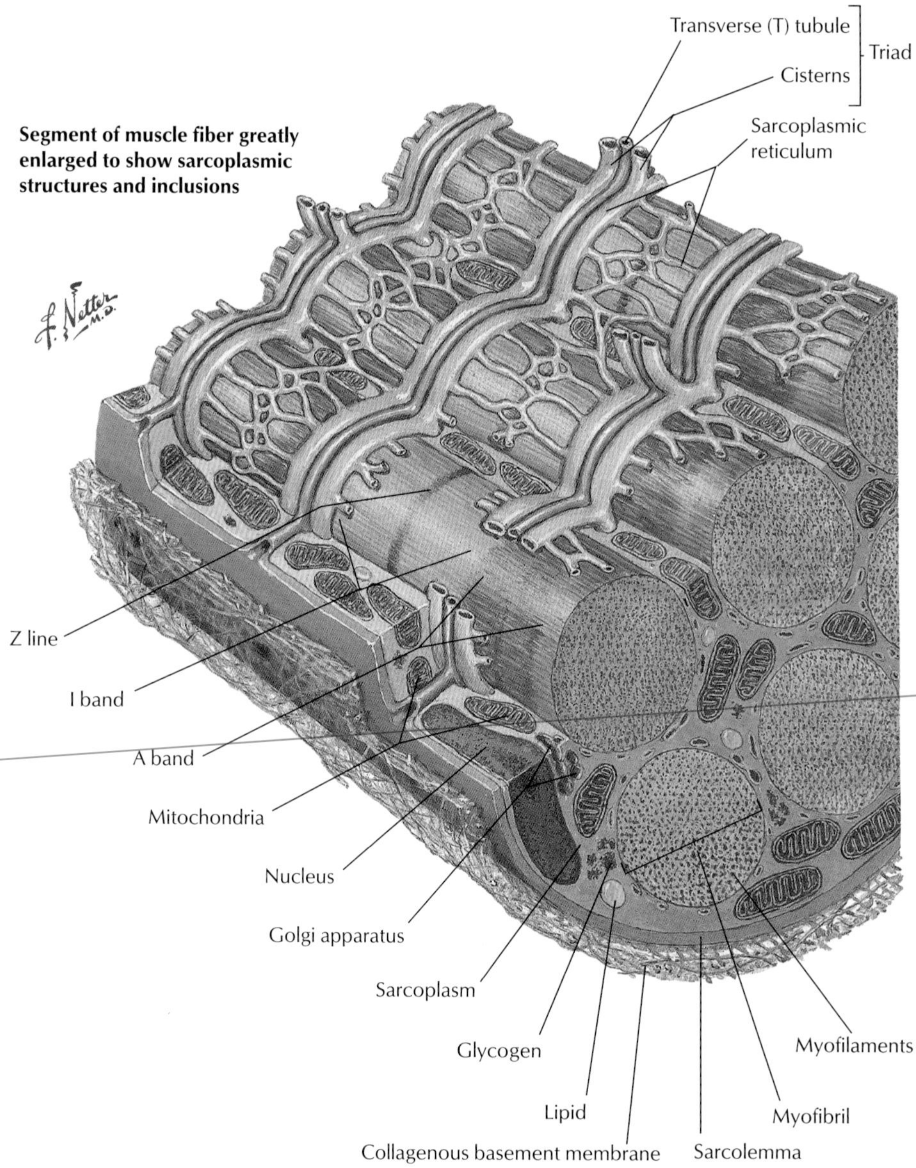

Segment of muscle fiber greatly enlarged to show sarcoplasmic structures and inclusions

Transverse (T) tubule

Cisterns

Triad

Sarcoplasmic reticulum

Z line

I band

A band

Mitochondria

Nucleus

Golgi apparatus

Sarcoplasm

Glycogen

Lipid

Collagenous basement membrane

Sarcolemma

Myofibril

Myofilaments

In general, the overall strength of a particular muscle is proportionate to its cross-sectional area. The strength or force developed during a muscle contraction depends on the number of muscle fibers that are activated at the same time, as well as the length of the muscle and its position and resultant moment arm.

Aerobic and anaerobic metabolism provide the energy necessary for the repetitive actin and myosin bridging required for muscle activity. The preferred route is *aerobic phosphorylation* by the oxidative metabolism of glucose from stored glycogen or fatty acids, because this reaction produces 34 ATP molecules per molecule of glucose, whereas

Figure 5-3: Biochemical Mechanics of Muscle Contraction

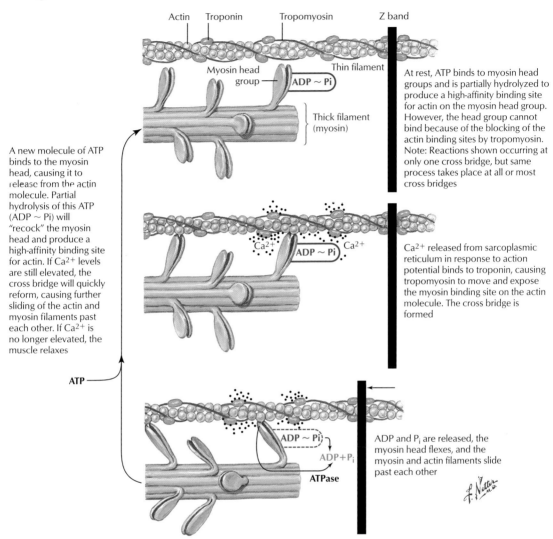

At rest, ATP binds to myosin head groups and is partially hydrolyzed to produce a high-affinity binding site for actin on the myosin head group. However, the head group cannot bind because of the blocking of the actin binding sites by tropomyosin. Note: Reactions shown occurring at only one cross bridge, but same process takes place at all or most cross bridges

Ca^{2+} released from sarcoplasmic reticulum in response to action potential binds to troponin, causing tropomyosin to move and expose the myosin binding site on the actin molecule. The cross bridge is formed

A new molecule of ATP binds to the myosin head, causing it to release from the actin molecule. Partial hydrolysis of this ATP ($ADP \sim Pi$) will "recock" the myosin head and produce a high-affinity binding site for actin. If Ca^{2+} levels are still elevated, the cross bridge will quickly reform, causing further sliding of the actin and myosin filaments past each other. If Ca^{2+} is no longer elevated, the muscle relaxes

ADP and P_i are released, the myosin head flexes, and the myosin and actin filaments slide past each other

the *anaerobic metabolism* of glycogen or glucose produces only 2 ATP molecules per molecule of glucose. Energy for high-intensity exercise of brief duration—for example, a short sprint of 50 to 200 yd—comes from stored high-energy phosphate compounds. For low-intensity exercise of long duration, aerobic metabolism takes care of most energy requirements. Greater amounts of anaerobic metabolism are required during more prolonged high-intensity exercise. Training increases the efficiency of the cardiovascular and metabolic pathways so that accumulation of lactic acid and fatigue are diminished.

Individual muscle groups contain three types of muscle fibers. *Type I myofibers* are "slow twitch," fatigue resistant, and relatively dark because of their higher concentration of cytochromes and enzymes that facilitate aerobic oxidative phosphorylation (**Figure 5-5**). *Type II myofibers* are "fast twitch," are more dependent on anaerobic glycolysis, and fatigue more rapidly. *Type IIa myofibers* are "fast twitch" and resistant to fatigue at an

Figure 5-4: Muscle Length–Muscle Tension Relationships

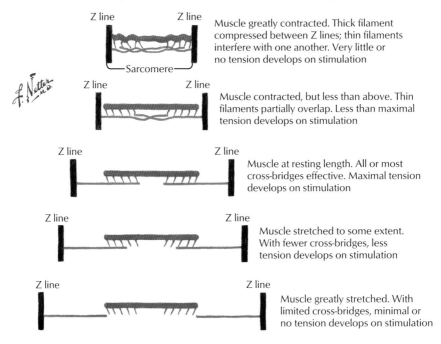

Muscle greatly contracted. Thick filament compressed between Z lines; thin filaments interfere with one another. Very little or no tension develops on stimulation

Muscle contracted, but less than above. Thin filaments partially overlap. Less than maximal tension develops on stimulation

Muscle at resting length. All or most cross-bridges effective. Maximal tension develops on stimulation

Muscle stretched to some extent. With fewer cross-bridges, less tension develops on stimulation

Muscle greatly stretched. With limited cross-bridges, minimal or no tension develops on stimulation

intermediate level between type I and *type IIb* fibers. The percentage of type I versus type II myofibers depends on a person's genetic makeup and varies according to the muscle observed. For example, muscles that perform quick, finely coordinated activities are made up of a predominance of type II fibers. People who "naturally" excel at these activities have a greater proportion of type II fibers; however, training can affect the interconversion of type IIa and IIb fibers. Endurance training increases the percentage of type IIa fibers relative to type IIb, and power lifting without emphasis on endurance increases the proportion of type IIb relative to type IIa fibers.

ANATOMY AND PHYSIOLOGY OF TENDONS AND LIGAMENTS

Tendons attach muscle to bone. Ligaments and their associated capsular tissues connect bone to bone. Tendons and ligaments are composed of fibroblasts, collagen, proteoglycan, glycoproteins, elastin, water, and connective tissue covering. The major constituent of tendons and ligaments is *type I collagen* (86% and 70% fat-free dry weight, respectively). The three chains of a type I collagen molecule are coiled in a triple helix that is held together by hydrogen and covalent bonds. Strength is greatly augmented at the microfibril level, where five collagen molecules are arranged in a parallel, quaternary pattern (quarter stagger), thus aligning oppositely charged amino acids. The surrounding *proteoglycan matrix* is hydrophilic and improves strength, probably by preventing fibrillar deformation.

Parallel orientation of the collagen bundles to their long axes allows tendons and ligaments to withstand high tensile loads. Thus, tendons can transmit the force of a strong muscular contraction, and ligaments can resist disruptive movement of a joint. Compared with tendons, ligaments typically are shorter and wider; they also have a lower percentage of collagen, a greater proportion

Figure 5-5: Muscle Fiber Types

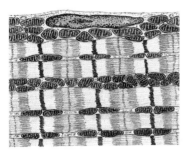 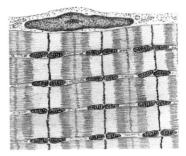

Type I: Dark or red fiber. Large profuse mitochondria beneath sarcolemma and in rows as well as paired in interfibrillar regions. Z lines wider than in type II

Type II: Light or white skeletal muscle fiber in longitudinal section on electron microscopy. Small, relatively sparse mitochondria, chiefly paired in interfibrillar spaces at Z lines

Histochemical classification		
Fiber type	**ATPase stain**	**SDH stain**
1. Fast-twitch, fatigable (IIb) Stain deeply for ATPase, poorly for succinic acid dehydrogenase (SDH), a mitochondrial enzyme active in citric acid cycle. Therefore, fibers rapidly release energy from ATP but poorly regenerate it, thus becoming fatigued.		
2. Fast-twitch, fatigue-resistant (IIa) Stain deeply for both ATPase and SDH. Therefore, fibers rapidly release energy from ATP and also rapidly regenerate ATP in citric acid cycle, thus resisting fatigue.		
3. Slow-twitch, fatigue-resistant (I) Stain poorly for ATPase but deeply for SDH. Therefore, fibers only slowly release energy from ATP but regenerate ATP rapidly, thus resisting fatigue.		

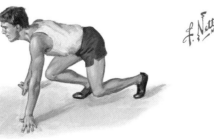

Cross section of skeletal muscle fibers stained for ATPase

Identical section stained for SDH

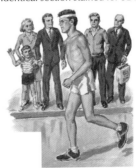

Sprinter
Training induces a greater proportion of type IIb fibers relative to type IIa

Marathon runner
Type IIa fiber is increased relative to type IIb

of proteoglycan, and slightly reduced longitudinal organization of the collagen fibers because of their more varied loading. Ligaments have nerve endings called *mechanoreceptors* that enhance joint stability by transmitting proprioception of joint position and stress. Some ligaments (eg, the anterior cruciate ligament) are organized into separate bundles that are taut at different joint positions, thereby providing a restraining force throughout the full arc of motion.

At the myotendinous junction, highly folded muscle membranes decrease stress by increasing the surface area; however, this region is a weak link at an area where muscle strains commonly occur. Bone-tendon and bone-ligament junctions are transitional areas where the collagenous fibers of tendon merge with the collagenous fibers of bone (Sharpey fibers).

Tendons that pull in a straight line are surrounded by a loose connective layer, called the *peritenon*. Tendons that undergo high bending movements, for example, flexor tendons of the hand, are enclosed by a synovial sheath that facilitates gliding movements of the tendon.

EFFECTS OF IMMOBILIZATION

Immobilization causes muscle atrophy, with declining size and weight of the muscle. Histologically, all myofibers atrophy. The rate of protein synthesis decreases within hours after immobilization begins, and the rate of muscle atrophy is greater in the initial days than in the subsequent period of immobilization. The decrease in muscle strength corresponds to the decrease in the muscle's cross-sectional area. Atrophy is greater in muscles immobilized in a shortened position compared with those in a stretched position.

Immobilization weakens ligaments in their midsubstance and at the bone-ligament insertion site. Insertion site weakness occurs secondary to changes in ligament substance and osteoclastic bone resorption. After resumption of joint motion, recovery of strength is slower at the insertion site than in the ligament substance. Even 12 months after mobilization, ligament insertion site strength is decreased, at 80% to 90% of normal. In a similar manner, immobilization decreases the tensile strength of tendons.

Immobilization causes joint stiffness. The resultant joint contractures are due primarily to synovial adhesions and the formation of new collagen fibrils that restrict the normal parallel sliding of ligament fibers. Another contributing factor is the decreased extensibility that occurs in muscles that have been immobilized in a shortened position.

MUSCLE STRENGTHENING AND CONDITIONING

Our sedentary lives have contributed to obesity becoming a national epidemic. Obesity is typically defined as an abnormal body mass index (BMI). BMI is weight in kilograms divided by height in meters squared (normal BMI is 18.5–24.9, underweight is <18.5 BMI, overweight is BMI of 25–29.9, and obesity is a BMI ≥30). Physicians and therapists should be proactive in counseling patients on the benefits of exercise. In addition to facilitating weight reduction, conditioning can lower blood pressure, decrease cholesterol levels, increase bone density, increase muscle mass, and promote emotional well-being.

A well-structured exercise program includes stretching, aerobic conditioning, and strength training. For the competitive athlete, the fitness program includes flexibility, strength training, and endurance training, but the regimen is sport specific to maximize the athlete's ability to withstand the demands of the sport.

Fitness training should start with a 5-minute light aerobic warmup and stretching. Stretching the connective tissues lessens the chance of injury because it results in doubling of energy before muscle-tendon tearing occurs. Static stretching is preferred. The most efficient technique is called *proprioceptive neuromuscular facilitation (PNF)*. This technique stretches the muscle to its pain-free physiologic limit for 10 seconds. After a few seconds of relaxation, the muscle is again stretched to its pain-free physiologic limit, which is held for 10 seconds. This procedure is repeated several times.

A complete exercise program includes aerobic conditioning such as walking, biking, or swimming. The American Heart Association recommends spending 30 to 40 minutes a session 4 to 5 times a week for maximum benefit. A more realistic approach for the busy person is to train for 12 to 20 minutes 3 to 4 times a week. The intensity of training should increase the heart rate to 60% to 85% of the maximum age-adjusted heart rate (calculated by 220 minus your age).

In general, strength training involves several repetitions to the point of fatigue, with exercises arranged so they work on several muscle groups in sequential fashion. Muscle strength improves through muscle hypertrophy and neurologic enhancement. In a poorly conditioned or untrained muscle, only 60% to 80% of myofibers can be activated simultaneously, but in a well-conditioned muscle, more than 90% of muscle fibers can fire simultaneously. With strength training, muscle size increases, but whether this increased muscle bulk results from an increase in the number or the size of myofibers is debatable. Strength training increases the contractile protein content in all myofibers, but type II fibers show greater hypertrophy. Muscle hypertrophy is particularly enhanced when exercises are done in a high-force, low-repetition mode; however, for the general population, a regimen of 2 to 3 sets of 15 to 20 repetitions of specific exercises for various upper and lower extremity muscles results in overload of the muscle without overtraining and fatigue.

Aerobic or endurance training, such as distance running, enhances the supply of energy rather than the size of the muscle. The cardiovascular system adapts to supply oxygen to the muscles at an increased rate. Muscle fibers in turn adapt by increasing the size and number of mitochondria, as well as the proportion of type IIa fibers. After exercise regimens, ligaments and tendons also develop increased tensile strength and greater resistance to failure.

The theory that older children should not participate in strength training has been disproved by several studies. With a supervised program that uses proper techniques, children have a low risk of injury and show increased strength. Boys 11 to15 years old and girls 10 to14 years old can do 12 to 20 repetitions, and older adolescents can participate safely in power lifting with proper spotting and supervision. Some adolescents are enamored with strength training and will do anything to enhance muscle bulk. These persons should be counseled about the adverse effects of anabolic steroid use, including testicular atrophy, gynecomastia, acne, alopecia, hepatic dysfunction, cardiomyopathy, premature closure of the physis, and heightened aggression.

EFFECTS OF AGING

When persons are in their mid-20s, skeletal muscle mass begins to decrease at a rate of 4% per decade; this continues until they reach their early 50s. Thereafter, the rate of loss accelerates to 10% of remaining skeletal muscle per decade. Age-related loss of mass and strength results primarily from decreases in the number and size of myofibers. Abnormal levels of growth hormone, testosterone, and thyroxine accentuate loss of muscle mass. In addition, the ability of muscle to maintain energy levels and sustain power with repeated contraction declines in older people. Older muscles also are more susceptible to injury—particularly from eccentric loads—and have reduced healing potential.

Strength training can increase muscle strength and size in older patients. Minor muscle injuries during exercise are more common among older people. Lower intensity strength training decreases the risk of these injuries. In addition, hormone replacement therapy may be indicated.

Tendons show degenerative changes that begin in the third decade. Decreased vascularity and cellularity lead to weaker, stiffer, and less compliant tendons because of an increased amount of insoluble collagen, reduced collagen turnover, and decreased proteoglycan and water content. These changes predispose tendons to spontaneous or low-energy-level tears, particularly in relatively avascular areas such as the shoulder rotator cuff, posterior tibialis, and Achilles tendon. Ligaments also have decreased tensile strength in older people. Some of this decreased strength is due to substance changes, and some is related to weakening of the bone-ligament insertion site.

MUSCLE INJURIES

Muscle injuries account for approximately 30% of sports medicine–related clinic visits. These injuries result from either an indirect overload mechanism or a direct injury, and they range from delayed muscle soreness (DMS) to complete laceration of the muscle.

An individual with DMS typically presents with pain and firmness in the muscle 1 to 3 days after an excessive workout. Stiffness and weakness also are common. DMS results from structural damage to the myofiber. The damage is reversible, but measurable deficits in strength last for up to 10 days. Athletes who use improper technique or who suddenly increase their training are susceptible to this problem. Thus, the popular "no pain, no gain" regimens can cause more harm than good.

A strain, which is commonly referred to as a "pulled muscle," is the partial tearing of a muscle-tendon unit. Muscle strain injuries result from indirect forces when the muscle is passively stretched or activated during stretch beyond its viscoelastic limits. The myotendinous junction is the most susceptible site, probably because terminal sarcomeres are stiffer than sarcomeres in the middle of the muscle. Muscles that cross two joints, including the hamstring, biceps brachii, rectus femoris, hip adductor, and gastrocnemius, are predisposed to muscle strain injuries because these muscles often function, and thus are overloaded, during eccentric, energy-absorbing activities. Fatigue and previous injury increase the risk of injury.

Muscle contusions usually result from non-penetrating blunt injury, whereas muscle lacerations usually result from penetrating sharp injury. Severe blunt trauma may progress to myositis ossificans (see Chapter 8).

After injury occurs, the repair of skeletal muscle progresses through four interrelated stages: necrosis/degeneration, inflammation, repair, and scar tissue formation. After injury, myofibers necrose and degenerate. Hematoma formation, with the subsequent arrival of inflammatory cells that secrete various cytokines and growth factors, occurs early and dominates the first 5 days. Muscle regeneration occurs via satellite cells that are activated by various growth factors to proliferate and differentiate into myofibers. Regeneration begins 7 to 10 days post injury, peaks at 2 weeks, and starts to fade 4 weeks after injury. With significant injury, the formation of scar (fibrous) tissue starts to predominate after 3 weeks. When scar tissue forms, the muscle can never completely regenerate. This fact is not significant with most strains, but with complete laceration of a muscle through its midsubstance, the muscle recovers only approximately 50% of its ability to produce tension.

Treatment for acute strains begins with rest, ice, compression, and elevation (RICE) to decrease hemorrhage, edema, and pain. By blocking the production of prostaglandins, nonsteroidal anti-inflammatory drugs (NSAIDs) decrease pain and may help the patient in beginning a rehabilitation program; however, the appropriate use of NSAIDs after muscle injury is still uncertain because reduced prostaglandin levels may interfere with the repair of regenerating muscle.

Muscle injury rehabilitation should be an incremental program that promotes regeneration and prevents recurrence. Stretching begins with gentle active motion and progresses to passive static stretching as pain allows. Strengthening starts with isometric and light resistance isotonic exercises. When motion is regained and pain is absent, the patient can progress to isokinetic, eccentric, and sports-specific strengthening. To prevent reinjury, the strained muscle should possess 90% of the strength of the muscle on the contralateral limb before the person is permitted to resume competitive sports activities.

Significant muscle lacerations are best treated by repair, perhaps augmented by tendon grafts or tissue scaffold substitutes.

ACUTE TENDON AND LIGAMENT INJURIES

Tendons and ligaments show similar patterns of elongation on tensile stress. Initial stress straightens the relaxed (crimped) collagen fibrils and orients the collagen bundles in a more parallel fashion but does not elongate the ligament (toe region of the stress/strain curve). Further stress into the linear region represents the modulus of elasticity (stiffness) of the tissue. If stress is not exceeded beyond the modulus of elasticity, the tendon or ligament will elongate but will resume its normal length when the tensile stress is stopped. However, with greater loads, the ultimate tensile strength is exceeded, with resultant permanent elongation or complete rupture of the tendon or ligament.

Individual muscle-tendon units and ligaments have different yield levels according to their size, anatomical location, and physiologic status. The substance of normal tendons has a much higher tensile strength and a much lower rate of injury compared with the musculotendinous junction, the muscle belly, or the bone-tendon junction (avulsion fracture). Indeed, normal tendons almost never rupture, and nearly all cases of acute tendon rupture occur in tissue that has been affected by degenerative tendinopathy, mucoid degeneration, tendolipomatosis, or calcifying tendinopathy. Ligament tears, however, are more often intrasubstance occurrences, resulting from the rupture of sequential series of collagen fiber bundles. When the ligament avulses from the bone, injury typically occurs between the transitional layers of the unmineralized and mineralized fibrocartilage layers. Laceration also may disrupt tendons and ligaments.

Aging, immobilization, corticosteroid injections, and some medications weaken tendons and ligaments and predispose these structures to rupture. Age and immobilization also weaken bone; therefore, bone may be the weak link, and the injuring force may cause a fracture. Glucocorticoids inhibit collagen synthesis, with subsequent reduction in collagen content, and documented cases of tendon rupture have occurred after glucocorticoid injections. Fluoroquinolone antibiotics cause tendinosis and tendinitis in a significant but low percentage of patients. The most common site is the Achilles tendon. Bilateral tendon ruptures have been reported in patients. Animal studies show cellular degeneration that is reversible with cessation of the drug.

Acute tendon ruptures require urgent assessment. The dynamic pull of the attached muscle causes loss of tendon continuity, which cannot be restored without surgery. With delay in treatment, the muscle gradually contracts, making the procedure more extensive and the result less reliable. Some partial tendon lacerations may be treated with immobilization. Some tendon ruptures—for example, proximal biceps tendon ruptures in most adults—do not cause functional disability and can be treated nonoperatively.

An acute ligament injury is called a *sprain.* The disruption may be partial or complete. Grade I sprains are partial tears with mild rupture or stretching of the collagen fibers and no apparent instability of the joint when the ligament is stressed. Grade II sprains are partial but more severe, and there is some laxity on stressing of the joint. Grade III sprains are complete ligament ruptures with complete instability of the ligament on stress maneuvers (**Figure 5-6**). Pain may be more severe with partial ligament tears, presumably because of stress and tension on nerves in the remaining intact portion of the ligament. Of note, pain and swelling may not permit adequate examination and stress maneuvers for accurate grading of acute sprains.

Similar to healing of other soft tissues, healing of tendons and ligaments progresses through four stages: inflammation, proliferation, remodeling, and maturation. In a paratenon-covered tendon and an extra-articular ligament, the initial healing stage brings hematoma, inflammatory cells, and

Figure 5-6: Grading of Ligament Sprains

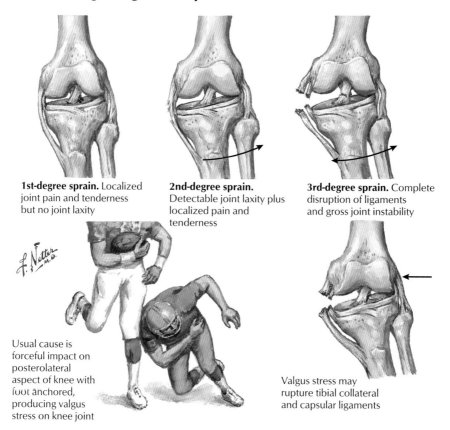

1st-degree sprain. Localized joint pain and tenderness but no joint laxity

2nd-degree sprain. Detectable joint laxity plus localized pain and tenderness

3rd-degree sprain. Complete disruption of ligaments and gross joint instability

Usual cause is forceful impact on posterolateral aspect of knee with foot anchored, producing valgus stress on knee joint

Valgus stress may rupture tibial collateral and capsular ligaments

fibroblasts to begin collagen synthesis, which can be detected as early as 3 days after injury. The second stage continues for 4 to 6 weeks and includes cellular and matrix proliferation. This stage transitions to the remodeling and maturation stages, which are characterized by a reduction in the mass of relatively disorganized fibrous tissue, a reorganization of collagen along the lines of tensile loading, an increase in cross-linking bonds between collagen fibers, and an increase in the tensile strength of the tendon or ligament over the first 4 to 6 weeks. The healing process of a complete tear continues for a year or longer.

The healing process is different for extrasynovial or tendinous sheath tendons. In a tendon enclosed by a sheath, healing is somewhat less predictable and differs in that intrinsic healing predominates, with fibroblasts coming directly from the epitenon and endotenon. In tendons that have been repaired and are undergoing controlled passive motion, intrinsic healing from the epitenon predominates. In tendons enclosed by a sheath that are treated by immobilization, initial granulation tissue develops from the epitenon and subsequent cellular proliferation from the endotenon.

Healing of the anterior cruciate ligament (ACL) and other intra-articular ligaments is often poor because the blood supply is limited, the synovial fluid interferes with hematoma formation and development of a fibrin clot scaffold, and mechanical shear does not allow the ends to stay approximated. Occasionally, the ACL will scar into the posterior cruciate ligament, providing some minimal stability; typically, though, neither nonoperative nor direct repair of the ligament results in successful healing of the ACL.

Prolonged immobilization in the treatment of tendon and ligament injuries leads to adhesions, reduced gliding, delayed increase in tensile strength, and poorer outcomes. Early, controlled motion and exercise lead to better collagen synthesis; earlier return of tensile strength of the innate ligament, tendon, or graft; and better range of motion and functional outcome. This is the preferred method of treatment, when feasible.

CHRONIC TENDINOPATHY

Chronic tendon problems account for more than half of occupational injuries. The etiology is multifactorial. Extrinsic cumulative trauma (overuse) is often a factor, but some people can do the same repetitive task without developing problems. Intrinsic causes include anatomical factors that increase stress on the muscle-tendon unit and local and systemic degenerative factors that weaken the tendon. Focal degenerative changes are often noted and are characterized by decreased vascular supply, degenerative changes in the tendon, and a paucity of inflammatory cells. Therefore, although these conditions were frequently labeled as *tendinitis* in the past, the terms *tendinosis* and *insertional tendinopathy* (bone-tendon junction) are usually more appropriate (**Figure 5-7**).

Inflammation, when present, is generally restricted to the tendon sheath. Thus, three clinical situations can occur in the same area. For instance, Achilles tendon problems may present as insertional tendinopathy, midsubstance tendinosis, or peritendinitis (inflammation of the paratenon). Progressive tendinopathy results in a dysfunctional muscle-tendon unit. The result is progressive weakness and functional disability. These tendons also are structurally weaker and at risk for rupture. Treatment of chronic tendinopathy varies according to the anatomic area involved. Initial treatment should consist of relative rest, avoidance of exacerbating activities, correction of associated mechanical factors, and physical therapy. NSAIDs are commonly prescribed but should be considered carefully because they may not benefit the degenerative process and may provide limited analgesia. If symptoms persist, cortisone injections can be used carefully. These injections are most useful in decreasing the inflammation of an associated bursitis. Reconstructive procedures are indicated for continued tendinopathy that is causing functional disability.

MYOPATHIC DISORDERS IN ADULTS

Primary muscle diseases may occur secondary to autoimmune, metabolic, congenital, and genetic disorders. These diseases cause muscle weakness, commonly affect proximal

Figure 5-7: Achilles Insertional Tendinopathy

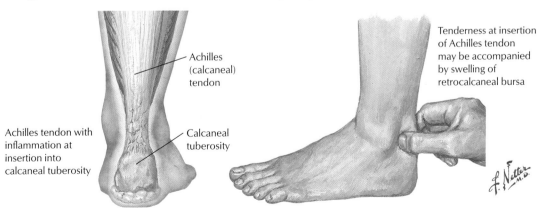

Achilles (calcaneal) tendon

Calcaneal tuberosity

Achilles tendon with inflammation at insertion into calcaneal tuberosity

Tenderness at insertion of Achilles tendon may be accompanied by swelling of retrocalcaneal bursa

muscles to a greater extent than distal groups, and may be progressive or self-limited.

Inflammatory Myopathies

Many diseases, such as rheumatoid arthritis, systemic lupus erythematosus, other collagen vascular diseases, postviral myositis, and granulomatous disease, may cause myopathic degeneration and regeneration with perivascular inflammation. With these conditions, muscle biopsy is helpful in confirming the diagnosis, thus leading to initiation of treatment.

Dermatomyositis and *polymyositis* are the collagen vascular disorders that affect muscle to the greatest degree. Any age group may be affected. Patients with these conditions present with symmetric proximal muscle weakness and tenderness. Weakness of the hip flexors, hip extensors, and quadriceps causes difficulty arising from the floor, getting out of a bathtub, or climbing up a high step. Loss of shoulder girdle strength is manifested by difficulty in performing overhead activities such as lifting an object off a shelf, or even combing one's hair. Eventually, the neck muscles become involved, causing difficulty in raising the head; in severe cases, dysphagia may occur. As the disease progresses, muscle pain, tenderness, and induration may develop (**Figure 5-8**).

These disorders are similar, except that dermatomyositis includes skin involvement, with a characteristic heliotrope rash around the eyes; periorbital edema; and elevated, dusky red patches and telangiectasias over the extensor surfaces of the elbows, knees, ankles, finger joints, and other areas exposed to sunlight.

The etiology is most likely an autoimmune response to a collagen vascular, infectious, or malignant process. Laboratory tests demonstrate elevations in acute phase protein level and erythrocyte sedimentation rate. As in other myopathies, the serum levels of enzymes that reside in skeletal muscle, such as transaminase, creatine phosphokinase, and aldolase, are elevated. Electromyographic (EMG) studies demonstrate myopathic patterns characterized by short duration, low amplitude, and polyphasic potentials.

Muscle biopsy confirms the diagnosis. Pathologic alterations include primary degeneration of muscle fibers, necrosis, basophilia with central positioning of nuclei, infiltrates of chronic inflammatory cells, and interstitial fibrosis. In patients older than 40 years, evaluation should exclude an underlying neoplasm. Removal of a tumor may lead to complete remission of the myositis. Most patients initially respond to high-dose corticosteroids; however, prognosis is variable.

Myopathies Associated with HIV Infection

Patients with human immunodeficiency virus (HIV) may display a wide range of disease processes, including pyomyositis, polymyositis, and drug-induced myopathy. Although manifestations tend to be seen in the later stages, these problems may be the first clinical signs of HIV infection. In fact, the differential diagnosis of sudden-onset arthralgia and myalgia with a compatible history of exposure should include HIV infection.

Metabolic Myopathies

Metabolic myopathy is a generic term that describes disorders of energy metabolism with resultant muscle deficiency in dynamic or routine activities. The enzyme deficiencies involve glycolysis, lipid metabolism, and the formation of ATP in the mitochondria. The clinical features of these diseases vary, but typically, pain develops after exercise because of muscle necrosis caused by an inadequate energy supply (**Figure 5-9**). Muscle necrosis causes an increase in serum muscle enzymes and a release of myoglobin in the urine, which can lead to acute renal tubular necrosis.

MYOPATHIC DISORDERS IN CHILDREN

Duchenne Muscular Dystrophy

Duchenne muscular dystrophy (DMD) is an X chromosome–linked recessive inherited disorder of muscle characterized by progressive loss of muscle mass and strength, with replacement of muscle by fibrofatty

Figure 5-8: Polymyositis/Dermatomyositis

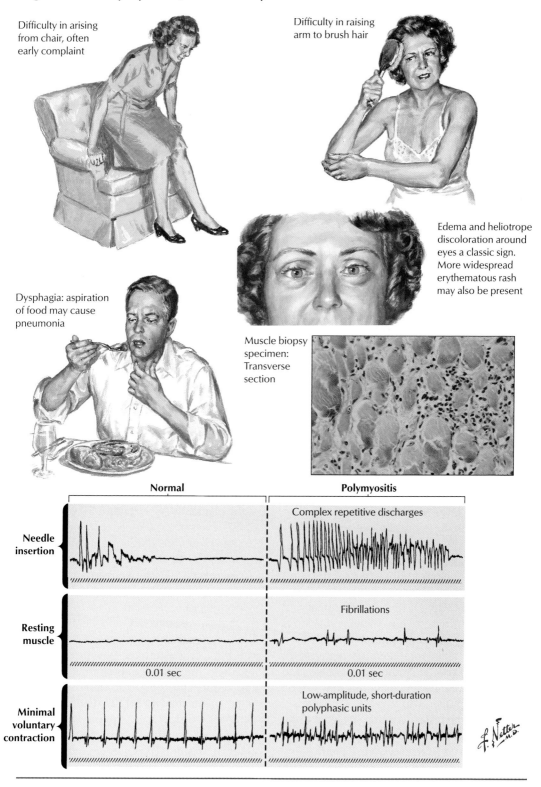

Difficulty in arising from chair, often early complaint

Difficulty in raising arm to brush hair

Edema and heliotrope discoloration around eyes a classic sign. More widespread erythematous rash may also be present

Dysphagia: aspiration of food may cause pneumonia

Muscle biopsy specimen: Transverse section

Normal	Polymyositis
Needle insertion	Complex repetitive discharges
Resting muscle	Fibrillations
0.01 sec	0.01 sec
Minimal voluntary contraction	Low-amplitude, short-duration polyphasic units

Figure 5-9: McArdle Disease

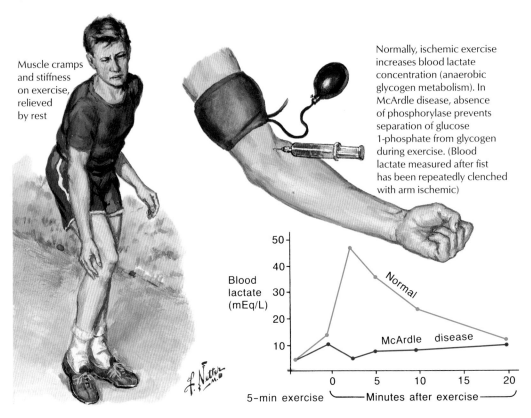

Muscle cramps and stiffness on exercise, relieved by rest

Normally, ischemic exercise increases blood lactate concentration (anaerobic glycogen metabolism). In McArdle disease, absence of phosphorylase prevents separation of glucose 1-phosphate from glycogen during exercise. (Blood lactate measured after fist has been repeatedly clenched with arm ischemic)

Blood lactate (mEq/L)

Normal

McArdle disease

5-min exercise — Minutes after exercise

tissue. The incidence is 2 to 3 per 10,000 live male births, and new mutations account for approximately 30% of cases. DMD results from an abnormality in the gene for dystrophin, a large protein that, with other proteins, stabilizes muscle cell membranes. In Becker muscular dystrophy (BMD), dystrophin is present in reduced amounts; therefore, the condition starts later and progresses more slowly.

Newborns with DMD appear normal, but because of progressive weakness, walking is delayed until 18 to 24 months. These children typically present for diagnosis because of difficulty walking and motor delays at age 2 to 3 years, but the correct diagnosis may not be made for another 1 to 2 years. At diagnosis, because of the proximal muscle weakness, the child is unable to climb steps and either cannot run or does a race-walk run. Patients stand with increased lumbar lordosis and the gait is wide-based. Examination shows a positive Gower sign, and pseudohypertrophy of the calves is caused by early fibrofatty infiltration of the plantar muscles (**Figure 5-10**). Creatine kinase levels are markedly elevated (7000 to 15,000 U/L). The diagnosis usually can be confirmed by DNA analysis of dystrophin.

Progressive muscle weakness causes cessation of walking at 8 to 12 years of age, development of scoliosis at 12 to 16 years, and respiratory insufficiency and death at 18 to 22 years. Medical management is controversial, but corticosteroids may prolong walking, delay the decline in pulmonary function, and reduce the need for scoliosis surgery. Night splints may retard the development of equinus contractures. Spinal stabilization procedures prevent severe deformities and associated sitting problems. Gene therapy

Figure 5-10: Duchenne Muscular Dystrophy

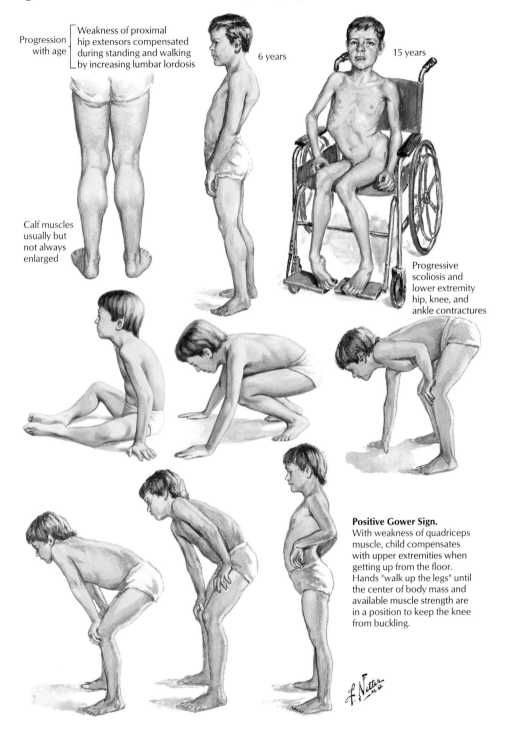

Progression with age — Weakness of proximal hip extensors compensated during standing and walking by increasing lumbar lordosis

6 years

15 years

Calf muscles usually but not always enlarged

Progressive scoliosis and lower extremity hip, knee, and ankle contractures

Positive Gower Sign.
With weakness of quadriceps muscle, child compensates with upper extremities when getting up from the floor. Hands "walk up the legs" until the center of body mass and available muscle strength are in a position to keep the knee from buckling.

research will alter the prognosis and increase the importance of early diagnosis.

Fascioscapulohumeral Muscular Dystrophy

Fascioscapulohumeral muscular dystrophy is an autosomal dominant disorder that is caused by a defect in *FRG1* on chromosome 4q35. Patients typically seek medical treatment when they are between 6 and 20 years of age because of weakness of the face, shoulders, and upper arms. Facial muscle weakness causes an apparent flat affect with pouting lips, transverse smile, absence of forehead wrinkles, and incomplete eye closure. Weakness of the serratus anterior, despite relatively good strength of the deltoid, leads to winging of the scapula and decreased shoulder elevation and abduction (**Figure 5-11**).

Muscle weakness progresses at a relatively slow, but variable, rate. Additional muscles, including the pelvic girdle and anterior tibialis, may become involved. Scoliosis is uncommon because of the later onset of disease, and life expectancy is good because cardiac muscle and the central nervous system are not involved.

Myotonic Disorders

Myotonic disorders are inherited conditions of muscle characterized by slow relaxation due to spontaneous discharge. Myotonia can be separated into two different types of disease. The first group includes ion disorders that affect calcium channels in skeletal muscle channels. This group can be subdivided into chloride and sodium channel diseases. Allelic disorders of the same ion may cause myotonia or periodic paralysis. *Myotonia congenita* is

Figure 5-11: Fascioscapulohumeral Muscular Dystrophy

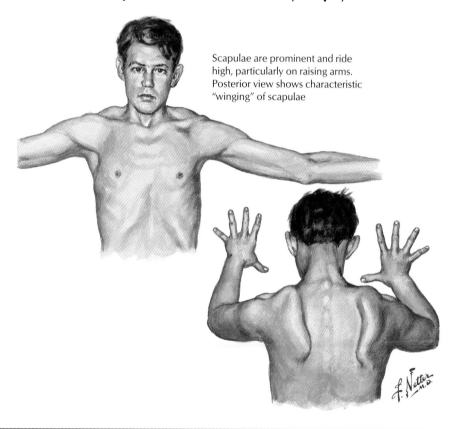

Scapulae are prominent and ride high, particularly on raising arms. Posterior view shows characteristic "winging" of scapulae

secondary to an autosomal dominant or autosomal recessive chloride channel mutation of the gene *ClC-1*. Patients develop stiffness and muscle cramps during the first 3 to 5 minutes of an activity, which improve with continued exercise and repetitive movement. Examination shows a "herculean" body with muscle hypertrophy, particularly in the buttocks, thighs, and calves (**Figure 5-12**). Life span is normal.

The second group of myotonic disorders comprises the myotonic dystrophies. My-otonic dystrophy type 1 (DM1) is the most common adult muscular dystrophy, with an incidence of 1 per 8000 live births. The molecular basis of DM1 is an unstable trinucleotide repeat CTG expansion in the 3ρ untranslated region of the gene that codes for myotonic dystrophy protein kinase. The severity of DM1 correlates with the size of the expansion. As a result, clinical manifestations are quite variable, ranging from asymptomatic, mild, moderate, or severe involvement associated with

Figure 5-12

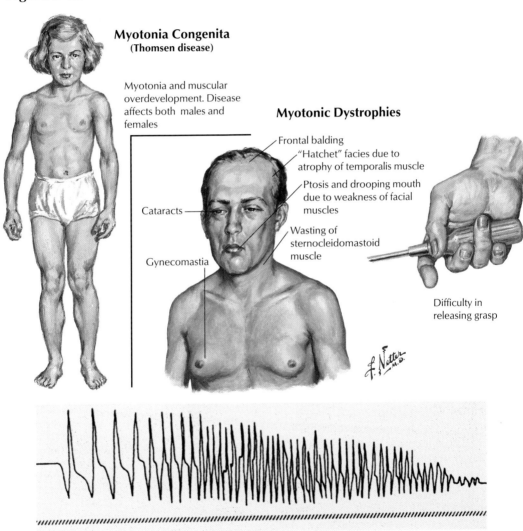

Myotonia Congenita
(Thomsen disease)

Myotonia and muscular overdevelopment. Disease affects both males and females

Myotonic Dystrophies

Frontal balding
"Hatchet" facies due to atrophy of temporalis muscle
Ptosis and drooping mouth due to weakness of facial muscles

Cataracts

Wasting of sternocleidomastoid muscle

Gynecomastia

Difficulty in releasing grasp

Electromyogram showing spontaneous myotonic discharge evoked by needle insertion.

Figure 5-13: Nemaline Myopathy

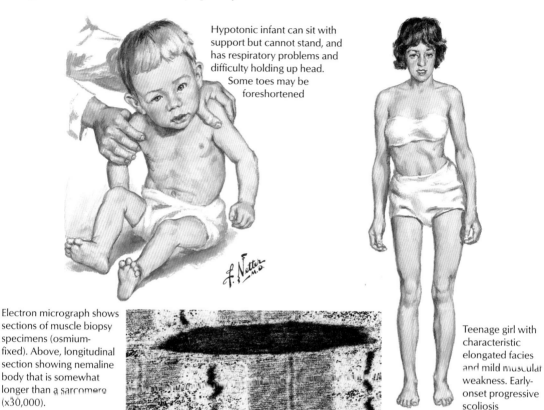

Hypotonic infant can sit with support but cannot stand, and has respiratory problems and difficulty holding up head. Some toes may be foreshortened

Electron micrograph shows sections of muscle biopsy specimens (osmium-fixed). Above, longitudinal section showing nemaline body that is somewhat longer than a sarcomere (x30,000).

Teenage girl with characteristic elongated facies and mild muscular weakness. Early-onset progressive scoliosis

congenital DM1. Mildly impaired patients have delay in their ability to relax a clenched fist and develop cataracts. Moderate involvement presents with progressive facial and distal muscle weakness, cardiac conduction defects, diabetes mellitus, testicular atrophy, and premature balding. Congenital DM1 is characterized by hypotonia, respiratory insufficiency, dysphagia, mental retardation, equinovarus foot deformities, and scoliosis.

Congenital Myopathies

The congenital myopathies constitute a group of different conditions that cause hypotonia at birth and in early infancy. They include central core disease, nemaline myopathy, myotubular myopathy, and congenital fiber type disproportion. Children present as "floppy babies" who have delayed motor milestones (**Figure 5-13**). Most patients improve with age, but

they are always somewhat clumsy. The condition of some patients deteriorates, and they die of respiratory failure. Possible skeletal abnormalities include pes planovalgus feet, hip subluxation, and scoliosis.

ADDITIONAL READINGS

Beredjiklian PK. Biologic aspects of flexor tendon laceration and repair. *J Bone Joint Surg Am.* 2003;85: 539–550.

Buckwalter JA, Einhorn TA, Simon SR, eds. *Orthopaedic Basic Science: Biology and Biomechanics of the Musculoskeletal System*, 2nd edition. Rosemont, Ill: American Academy of Orthopaedic Surgeons; 2000.

Huard J, Yong LI, Fu FH. Muscle injuries and repair: current trends in research. *J Bone Joint Surg Am.* 2002;84: 822–832.

Sharma P, Maffulli N. Tendon injury and tendinopathy: healing and repair. *J Bone Joint Surg Am.* 2005;87: 187–202.

Sussman MD. Muscular dystrophy. In: Fitzgerald RH, Kaufer H, Malkani AL, eds: *Orthopaedics*. Philadelphia, Pa: Mosby; 2002:1573–1583.

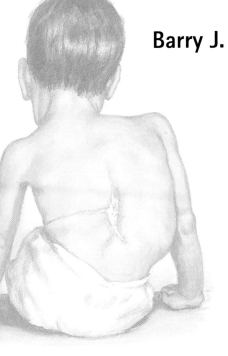

six

Disorders of
Nerves

Barry J. Gainor, MD

ANATOMY AND PHYSIOLOGY

The peripheral nervous system is the circuitry that connects the end organs of the musculoskeletal system to the central nervous system. It is composed of 12 pairs of cranial nerves and 31 pairs of spinal nerves. The latter are grouped into the following pairs: 8 cervical, 12 thoracic, 5 lumbar, 5 sacral, and 1 coccygeal. *Spinal nerves* are mixed nerves that include motor, sensory, and autonomic fibers. Sensory impulses travel from the periphery on axons that terminate at cell bodies (neurons) in the dorsal root ganglion. *Lower motor neurons*

are located in the ventral horn of the spinal cord; their axons exit the spinal cord as ventral roots that connect with the *dorsal root ganglion*, then continue as mixed spinal nerve roots. In the cervical and lumbosacral regions, the spinal nerve roots are grouped as a *plexus* that then forms the peripheral nerves. Parasympathetic and sympathetic fibers exit the spinal cord with the motor axons.

Schwann cells line most peripheral nerves at intervals of 0.1 to 1.0 mm, and these cells insulate the nerves by forming a *myelin sheath* around the axon (**Figure 6-1**). The myelin

Figure 6-1: Anatomy of Peripheral Nerve

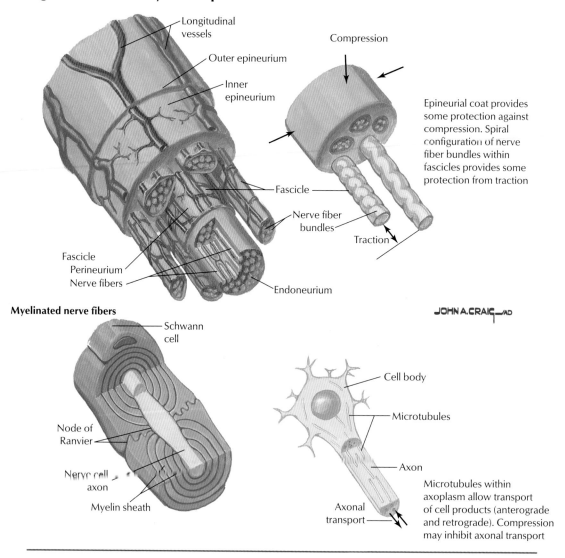

Longitudinal vessels

Compression

Outer epineurium

Inner epineurium

Epineurial coat provides some protection against compression. Spiral configuration of nerve fiber bundles within fascicles provides some protection from traction

Fascicle

Nerve fiber bundles

Traction

Fascicle
Perineurium
Nerve fibers

Endoneurium

Myelinated nerve fibers

JOHN A. CRAIG — AD

Schwann cell

Cell body

Microtubules

Node of Ranvier

Nerve cell axon

Myelin sheath

Axon

Axonal transport

Microtubules within axoplasm allow transport of cell products (anterograde and retrograde). Compression may inhibit axonal transport

sheath is composed of a double membrane, with alternating protein and lipid layers that spiral around the axon in concentric layers. *Nodes of Ranvier* make up the intervals between Schwann cells.

Myelinated axons conduct electrical impulses faster and more efficiently than do nonmyelinated axons. Diseases that damage the myelin sheath can markedly slow conduction of action potentials, with resultant muscle weakness and/or sensory disturbance. Although the myelin sheath provides rapid, passive propagation of a nerve impulse, its structure interferes with initiation of an action potential. This process is evoked at the nodes of Ranvier, where a high concentration of voltage-gated Na^+ channels allows an exchange of ions between the axon and the surrounding extracellular fluid.

The *epineurium* is the relatively thick connective tissue that surrounds and protects peripheral nerves (see **Figure 6-1**). The *endoneurium* is a relatively thin layer of connective tissue that provides support for individual nerve fibers. A *fascicle* is a group of nerve fibers that is surrounded by *perineurium*.

An electromyogram (EMG) evaluates the electrical activity of individual motor units. An EMG can assist in determining whether a condition that causes muscle weakness stems from a peripheral nerve, a neuromuscular junction, or a muscular condition. A nerve conduction study measures the velocity of nerve conduction along peripheral nerves. Nerve conduction may be slowed by localized compression of the nerve or by demyelinating disorders (**Figure 6-2**).

MOTOR AND SENSORY EXAMINATION

Nerve root function should be evaluated if the patient's presenting symptoms suggest a neck or back problem. Peripheral nerve function should be assessed if the problem is localized to the extremities. To make the examination thorough and efficient, evaluate one muscle and one area of sensation that is innervated by the distal portion of the nerve root or peripheral nerve (**Table 6-1**). Because

no muscle is entirely innervated by one nerve root, the clinician, when evaluating spinal conditions, should select a muscle that is mostly innervated by that nerve root, or that will have at least grade 3 strength if that nerve root is intact. Likewise, sensation should be assessed in an area that is always innervated by the nerve root but that is distal enough that overlap from more proximal nerve roots is prevented (**Table 6-2**).

UPPER MOTOR NEURON DISORDERS THAT CAUSE STATIC ENCEPHALOPATHY

Disorders of the central nervous system may be progressive or static. Static encephalopathies frequently cause musculoskeletal disorders that can be improved, although not cured, by appropriate intervention. The clinical manifestations of a static encephalopathy vary according to the extent and site of the upper motor neuron lesion. Spasticity is common and is due to injury of the upper motor neurons in the extrapyramidal tract. Subsequent disruption of upper motor neuron inhibitory pathways results in variable degrees of increased muscle tone and increased deep tendon reflexes when the muscle is put on stretch (spasticity). Clonus, clasp-knife reflexes, and Babinski and Hoffmann signs are other manifestations of extrapyramidal dysfunction. Lesions in the pyramidal motor system cause dysfunction of the corticospinal tracts and result in hypotonia and palsy (muscle weakness). Lesions in the cerebellum affect balance and proprioception.

Cerebral palsy (CP) is a static encephalopathy caused by a lesion in the immature brain that results in abnormal posture and movement. The lesion commonly develops before birth or during the early neonatal period, but it may occur during delivery or up to 18 months of age (the upper age limit is arbitrary, but 18 months is generally accepted). Cerebral palsy is the most common cause of physical disability among children in developed countries. Risk factors for CP include prematurity, infection, and trauma. Prema-

Figure 6-2: Electrodiagnostic Studies of Nerves

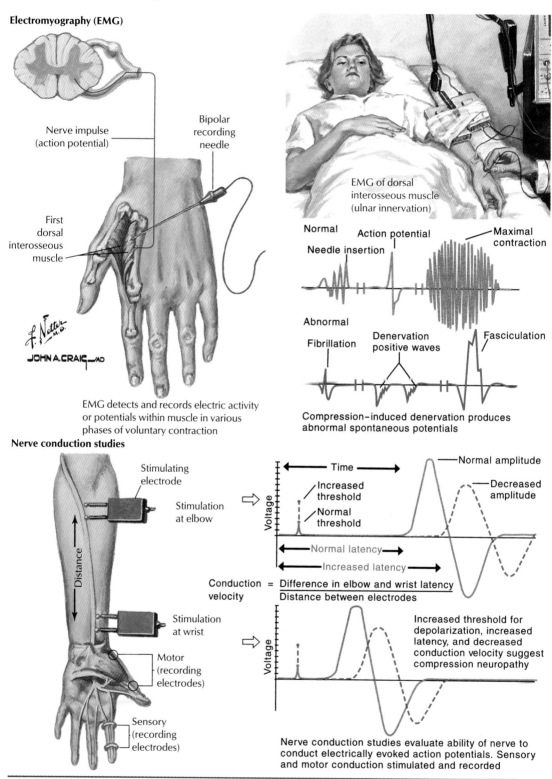

Electromyography (EMG)

Nerve impulse
(action potential)

Bipolar
recording
needle

First
dorsal
interosseous
muscle

EMG of dorsal
interosseous muscle
(ulnar innervation)

Normal — Action potential — Maximal contraction

Needle insertion

Abnormal

Fibrillation — Denervation positive waves — Fasciculation

EMG detects and records electric activity
or potentials within muscle in various
phases of voluntary contraction

Compression–induced denervation produces
abnormal spontaneous potentials

Nerve conduction studies

Stimulating
electrode

Stimulation
at elbow

Distance

Stimulation
at wrist

Motor
(recording
electrodes)

Sensory
(recording
electrodes)

Time — Normal amplitude

Increased threshold

Normal threshold

Decreased amplitude

Normal latency

Increased latency

$$\text{Conduction velocity} = \frac{\text{Difference in elbow and wrist latency}}{\text{Distance between electrodes}}$$

Increased threshold for
depolarization, increased
latency, and decreased
conduction velocity suggest
compression neuropathy

Nerve conduction studies evaluate ability of nerve to
conduct electrically evoked action potentials. Sensory
and motor conduction stimulated and recorded

Table 6-1
Evaluation of Peripheral Nerves

Nerve	Muscle	Sensory
Upper Extremity		
Axillary	Deltoid—shoulder abduction	Arm, lateral aspect
Musculocutaneous	Biceps—elbow flexion	Lateral proximal forearm
Median	Flexor pollicis longus—thumb flexion*	Tip of thumb, palmar aspect
	Opponens pollicis—thumb opposition†	Tip of thumb, palmar aspect
Ulnar	First dorsal interosseous—adduction index finger (palpate in thumb web space)	Tip of little finger, palmar aspect
Radial	Extensor pollicis longus—thumb extension	Dorsum, proximal phalanx thumb
Lower Extremity		
Femoral	Quadriceps—knee extension	Proximal to medial malleolus
Obturator	Adductors—hip adduction	Medial aspect, midthigh
Peroneal		
Deep branch	Extensor hallucis longus—great toe	Dorsum, first web space
Superficial branch	Peroneus brevis—foot eversion	Dorsum, lateral forefoot
Tibial	Flexor hallucis longus—great toe flexion	Forefoot, plantar aspect forefoot

*If injury at or proximal to proximal forearm.
†If injury distal to proximal forearm.

ture, low birth weight infants are susceptible to intraventricular hemorrhage that may cause anoxia and necrosis of upper motor neurons. Infection and trauma causing anoxia and upper motor neuron necrosis may be prenatal or postnatal events.

Encephalopathy is static in CP, and musculoskeletal abnormalities are rarely present at birth; however, musculoskeletal deformities frequently develop in patients with CP because growth, combined with underlying muscle imbalance, causes muscle contractures and concomitant bony deformities, joint subluxations and dislocations, and scoliosis. As in other static encephalopathies, the CP cannot be cured, but the secondary effects may be minimized by therapy programs that prevent or delay progression of muscle contractures, by medications or operations that alter muscle tone, and by operations that correct fixed contractures or bony abnormalities.

Static encephalopathies may be classified on an anatomic or neurophysiologic basis (**Table 6-3**). Patients with CP typically are described with both systems (eg, spastic hemiplegic). Spasticity is the most common movement disorder; 85% of persons with CP have spasticity or a mixed spastic-dyskinetic disorder. Children with CP with spastic hemiplegia walk independently, most with spastic diplegia walk to some degree but may require crutches or a walker, and those with quadriplegia uncommonly achieve functional walking status (**Figure 6-3**). Deficits in balance and proprioception often occur in persons with CP or other upper motor neuron diseases; these deficits may complicate and limit the

Table 6-2
Evaluation of Nerve Root Function

Level	Motor Function	Sensation
C3	Facial, some neck muscles	
C4	Diaphragm, some neck muscles	
C5	Deltoid (shoulder abduction) Biceps, brachialis (elbow flexion)	Lateral aspect of arm Lateral aspect of proximal forearm
C6	Radial wrist extensors, brachioradialis	Palmar tip of thumb
C7	Finger extensors, triceps (elbow extension), wrist flexion, forearm pronation	Palmar tip of long finger
C8	Finger flexion flexor digitorum profundis IV	Palmar tip of little finger
T1	Hand intrinsic , 1st dorsal interosseus	Medial aspect of arm
T4	T4 intercostal and paraspinal muscles	Nipple area
T10	T10 intercostal, paraspinal, and abdominal muscles	Umbilicus
L1	Weak hip flexion	Anterior, proximal thigh
L2	Hip adductors and flexors	Anterior, middle thigh
L3	Quadriceps (knee extension)	Inferior aspect of patella
L4	Anterior tibialis (ankle dorsiflexion) and medial hamstrings	Medial leg, proximal to medial malleolus
L5	Extensor hallucis longus (great toe extension) and hip abductors, lateral hamstrings, peroneals, other toe extensors	Dorsum first web space
S1	Flexor hallucis longus (great toe flexion) and hip extensors, other ankle plantar flexors	Lateral border of the foot

results of treatment. Seizures, learning defects, and mental retardation are also associated with CP.

Stroke is the third leading cause of death in the United States and the leading cause of hemiplegia in adults. Cerebral thrombosis is the cause of nearly three fourths of cerebrovascular accidents, and arteriosclerosis is a significant predisposing factor. Intracerebral or subarachnoid bleeding causes about one sixth of all cerebrovascular accidents, and hypertension is often a cofactor. Cerebral emboli cause less than 10% of strokes (**Figure 6-4**).

The leading cause of acquired mental retardation and spasticity of the limbs in young adults is traumatic brain injury (TBI). Young men between the ages of 15 and 25 years account for most of the patient population, and TBI is the cause of death in more than half of polytrauma patients. When caused by a direct blow, TBI results in local disruption of cerebral tissues, which may be further damaged by a subdural or epidural hematoma. Anoxic injuries usually damage the brain in a global fashion, resulting in spastic quadriplegia and severe loss of function. A near-drowning accident is the most common cause of anoxic brain injury in young children. Chemical asphyxia, drug overdose, and myocardial infarction may cause cerebral anoxia and static encephalopathies in young and older adults.

Table 6-3	
Classification of Cerebral Palsy	

Anatomic Pattern

Hemiplegic: affects ipsilateral upper and lower extremities

Diplegic: primarily affects both lower extremities, but upper extremities often show mild spasticity and loss of coordination

Quadriplegic: affects all four limbs, as well as the trunk muscles. Swallowing, speech, and vision may be affected

Neurophysiologic Pattern

Spasticity: involves increased excitability of muscle to stretch, which results from loss of inhibitory effect of spinal proprioceptive reflexes

Dyskinesia: abnormal movement patterns that can be subdivided into athetosis, ataxia, and dystonia

Figure 6-3: Cerebral Palsy

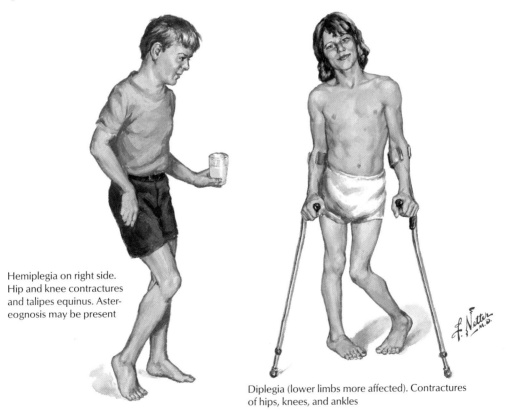

Hemiplegia on right side. Hip and knee contractures and talipes equinus. Astereognosis may be present

Diplegia (lower limbs more affected). Contractures of hips, knees, and ankles

Figure 6-4: Passive Range-of-Motion Exercises After Stroke

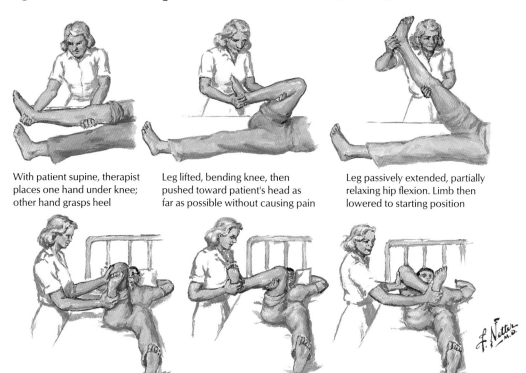

With patient supine, therapist places one hand under knee; other hand grasps heel

Leg lifted, bending knee, then pushed toward patient's head as far as possible without causing pain

Leg passively extended, partially relaxing hip flexion. Limb then lowered to starting position

Hip flexion rotation exercises with patient supine. Hip and knee passively flexed, then limb rotated laterally and medially as pain permits

Patients with stroke or TBI also may develop contractures from spastic muscles that adversely affect walking or upper extremity function. Because growth in these persons is usually complete, they are less likely to develop bony deformities or dislocations. Treatment principles are similar to those used in CP.

DISORDERS OF THE SPINAL CORD

Myelomeningocele is an embryologic defect of the dorsal vertebral elements and spinal cord typified by failure of fusion between the vertebral arches and dysplasia of the spinal cord and its enveloping membranes. The cause of myelomeningocele remains unclear but probably is multifactorial To prevent meningitis, the lesion should be closed immediately and associated hydrocephalus controlled by ventriculoperitoneal shunting procedures (**Figure 6-5**).

Myelodysplasia typically causes complete paralysis distal to the site of the lesion, and patients are typically classified by their neurologic status into thoracic (no L1 to S4 function), upper lumbar (intact to L1 or L2), midlumbar (intact to L3 or L4), or lumbosacral level (intact to L5 or S1). A comprehensive team approach is optimal because patients frequently have multisystem pathology that involves developmental delay, bowel and bladder dysfunction, and progressive joint contractures and bony deformities.

Friedreich ataxia, or *hereditary spinocerebellar ataxia*, is a progressive, degenerative disorder of the spinocerebellar tracts, the corticospinal tracts, and the posterior column. It is the most common early-onset inherited ataxia and results from autosomal recessive transmission of a mutation in gene *X25* that is encoding frataxin. An expanded GAA

Figure 6-5: Myelodysplasia

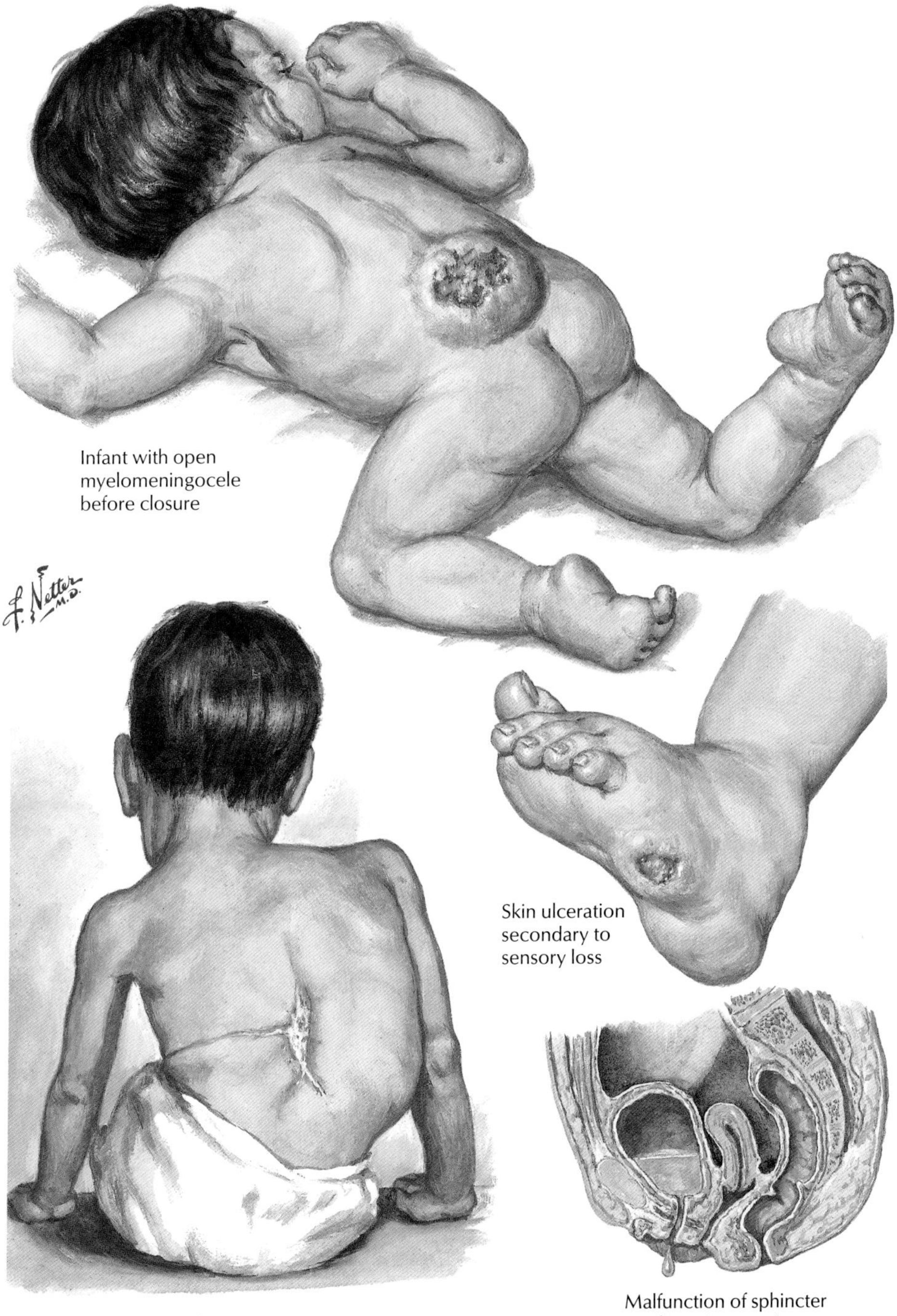

Infant with open
myelomeningocele
before closure

Skin ulceration
secondary to
sensory loss

Progressive scoliosis common
in myelomeningocele

Malfunction of sphincter
predisposing to urinary
tract infection is common
complication

trinucleotide repeat that occurs in the first intron of both alleles accounts for 95% of the mutations and causes reduced or complete absence of frataxin.

Onset of symptoms occurs before 20 years of age, and patients typically present for medical evaluation at between 7 and 15 years because of ataxia and an unsteady gait. Examination shows absent deep tendon reflexes and a positive Babinski sign. Position sense, vibration sense, and two-point discrimination demonstrate progressive deterioration; however, touch, pain, and temperature sensitivity are preserved. Anterior horn cells usually are uninvolved, but weakness may result from involvement of the pyramidal tracts. Progressive dysarthria characterized by slow, jerky speech with sudden utterances appears shortly after onset. In the second decade, most patients lose the ability to walk and sit without support. Diabetes mellitus and seizures may develop. Hypertrophic cardiomyopathy and conduction disturbances may cause death in the third or fourth decade.

Typical musculoskeletal abnormalities include symmetric cavus deformity of the feet, with marked elevation of the arch, equinus posturing of the forefoot, and clawing of the toes. Scoliosis is common and, when onset of curvature is before 10 years of age, it usually progresses to require surgical stabilization.

Traumatic spinal cord injury results in paralysis of different groups of muscles, depending on the level of injury (see **Table 6-2**). Patients are categorized by the level of preserved sensation and voluntary functioning muscles rather than by the location of the spinal fracture. For example, a C6 tetraplegic patient typically has deltoid, biceps, brachialis, radial wrist extensor, and brachioradialis function. The C6 level of function is the most proximal level of spinal cord injury that is compatible with independence. Patients often require assistance with transfers, but they can use a manual wheelchair, can operate a motor vehicle equipped with hand controls, and, with appropriate splints and tendon transfers, can hold a fork, pen, and cup.

DISORDERS OF THE LOWER MOTOR NEURONS

Poliomyelitis is an acute viral disease that has special affinity for the lower motor neurons of the spinal cord and certain motor nuclei of the brain. Most patients have a subclinical infection characterized by nonspecific febrile illness. Approximately 5% to 10% develop flaccid paralysis, with the severity dependent on the number of infected cells. The acute phase of the disease lasts from 5 to 10 days. The convalescent phase may be as long as 16 months, during which some degree of muscle strength returns through recovery of anterior horn cells that were damaged, but not destroyed, by the viral infection. The chronic phase of the disease is marked by residual muscle weakness and resultant contractures and deformities. Fortunately, development of effective vaccinations in the mid-1950s largely eliminated wild virus infection, and worldwide eradication of poliomyelitis should occur during the coming decade.

Treatment of poliomyelitis during the acute phase is supportive and may require ventilatory assistance if respiratory paralysis has occurred. During the convalescent phase, physical therapy and braces are used to aid rehabilitation and minimize development of contractures. In the chronic phase, operations such as tendon transfer, osteotomy, and arthrodesis may prove helpful in improving limb alignment and function.

Postpoliomyelitis syndrome, which may develop 30 to 40 years after disease onset, is characterized by fatigue, weakness, and aching pain that is variable in location and involves previously affected sites. Evidence supports the concept that this syndrome is an acceleration of the normal aging process. A limited number of muscle fibers have been "overworked" for many years and may degenerate at an early age. In these patients, loss of relatively few fibers may significantly affect function and may stress other supporting structures. Treatment includes evaluation for other disorders, patient education, judicious use of medications, and the performance of selective reconstructive procedures. Although they lack specific names, other neuromuscular disorders may cause similar problems during the middle adult years. Treatment principles are the same.

Spinal muscular atrophy of childhood (SMA) is the most common hereditary motor neuronopathy, with an incidence of 1 in 6000 to 10,000 live births. This autosomal recessive disorder is caused by mutations in the survival motor neuron 1 gene. Resultant degeneration of anterior horn cells causes symmetric, and often severe, muscle weakness and atrophy that is greater in the proximal muscle groups. Sensation is intact, and findings of motor conduction studies are normal.

Although clinical heterogeneity is observed, classification of patients with SMA is helpful. Patients with SMA type I, sometimes called *Werdnig-Hoffmann disease*, have severe weakness at birth and do not attain the ability to sit. Most patients with SMA type I die from respiratory failure during the first 2 years of life. Patients with SMA type II achieve the ability to sit unaided but never stand. In SMA type III, sometimes called *Kugelberg-Welander disease*, the child achieves the ability to walk unassisted. In type IIIa, muscle weakness begins before age 3 years, and in type IIIb, the onset of symptoms occurs after age 3 years. The ability to continue to walk 40 years after diagnosis is approximately 20% in type IIIa and 60% in type IIIb disease.

Scoliosis develops in virtually all persons with type II and type IIIa SMA, and in approximately half of patients with type IIIb SMA. The scoliosis pattern is typically a long, C-shaped, thoracolumbar curvature that extends to the pelvis. Appropriate treatment includes early stabilization with a fusion that extends from the upper thoracic spine to the pelvis. Lower extremity problems include flexion, abduction, and external rotation contractures at the hips; flexion contractures at the knees; and equinus contractures at the ankles.

Arthrogryposis multiplex congenita is characterized by contractures of multiple joints present at birth. Some patients have a chromosomal or central nervous system disorder, but in most cases, the etiology is uncertain. In these patients, the condition is not hereditary and the arthrogryposis may result from a viral infection causing variable necrosis of anterior horn cells during early fetal development. The resultant fetal akinesia, combined with muscle weakness and imbalance during a time of rapid embryologic growth, causes the severe contractures that are present at birth. These patients have normal sensation and normal intelligence. Treatment includes bracing and appropriate surgeries to position the extremities in a more functional position. Despite severe physical involvement, these patients develop unique ways of manipulating their environment and function surprisingly well (**Figure 6-6**).

DISORDERS OF PERIPHERAL NERVES: HEREDITARY SENSORY MOTOR NEUROPATHIES

The hereditary sensory motor neuropathies (HSMNs) are a heterogenous group of inherited neuropathies that disrupt myelination and Schwann cell function in a variety of complex and still poorly understood ways. *Charcot-Marie-Tooth* (CMT) disease is the former and still often used name for HSMNs. The incidence is approximately 1 in 2500 people. HSMNs have a broad range of disease expression, sometimes even within the same family. Common features include symmetric weakness that is greater in the distal portion of the extremity, weakness that is greater in the lower extremities than in the upper extremities, and stocking/glove sensory deficits that affect all modalities; however, patients are usually less symptomatic from the sensory loss.

To date, at least eight different proteins and significantly more abnormal gene mutations have been found in the HSMNs. As a result, classification of HSMNs is in a state of transition. Present systems are based on nerve conduction velocity and inheritance patterns, but genetic heterogeneity causes overlap and classification difficulties in some patients. A simple classification of CMT is useful for most patients (**Table 6-4**).

Figure 6-6: Arthrogryposis Multiplex Congenita

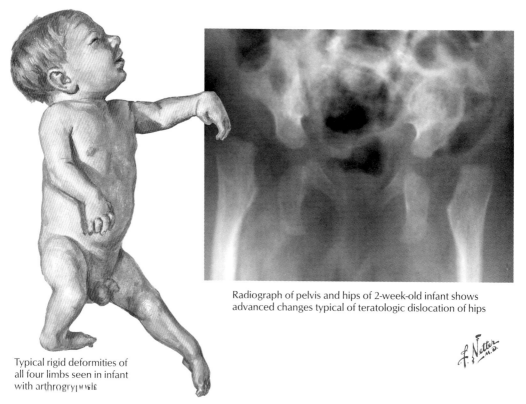

Radiograph of pelvis and hips of 2-week-old infant shows advanced changes typical of teratologic dislocation of hips

Typical rigid deformities of all four limbs seen in infant with arthrogryposis

CMT 1A is the most common HSMN disorder and 70% to 80% of CMT 1A cases are secondary to duplication of a 1.5-megabase DNA fragment on chromosome 17 that results in three copies of peripheral myelin protein 22 (PMP22). Resultant excess of PMP22 disrupts Schwann cell function and the myelination process. CMT 1A patients typically experience symptoms in the second decade, and age at onset of symptoms correlates with eventual severity. Most often, patients present with difficulty walking and frequent tripping, particularly on uneven ground. Some patients describe difficulty wearing shoes, foot pain, or calf cramps. Typical findings include symmetric muscle weakness, particularly in the intrinsic muscles of the foot and the peroneal muscles of the calf. The foot shows clawing of the toes, cavus of the midfoot, and varus of the heel. Calf atrophy is usually noted (**Figure 6-7**).

Examination reveals distal muscle weakness, decreased deep tendon reflexes, and sensory changes, with impairment of light touch, proprioception, and vibration, and relative preservation of pain and temperature sensation. The family history is often positive, and nerve conduction velocities are slowed.

Atrophy of the intrinsic hand muscles begins at a later stage with mild clawing of the fingers. The patient loses fine motor skills. The shoulder and pelvic girdle musculature usually are not involved, and trunk and face muscles are usually spared. Ataxia is not present, and intelligence is not affected.

Early treatment consists of therapy and bracing or shoe modifications to alleviate and minimize progression of flexible deformities. The goal in surgical management of fixed deformities of the foot and ankle is to use tendon transfers and realignment osteotomies that will correct the deformities and provide

Table 6-4		
Classification of Charcot–Marie–Tooth Disease*		
Type	**Incidence**	**Characteristics**
CMT 1	Approximately 50%	Mostly autosomal dominant, slow NCV
CMT 2	20% to 40%	Mostly autosomal dominant, normal or near-normal NCV
CMT 4	Rare	Autosomal recessive, very low NCV, severe disability
CMT X	10% to 20%	X-linked, defect in connexin 32

*CMT, Charcot-Marie-Tooth disease; NCV, nerve conduction velocity.

cellular matrix. These lesions may occur at any site at which cranial, spinal, or peripheral nerves are present. *Cutaneous neurofibromas* are slightly raised lesions that have a soft and somewhat gelatinous consistency (**Figure 6-8**). *Plexiform neurofibromas* are characterized by diffuse hypertrophy of the involved nerves but with preservation of the fascicular organization of the nerves. Dermal lesions feel like a "bag of worms" and may cause disfigurement and hyperpigmentation of the overlying skin. Deeper plexiform neurofibromas may cause diffuse hypertrophy of the soft tissue and bone, with resultant leg-length discrepancy or macrodactyly, or even gigantism of the entire extremity. Enlargement of a plexiform neurofibroma may cause neurologic dysfunction with motor and sensory abnormalities. Malignant peripheral nerve sheath tumors (MPNSTs) result

Figure 6-7: Charcot-Marie-Tooth Disease Type 1A

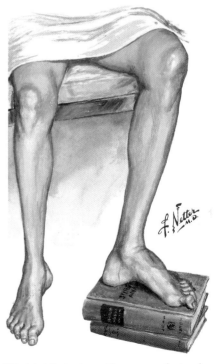

Thin (storklike) calves with cavovarus foot and claw toes with primary weakness of peroneal and intrinsic foot muscles

improved walking function. If possible, triple arthrodesis of the hindfoot is avoided because severe ankle arthritis often develops, with further loss of proprioception.

NEUROFIBROMATOSIS

Neurofibromatosis type 1 (NF1), with an incidence of 1 in 4000 people, is the most common single gene disorder to affect the nervous system. The molecular basis of this autosomal dominant disorder is a mutation in the *NF1* gene and subsequent abnormal production of neurofibromin. The function of neurofibromin is not well understood, but it has a role in the regulation of ras proteins that are critical for cell proliferation; the *NF1* gene also affects tumor suppression. Clinical manifestations of NF1 are protean and progress with age; their severity varies greatly, even within families (**Table 6-5**).

Neurofibromas are benign tumors composed of fibroblasts, axons, Schwann-like cells, perineural cells, mast cells, and extra-

Table 6-5
Classification of Neurofibromatosis

Manifestation	Approximate Percentage
Major Disease Features	
>6 café au lait spots	95
Axillary freckling	80
Cutaneous neurofibroma	90
Lisch nodules	95
Minor Disease Features	
Plexiform neurofibroma	20-40
Malignant peripheral nerve sheath tumors	2-4
Learning disabilities	30-65
Hypertension Adults: essential Children: renal artery stenosis	Common
Short stature	Mean is 5%-10% normal
Malignant neoplasms	2-3 times normal
Scoliosis	20-25
Pseudarthrosis, long bones	2-4

from malignant degeneration of a plexiform neurofibroma.

Medical management of NF1 requires an understanding of the numerous associated potential problems. Scoliosis is the most common musculoskeletal disorder associated with NF1. Dystrophic curves are common and may be difficult to stabilize. In addition to MPNSTs, other malignant neoplasms are two to three times more common in NF1; their incidence increases with age.

NERVE ENTRAPMENT SYNDROMES

Nerve entrapment is compression of a peripheral nerve at a specific anatomic location.

Most entrapment neuropathies occur at locations at which the nerve normally passes through a relatively confined space (**Figure 6-9**). Additive pathomechanical factors include adjacent inflammation, anatomic anomalies, tumors, scar formation, and arthritic or degenerative changes. Degree of magnitude and duration of pressure are important factors, but intraneural transport and microvascular changes can occur at relatively low pressure levels (<30 mm Hg). Pathologic findings at the site of compression include demyelination, remyelination, and loss of large myelinated fibers (**Figure 6-10**). With advanced disease, the nerve develops a "wasp band" appearance caused by thinning of the nerve beneath the area of compression and proximal enlargement from venous congestion and edema.

Typical symptoms include pain and paresthesia in the anatomic distribution of the peripheral nerve. Weakness of distally innervated muscles also may be noted. Examination shows motor and sensory deficits distal to the area of compression. Muscle atrophy may be present. A positive Tinel sign (percussion on the affected nerve causing distal tingling and paresthesia) is often present. Diagnostic maneuvers that accentuate nerve compression may be helpful. Entrapment of a nerve at two separate anatomic sites—the double crush syndrome—may cause overlap of symptoms and diagnostic problems.

Carpal tunnel syndrome is compression of the median nerve at the wrist and is the most common nerve entrapment (**Figure 6-11** and Chapter 16). Presenting symptoms usually include paresthesias, especially at night; aching of the wrist with prolonged positioning of the wrist in marked flexion or extension; and clumsiness of the hand. Examination usually reveals diminished sensation in the radial three and a half digits and a positive Tinel sign over the median nerve at the wrist. The Phalen test, performed through maximal flexion of the wrist for 60 seconds, is typically positive, with reproduction of the paresthesias. Electrodiagnostic studies may

Figure 6-8: Neurofibromatosis

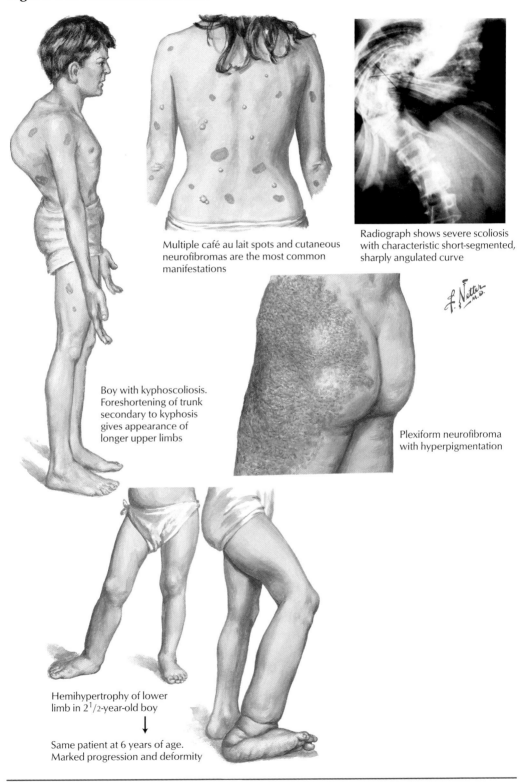

Multiple café au lait spots and cutaneous neurofibromas are the most common manifestations

Radiograph shows severe scoliosis with characteristic short-segmented, sharply angulated curve

Boy with kyphoscoliosis. Foreshortening of trunk secondary to kyphosis gives appearance of longer upper limbs

Plexiform neurofibroma with hyperpigmentation

Hemihypertrophy of lower limb in 2^1/$_2$-year-old boy

Same patient at 6 years of age. Marked progression and deformity

Figure 6-9: Predisposing Factors to Compression Neuropathy

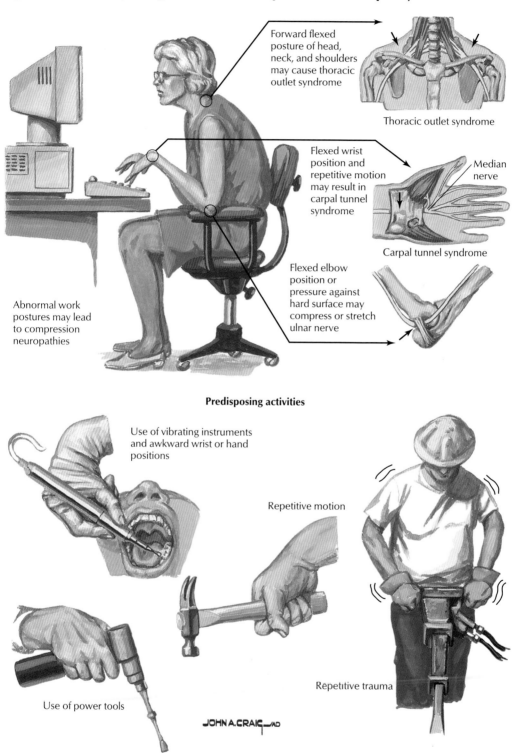

Forward flexed posture of head, neck, and shoulders may cause thoracic outlet syndrome

Thoracic outlet syndrome

Flexed wrist position and repetitive motion may result in carpal tunnel syndrome

Median nerve

Carpal tunnel syndrome

Flexed elbow position or pressure against hard surface may compress or stretch ulnar nerve

Abnormal work postures may lead to compression neuropathies

Predisposing activities

Use of vibrating instruments and awkward wrist or hand positions

Repetitive motion

Use of power tools

Repetitive trauma

JOHN A. CRAIG—AD

Figure 6-10: Nerve Injury in Compression Neuropathy

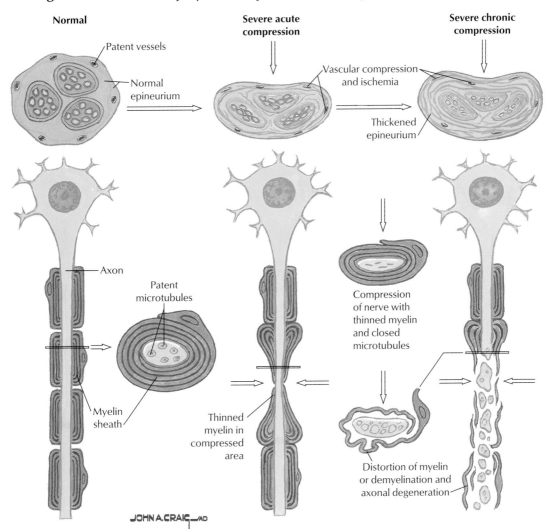

be helpful in confirming the diagnosis but are sometimes false negative.

Nonoperative treatment usually begins with splinting or a local steroid injection. In patients who do not respond to these simple measures, surgical release is usually an effective treatment modality. The median nerve is sometimes entrapped in the elbow region by the pronator teres muscle, or under the lacertus fibrosus.

The ulnar nerve may become entrapped within the cubital tunnel at the elbow and also at the ulnar tunnel (Guyon canal) at the wrist. Findings include paresthesias, especially at night; loss of sensation in the ulnar one and a half digits; diminished intrinsic strength; and associated difficulty with activities such as turning a key in a door. A positive Tinel sign and provocative maneuvers may differentiate the site of compression. A positive Phalen test suggests entrapment at the ulnar tunnel. A positive "bend test," performed by hyperflexion of the elbow and compression of the ulnar nerve in the cubital tunnel, indicates

Figure 6-11: Common Sites of Upper Extremity Nerve Entrapment

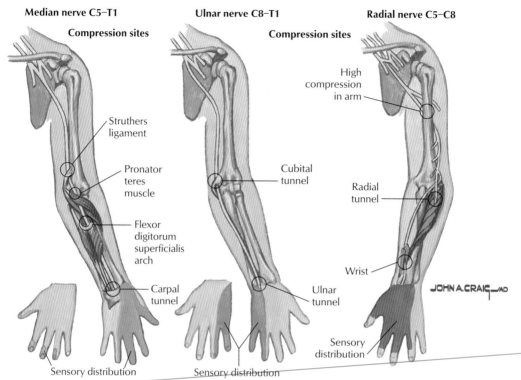

Median nerve C5–T1

Compression sites

Struthers ligament

Pronator teres muscle

Flexor digitorum superficialis arch

Carpal tunnel

Sensory distribution

Ulnar nerve C8–T1

Compression sites

Cubital tunnel

Ulnar tunnel

Sensory distribution

Radial nerve C5–C8

High compression in arm

Radial tunnel

Wrist

Sensory distribution

JOHN A.CRAIG_AD

Motor and sensory functions of each nerve assessed individually throughout entire upper extremity to delineate level of compression or entrapment

entrapment at the elbow. For significant symptoms, surgical treatment at the wrist would involve decompression of the ulnar tunnel. Anterior transposition of the ulnar nerve at the elbow is a common surgical option for entrapment of the ulnar nerve within the cubital tunnel.

Radial tunnel syndrome involves compression of the posterior interosseous branch of the radial nerve as it passes through the substance of the supinator muscle just distal to the elbow. Because the posterior interosseous nerve is purely motor, this condition causes no sensory disturbance but affects motor function of the thumb and finger extensors and the extensor carpi ulnaris. However, symptoms and signs of motor weakness are often vague in the early phases of the condition. Furthermore, radial tunnel syndrome sometimes masquerades as

a resistant lateral epicondylitis. Electrodiagnostic studies are seldom useful. Diagnosis is made on the basis of history and physical examination that typically shows tenderness at the two heads of the supinator muscle (about 5 cm distal to the lateral epicondyle). Surgical decompression with release of the impinging fibrous bands of the supinator muscle is usually helpful.

Thoracic outlet syndrome (TOS) involves compression of the brachial plexus and/or subclavian vessels in the superior thoracic outlet. Causative factors include fibrotic changes in the anterior scalene muscle, a cervical rib, and a long transverse process of C7. Confirmation of the diagnosis can be a challenge for the clinician because symptoms are often vague and inconsistent. Commonly affected is the medial cord (C8 and T1) of the brachial plexus, which supplies the medial brachial, medial antebrachial, and ulnar nerves, with resultant weakness of the hand intrinsics and paresthesias involving the medial aspects of the arm, forearm, and hand. Vascular compression causes pain, coldness, and cyanosis or pallor in the arm and hand. Neurogenic and vascular symptoms are exacerbated by overhead activities. Provocative maneuvers such as the Adson test and costoclavicular tests are variable in usefulness. The elevated arm stress test (EAST) is the simplest and most reliable measure. This test involves abduction and external rotation of the arm to the horizontal level at the shoulder while the fist is opened and closed repeatedly for 1 minute; results are positive if this movement reproduces the patient's symptoms. Most patients can be treated nonoperatively by posture and strengthening exercises.

Meralgia paresthetica is entrapment of the lateral femoral cutaneous nerve by the inguinal ligament as the nerve exits the pelvis medial to the anterior superior iliac spine. This disorder is associated with obesity, intrapelvic disorders, or prolonged compression caused by leaning against workbenches or wearing tight-fitting garments or belts. Characteristic symptoms include paresthesias, hypesthesias, or dysesthesias over the lateral thigh area. Examination reveals decreased sensation in the area of the lateral femoral cutaneous nerve and usually a positive Tinel sign. Appropriate nonoperative methods such as weight reduction or removal of the offending belt can eliminate symptoms and obviate the need for surgical decompression.

Compression of the posterior tibial nerve or its terminal medial and lateral plantar branches at the ankle results in *tarsal tunnel syndrome*. This disorder is sometimes seen in patients with valgus hindfoot deformities, which suggests that postural functions of the foot may be an important factor. Paresthesia and pain radiating from the medial aspect of the heel to the sole of the foot are typical symptoms. A positive Tinel sign just posterior to the medial malleolus is suggestive of tarsal tunnel syndrome. A useful diagnostic test is exacerbation of symptoms by placing the foot in a position of maximum ankle dorsiflexion, heel valgus, and toe extension. Electrodiagnostic studies are sometimes helpful when results are correlated with clinical examination findings. The results of surgical decompression for tarsal tunnel syndrome are unpredictable, and patients with mild symptoms should be observed.

INJURY AND REPAIR OF PERIPHERAL NERVES

Peripheral nerves may be injured by blunt or penetrating trauma or by prolonged compression and ischemia. Classification of injury includes neurapraxia, axonotmesis, and neurotmesis.

Neurapraxia refers to a local and temporary demyelinating block that typically occurs after a compression injury (**Figure 6-12**). The continuity of the axons is not interrupted. Local myelin repair occurs, and recovery is seen within weeks to months after injury. *Axonotmesis* is disruption of axonal continuity with preservation of the endoneural sheath. It occurs with an advanced compression injury or results from blunt trauma or a traction mechanism that interrupts axonal continuity. The timetable for functional recovery corresponds with the schedule required for axons to regenerate and reinnervate distal target organs. Because the endoneural tubes are preserved, the prognosis for reinnervation is favorable but not universal. *Neurotmesis* is disruption of the axon and endoneural tubes. The degree of injury with neurotmesis ranges from an intact perineurium (third degree) to complete loss of nerve continuity (fifth degree). Severe traction injuries and penetrating trauma cause neurotmesis injuries.

Injuries that disrupt the axon cause *Wallerian degeneration*, with the axon and myelin sheath degenerating over the entire distance distal to the injury and over a variable distance proximal to the injury. After a time, the proximal axon develops sprouts of new growth. If the endoneural tubes are preserved (axonotmesis), the prognosis for reinnervation and recovery of function is favorable. The timetable for functional recovery is influenced

Figure 6-12: Sunderland Classification of Nerve Injury

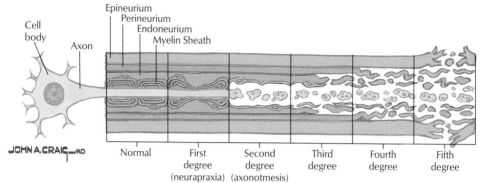

Classification of nerve injury by degree of involvement of various neural layers

by the severity and location of the injury, but once initiated, reinnervation typically progresses at 1 mm per day. The chance of spontaneous recovery is much less with disruption of the endoneural tubes (neurotmesis) because, when regenerating axons reach the area of disruption, the sprouts of new growth commonly grow in a misdirected manner into surrounding tissue. A bulbous neuroma forms at the site of disruption.

Electrodiagnostic studies may be helpful in differentiating among types of nerve injuries. With neurapraxia, conduction blocks occur across the injury, but no fibrillation or denervation changes are noted. Fibrillation potentials, characterized by increased and spontaneous muscular activity on insertion of the EMG needle 2 to 5 weeks after injury, are characteristic of axonotmesis and neurotmesis. Reinnervation potentials, observed primarily with axonotmesis, are typically observed 6 to 8 weeks after injury.

With neurotmesis, surgical repair is necessary to alter the poor prognosis. Repair of peripheral nerves is enhanced by microsurgical technique that emphasizes atraumatic handling of tissues, realignment of individual fascicles, and coaptation of the gaps between nerve stumps. If muscle units are not reinnervated within about 18 months of denervation, the affected muscle will irreversibly atrophy, and recovery will not occur. Sensory end organs will respond to reinnervation years after

a peripheral nerve has been transected and then repaired by late secondary neurorrhaphy or nerve grafting.

CHARCOT ARTHROPATHY

Neuropathic arthropathy, commonly called *Charcot arthropathy*, develops in neurologic conditions that involve altered sensation, particularly loss of light touch and pain. Conditions commonly associated with Charcot arthropathy include syringomyelia, leprosy, myelomeningocele, spinal cord injury, congenital indifference to pain, and peripheral neuropathies secondary to diabetes mellitus or alcoholism. The common feature in patients with Charcot arthropathy is deficient sensation but motor function that permits continued use, and therefore, unperceived overload, of a joint. An injury or even subtle malalignment of the joint is a predisposing factor. With repetitive overload of the joint, the ligaments and capsule become stretched. Ultimately, the synovium becomes impressively inflamed, joint alignment is markedly altered, and severe erosion of cartilage and subchondral bone occurs.

Diabetes mellitus is the most common cause of Charcot arthropathy. It most often affects the foot and ankle joints but may also cause severe knee dysfunction (**Figure 6-13**). Shoulder arthropathy is associated with syringomyelia. Patients present with swelling, altered alignment of the joints, ulceration of

Figure 6-13: Charcot Arthropathy

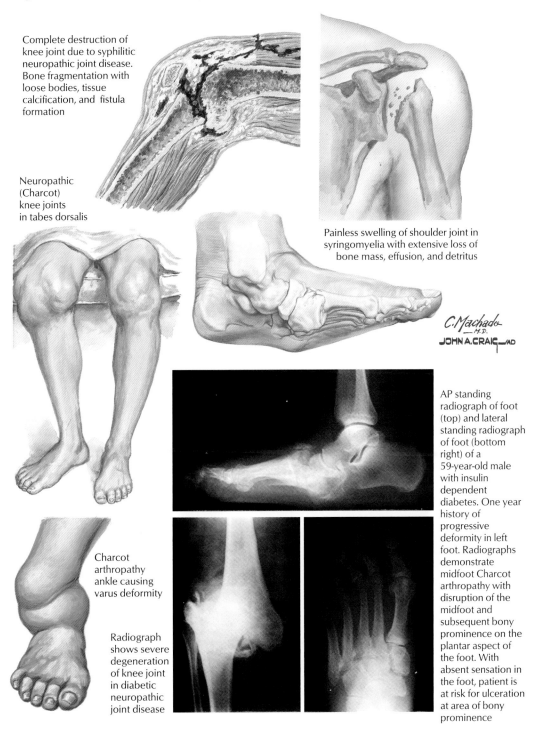

Complete destruction of knee joint due to syphilitic neuropathic joint disease. Bone fragmentation with loose bodies, tissue calcification, and fistula formation

Neuropathic (Charcot) knee joints in tabes dorsalis

Painless swelling of shoulder joint in syringomyelia with extensive loss of bone mass, effusion, and detritus

C.Machado
—M.D.
JOHN A.CRAIG—AD

Charcot arthropathy ankle causing varus deformity

Radiograph shows severe degeneration of knee joint in diabetic neuropathic joint disease

AP standing radiograph of foot (top) and lateral standing radiograph of foot (bottom right) of a 59-year-old male with insulin dependent diabetes. One year history of progressive deformity in left foot. Radiographs demonstrate midfoot Charcot arthropathy with disruption of the midfoot and subsequent bony prominence on the plantar aspect of the foot. With absent sensation in the foot, patient is at risk for ulceration at area of bony prominence

Figure 6-14: Diabetes

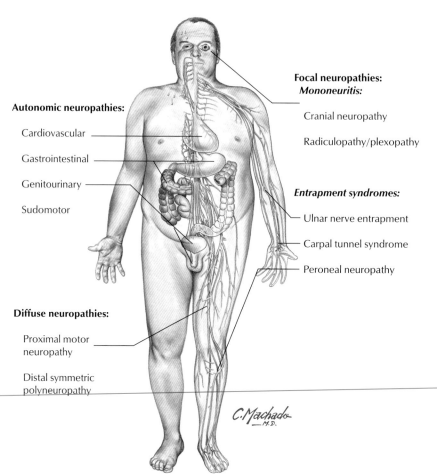

Focal neuropathies:
Mononeuritis:

Cranial neuropathy

Radiculopathy/plexopathy

Autonomic neuropathies:

Cardiovascular

Gastrointestinal

Genitourinary

Sudomotor

Entrapment syndromes:

Ulnar nerve entrapment

Carpal tunnel syndrome

Peroneal neuropathy

Diffuse neuropathies:

Proximal motor
neuropathy

Distal symmetric
polyneuropathy

C. Machado
—M.D.

the feet, and sometimes pain. The pain is not as intense as one would expect, but it is noted with a markedly distended joint when there is some sensation. Radiographs show marked destruction and altered alignment of the joint.

Treatment of Charcot arthropathy includes activity modification and protective measures to permit reduction of synovial inflammation. In the foot, initial treatment often requires a cast, which provides the best support to the ligamentous structures while minimizing continued erosions that stimulate further synovial inflammation. When the swelling decreases, an appropriate orthotic can be prescribed. Operative treatment by arthrodesis, realign-ment osteotomy, or joint replacement has a high rate of complications.

DIABETIC NEUROPATHY

Diabetes mellitus is a metabolic disorder characterized by elevated glucose levels. With increasing obesity, the incidence of diabetes and its associated complications is increasing. In the United States, one out of every seven dollars spent for health care is related to diabetes.

Neuropathy is common in diabetes, with clinical manifestations present in one half of the patients who have had diabetes for more than 25 years and specialized test evidence

Table 6-6
Classification of Diabetic Neuropathy

Focal Neuropathies

Mononeuritis
   Cranial neuropathy
   Plexus radiculopathy

Entrapment syndromes
   Carpal tunnel syndrome
   Ulnar nerve entrapment at the elbow
   Peroneal nerve entrapment at the fibular head

Diffuse Neuropathies

Proximal motor neuropathy

Distal symmetric polyneuropathy

Autonomic

Cardiovascular

Gastrointestinal

Genitourinary

Sudomotor

immune system function. The neuropathy can cause loss of motor, sensory, and autonomic function with resultant pain syndromes (mononeuritis and focal entrapment syndromes), weakness, cardiovascular dysfunction, gastrointestinal complaints, erectile dysfunction, and foot ulceration (see Chapter 11 and **Figure 6-14**).

The foot is the extremity region most often affected by diabetic neuropathy. Loss of sensation is the major factor leading to ulceration, infection, and amputation. Other contributing factors are autonomic dysfunction that causes dry and crackling skin, vascular insufficiency, and motor weakness. Motor insufficiency primarily affects the intrinsic muscles, with subsequent development of claw toes and increased pressure on the forefoot by the abnormal plantar position of the metatarsal heads.

ADDITIONAL READINGS

Gelberman RH, ed. *Operative Nerve Repair and Reconstruction*. Philadelphia, Pa: JB Lippincott; 1991.

Green DP, Hotchkiss RN, Pederson WC, Scott WW, eds. *Green's Operative Hand Surgery*, 5th edition. New York, NY: Churchill Livingstone; 2005.

Greene WB. Neurofibromatosis type I. In: Fitzgerald RH, Kaufer H, Malkani AL, eds. *Orthopaedics*. Philadelphia, Pa: Mosby; 2002:1584–1588.

Trumble TE, McCallister WV. Nerve physiology and repairs. In: Fitzgerald RH, Kaufer H, Malkani AL, eds. *Orthopaedics*. Philadelphia, Pa: Mosby; 2002:1929–1936.

of nerve dysfunction in many others. The pathogenesis of diabetic neuropathy is mutifactorial and includes alterations in metabolic, vascular, growth factors, and

seven

Osteomyelitis and Septic Arthritis

Walter B. Greene, MD

Although a delay in diagnosis does not cause harm in many musculoskeletal conditions, that is not the case in bone and joint infections. Indeed, even a 24- to 48-hour delay in instituting the proper treatment for bone and joint infections may significantly increase the risk of prolonged or permanent disability. Furthermore, musculoskeletal infections have unique features. In particular, the pattern of skeletal blood flow during childhood markedly influences the incidence and type of infection.

Osteomyelitis is an infectious process that involves bone and its medullary cavity. Septic arthritis is an infection in a joint. Bacteria are the usual causes of osteomyelitis and septic arthritis. Fungal infections in bones and joints are uncommon and typically occur in patients with compromised immune status (eg, neonates and patients with immune deficiencies). Primary viral infections have not been observed in the musculoskeletal system.

Infecting organisms may enter bones or joints in the following ways: (1) by hematogenous spread; (2) through external inoculation from a penetrating wound, such as an open fracture, or after certain operations; or (3) by extension from an adjacent structure that is infected (**Figures 7-1** and **7-2**). The route of entry is an important factor in the patient's presentation and treatment.

HEMATOGENOUS OSTEOMYELITIS
Causes and Pathogenesis

Bacteremia occurs daily from such simple acts as brushing our teeth. The load of bacteria present in the circulating blood may be significantly increased through another source of infection, such as impetigo, otitis media, pharyngitis, or pneumonia. Fortunately, bacteria in the bloodstream usually are destroyed by reticuloendothelial tissue in organs such as the lung, liver, and spleen; if these defense mechanisms fail, however, bacteria may gain access to bone. In experimental studies, previous trauma enhances the likelihood of hematogenous osteomyelitis, but the importance of a preceding traumatic event is less clear in the clinical setting.

Hematogenous osteomyelitis is much more common in children. The growth plate (physis) is a barrier to the terminal branches of the metaphyseal arteries. Therefore, vascular flow must make a U-turn at the physis. The resultant sluggish circulation, in combination with transient bacteremia, creates a setup for bacteria to gain a foothold in the metaphysis (**Figure 7-3**).

Osteomyelitis that starts in the metaphysis spreads in two directions: (1) down the

Figure 7-1: Direct Causes of Osteomyelitis

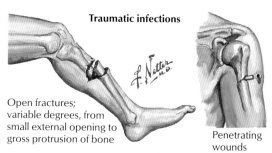

Traumatic infections

Open fractures; variable degrees, from small external opening to gross protrusion of bone

Penetrating wounds

Operative infections

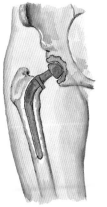
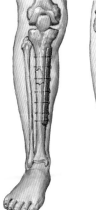
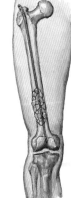

Total joint replacement (loosening of prosthesis usually occurs but does not necessarily indicate infection)

Internal fixation of fractures

Tumor resection with bone graft for limb salvage

Figure 7-2: Direct Causes of Osteomyelitis (continued)

Secondary to contiguous focus of infection

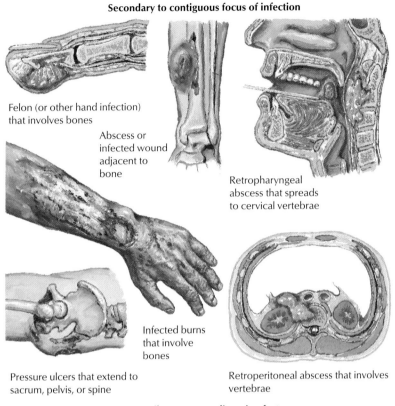

Felon (or other hand infection) that involves bones

Abscess or infected wound adjacent to bone

Retropharyngeal abscess that spreads to cervical vertebrae

Infected burns that involve bones

Pressure ulcers that extend to sacrum, pelvis, or spine

Retroperitoneal abscess that involves vertebrae

Contributory or predisposing factors

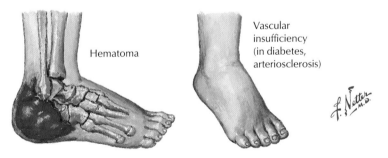

Hematoma

Vascular insufficiency (in diabetes, arteriosclerosis)

medullary cavity, and (2) through the relatively thin metaphyseal cortex (**Figure 7-4**). Fortunately, the cartilaginous growth plate is a barrier, and the physis and adjacent epiphysis are typically spared. When the infectious process penetrates the metaphyseal cortex, pus elevates the loosely adherent periosteum, and a *subperiosteal abscess* may form. The periosteum, however, remains viable and attempts to limit the spread of infection by laying down new bone—a process that is visible on radiographs after 7 to 14 days.

Periosteal new bone formation typically is observed only in the metaphysis; however, with a delay in diagnosis and a relatively virulent organism, the periosteum of the entire shaft may become elevated. The resultant new bone formation encircling the cortical shaft forms an *involucrum*. Likewise, with delay in diagnosis, blood flow may be compromised to the extent that segments of bone become necrotic. An isolated segment of dead bone surrounded by pus or scar tissue is called a *sequestrum*. In certain locations, insertion of the joint capsule occurs below (distal to) the physis (see **Figures 7-4** and **7-5**). At these sites, pus perforating the metaphyseal cortex causes *concomitant septic arthritis* (see the discussion later in the chapter). This situation most commonly occurs with the spread of osteomyelitis from the proximal femur into the hip joint, but it also may occur at the proximal humerus, distal lateral tibia, and proximal radius.

A striking inflammatory response is initiated in response to bacterial antigens and toxins. Hoards of neutrophils and lymphocytes migrate to the metaphysis (**Figure 7-6**). While battling the infection, these cells release interleukins and other cytokines. These enzymes, coupled with thrombosis of terminal vessels, may cause dramatic necrosis and osteolysis. In experimental studies, necrosis of osteocytes and resorption of bony trabeculae are observed as early as 12 to 24 hours after the induction of osteomyelitis. However, radiographic demonstration of osteolysis (seen as mottled areas of radiolucency) is not apparent until 10 to 14 days after disease onset; indeed, osteolysis may never be apparent on routine radiographs if the infection is promptly diagnosed and appropriately treated.

Acute Hematogenous Osteomyelitis

Osteomyelitis may be classified as acute, subacute, or chronic. *Acute hematogenous osteomyelitis* is an infection that is diagnosed within 2 weeks of the onset of symptoms. It is more common in males (2:1 ratio), is most often monostotic (>90%), and usually involves the lower extremity (90%). Parents of children with this condition commonly report that their children walk with a limp, or that they refuse to walk.

Although differentiation is not always clear, it is helpful for the clinician to classify acute hematogenous osteomyelitis as either early acute or late acute. The typical patient with *early acute osteomyelitis* seeks medical care within 24 to 48 hours' of symptom development. Characteristic signs and symptoms include febrile illness of 24 to 48 hours' duration, malaise, avoidance of use of the extremity, and localized tenderness and swelling. Even with a virulent bacterium, an infection of only 24 to 48 hours' duration will most likely be confined to the medullary cavity and will involve limited thrombosis of terminal vessels and necrosis of bone. In essence, early acute osteomyelitis can be likened to a *cellulitis of bone*, and most patients readily respond to antibiotic therapy.

Late acute hematogenous osteomyelitis typically occurs in children who present for medical care 4 to 5 days after the onset of symptoms. Patients typically have a subperiosteal abscess and many require surgical drainage, in addition to antibiotic therapy. Because the history may be vague and bacterial strains differ, it is not possible for the clinician to determine optimal treatment solely from the duration of symptoms.

Figure 7-3

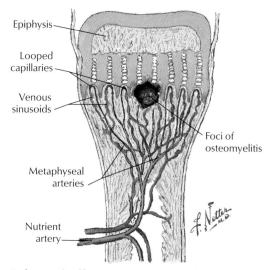

Epiphysis

Looped capillaries

Venous sinusoids

Foci of osteomyelitis

Metaphyseal arteries

Nutrient artery

Pathogenesis of hematogenous osteomyelitis.
Terminal branches of metaphyseal arteries form loops at growth plate and enter irregular afferent venous sinusoids. Blood flow slowed and turbulent, predisposing to bacterial seeding. In addition, lining cells have little or no phagocytic activity. Area is catch basin for bacteria, and foci of osteomyelitis may form.

Figure 7-4: Spread of Hematogenous Osteomyelitis

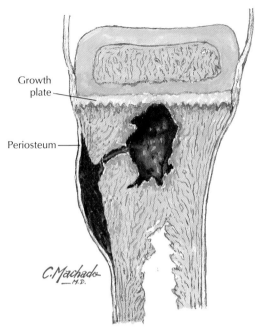

Growth plate

Periosteum

C. Machado —M.D.

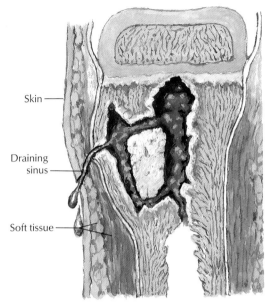

Skin

Draining sinus

Soft tissue

Abscess, limited by growth plate, spreads transversely along Volkmann canals and elevates periosteum; extends subperiosteally and may invade shaft. In infants under 1 year of age, some metaphyseal arterial branches pass through growth plate, and infection may invade epiphysis and joint.

Infectious process may erode periosteum and form sinus through soft tissues and skin to drain externally. Process influenced by virulence of organism, resistance of host, administration of antibiotics, and fibrotic and sclerotic responses.

Figure 7-5

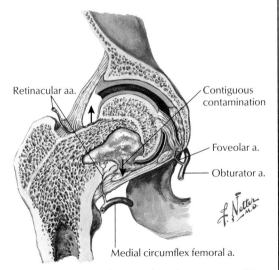

Retinacular aa.

Contiguous contamination

Foveolar a.

Obturator a.

f. Netter m.d.

Medial circumflex femoral a.

Septic arthritis secondary to concomitant osteomyelitis
Primary routes of contamination of joint space

Figure 7-6

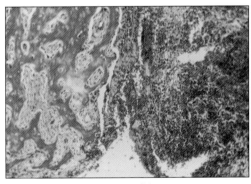

Acute hematogenous osteomyelitis

Right slide of slide demonstrates inflammatory response with proliferative neutrophils and lymphocytes. Left side of slide demonstrates "new" woven bone formation.

Late acute osteomyelitis is more likely to occur in three groups of children: neonates, older children, and premature infants. The delay in diagnosing this condition in neonates and infants occurs because of their inability to verbalize symptoms and because they are not walking (and therefore not limping). In children older than 9 years, the diagnosis may be delayed because children at this age have good coordination and minimal limping during the early stage of the infectious process. Predisposing factors in premature infants include an immature immune system and the frequent need for long-term intravenous catheters. In these patients, the appearance of a mass from a large subperiosteal abscess that has spread into the adjacent soft tissues may be the initial diagnostic clue. *Multifocal osteomyelitis* is more common in premature infants.

Physical findings vary according to the location, duration, and severity of infection (**Figure 7-7**). Osteomyelitis in locations that are relatively superficial (eg, the distal femur and proximal tibia) is likely to cause obvious swelling and localized tenderness. In deeper locations, such as the proximal femur and proximal humerus, physical findings are limited to restriction of hip or shoulder motion, but the motion is not as severely limited as that observed in septic arthritis. A temperature of 38°C to 39°C is typical in late acute osteomyelitis, but the temperature may be only slightly elevated in patients with early acute osteomyelitis.

Evaluation and Treatment of Acute Osteomyelitis

Routine laboratory studies include a complete blood cell count (CBC), erythrocyte sedimentation rate (ESR) and/or C-reactive protein (CRP), anteroposterior and lateral radiographs of the affected area, blood culture, and aspiration of the affected area. The white blood cell count is most often elevated in late acute osteomyelitis but may be within normal limits. ESR and CRP levels are usually elevated but may be normal in early acute osteomyelitis. Initial radiographs are usually normal but may demonstrate contiguous soft tissue swelling. Ten to 14 days after the onset of symptoms, periosteal elevation and irregular radiolucent patches surrounded by a faint rim of reactive bone formation in the metaphysis are often apparent (**Figure 7-8**). Blood culture and bone aspiration should be performed. Blood cultures identify the causative organism approximately 50% of the time in late acute hematogenous osteomyelitis. Aspiration of the bone or a subperiosteal abscess, in combination with blood culture, identifies the causative organism 70% of the time.

Special imaging studies may be useful when the diagnosis is unclear and when the results would alter treatment. A technetium Tc 99m

Figure 7-7: Clinical Manifestations of Hematogenous Osteomyelitis

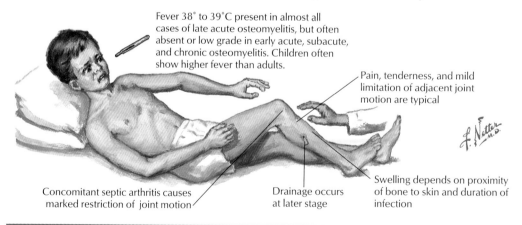

Fever 38° to 39°C present in almost all cases of late acute osteomyelitis, but often absent or low grade in early acute, subacute, and chronic osteomyelitis. Children often show higher fever than adults.

Pain, tenderness, and mild limitation of adjacent joint motion are typical

Concomitant septic arthritis causes marked restriction of joint motion

Drainage occurs at later stage

Swelling depends on proximity of bone to skin and duration of infection

Figure 7-8: Radiographic Changes in Healing Phase of Late Acute Hematogenous Osteomyelitis

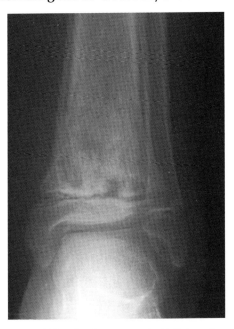

9-year-old female who presented with 7 days of increasing pain in the ankle region. Patient treated by drainage of soft tissue abscess (see Figure 7-10) and 6 weeks of intravenous antibiotics. AP radiograph 6 weeks after initiation of treatment shows radiolucent changes in the tibial metaphysis from the bone resorption as well as areas of sclerosis from new bone forming on existing trabeculae. Bone formation is also noted beneath the periosteum that was elevated by the infectious process breaking through the metaphysis.

ation, antibiotics should be promptly started after routine laboratory study results are obtained, even if aspiration does not yield purulent material. With response to treatment and subsequent radiographic evidence of metaphyseal lytic patches, the diagnosis is secured. A bone scan, however, is useful when the diagnosis is unclear, as frequently occurs with osteomyelitis in atypical locations, such as the clavicle, pelvis, or fibula (**Figure 7-9**). Magnetic resonance imaging (MRI) is the most specific and sensitive study for demonstrating osteomyelitis (**Figure 7-10**). Because of its cost and the frequent need for general anesthesia in children, MRI should be reserved for diagnostic purposes in unusual cases. Ultrasonography may be a good method for defining the size and location of a subperiosteal abscess. Whether ultrasonography should be used routinely in acute hematogenous osteomyelitis is unclear at present.

The differential diagnosis includes cellulitis, septic arthritis, fracture, neoplasm, and bone infarction. *Cellulitis* may restrict movement and

Figure 7-9: Bone Scan in Acute Osteomyelitis

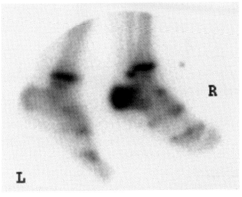

Bone scan showing increased uptake in right calcaneus. 11-year-old male with 3 day history of pain in the region of the right ankle and 1 day history of limping. Ankle held in plantarflexion and heel in varus but there was no obvious swelling. Plain radiographs were normal. MRI was not diagnostic but four phase technetium bone scan markedly positive and consistent with osteomyelitis of the calcaneus. Patient was treated with 6 days of intravenous antibiotics and additional 5 weeks of oral antibiotics.

bone scan is a very sensitive and specific test for acute osteomyelitis; however, the test is not infallible. In most cases of acute hematogenous osteomyelitis, a bone scan is not needed because results of this study would not alter treatment. For example, a 2-year-old who presents with a temperature of 38°C, refusal to walk, tenderness in the distal thigh, and no other obvious condition (such as a tumor or fracture) is considered to have osteomyelitis until proven otherwise. In this situ-

Figure 7-10: MRI Early and Late Acute Osteomyelitis

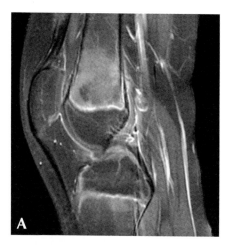

(A) Lateral T2 weighted MRI of distal femur with early acute osteomyelitis. 10-year-old female with progressive pain left knee region and difficulty walking. Plain radiographs normal. MRI showed signal changes distal femur metaphyseal region consistent with osteomyelitis.

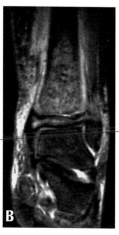
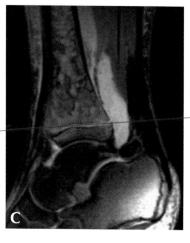

AP (B) and lateral (C) of T2 weighted MRI of the distal tibia with late acute osteomyelitis. Note the inflammatory changes in the distal tibia metaphysis, the signal changes beneath the elevated periosteum, and the large posterior abscess from pus breaking through the periosteum.

cause limping; however, in most cases, swelling and marked erythema of the skin differentiate cellulitis from osteomyelitis. *Septic arthritis* causes swelling and severely restricts joint motion. The swelling is obvious in superficial locations, but in locations such as the hip, aspiration of the joint may be required to differentiate osteomyelitis from septic arthritis. A history of an injury followed by acute pain usually indicates a *fracture*. However, in patients with insensate extremities (caused by myelomeningocele, for example), fractures may cause a clinical picture that simulates osteomyelitis. *Leukemia* proliferates in the hematopoietic marrow and may cause children to exhibit pain, limping, lethargy, and even fever. In acute leukemia, ra-

diographs also may demonstrate osteopenia and radiolucent lesions. The diagnosis of leukemia is suggested by gradual onset of symptoms, and by additional symptoms such as easy bruising, night pain, pain at multiple sites, and a low leukocyte count. Likewise, *Ewing sarcoma* may cause periosteal elevation or radiolucent lesions. A biopsy provides an accurate diagnosis.

Treatment and Complications of Acute Osteomyelitis

Intravenous antibiotics should be started promptly in acute osteomyelitis. The initial selection of antibiotics is empiric and varies with the patient's age. In a child younger than 1 year, *Staphylococcus aureus* is the most common infecting agent, but group B streptococci and enteric organisms such as *Escherichia coli* are common enough that these organisms also should be covered by treatment pending a positive culture. For children at least 4 years of age, initial antibiotic coverage is restricted to *S aureus* because this organism accounts for more than 90% of cases of osteomyelitis in this particular age group. For a child between the ages of 1 and 4 years who has received immunization for *Haemophilus influenzae,* antibiotic coverage may be restricted to *S aureus.* The emergence of community-acquired, methicillin-resistant *S aureus* (MRSA) has caused increasing concern in the initial antibiotic coverage of acute osteomyelitis in children. At present, MRSA is more prevalent in soft tissue infections and current recommendations for antibiotic coverage in acute hematogenous osteomyelitis in children are for an antibiotic that covers methicillin-sensitive *S aureus.*

Hematogenous osteomyelitis in adults is more likely to occur in the vertebrae and/or in immunocompromised patients. The causative agent in these situations is likely to be Gram-negative organisms, so initial antibiotic coverage should include agents effective against both *S aureus* and Gram-negative organisms.

Surgical intervention usually is not needed for early acute osteomyelitis. Surgical drainage should be done on an urgent basis in children with late acute osteomyelitis and an obvious subperiosteal abscess. Children who have no definitive evidence of a significant subperiosteal abscess may be treated with intravenous antibiotics for 24 to 48 hours. If persistent fever and swelling occur, the bone should be examined and any subperiosteal abscess drained.

Complications that may occur during treatment include recurrent osteomyelitis, distant seeding, concomitant septic arthritis, pathologic fracture, and growth arrest. To minimize the risk of *recurrent osteomyelitis,* antibiotics are typically continued for 6 weeks. *Distant seeding,* the hematogenous spread of the bone infection to another location, is a complication that is more likely to occur in late acute osteomyelitis but is fortunately uncommon. Children with *concomitant osteomyelitis* and *septic arthritis* typically present with symptoms and signs more consistent with septic arthritis. The diagnosis of osteomyelitis is typically made when lytic areas are subsequently seen in the proximal femur.

Pathologic fractures occur because osteomyelitis causes osteonecrosis, bone resorption, and subsequent new bone formation. Fractures typically occur during the early phase of bone formation. At this time, the child is feeling better and is more mobile because infectious symptoms have for the most part resolved. However, at this time, the bone is relatively weak and is susceptible to fracture, unless it is appropriately protected.

Damage to the growth plate with subsequent early closure is surprisingly uncommon, considering its proximity to the physis. If the physeal bar is central, growth is symmetrically tethered, and a leg-length discrepancy develops. If the physeal bar has a peripheral location, asymmetric growth and an angular deformity develop.

Subacute Hematogenous Osteomyelitis

Subacute hematogenous osteomyelitis occurs secondary to infection by a less virulent organism coupled with a more effective response of the immune system. By definition, patients with subacute hematogenous osteomyelitis seek medical care after at least 2 weeks of symptoms, but generally, their symptoms have begun at least 1 month earlier. Children who develop subacute osteomyelitis are typically older, ranging in age from 2 to16 years. The sex ratio is equivalent in subacute osteomyelitis. The onset of symptoms is indolent, with neither the parents nor the child being able to pinpoint the exact date. Systemic signs such as fever are mild or absent. Physical examination findings often are within normal limits, or they may demonstrate mild localized tenderness and swelling.

The white blood cell count is usually normal. The erythrocyte sedimentation rate may be elevated or normal.

Histologically, subacute osteomyelitis is characterized by a large amount of granulation tissue, chronic inflammatory cells, and new bone formation. Subacute osteomyelitis is observed as a cavitary or neoplastic-like lesion. *Cavitary lesions* usually occur in the metaphysis and/or epiphysis. Radiographs show a radiolucent area surrounded by a thin rim of reactive bone formation. *Neoplastic-like subacute osteomyelitis* is most often seen in the diaphysis of long bones or in atypical locations such as the clavicle (**Figure 7-11**). Radiographs show periosteal elevation and new bone formation.

In subacute osteomyelitis, the incidence of positive culture is only 30%, even with bone biopsy, and it is now recognized that most children with cavitary subacute osteomyelitis may be empirically treated with a 6-week trial of oral antibiotic therapy effective against *S aureus*. If the cavitary lesion does not respond to treatment, operative débridement and curettage should be done. A biopsy is required in neoplastic-like subacute osteomyelitis. Pending culture and biopsy results of an aggressive-appearing lesion, antibiotic therapy should include a drug that is effective against *S aureus*. If cultures show no growth, then oral antibiotics should be continued for 6 weeks.

Chronic Hematogenous Osteomyelitis

Patients with chronic hematogenous osteomyelitis typically have had symptoms for several weeks to several months. Sequestra often are present. A sinus tract to the skin may occur. This tract decompresses purulent drainage from the osteomyelitis but also is a portal for secondary seeding of the bone.

In less developed countries, chronic hematogenous osteomyelitis in children is relatively common and typically follows a delay in treatment. In industrialized countries, the condition is uncommon in children and most often occurs in adults, either secondary to open fracture or by direct extension from foot ulcer in patients with diabetes mellitus (**Figure 7-12**). Typical radiographic findings include areas of radiolucency that indicate bone destruction and radiodense sequestra surrounded by a radiolucent area of fibrous tissue.

Chronic osteomyelitis has a variable presentation. Patients typically note increasing pain and swelling. Purulent drainage from the sinus tract is often contaminated by skin surface organisms; therefore, biopsy of the bone is often necessary if reliable culture material is to be obtained.

The treatment of chronic osteomyelitis requires aggressive débridement of all necrotic bone and marginally vascularized tissue, such as the fibrous scar tissue surrounding a sinus tract or sequestrum. After excision of all infected tissue, the wound may be closed with the use of a local muscle flap or free tissue transfer (**Figure 7-13**). These procedures decrease recurrence by minimizing the risk of secondary contamination with another organism and improving the local, on-site delivery of antibiotics and immune cells. In patients who have chronic osteomyelitis at sites not amenable to the use of a local muscle flap, or who have peripheral vascular disease that precludes free tissue transfer, surgical débridement may be followed by the application of wet-to-dry or vacuum-assistance dressings until granulation tissue covers the exposed surfaces. If a significant bony defect remains after surgical debridement, then cancellous bone graft material is packed into the wound. With coverage of the wound by granulation tissue, skin coverage may occur by secondary epithelialization or by placement of a split-thickness skin graft.

Initial antibiotic coverage pending culture results in chronic osteomyelitis varies according to the clinical situation. If the osteomyelitis occurs secondary to a previous operation and placement of an implant, MRSA should be covered. In patients with diabetes mellitus and open fracture, Gram-negative bacteria are common; thus, these organisms, as well as MRSA, should be covered pending culture results. Intravenous antibiotic therapy is often continued for 6 to 12 weeks.

Figure 7-11: Subacute Osteomyelitis

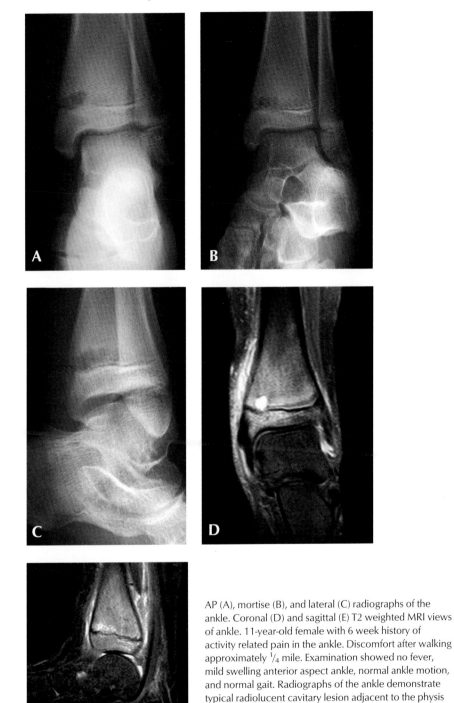

AP (A), mortise (B), and lateral (C) radiographs of the ankle. Coronal (D) and sagittal (E) T2 weighted MRI views of ankle. 11-year-old female with 6 week history of activity related pain in the ankle. Discomfort after walking approximately $1/4$ mile. Examination showed no fever, mild swelling anterior aspect ankle, normal ankle motion, and normal gait. Radiographs of the ankle demonstrate typical radiolucent cavitary lesion adjacent to the physis in the posteriomedial aspect of the metaphysis. Coronal and sagittal T2 MRI views demonstrate inflammatory response in the metaphysis and subperiosteal tissue.

Figure 7-11: Subacute Osteomyelitis (continued)

Cavitary subacute osteomyelits is progressing to septic arthritis. AP radiographs of distal femur at presentation (F) and at completion of 6 weeks of treatment (G). 12-month-old female with 1 month history of progressive discomfort right knee and refusal to stand. Two days prior to evaluation developed mild swelling of the knee. Exam showed knee motion from 10° to 80° of flexion. The WBC was 8600 and the erythrocyte sedimentation rate was 50 mm/hr. Under general anesthesia, 10 ml. of purulent fluid was aspirated from the knee. Metaphyseal cavity aspirated but no fluid obtained. Patient treated with 3 days of intravenous and 6 weeks of oral antibiotics. AP radiograph at presentation shows radiolucent metaphyseal cavitary lesion. AP radiograph at completion of treatment shows new bone formation and the cyst to be resolving.

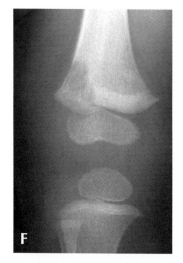 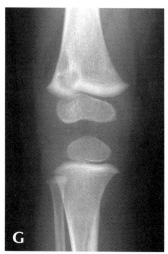

AP radiograph of clavicle demonstrating subacute osteomyelitis imitating neoplastic process (H). 11-year-old female with progressive discomfort and swelling over right clavicle. Radiograph demonstrates sclerosis and expansion of clavicle consistent with

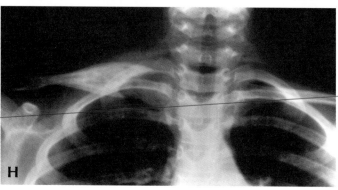

neoplastic process. Biopsy demonstrated chronic inflammatory process and no evidence of neoplastic cells. Culture was negative. Patient responded well to 6 week course of oral antibiotics.

SEPTIC ARTHRITIS
Causes and Pathogenesis

Septic arthritis, or infection of a joint, can occur at any age but, like osteomyelitis, is more common among children younger than 5 years. Septic arthritis in adults is likely to involve joints with preexistent degenerative changes. The incidence is increased in the elderly and other population groups that have decreased function of the immune system. The explanation for the high incidence in young children is unclear but is probably related to the combination of a developing immune system, frequent falls (experimental studies confirm the association of septic arthritis with preexistent trauma), and the proclivity of certain organisms to infect joints. These organisms include *S aureus*, the most common cause of septic arthritis at all ages, and *H influenzae* type B, which accounted for 30% of septic arthritis in children younger than 5 years before the development of effective vaccinations.

Septic arthritis involves a single joint in more than 95% of cases. Bacteria may enter a joint by hematogenous means, by direct inoculation (eg, lacerations, puncture wounds, surgery), or by extension from

Figure 7-12: Lesions in Diabetic Foot

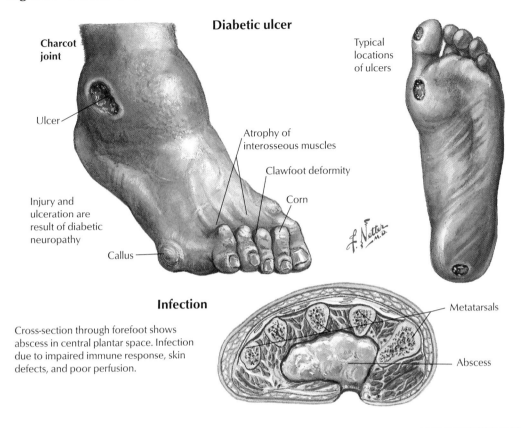

Diabetic ulcer

Charcot joint

Typical locations of ulcers

Ulcer

Atrophy of interosseous muscles

Clawfoot deformity

Corn

Injury and ulceration are result of diabetic neuropathy

Callus

Infection

Metatarsals

Cross-section through forefoot shows abscess in central plantar space. Infection due to impaired immune response, skin defects, and poor perfusion.

Abscess

Figure 7-13: Chronic Osteomyelitis

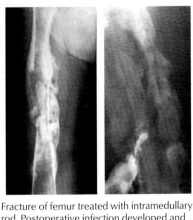

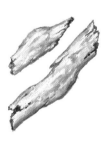

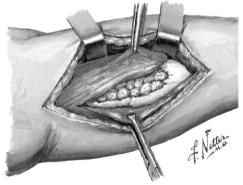

Fracture of femur treated with intramedullary rod. Postoperative infection developed and rod was removed. Persistent drainage and sinus tract developed. Radiograph at left shows sequestra and radiolucent lesions consistent with chronic osteomyelitis. Sinogram at right reveals sinus tract extending to site of fracture.

Sequestra surgically removed, sinus tract excised, and all dead and infected tissue thoroughly debrided.

Bone defect packed with cancellous bone autograft from ilium overlaid with muscle flap from vastus lateralis muscle. Patient remained free of pain and drainage.

adjacent tissue (eg, osteomyelitis, septic bursitis). The most common site of hematogenous septic arthritis is the knee (41% of cases), followed by the hip (23%), ankle (14%), elbow (12%), wrist (4%), and shoulder (4%). Other joints of the hands and feet, as well as the sacroiliac and acromioclavicular joints, account for a small percentage of septic arthritis cases.

Bacterial proliferation in the joint produces hyperemia and a marked inflammatory response. In septic arthritis, articular cartilage may be rapidly eroded by the large quantity of various destructive enzymes released by inflammatory cells and bacterial toxins (**Figure 7-14**). In experimental studies, breakdown of glycosaminoglycans can be demonstrated as early as 8 hours after initiation of the infectious process.

Clinical Features and Diagnostic Approach

Typical symptoms of septic arthritis include acute onset of swelling and pain in the affected joint accompanied by malaise and fever (temperature of 38°C–39°C). Children with the condition frequently limp, stop walking, or refuse to move the upper extremity (pseudoparalysis). Patients hold the affected joint in a comfortable position that accommodates maximum distention, and attempts to move the joint cause intense pain and guarding. Typical postures of involved joints include the hip held in flexion, abduction, and external rotation; the knee in 20° to 40° flexion; the ankle in 10° to 20° equinus; and the elbow in 40° to 60° flexion (**Figure 7-15**). The differential diagnosis of septic arthritis is outlined in **Table 7-1**.

Routine studies include CBC, ESR, anteroposterior and lateral radiographs of the affected joint, blood culture, and, most important, joint aspiration (**Figure 7-16**). Plain radiographs are used primarily to rule out other conditions, but they may show soft tissue swelling and, with delayed diagnosis in a young child, subluxation or dislocation of the joint. The CBC may be normal. The ESR is frequently elevated but is an unreliable guide in neonates, persons with sickle cell anemia, and patients who have early-onset disease. Synovial fluid should be analyzed for its appearance, Gram stain, cell count, and glucose level, and it should be cultured. Synovial fluid is turbid in septic arthritis and ranges in color from cloudy yellow to creamy white pus. The

Figure 7-14: Septic Arthritis

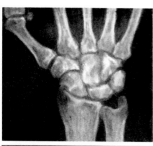
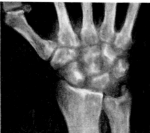
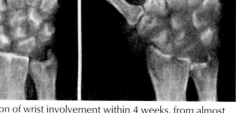

Rapid progression of wrist involvement within 4 weeks, from almost normal (left) to advanced destruction of articular cartilages and severe osteoporosis (right)

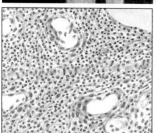

Biopsy specimen of synovial membrane shows infiltration with polymorphonuclear cells, lymphocytes, and mononuclear cells, and tissue proliferation with neovascularization

Figure 7-15

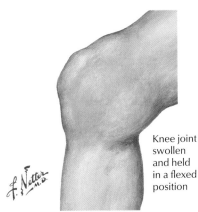

Knee joint swollen and held in a flexed position

white blood cell count in the synovial fluid is higher than 50,000/mm^3 and commonly ranges from 100,000 to 200,000/mm^3. Glucose levels are decreased, and the mucin clot is thin. In septic arthritis caused by *Neisseria gonorrhoeae*, the synovial fluid is less turbid, and its white blood cell count is typically lower (mean, approximately 45,000/mm^3; range 20,000 to 100,000 mm^3).

The likelihood that a positive culture will be obtained in septic arthritis (blood plus joint aspirate) is approximately 70%. The yield is lower for infection caused by *N gonorrhoeae*. To improve the positive culture rate, it is important that the aspirate be transported immediately to the laboratory for appropriate plating. Injecting part of the sample into blood culture tubes may increase the likelihood of a positive identification. Chocolate agar plating optimizes the possibility that a gonococcal infection will be identified. Gram stain provides

Table 7-1
Differential Diagnosis of Septic Arthritis

Condition	Differential Diagnosis From Septic Arthritis
Appendicitis	Possible psoas muscle irritation that may result in flexion of the right hip, abdominal tenderness
Bursitis	No joint effusion, swelling in the area of affected bursa
Cellulitis	No joint effusion, marked erythema of skin
Gout	Intense pain, great toe common involvement, crystals seen on joint aspiration
Hemarthrosis	History of trauma, bloody fluid on aspiration
Juvenile rheumatoid arthritis	Gradual onset of symptoms, morning stiffness, better joint motion
Lyme disease	Indolent onset, boggy synovium
Osteomyelitis	No joint effusion, better range of motion
Rheumatic fever	Less effusion, arthralgia
Reactive arthritis	Less pain and effusion, joint fluid white blood cell count 10,000 to 20,000/mm^3
Transient synovitis	Hip involvement only, no systemic symptoms, better range of motion, may require aspiration to differentiate septic arthritis

Figure 7-16: Septic Joint Aspiration

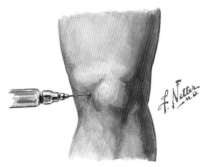

Sample of joint fluid aspirated for culture

useful information in 30% of cases and may help in diagnosis when the cultures are negative, particularly if Gram-negative intracellular diplococci are observed.

Treatment

To prevent erosion of the cartilage and early arthritis, prompt treatment with intravenous antibiotics must be instituted as soon as the joint has been aspirated and a provisional diagnosis has been made. Guidelines for antibiotic use in children with septic arthritis are similar to the suggestions given for treatment of osteomyelitis. In the adolescent or young adult with septic arthritis, initial therapy should include antibiotics that treat *N gonorrhoeae* and *S aureus*.

Surgical irrigation and drainage are uncommonly needed for gonococcal arthritis, but this therapy should be strongly considered for other cases, unless the septic arthritis is of limited duration. Septic arthritis of the hip is routinely decompressed because pus in this joint may occlude circulation to the femoral head, resulting in osteonecrosis (**Figure 7-17**).

Repeated aspiration is another technique for managing septic arthritis, but this method is not as effective and can be difficult for the patient because the aspirations are repeated daily for several days. Daily aspirations are used primarily in elderly patients who have less severe joint effusion and whose medical condition makes general or spinal anesthesia problematic.

Another treatment involves open arthrotomy through a small incision. The joint can be débrided and thoroughly irrigated and a drain left in place to maintain decompression. Arthroscopic debridement and irrigation also can be effective.

The treatment of neonates with septic arthritis of the hip may be complicated. Frequent delay in diagnosis, coupled with a normally shallow acetabulum, makes this age group susceptible to dislocation and osteonecrosis. In addition to undergoing prompt surgical decompression, patients should be splinted so that the risk of chronic instability is minimized.

SPECIAL CONDITIONS
Diskitis

Diskitis in children, sometimes called *benign diskitis* because the condition may resolve without intervention, typically occurs in the lumbar or lower thoracic spine. This condition is now understood to be a bacterial infection that begins as osteomyelitis in the anterior corner of a vertebral body. Infection spreads to the disc via the terminal vessels. Because of its limited circulation and regenerative capacity, disc narrowing is the most common radiographic finding. However, MRI consistently shows extensive inflammatory changes at the anterior corner of one or both adjacent vertebrae.

The typical age of children with diskitis (2 to 6 years), coupled with the insidious onset of symptoms, commonly leads to a delay in diagnosis. The problem may be perceived as back pain or abdominal or lower limb discomfort. The child may refuse to walk or may splint the spine (decreased lumbar lordosis) and walk by leaning forward. Percussion of the spine elicits tenderness. Anteroposterior and lateral radiographs of the spine eventually demonstrate irregularity and narrowing of the disc, but these findings may not be apparent upon initial presentation. The CBC is often normal, but the ESR and CRP are usually elevated. Leukemia should be included in the differential diagnosis. If radiographs are normal, an MRI can best confirm the diagnosis. Blood

Figure 7-17: Osteonecrosis and Hip Arthropathy Following Septic Arthritis

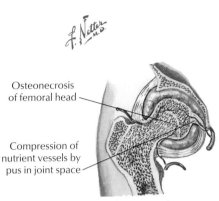

Osteonecrosis of femoral head

Compression of nutrient vessels by pus in joint space

Septic joint requiring decompression. Some joints, such as hip, require prompt surgical decompression to avoid damage to vascular supply

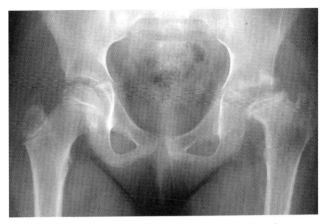

Radiograph of pelvis showing subluxation, osteonecrosis, and subsequent incongruity of the left femoral head. Patient developed septic arthritis of the hip 9 months prior to radiograph but had inadequate early treatment. Underwent arthrotomy and drainage of the hip and institution of adequate antibiotic therapy 6 weeks after onset of symptoms.

cultures should be obtained as well. Aspiration of the disc is usually not done because of the low yield and greater potential morbidity noted in patients of this age.

Children with diskitis are treated for 6 weeks with oral antibiotics that cover *S aureus.* Casting or prolonged bed rest usually is not necessary.

Vertebral Osteomyelitis

In older children and adults, osteomyelitis of the spine has a similar pathophysiology and presentation. Hematogenous seeding occurs at the termination of the vertebral body arterial circulation (bony end plates, particularly the anterior superior and inferior corners). Risk factors include immunodeficiency conditions, surgical procedures that involve the genitourinary or gastrointestinal system, and intravenous drug abuse.

Similar to diskitis in young children, vertebral osteomyelitis is characterized by the following: typical location in lower thoracic or lumbar vertebrae; indolent onset of symptoms that initially may suggest an abdominal, genitourinary, or chest problem; and frequent delay in diagnosis. Back pain, low-grade fever,

malaise, and even weight loss are common symptoms. Pain may remain unrelieved by bed rest and may occur at night.

Examination reveals localized tenderness to percussion and limited spine motion. Neurologic deficits are uncommon. The white blood cell count (WBC) is often normal, but the ESR and CRP are elevated in most patients. Blood cultures should be obtained but are positive in less than 30% of cases. Plain radiographs may be normal at the patient's initial visit but eventually will show lytic changes in the anterior metaphyseal region and narrowing of the disc space. MRI is the best imaging modality for confirming the diagnosis. Computed tomography (CT) or fluoroscopically assisted needle aspiration of the vertebral body and/or disc should be performed to identify the causative organism, because in this population, the positive culture rate is high, and aspiration may be performed with intravenous sedation.

Treatment includes intravenous antibiotics for 6 weeks, possibly followed by supplemental oral antibiotics. Bracing may reduce pain while the infection and osteolysis are resolving. Most patients can be managed nonoper-

Figure 7-18: Tuberculous Arthritis

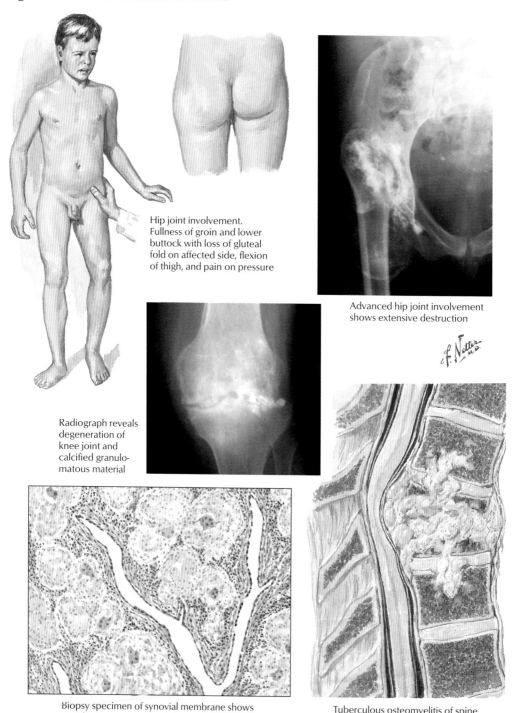

Hip joint involvement. Fullness of groin and lower buttock with loss of gluteal fold on affected side, flexion of thigh, and pain on pressure

Advanced hip joint involvement shows extensive destruction

Radiograph reveals degeneration of knee joint and calcified granulomatous material

Biopsy specimen of synovial membrane shows conglomerate caseating tubercles

Tuberculous osteomyelitis of spine (Pott disease) with angulation and compression of spinal cord

atively, but surgical treatment is required under the following circumstances: progressive vertebral collapse and kyphosis, development of a significant paraspinal or epidural abscess, significant or progressive neurologic deficits, and persistent pain with resultant instability.

Tuberculosis

Tuberculosis is uncommon in the United States but endemic in many Third World countries. Musculoskeletal manifestations of tuberculosis include dactylitis (painful swelling of the hands, feet, or both), septic arthritis, and osteomyelitis (**Figure 7-18**). Bone and joint infections secondary to tuberculosis have a more indolent onset than do their bacterial counterparts.

The most common site of skeletal involvement in tuberculosis is the spine. Similar to vertebral osteomyelitis, tuberculosis of the spine (Pott disease) is more common in the thoracolumbar spine and typically begins in an anterior corner of the vertebral body. Because of the indolent onset, a paravertebral abscess may be noted at the time of diagnosis. With progressive destruction of the anterior portion of the vertebral body, patients may develop a progressive kyphosis or gibbous deformity.

Diagnosis involves obtaining specimens for culture and diagnosis. Three- or four-drug therapy is initiated. Surgery is usually an adjunct to medical management and is typically reserved to correct resultant spinal deformities.

Sickle Cell Disease

Young children with sickle cell disease may develop dactylitis. Indeed, dactylitis may precede the diagnosis of sickle cell disease. The pathophysiology is infarction of hematopoietic marrow, which, in young children, extends to the bones of the hands and feet.

The incidence of osteomyelitis is increased in patients with sickle cell disease, and the diagnosis can be difficult, because the presenting signs and symptoms are similar to a sickle cell crisis (bone marrow infarction). The infection actually may start as a crisis that evolves into osteomyelitis. Laboratory studies provide limited information to differentiate osteomyelitis from sickle cell crisis. Patients with sickle cell disease have a falsely low ESR. Results of CBC, early routine radiographs, and bone scans, and MRI findings frequently overlap in these conditions. Recent studies indicate that sequential radionuclide bone marrow and bone scans may be helpful in differentiating osteomyelitis from bone infarction in patients with sickle cell disease.

If clinical signs and laboratory results suggest osteomyelitis, a biopsy should be performed to confirm the diagnosis and to obtain cultures for identification of the causative bacteria. *S aureus* and salmonellae are common causes of osteomyelitis in sickle cell disease. Initial antibiotic therapy should cover both organisms until culture analysis establishes the causative agent.

Nail Puncture Wounds

Nail puncture wounds of the foot are common. Fortunately, most respond to superficial débridement of the skin and foreign body removal. If a patient returns 1 to 7 days after injury with increased swelling and pain, the most likely problem is a cellulitis or superficial abscess that is secondary to infection with *S aureus* or streptococci. If the patient presents later, the most likely diagnosis is osteomyelitis and/or septic arthritis caused by *Pseudomonas aeruginosa*. These infections require surgical débridement and removal of all necrotic tissue. With adequate débridement, antibiotic treatment is limited to 7 to10 days of intravenous therapy.

ADDITIONAL READINGS

Gorbach AL, Bartlett JG, Blacklow NR, eds. *Infectious Disease*, 3rd edition. Philadelphia, Pa: Lippincott Williams and Wilkins; 2003.

Greene WB. Osteomyelitis. In: Staheli LT, ed. *Pediatric Orthopaedic Secrets*, 2nd edition. Philadelphia, Pa: Hanley and Belfus; 2003:354–360.

Lahiji A, Esterhai JL. Principles of treatment of infection and antimicrobial therapy. In: Chapman MW, ed. *Chapman's Orthopaedic Surgery*, 3rd edition. Philadelphia, Pa: Lippincott Williams and Wilkins; 2001:3505–3532.

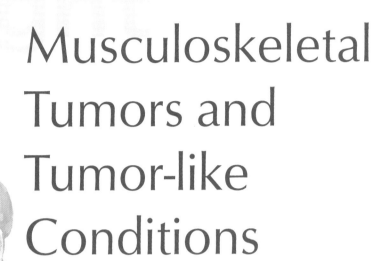

Musculoskeletal Tumors and Tumor-like Conditions

Walter B. Greene, MD

T umors and tumor-like conditions of bone and associated soft tissues are uncommon, but their timely identification and appropriate management are critical. Tumors are classified by their tissue of origin and as either benign or malignant (**Tables 8-1** and **8-2**). In certain neoplasms, the tissue of origin is unknown (giant cell tumors) or controversial (Ewing sarcoma). Tumor-like conditions that result in space-occupying lesions, although routinely grouped with tumors, are non-neoplastic and may resolve without treatment.

Table 8-1
Tumors of Bone

Tissue of Origin	Benign Tumor	Malignant Tumor

Osseous	Osteoid osteoma
	Osteoblastoma
		Osteosarcoma
		  Classic
		  Periosteal osteosarcoma
		  Periosteal secondary osteosarcoma

Chondroid	Osteochondroma Enchondroma Chondroblastoma Chondromyxoid fibroma	Chondrosarcoma
Fibrous	Nonossifying fibroma Fibrous dysplasia	Fibrosarcoma of bone Malignant fibrous histiocytoma
Marrow/hematopoietic	Langerhans cell histiocytosis	Leukemia Lymphoma Plasma cell myeloma Granulocytic sarcoma
Vascular	Hemangioma Epithelioid hemangioma	Hemangioendothelioma Angiosarcoma
Neural	Schwannoma Neurofibroma	Primitive neuroectodermal tumor Ewing sarcoma
Notochord	Notochord remnant	Chordoma
Epithelial		Adamantinoma
Adipose	Lipoma	Liposarcoma
Unknown	Giant cell tumor	Malignant giant cell tumor
Tumor-like condition	Simple bone cyst Aneurysmal bone cyst Bone island	

Table 8-2
Common Soft Tissue Tumors in the Extremities

Tissue of Origin	Benign Tumor	Malignant Tumor
Osseous	Myositis ossificans	Extraosseous osteosarcoma
Chondroid	Extraskeletal chondroma Synovial chondromatosis	Extraosseous chondrosarcoma
Fibrous	Fibroma Nodular fasciitis Fibrous histiocytoma Xanthoma	Fibrosarcoma Malignant fibrous histiocytoma
Synovial	Giant cell tumor of tendon sheath Localized Diffuse	Synovial sarcoma Malignant giant cell tumor of tendon sheath
Vascular	Hemangioma Lymphangioma Glomus	Angiosarcoma Hemangioendothelioma Hemangiopericytoma
Neural	Neurilemoma Neurofibroma	Malignant peripheral nerve sheath tumor
Adipose	Lipoma Angiolipoma	Liposarcoma
Muscle	Rhabdomyoma Leiomyoma	Rhabdomyosarcoma Leiomyosarcoma
Unknown	Myxoma	
Tumor-like condition	Myositis ossificans Ganglion cyst Pigmented villonodular synovitis Palmar fibromatosis (Dupuytren contracture and plantar fibromatosis)	

BONE TUMORS

Pathogenesis and Clinical Features

Bone tumors destroy surrounding osseous tissue. Malignant tumors characteristically grow more rapidly than do benign lesions, so the response of the surrounding native bone to malignant tumor expansion is unlikely to be effective. In benign lesions, a *sclerotic, reactive rim of bone* often forms to buttress the weakening effect of the tumor. Malignant lesions, in contrast, are characterized by *permeative growth* that causes necrosis of surrounding osseous tissue and *ill-defined osteolysis*. Such lesions have an ill-defined, moth-eaten appearance on radiographs (**Figure 8-1**). Slowly growing malignant tumors or rapidly growing benign tumors show a combination of permeative osteolysis that appears moth-eaten and other areas of reactive sclerosis (**Figure 8-2**).

Figure 8-1

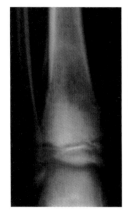

Bone destruction in osteosarcoma
Osteolytic, permeative bone destruction in an osteosarcoma. The lack of any areas of coarse radiodensity is somewhat atypical.

Malignant tumors often erode the cortex. Rapid growth spills into adjacent soft tissue, and reactive bone formation is absent on radiographs. More moderate growth creates Codman triangle or an "onion skin" arrangement on radiographs (see **Figure 8-2**). *Codman triangle* is a triangle of reactive bone formation found at the proximal and distal extremes of the elevated periosteum. *"Onion skin" layers* of reactive bone formation represent a more competent response; successive waves of tumor expansion create layers of reactive bone formation.

Tumors that produce an osseous matrix characteristically create coarse *linear radiodensities* or diffuse radiodensities that resemble *cotton patches*. If the tumor produces cartilage, the resultant cartilaginous nodules eventually may undergo calcification and enchondral ossification, similar to normal replacement of cartilage by bone. The resultant calcified cartilage appears as *stippled "popcorn"* or *ringlike marbles* on plain radiographs (see **Figure 8-2**).

Symptoms of bone tumor include pain, presence of a mass, deformity, impairment of joint function, and pathologic fracture. Most malignant bone tumors cause pain, but benign lesions may or may not be painful. Pain associated with bone tumors is typically deep, aching, and only mildly increased by activity. Pain consistently present at rest or during the night suggests a malignant tumor; however, some benign tumors (eg, osteoid osteoma) cause nocturnal pain.

The patient's initial concern may be the appearance of a mass. If the mass is associated with pain, the lesion is likely to be malignant. Deformity and loss of joint function result from weakening of the bone by the tumor. Preexistent pain suddenly increased by trivial trauma suggests a pathologic fracture, such as compression fracture of a vertebra that has been infiltrated by metastatic cancer. Marked pain occurring with routine activities suggests an impending fracture.

Musculoskeletal tumors affect patients of all ages, but certain tumors are associated with specific age groups. In general, primary bone tumors are more common in the first and second decades. Exceptions are chondrosarcoma and osteogenic sarcoma associated with other conditions. Metastatic bone cancer typically occurs in older patients.

Diagnostic Approach

The location of a tumor is an important clue in its diagnosis. For example, osteosarcoma usually arises in the metaphysis of rapidly growing bones and, therefore, most commonly occurs in the distal femur and proximal tibia during adolescence. Giant cell tumor occurs in young adults after closure of the growth plate and involves the epiphysis and the metaphysis. The unique chondroblastoma typically arises in the epiphysis or the apophysis.

Figure 8-2: Neoplasms in Bone

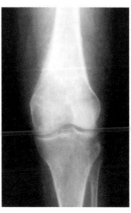

AP radiograph of osteogenic sarcoma of the distal femur demonstrating areas of sclerosis and radiolucency in the metaphysis. Tumor has spread into the soft tissues causing periosteal new bone formation and sunburst appearance.

Tumor therapy is based on the specific diagnosis and on staging of the extent and histologic grade of the tumor. The *Enneking system* is widely used for staging primary malignant tumors of bone (**Figure 8-3**). Histologic grades are benign (G_0), *low-grade malignant* (G_1), and *high-grade malignant* (G_2). Local extent of disease includes intracapsular (T_0, surrounded by an intact capsule of fibrous tissue or reactive bone), *extracapsular but intracompartmental* (T_1, remaining within an intraosseous, intramuscular compartment), and *extracapsular* and *extracompartmental* (T_2, extending beyond its compartment of origin or arising within incompletely bounded spaces, such as the popliteal fossa, axilla, or groin). Grades of metastasis include no *known metastases* (M_0) and *metastases present* (M_1).

A biopsy is performed after appropriate staging studies (**Figure 8-4**). Alternatives include fine needle aspiration (FNA), core needle biopsy, and open biopsy. Each technique has advantages and disadvantages. FNA is a simple procedure that can be done using local anesthesia. It is most helpful in diagnosing soft tissue tumors and bony tumors with homogenous cell types; however, FNA biopsy obtains the least amount of material. Core needle biopsy may be aided by ultrasonography, fluoroscopy, computed tomography (CT), and magnetic resonance imaging (MRI). The surgeon obtains a core of tissue that measures 10 mm by 2 mm. An open, or incisional, biopsy is a surgical procedure that provides the largest amount and the best sampling of tissue for pathologic identification. All biopsies should be planned and performed carefully so that compromise of subsequent limb salvage operations is avoided.

Treatment

The goal in treatment of benign bony tumors is complete excision to minimize the risk of recurrence while avoiding injury to adjacent tissues. Excision of some lesions, however, creates a large defect that necessitates bone grafting.

For a malignant tumor, chemotherapy may be the only therapy, but the role of chemo-

Figure 8-3: Staging of Musculoskeletal Tumors

BENIGN

Stages 1–3. Histologically benign (G_0); variable clinical course and biologic behavior

Stage 1. Remains static or heals spontaneously with indolent clinical course. Well encapsulated

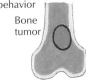

Bone tumor

Stage 2. Active; progressive, symptomatic growth. Remains intracapsular. Limited by natural boundaries but may often deform them

Stage 3. Aggressive; locally aggressive but not limited by capsule or natural boundaries. May penetrate cortex or compartment boundaries. Higher rate of recurrence

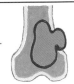

MALIGNANT

Stage I. Histologically low grade (G_1); well differentiated; few mitoses; moderate nuclear atypia. Tends to recur locally. Radioisotope uptake moderate

Intraosseous or intracompartmental

Extraosseous or extracompartmental; penetrates cortex or compartment boundaries

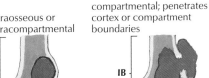

IA

IB

Stage II. Histologically high grade (G_2); poorly differentiated; high cell-to-matrix ratio; many mitoses; much nuclear atypia, necrosis, neovascularity; permeative. Radioisotope uptake intense. Higher incidence of metastases

Intraosseous or intracompartmental

Extraosseous or extracompartmental; penetrates cortex or compartment boundaries

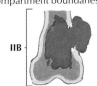

IIA

IIB

Stage III. Metastases; regional or remote (visceral, lymphatic, or osseous)

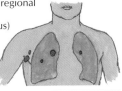

Figure 8-4: Tumor Biopsy

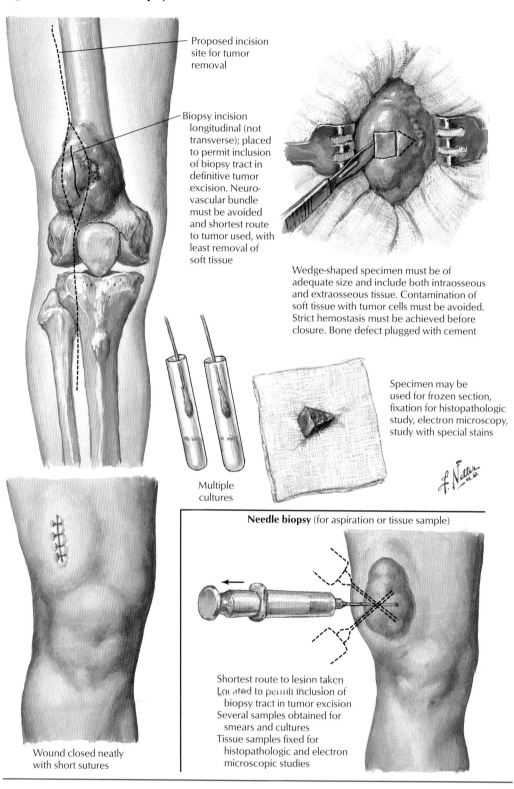

Proposed incision site for tumor removal

Biopsy incision longitudinal (not transverse); placed to permit inclusion of biopsy tract in definitive tumor excision. Neurovascular bundle must be avoided and shortest route to tumor used, with least removal of soft tissue

Wedge-shaped specimen must be of adequate size and include both intraosseous and extraosseous tissue. Contamination of soft tissue with tumor cells must be avoided. Strict hemostasis must be achieved before closure. Bone defect plugged with cement

Specimen may be used for frozen section, fixation for histopathologic study, electron microscopy, study with special stains

Multiple cultures

Wound closed neatly with short sutures

Needle biopsy (for aspiration or tissue sample)

Shortest route to lesion taken
Located to permit inclusion of
   biopsy tract in tumor excision
Several samples obtained for
   smears and cultures
Tissue samples fixed for
   histopathologic and electron
   microscopic studies

Figure 8-5: Surgical Margins for Musculoskeletal Tumors

Limb salvage procedures

Tumor zones →

Tumor
Capsule
Reactive zone

Soft tissue tumor

Radical resection
En bloc removal of entire muscle compartment

Wide excision
En bloc removal of tumor and reactive zone plus margin of normal tissue

Marginal excision
En bloc removal of tumor within reactive zone

Intracapsular excision
Debulking or piecemeal

Bone tumor

Radical resection
En bloc removal of entire bone

Wide excision
En bloc removal of tumor, reactive zone, and surrounding margin of normal bone

Marginal excision
En bloc removal of tumor through reactive zone

Intracapsular excision
Piecemeal or curettage

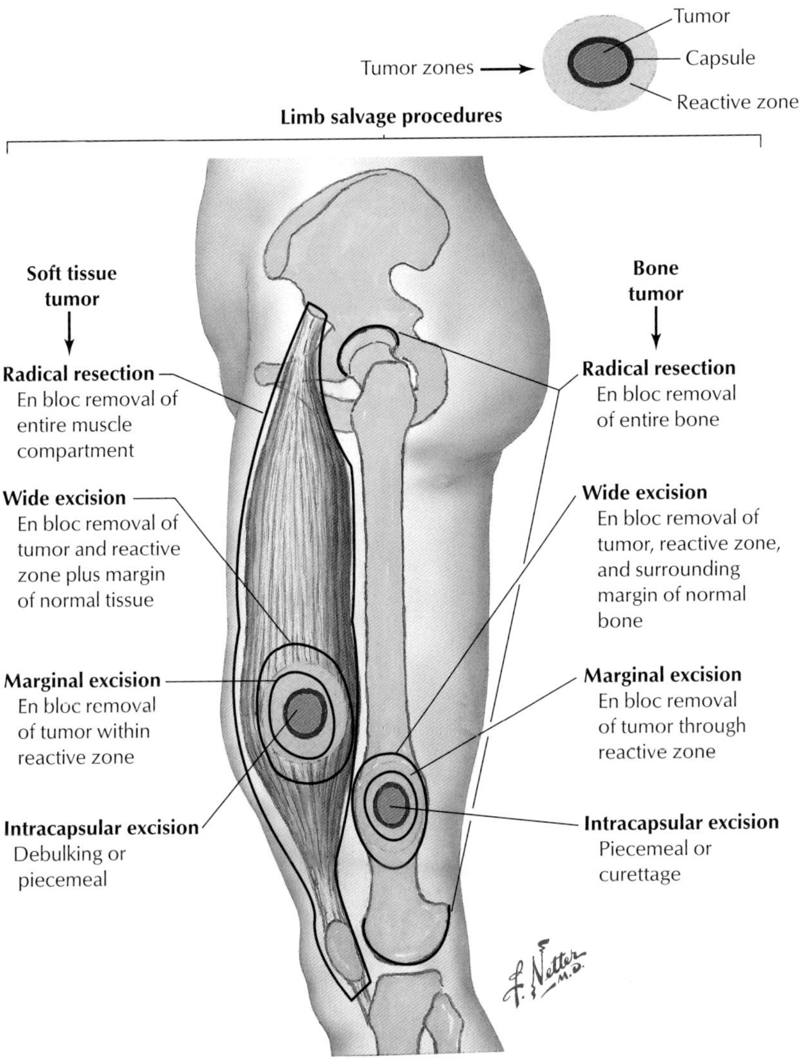

therapy in most musculoskeletal tumors is to achieve systemic control. The goal of surgery is achievement of local control. Radiation therapy may be used as an adjunct in both achieving local control and avoiding metastatic spread. To increase the probability that not even a single malignant tumor cell is left behind, a wide margin of normal tissue must be removed along with the underlying obvious malignancy (**Figure 8-5**). In general, a wide surgical margin in a malignant bone tumor includes 5 cm of uninvolved bone and 1 cm of soft tissue. However, some variability

in management is acceptable, according to whether the tumor is of low or high grade.

The surgeon who treats a malignant lesion must determine whether a limb salvage operation or an amputation will provide the best outcome in terms of postoperative function and local control. Amputation usually provides better postoperative function and reduced risk of recurrence for tumors located in the distal leg, particularly when resection of the posterior tibial nerve would be required after a limb salvage operation. Limb salvage surgery should be considered for treatment of tumors in the more proximal aspect of an extremity, because an amputation at this level would be very disabling.

Benign Bone Tumors

Osteoid Osteoma

An osteoid osteoma is a unique and relatively common benign bone tumor (**Figure 8-6**). The typical age at presentation is 5 to 25 years, with peak incidence in the second decade. The male-to-female ratio is 3:1. Although osteoid osteoma has been detected in virtually every bone, approximately half of cases involve the femur or tibia. Histologic examination reveals a small (1.0–1.5 cm) nidus that is composed of a vascular stroma, woven trabecular bone, and numerous osteoblasts and osteoclasts. Surrounding the nidus is a sclerotic zone of reactive bone. Therefore, radiographs show a radiolucent zone (the nidus) surrounded by a halo of increased density. CT scanning or MRI may be necessary for visualizing lesions in certain locations, such as the spine, pelvis, or foot.

Pain associated with an osteoid osteoma is frequently worse at night and often is dramatically relieved by nonsteroidal anti-inflammatory drugs (NSAIDs). Lesions in the spine may cause a painful scoliosis. This intense pain is thought to be secondary to high levels of tumor cyclooxygenase-2 (COX-2), prostaglandin E_2, and prostacyclin.

Treatment options include observation, surgical excision, and CT-guided radiofrequency ablation (RFA). Because osteoid osteoma eventually resolves spontaneously, patients with mild symptoms may be treated

Figure 8-6: Osteoid Osteoma

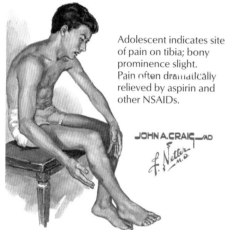

Adolescent indicates site of pain on tibia; bony prominence slight. Pain often dramatically relieved by aspirin and other NSAIDs.

JOHN A. CRAIG—MD

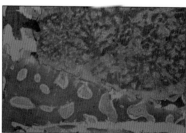

Section reveals osteoblastic nidus sharply demarcated from dense, reactive cortical bone (H and E stain)

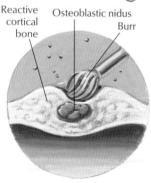

Reactive cortical bone   Osteoblastic nidus   Burr

High-speed burr utilized to remove thickened reactive cortical bone and expose osteoblastic nidus

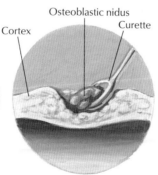

Osteoblastic nidus   Curette   Cortex

Curette used to remove the hypervascular osteoblastic nidus

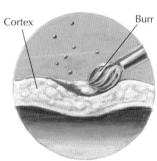

Cortex   Burr

Burr used to smooth edges of cortex after removal of osteoblastic nidus

Figure 8-6: Osteoid Osteoma

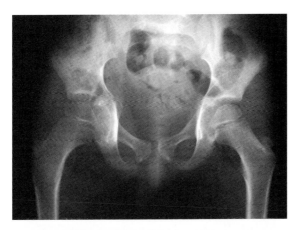

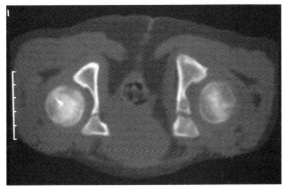

6-year-old male with several month history of pain in region of right hip that is often worse at night. AP radiograph of pelvis (top) shows sclerosis in the region of the right acetabulum but no definitive lesion. CT scan diagnostic (bottom) and shows typical nidus of osteoid osteoma posterior to the triradiate cartilage in the ischium.

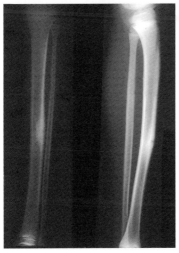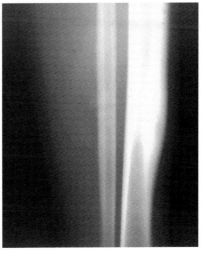

Lateral radiograph of the tibia in a girl with typical symptoms of osteoid osteoma. Radiographs show nidus with surrounding reactive bone formation.

with NSAIDs and observation. However, spontaneous resolution often does not occur for several years, and the intense pain usually warrants resection. Surgical excision includes a "burr down" technique to expose the nidus, and subsequent thorough curettage of the nidus. The surrounding sclerotic bone is burred back to healthy bone, with enough reactive bone retained that supplemental bone grafts and prolonged restriction of activities can be avoided. Treatment by RFA includes placement of a needle into the nidus under CT guidance and thermal necrosis of the tumor with high-frequency radio waves. Because tissue necrosis may injure surrounding structures, RFA is not recommended for tumors in the spine or other areas adjacent to critical neurovascular structures.

Recurrence of osteoid osteoma is associated with incomplete excision of the nidus. The recurrence rate after RFA treatment is higher than after surgical excision; however, RFA is associated with lower morbidity because this procedure obviates surgical dissection and minimizes disruption of the surrounding reactive bone.

Figure 8-7: Solitary Osteochondroma

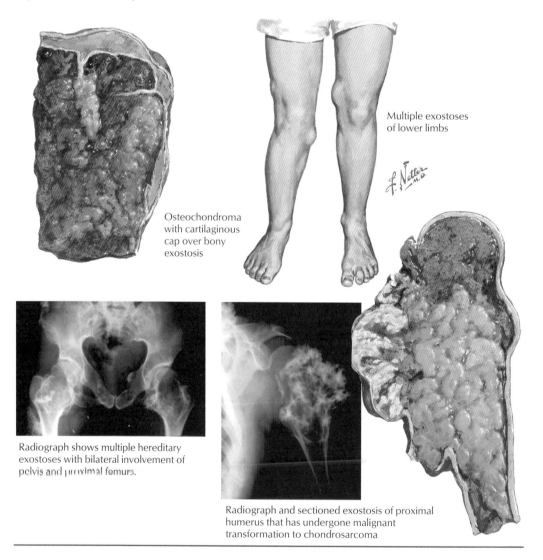

Multiple exostoses of lower limbs

Osteochondroma with cartilaginous cap over bony exostosis

Radiograph shows multiple hereditary exostoses with bilateral involvement of pelvis and proximal femurs.

Radiograph and sectioned exostosis of proximal humerus that has undergone malignant transformation to chondrosarcoma

Osteoblastoma

Osteoblastoma is an uncommon benign tumor with histologic and radiographic similarities to osteoid osteoma. Compared with osteoid osteoma, osteoblastoma occurs in a slightly older population, frequently involves the posterior elements of the vertebrae, and usually does not cause night pain. Patients with osteoblastoma do not report the striking relief of pain with NSAIDs that is frequently seen in patients with osteoid osteoma. Osteoblastomas have giant cells, a greater amount of stromal tissue, and broader osteoid seams compared with osteoid osteoma. Radiographs show a radiolucent zone and a thin margin of reactive bone. Treatment is en bloc marginal excision. The risk of recurrence varies according to the activity of the tumor and ranges from 10% to 30%.

Osteochondroma

Osteochondroma is the most common benign bony tumor (**Figure 8-7**). Most osteochondromas are located at the metaphyseal portion of long bones, particularly the distal femur and proximal tibia. These lesions, however, also occur in other areas, such as the scapula and pelvis. An osteochondroma may be solitary and idiopathic or multiple and genetic (called *hereditary multiple exostosis*).

Figure 8-7: Solitary Osteochondroma (continued)

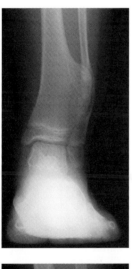
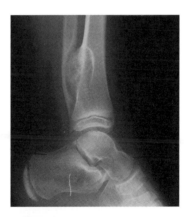
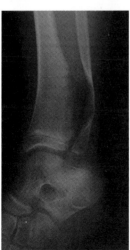
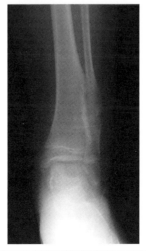

Standing preoperative AP and lateral radiograph of ankle (top) in an 8-year-old female with 2 year history of progressive pain and swelling of lateral aspect of distal tibia. Radiographs show large sessile osteochondroma of distal tibia that has caused 9° of ankle varus and bowing of the fibula. Patient had negative family history and exam for multiple hereditary exostosis.

Intraoperative AP radiograph (bottom left) after removal of the osteochondroma shows the marked bowing and thinning of the distal fibula. Osteotomy of the fibula with closure of the periosteum was performed to enhance remodeling.

AP radiograph (bottom right) 6 weeks after operation shows early healing and remodeling response of the fibula.

Solitary osteochondroma has a male-to-female ratio of 2:1. Patients are generally in the second decade and seek medical advice because of a bony mass. Activity-related pain occurs because the mass irritates surrounding muscles. Compression of an adjacent nerve causes radicular pain or paresthesia.

Histologic examination demonstrates a bony stalk covered by a cartilaginous cap. In children, the cartilage is similar to, but less organized than, the normal growth plate. Chondrocyte growth in the cap undergoes ossification. The resultant trabecular bone makes up the main portion of the osteochondroma—the bony stalk. Cortical bone and trabecular bone of the osteochondroma merge into the host bone.

An osteochondroma may undergo malignant transformation, usually to a chondrosarcoma. This transformation occurs primarily in patients with hereditary multiple exostosis during the adult years. The incidence is low and probably in the range of 1% to 2%. Signs suggestive of malignant transformation include pain and continued growth of the osteochondroma after skeletal maturity.

Treatment for a symptomatic osteochondroma is marginal excision that includes the cartilaginous cap and the overlying perichondrium. Recurrence is uncommon.

Enchondroma

Enchondroma is a relatively common benign tumor that may occur at any age. More than half of cases involve the small bones of the hands and feet. Other common sites are the metaphysis of the distal femur and the proximal humerus.

Many enchondromas are asymptomatic and are discovered by chance on radiographs taken for other reasons. In the hands and feet, symptoms may include swelling of the involved bone or a pathologic fracture. Any patient with pain and a lesion in a long bone that simulates an enchondroma should be evaluated for a possible malignancy.

An enchondroma is composed of chondrocytes and chondroid matrix that is more disorganized than normal cartilage. However, differentiating an enchondroma from a low-grade malignant chondrosarcoma may be challenging. Radiographs of enchondromas in the hands show a central radiolucent lesion and scant stippled calcification. The surrounding cortex is frequently thinned and expanded. In long bones, enchondromas show variable mineralization with stippled or popcorn ball radiodensities.

Asymptomatic solitary enchondroma may be treated with observation. Large lesions in the hand that are expanding the cortex or that have caused a pathologic fracture can be treated by curettage with or without bone grafting. Long bone lesions associated with pain should be evaluated by a CT scan, MRI, or both, so their full extent can be delineated. Findings of endosteal scalloping and focal lytic areas within an otherwise well-mineralized lesion suggest malignant transformation.

Multiple enchondromas occur in Ollier syndrome and Maffucci disease. Ollier syndrome is characterized by unilateral predominance of enchondromas, angular deformities, and limb-length discrepancy. Maffucci disease is characterized by multiple enchondromas and soft tissue hemangiomas. In both conditions, the chance that a secondary chondrosarcoma may develop later in life is approximately 25%.

Chondroblastoma

Chondroblastoma is an uncommon but unique benign tumor that occurs in children. It is almost always located in the epiphysis of long bones, particularly the distal femur, proximal tibia, proximal humerus, and proximal femur. Patients are generally adolescents whose presenting symptom is periarticular pain.

Histologic examination demonstrates a "cobblestone" pattern, with plump chondroblasts surrounded by a thin chondroid matrix and scattered giant cells. Radiographs demonstrate a lytic lesion in the epiphysis that is surrounded by a thin margin of sclerotic reactive bone. Fine, "chicken-wire" calcification also may be observed. Chondroblastomas may spread into the metaphysis or may even break through the cortex into the articular cartilage.

Most patients can be treated with curettage and bone grafting (marginal excision). The growth plate is usually perforated by the tumor or by the curettage; curettage of the entire physis will prevent angular deformities and provide a more complete margin of excision. Because most patients are nearing completion of growth, the resultant epiphysiodesis usually has minimal consequences on shortening of the extremity. Recurrent lesions require a wide-margin resection.

Nonossifying Fibroma

Nonossifying fibroma is very common (**Figure 8-8**). It usually causes no symptoms and rarely requires treatment. Most lesions are discovered incidentally during radiography for an unrelated injury. Nonossifying fibromas typically occur in the metaphysis of the femur or tibia.

Histologic examination shows dense areas of spindle-shaped cells in a whorled pattern. Multinucleated giant cells and foci of xanthomatous tissue are common. Radiographs show a radiolucent lesion that is eccentric (abutting one cortex) and surrounded by a rim of sclerotic, reactive bone.

Most nonossifying fibromas regress spontaneously during puberty or shortly thereafter and do not require treatment. Large lesions that cause pain or that are large enough to cause concern about fracture should be treated by curettage and bone grafting. When a pathologic fracture occurs because of a nonossifying fibroma, initial treatment should include care of the fracture and observation,

Figure 8-8: Nonossifying Fibroma

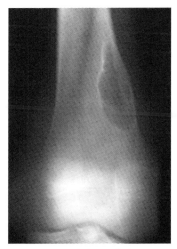

Eccentric radiolucent lesion with margin of reactive bone in metaphysis of distal femur

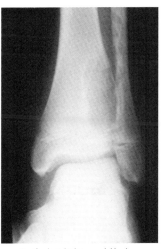

Both distal tibia and fibula involved; fibula fractured

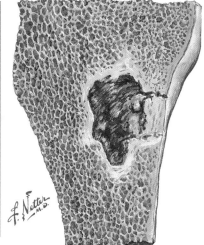

Sectioned proximal tibia with tumor. Reddish tan fibrous core and margin of reactive bone. En bloc excision not usually required as lesions heal eventually, either spontaneously or after curettage.

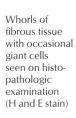

Whorls of fibrous tissue with occasional giant cells seen on histopathologic examination (H and E stain)

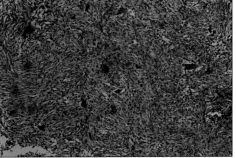

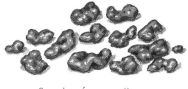

Scrapings from curettage

because the injury often promotes regression of the nonossifying fibroma.

Fibrous Dysplasia

Fibrous dysplasia is a developmental abnormality of bone characterized by lesions of fibrous tissue proliferation among scattered trabeculae of woven bone. Approximately 85% of patients with fibrous dysplasia have involvement of only one bone. Many of these *monostotic* patients are asymptomatic, and the lesion is detected during radiography conducted to study an unrelated condition. The rib is the most common location, but any bone may be involved. On occasion, an adolescent with monostotic fibrous dysplasia seeks medical care because of either a pathologic fracture or an angular deformity of the limb.

Polyostotic fibrous dysplasia may range from only two or three areas of limited involvement, or it may include extensive skeletal abnormalities. Some patients with severe polyostotic involvement have *McCune-Albright syndrome* (MAS) with associated skin lesions, precocious puberty, and hyperfunction of multiple endocrine glands. The skin abnormalities in MAS are characterized by café au lait spots with irregular borders ("coast of Maine" café au lait spots) that differ from the smooth border ("coast of California") café au lait spots found in those with neurofibromatosis. Mutations in the α subunit of Gs proteins that link receptors to adenyl cyclase activity have been demonstrated in MAS and lesions of monostotic fibrous dysplasia.

Patients with polyostotic fibrous dysplasia usually develop a limp during the childhood years because of shortening or angulation of the bone. Severe coxa vara, the so-called shepherd crook deformity, is caused by a characteristic lesion that causes deficient hip mechanics and shortens the limb. Treatment of this deformity is challenging because the severe coxa vara creates extreme tensile forces that retard bone healing, and because bone grafts frequently resorb in fibrous dysplasia. Best results are obtained with a combination of curettage, bone grafting, realignment valgus osteotomy, and rigid internal fixation.

Langerhans Cell Histiocytosis

Langerhans cell histiocytosis (LCH) is a disease complex characterized by infiltration of one or more organs by large mononuclear cells (Langerhans cell histiocytes). Electron microscopy reveals that these histiocytes have unique tubular or rocket-shaped granules. Between 2% and 79% of the histiocytes in LCH lesions are Langerhans cells; other histiocytic cell types found in LCH include lymphocytes, eosinophils, neutrophils, and, on occasion, multinuclear giant cells.

The pathogenesis of LCH is still speculative. Because patients with LCH develop cystic bony lesions, the disease often is included in discussions of tumors; however, LCH is not a classic neoplasm, and studies suggest that it may be a reactive immunologic process.

LCH is more common among children, and in this group, the median age of onset is 2 to 3 years. Clinical manifestations are protean. The initial evaluation should include a complete examination as well as radiographic and laboratory studies. The classification of disease extent is solitary bone involvement only, multiple bone lesions without soft tissue involvement, bone and soft tissue lesions, or soft tissue involvement alone.

At the first visit, the majority (50% to 75%) of pediatric cases involve a bony lesion without soft tissue involvement. Children with solitary bone involvement at disease onset have the best prognosis; no deaths have been reported in this group. In comparison, children with organ dysfunction at disease onset have a mortality rate of 30% to 70%. Between 30% and 70% of cases evolve from solitary to multiple bone lesions, but many of the subsequent lesions are asymptomatic.

Children with a solitary bony lesion may be asymptomatic, and their condition may have been diagnosed from radiographs obtained for unrelated reasons. However, these children typically present for care with localized swelling, pain, or limping.

Skeletal lesions occur in 80% to 97% of patients with LCH. Common sites of bony lesions include the skull, spine, pelvis, ribs, and femur.

Other long bones may be involved, but lesions in the hands and feet are rare. Skull lesions have a well-defined, punched-out appearance on radiographs. *Vertebra plana*, the typical spinal lesion, is characterized by marked collapse of the vertebral body; however, in contrast to an infectious process, adjacent discs are preserved in LCH. Long-bone lesions typically are lytic and are found in the diaphysis or metaphysis. Other radiographic features include endosteal scalloping, cortical thinning, and widening of the medullary cavity.

Common sites of soft tissue involvement include the skin, lymph nodes, lungs, liver, and pituitary stalk. Skin involvement may vary from a few discrete pinhead lesions to a generalized pustular eczematous eruption. *Diabetes insipidus* occurs in 12% to 50% of children with multiple system involvement.

Treatment options for a child with a solitary bony lesion include observation, steroid injection, medical management, and curettage. Most children with solitary bone involvement may be treated with observation because many lesions resolve spontaneously. Chemotherapy is required with extensive soft tissue involvement and organ dysfunction.

Giant Cell Tumor of Bone

Although many bone tumors contain multinucleated giant cells, a true giant cell tumor is a distinct, benign, but locally aggressive lesion of unknown origin (**Figure 8-9**). It occurs in young adults after closure of the growth plate. A slight female predominance has been noted. Common locations include the distal femur, proximal tibia, and distal radius.

Histologic examination shows numerous multinucleated giant cells, slightly elongated stromal cells with oval nuclei, and areas of vascular channels and free blood. Radiographic features include a lytic, eccentric lesion that involves the epiphysis and metaphyseal region of bone. The cortex is frequently thin and often expanded. The subchondral bone may be eroded. Typical presenting symptoms include localized pain, swelling, and reactive joint effusion. Giant cell tumors are unpredictable; however, the local aggressiveness of the lesion correlates with the histologic appearance. Occasionally, malignant transformation occurs.

Treatment options include curettage and bone grafting, as well as filling of the defect with cement. Recurrent lesions or lesions that have extended into the joint require wide-margin excision and reconstruction.

Solitary Bone Cyst

A solitary bone cyst is a relatively common pediatric bony lesion with a male-to-female ratio of 2:1 (**Figure 8-10**). Common locations include the proximal humerus and proximal femur. Patients typically experience pain after a pathologic fracture occurs.

The cyst is filled with a clear yellow fluid unless a recent fracture has occurred. The cavity is lined with a thin layer of fibrous tissue that frequently includes giant cells. Radiographs show a metaphyseal lytic lesion with thinning of the cortex. *Active cysts* abut the growth plate, occur more often in patients younger than 10 years, and are associated with a higher recurrence rate. *Latent cysts*, which are seen in older children, are separated from the physis by a margin of normal bone. Their thicker bony cortex further indicates progressive ossification and healing. The *"falling-leaf" sign* is a fragment of the eggshell-thin cortex that was displaced into the cavity after a pathologic fracture.

Treatment of active lesions or lesions at risk of fracture includes injection therapy with steroids, autologous bone marrow, or another substance with the goal of promoting bone formation and healing. Lesions of the proximal femur are at greater risk for a disabling fracture. Flexible intramedullary nails or other fixation devices may be used as internal struts. The perforation of a cyst by these devices stimulates the healing process.

Aneurysmal Bone Cyst

An aneurysmal bone cyst (ABC) is an expansile, blood-field, multilocular lytic lesion of bone. Peak incidence is noted in the second decade; 80% of these cysts occur in patients younger than 20 years. Any bone

Figure 8-9: Giant Cell Tumor of Bone

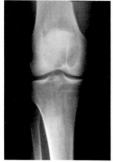
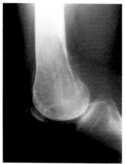

Anteroposterior radiograph shows giant cell tumor of epiphysis and metaphysis of distal femur extending into but not penetrating subchondral plate

Lateral view reveals radiolucent lesion bulging posteriorly into popliteal fossa

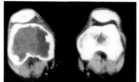

CT scan of right femur reveals marked endosteal erosion by intraosseous lesion

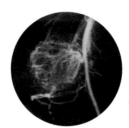

Angiogram demonstrates intense vascularity of tumor area

Pathologic fracture through giant cell tumor of distal femur

Bone scan demonstrates characteristic "doughnut sign" (also typical of aneurysmal bone cyst)

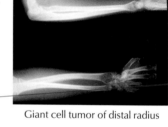

Giant cell tumor of distal radius

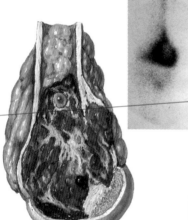
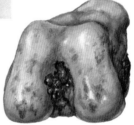
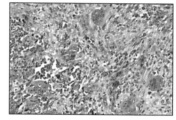

Sectioned distal femur shows meaty, hemorrhagic tissue with lighter, dense, fibrous areas, small cysts and blood clots, and thin margin of reactive bone with Codman triangle. Tumor has infiltrated soft tissue.

View of femoral condyles. Tumor apparent in spots through thin subchondral plate and articular cartilage; also in intercondylar notch covered by synovial membrane.

Section shows stroma of spindle-like cells with pale-staining cytoplasm and nuclei, many multinucleated giant cells, vascular channels, and free blood (H and E stain)

may be affected, but common sites are the proximal femur, proximal tibia, and spine. In long bones, the metaphysis is the typical site, whereas in the spine, the posterior elements are more commonly involved.

Clinical presentation includes pain, swelling, and often a pathologic fracture. Histologic examination reveals lakes of blood surrounded by loose fibrous tissue septa, giant cells, and inflammatory cells. The classic radiographic finding is a lytic lesion that has a "ballooned out" thin cortex and a "soap bubble" multilocular pattern.

Treatment requires excision with curettage of the lining. Bone loss may be excessive in large ABCs, and preoperative embolization should be considered in such cases for control of surgical blood loss. The lesion may be

Figure 8-10: Pathologic Fracture through Solitary Bone Cyst

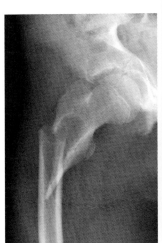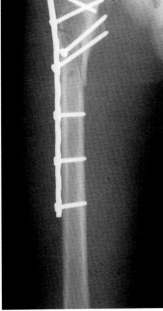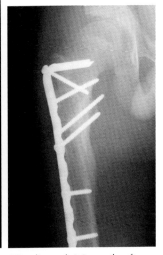

| AP radiograph of proximal femur at time of injury | AP radiograph 9 days after curettage and internal fixation of fracture | AP radiograph 3.3 months after operation |

13-year-old male with approximately 1 month history of activity related anterior thigh pain. Patient fell off his bike with immediate onset of pain, deformity, and inability to walk. Radiograph (left) shows displaced subtrochanteric femur fracture through large cyst in the proximal femur. Findings at operation were a large hole in the bone that had only a scant lining. Patient treated with curettage of the lesion and internal fixation with a blade plate (middle). Radiograph 3.3 months after operation (right) reveals interval healing of the fracture and obliteration of the cyst.

packed with an autograft, an allograft, or cement. The rate of recurrence is 20% to 30%, and is higher among young children and patients with large lesions.

Malignant Bone Tumors

Osteosarcoma

Osteosarcoma represents only 0.2% of all malignancies, but it is the most common primary malignant bone tumor (excluding multiple myeloma, which arises in bone but is considered a systemic malignancy of bone marrow rather than a bone tumor). The condition usually develops during adolescence and affects males more often than females. Another group at risk includes older adults with previous irradiation, Paget disease, or another preexisting lesion. Osteosarcoma may arise anywhere, but 70% of these lesions develop in the metaphysis of the distal femur, proximal tibia, or proximal humerus (**Figure 8-11**).

Histologic findings vary, but the characteristic feature is large, pleomorphic, high-grade sarcomatous cells that produce osteoid and woven bone. The sarcoma invades the marrow spaces, entrapping normal trabecular bone, and also penetrates the cortex, with resultant elevation of periosteum and devel-

Figure 8-11: Osteosarcoma

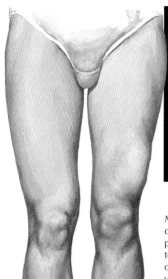

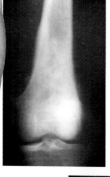

AP and lateral radiograph shows dense lesion and periosteal elevation

Mass on left distal femur palpable and tender but only slightly visible

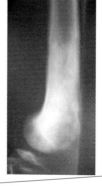

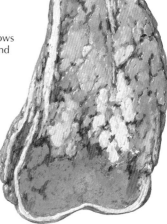

Tumor occupies entire metaphysis of distal femur and has extended into the soft tissues

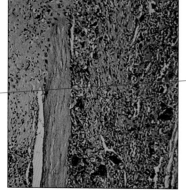

Highly malignant stroma with cartilaginous and osteoid components (H and E stain)

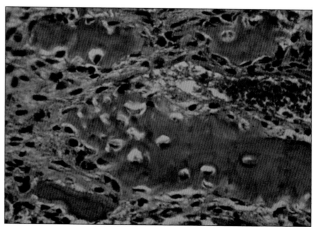

Masses of tumor cells with hyperchromatic nuclei interspersed with foci of malignant osteoid are typical histopathologic findings (H and E stain)

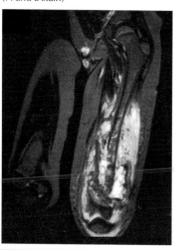

Osteosarcoma
MRI of thigh showing pathologic fracture of distal femur and extensive soft tissue spread of osteogenic sarcoma into both anterior and posterior thigh compartments.

opment of Codman triangle. Radiographs typically show a permeative destructive lesion that may be predominantly dense or osteoblastic, purely osteolytic, or of mixed radiographic pattern.

Pain is the characteristic early symptom. Later symptoms include a mass and decreased joint motion. Pathologic fracture also may occur.

Staging studies include MRI of the lesion to define the local extent of disease, CT scan of the lungs to define metastasis, and bone scan to detect possible skip lesions or other areas of metastasis. At presentation, 5% of osteosarcomas are stage IIA, 80% are stage IIB, and 15% are stage III (see **Figure 8-3**).

Before effective chemotherapy was developed, approximately 80% of patients died of metastases, even after prompt amputation. Standard treatment now includes biopsy confirmation of diagnosis, staging studies, preoperative chemotherapy for 11 weeks, surgical resection, and postoperative chemotherapy for several more weeks. It is thought, but has not definitely been proved, that preoperative chemotherapy improves survival and the potential for limb salvage surgery. Most chemotherapy protocols include doxorubicin, high-dose methotrexate, and cisplatin. Improved reconstructive techniques have increased the number of limb-sparing operations to approximately 80%. With current treatment, the 5-year disease-free survival rate for persons with stage II osteosarcoma is approximately 70%.

Chondrosarcoma

Chondrosarcoma is less common and grows more slowly than osteosarcoma (**Figure 8-12**). *Primary chondrosarcomas* are located centrally within the medullary canal, are more common among males, and have a peak incidence at between 30 and 60 years of age. Frequent sites include the proximal femur, pelvis, proximal humerus, and scapula. *Secondary chondrosarcomas* are typically associated with a previous osteochondroma and are located on the periphery of bone, but they may occur in an extraosseous soft tissue location.

Persistent, dull aching pain is the most common symptom of a central chondrosarcoma. Histologic findings include chondrocytes with varying degrees of malignant changes. Low-grade chondrosarcomas may be difficult to differentiate from benign osteochondromas or enchondromas. Radiographs show a permeative radiolucent lesion with areas of calcification that may be diffuse ("salt and pepper" pattern) or more discrete ("popcorn" pattern). The incidence of distant metastases is related to the degree of malignancy.

Chondrosarcoma is treated by surgical resection. Radiation therapy is not helpful, and chemotherapy is reserved for patients with metastases.

Malignant Fibrous Histiocytoma and Fibrosarcoma

Malignant fibrous histiocytoma (MFH) and fibrosarcoma (FS) develop less often in bone than in soft tissue (**Figure 8-13**). MFH may be associated with bone that is atypical (because of infarct, irradiation, or chronic osteomyelitis, for example). These tumors develop throughout the adult years, but MFH tends to occur in older adults.

Histologic studies usually reveal fibroblastic cells arranged in a storiform growth pattern ("rope-mat" pattern). Histiocytic cells with striking pleomorphism and giant cells may be scattered throughout the tumor. Radiographs show a permeative lytic metaphyseal lesion with cortical destruction and soft tissue extension.

The typical presenting symptom is pain, but pathologic fracture also may occur. Swelling may be evident if the tumor is superficial. Treatment is similar to that for osteosarcoma.

Ewing Sarcoma

Ewing sarcoma is the second most common malignant bone tumor, after osteosarcoma (**Figure 8-14**). The age range is 5 to 25 years, with peak incidence at between 10 and 20 years. Ewing sarcoma is more common among males. The most common site is the fe-

Figure 8-12: Chondrosarcoma

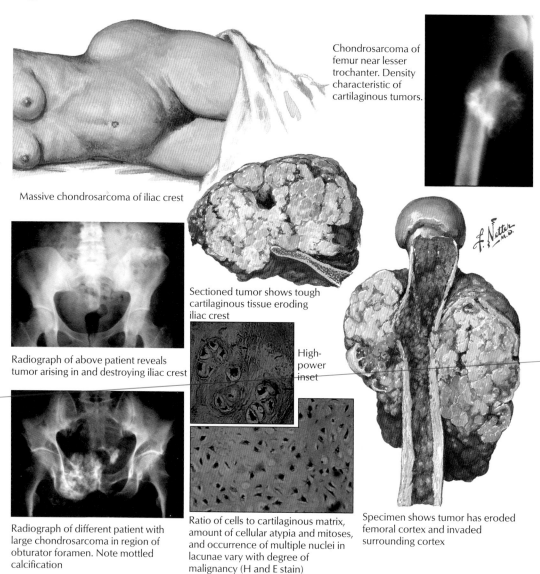

Chondrosarcoma of femur near lesser trochanter. Density characteristic of cartilaginous tumors.

Massive chondrosarcoma of iliac crest

Sectioned tumor shows tough cartilaginous tissue eroding iliac crest

High-power inset

Radiograph of above patient reveals tumor arising in and destroying iliac crest

Radiograph of different patient with large chondrosarcoma in region of obturator foramen. Note mottled calcification

Ratio of cells to cartilaginous matrix, amount of cellular atypia and mitoses, and occurrence of multiple nuclei in lacunae vary with degree of malignancy (H and E stain)

Specimen shows tumor has eroded femoral cortex and invaded surrounding cortex

mur, followed by the tibia, humerus, pelvis, and fibula. In Ewing sarcoma tissue, the reciprocal translocation (11:22) (q24:q12) is virtually always present. This translocation produces a fusion transcription factor that can transform fibroblasts. This cytogenic translocation is also found in peripheral neuroectodermal tumors (PNETs). Currently, Ewing sarcoma is considered part of the PNET family,

and the cell of origin for Ewing sarcoma is probably neuronal.

Pain is the most common presenting symptom. In advanced cases, systemic symptoms such as fever and malaise may be noted, and the condition may mimic osteomyelitis.

Histologic examination demonstrates densely packed areas of small, round cells. Radiographs show a permeative pattern of

Figure 8-13

Malignant Fibrous Histiocytoma of Bone

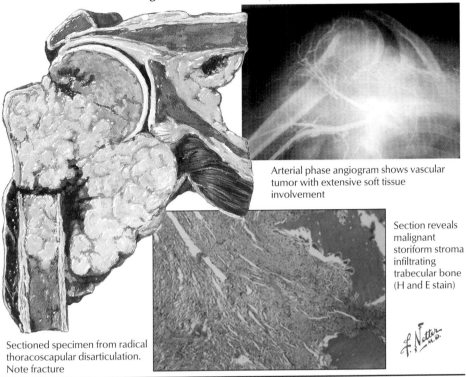

Arterial phase angiogram shows vascular tumor with extensive soft tissue involvement

Section reveals malignant storiform stroma infiltrating trabecular bone (H and E stain)

Sectioned specimen from radical thoracoscapular disarticulation. Note fracture

Fibrosarcoma of Bone

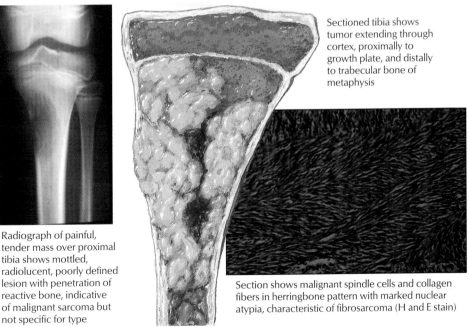

Sectioned tibia shows tumor extending through cortex, proximally to growth plate, and distally to trabecular bone of metaphysis

Radiograph of painful, tender mass over proximal tibia shows mottled, radiolucent, poorly defined lesion with penetration of reactive bone, indicative of malignant sarcoma but not specific for type

Section shows malignant spindle cells and collagen fibers in herringbone pattern with marked nuclear atypia, characteristic of fibrosarcoma (H and E stain)

Figure 8-14: Ewing Sarcoma

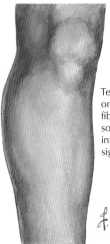

Tender bulge on proximal fibula with some inflammatory signs

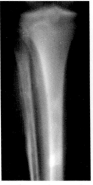

Radiograph reveals mottled, destructive, radiolucent lesion

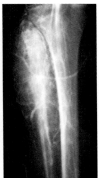

Angiogram shows vascular blush extending into soft tissue

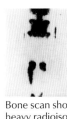

Bone scan shows heavy radioisotope uptake in tumor area. Other hot spots related to normal bone growth

Infiltrative, destructive tumor extending into soft tissue seen in sectioned proximal fibula

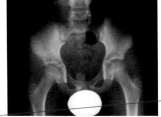

Lesion of mottled density involves anterior superior iliac spine

Sectioned femur shows highly vascular intraosseous and soft tissue tumor components with much reactive bone

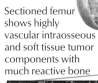

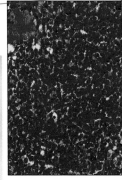

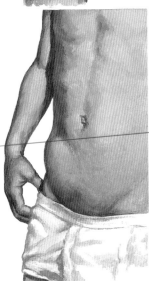

Ewing sarcoma of pelvis. Scarcely visible but palpable mass in right lower quadrant

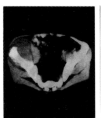

CT scan defines mass filling right iliac fossa

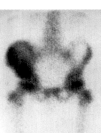

Bone scan shows heavy radioisotope uptake in right iliac wing

Section shows masses of small, round cells with uniformly sized hyperchromatic nuclei (H an E stain)

destruction in the diaphysis or the metaphyseal portion of bone. Thinning and erosion of the cortex is common and a Codman triangle, or "onion skin" periosteal reaction, may be seen (see **Figure 8-2**).

After appropriate staging and biopsy have been performed, the patient is treated with inductive chemotherapy. The tumor then is further evaluated for treatment with wide-margin surgical resection or irradiation. The survival rate is approximately 70% for patients without metastases.

Adamantinoma

Adamantinoma is a rare tumor that occurs primarily in males at between 10 and 30 years of age. This lesion occurs in the diaphysis of the tibia in 80% of cases. Histologic examina-

Figure 8-14: Ewing's Sarcoma (continued)

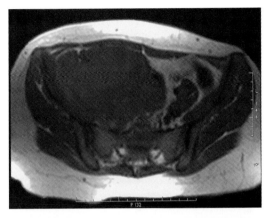

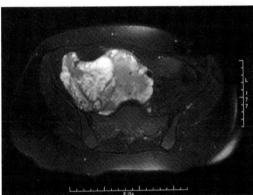

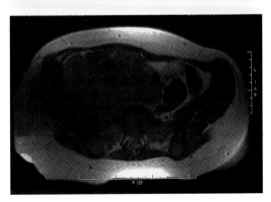

MRI of 19-year-old female who presented with progressive and severe radicular pain in the right lower extremity associated with femoral nerve palsy. (Top) T1 weighted image of pelvis. (Middle) T2 weighted image and (bottom) gadolinium enhanced T1 image. MRI shows extensive soft tissue mass anterior to the ilium that has displaced the iliopsoas muscle and femoral nerves and vessels. Gadolinium enhanced views confirm some central necrosis within the sarcoma.

tion shows aggregates of epithelial-type cells surrounded by fibro-osseous stroma. Radiographs typically show a radiolucent lesion with a "soap bubble" appearance.

SOFT TISSUE TUMORS

Benign Soft Tissue Tumors

Lipoma

Lipoma is the most common mesenchymal neoplasm (**Figure 8-15**). The typical age of presentation is 40 to 60 years. Patients typically seek medical care because of a mass that is not painful. Superficial lipomas are commonly found on the back, thorax, shoulder, abdomen, and neck. Deeper lipomas are usually detected at a later stage.

The classic histologic feature of lipomas is mature lipocytes (fat cells) that are usually slightly larger than normal fat cells. Lipomas gradually enlarge over time but may remain unchanged for several years. Lesions of significant size are treated by marginal excision.

Angiolipoma is a relatively rare tumor that commonly develops in young adult men. Palpation elicits tenderness. Common sites are the forearm, trunk, and upper arm. Histologic examination shows fat lobules with interspersed areas of capillary networks.

Myositis Ossificans

Myositis ossificans is not a tumor but a reparative response of reactive ossification in the soft tissue after blunt trauma (**Figure 8-16**). The typical patient is a male adolescent who has received a direct blow and who subsequently develops an enlarging mass in the thigh, buttock, or upper arm.

Fibrous Histiocytoma

Fibrous histiocytoma, a relatively common tumor, has a peak incidence in persons 20 to 40 years of age. It is most commonly located in subcutaneous tissue.

Histologic examination demonstrates spindle-shaped fibroblastic cells in a storiform pattern. Subcutaneous lesions are usually smaller than 3 cm in diameter, but they may

Figure 8-15: Lipoma

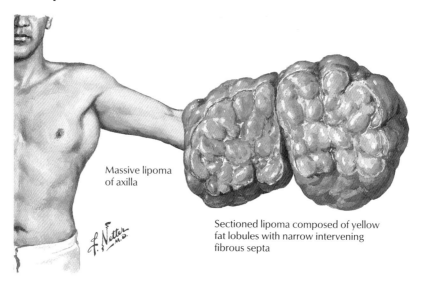

Massive lipoma of axilla

Sectioned lipoma composed of yellow fat lobules with narrow intervening fibrous septa

Figure 8-16: Myositis Ossificans

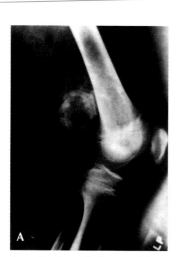

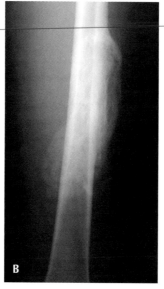

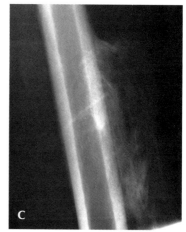

Lateral radiograph shows nodule with peripheral maturation in soft tissue of posterior distal thigh

AP and lateral radiograph of a femur of a 40-year-old male whose thigh was struck by heavy metal drum approximately 7 months prior. The patient noted pain, swelling, and discomfort after the injury. The thigh stayed warm for a long period of time, gradually started to cool down, but then patient noted increasing difficulty in moving his leg. The patient noted particular problems in going up and down stairs.

Examination revealed a 20 x 9 cm firm mass in the thigh and knee flexion limited to 30°. Radiographs demonstrate mature myositis ossificans.

become very large. Deeper tumors are usually larger than 5 cm in diameter at diagnosis.

Hemangioma

Hemangiomas are relatively common and typically develop in children. Most lesions are located in subcutaneous tissue, but hemangiomas may develop in muscle and internal organs. Capillary (small-vessel) hemangiomas are noninvasive and are red when viewed from the skin's surface. Cavernous hemangiomas are likely to be invasive; they contain calcifications that may be seen on radiographs, and they are bluish when subcutaneous. Histologic evaluation reveals bundles of capillaries or dilated vascular channels.

Malignant Soft Tissue Tumors

Malignant tumors of soft tissue are uncommon and slightly more prevalent among males than among females. These tumors develop in persons of all ages, but in general, their incidence increases with advancing age. The typical symptom is an expanding, but often painless, mass. Patients who have pain frequently note that the symptom is worse at night and is inconsistently relieved by NSAIDs. Patients may experience radicular pain if the tumor is pressing on an adjacent nerve.

Physical examination includes noting the location and size of the mass, associated skin changes, and the status of adjacent lymph nodes, nerves, and vessels. Results of laboratory studies may allow the clinician to exclude an infectious process. Although plain radiography should be used as a screening test, compared with MRI it provides limited information concerning tumor size, relationship to adjacent structures, and characteristics. Malignant sarcomas, for example, often demonstrate heterogenous changes on MRI because of pleomorphism of cell types and areas of tissue necrosis and mineralization.

A needle biopsy is a practical diagnostic tool used in the evaluation of soft tissue sarcomas. In performing a needle or an open biopsy, it is important to confine the needle placement or incision location to one compartment, and to avoid tissue contamination

that would compromise subsequent surgical resection (see **Figure 8-4**). The histologic grade and size of the lesion are the most significant factors in predicting risks for metastasis and survival.

The goal of surgical excision is to obtain margins that are free of tumor while preserving limb function as much as possible. The biopsy track should be completely excised. Margins should be wide for a low-grade soft tissue sarcoma and, if possible, radical for a high-grade soft tissue sarcoma (see **Figure 8-5**). In a radical procedure, the entire anatomic compartment containing the tumor is removed.

Postoperative radiation therapy is frequently used to reduce the risk of local recurrence. Chemotherapy has a more limited role in the treatment of soft tissue sarcoma, and its use is frequently limited to patients with metastatic disease.

Liposarcoma

Liposarcomas have variable histologic characteristics but generally occur as low-grade myxoid liposarcomas, which are more common in young adults, or high-grade pleomorphic liposarcomas, which are more common in older patients (**Figure 8-17**). Common locations include the buttocks, thigh, and upper arm.

Synovial Cell Sarcoma

The term *synovial cell sarcoma* derives from the condition's cellular characteristics that are suggestive of primitive synovial cells. Contrary to what its name implies, synovial cell sarcoma does not develop in joints. Compared with other soft tissue sarcomas, synovial cell sarcomas occur more often in the hands and feet. Patients often note bothersome pain for some time before a mass can be palpated (**Figure 8-18**). The typical age range for persons with synovial cell sarcoma is 15 to 35 years.

Histologic findings include clusters of epithelioid or glandular tissue intermixed with areas where spindle cells predominate. Some synovial cell sarcomas are monophasic and have only spindle cell tissue. Plain radiographs often

Figure 8-17: Liposarcoma

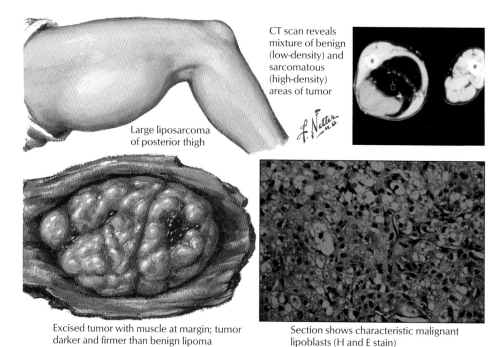

CT scan reveals mixture of benign (low-density) and sarcomatous (high-density) areas of tumor

Large liposarcoma of posterior thigh

Excised tumor with muscle at margin; tumor darker and firmer than benign lipoma

Section shows characteristic malignant lipoblasts (H and E stain)

show small, irregular areas of calcification. The SYT-SSX1 translocation is often found.

Rhabdomyosarcoma

Rhabdomyosarcoma is the most common malignant soft tissue tumor in children. Its four histologic patterns are embryonal, botryoid, alveolar, and pleomorphic. Embryonal rhabdomyosarcoma, the most common type, is characterized by poorly differentiated rhabdomyoblasts and a limited collagen matrix.

Common locations of embryonal rhabdomyosarcoma include the head, neck, genitourinary tract, and retroperitoneum. The histology of botryoid-type lesions is similar to that of embryonal tumors, but the botryoid lesions are in a hollow viscus.

Alveolar rhabdomyosarcoma is characterized by small, round or oval tumor cells loosely arranged in groups surrounded by collagen bundles. Alveolar lesions are more common in the extremities and in older chil-

Figure 8-18: Synovial Cell Sarcoma

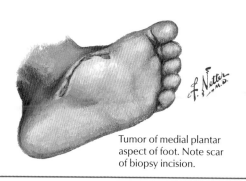

Tumor of medial plantar aspect of foot. Note scar of biopsy incision.

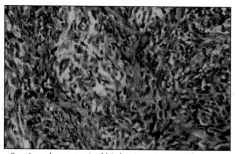

Section shows typical biphasic pattern with accumulation of eosinophilic mucinous material (H and E stain)

dren. A typical presentation is an enlarging mass that causes very little pain even though it may be very large.

Pleomorphic rhabdomyosarcoma, the least common pattern, occurs more frequently in adults. Many previously diagnosed pleomorphic lesions are now classified as malignant fibrous histiocytoma.

Translocation between chromosomes 2 and 13 occurs in 70% of patients with alveolar rhabdomyosarcoma. The other types feature translocation between chromosomes 1 and 13.

Treatment of rhabdomyosarcoma involves a combination of chemotherapy and surgical excision.

Malignant Fibrous Histiocytoma

Malignant fibrous histiocytoma (MFH) is the most common sarcoma of soft tissue in adults (**Figure 8-19**). The condition is more often found in older adults, in males, and in the lower extremity. Presenting symptoms include a mass, pain, or both.

Morphology varies, but histologic studies most commonly show spindle-shaped fibroblasts in a storiform pattern. Areas of myxoid, giant, inflammatory, histiocytic, and angiomatoid cells may be observed. Deeper lesions are often larger at diagnosis and, therefore, have a worse prognosis. The 5-year survival rate is approximately 60% for patients without metastasis at presentation.

Figure 8-19: Malignant Fibrous Histiocytoma of Soft Tissue

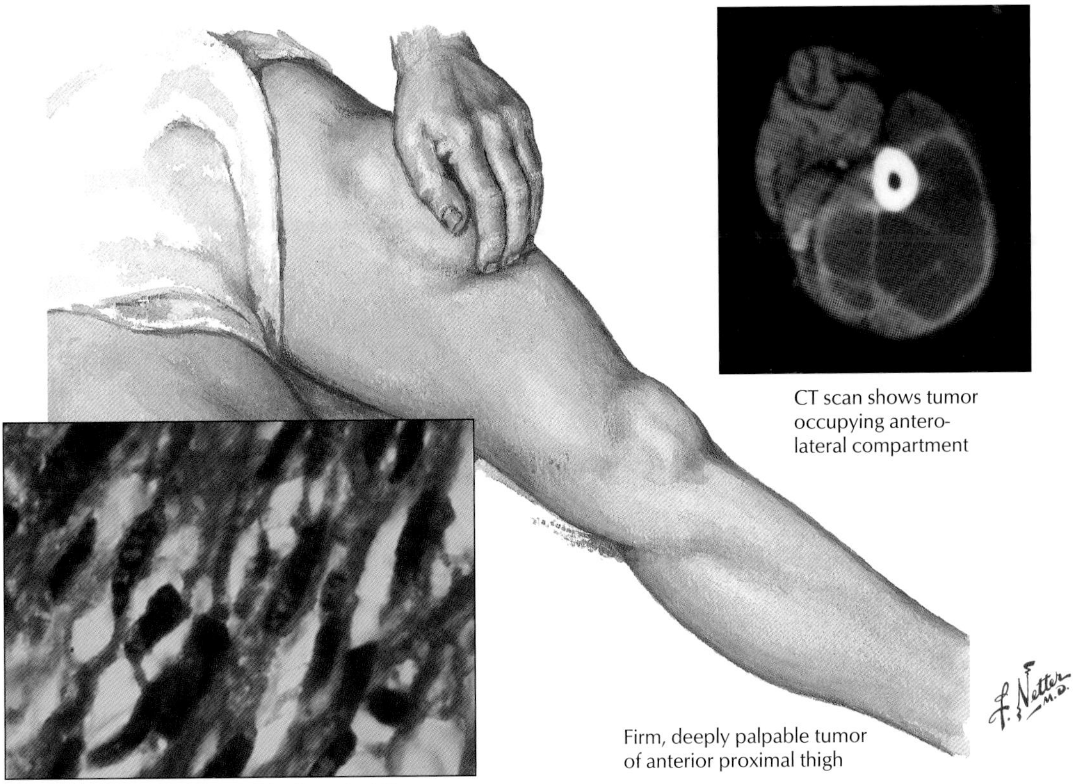

CT scan shows tumor occupying antero-lateral compartment

Firm, deeply palpable tumor of anterior proximal thigh

High-power section reveals characteristic pattern of malignant fibrous stroma and histiocytes (H and E stain)

METASTATIC BONE TUMORS

Metastatic bone tumors are far more common than are primary malignant bone tumors (**Figure 8-20**). Breast, prostate, lung, kidney, and thyroid malignancies are particularly prone to involve bone; however, virtually all patients who die of cancer develop at least microscopic foci of bony metastases during the course of their disease. The spine and pelvis are the most frequent sites of bony metastases, followed by the proximal femur and proximal humerus. Metastases distal to the elbow and knee are uncommon, although lung cancer may involve the hands and, less often, the feet.

Most metastatic bone disease is osteolytic (ie, causes bone dissolution and destruction).

Figure 8-20: Tumors Metastatic to Bone

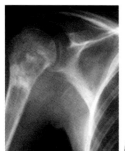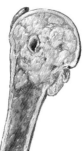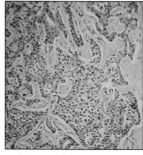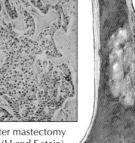

From breast. Tumor of proximal humerus appeared 3 years after mastectomy for carcinoma. Pathology typical of adenocarcinoma of breast (H and E stain).

From thyroid gland. Tumor of distal femur was radiolucent on radiograph. Biopsy findings of colloid-containing follicles typical of thyroid carcinoma (H and E stain).

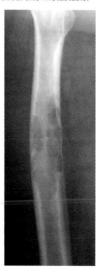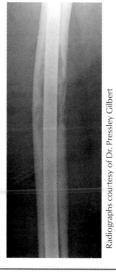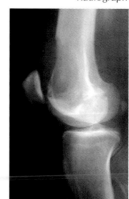

From lung. Initial symptom was painful, erythematous swelling of 5th ray of hand. Chest radiograph showed hilar densities that proved to be source of this unusual site metastasis.

From multiple myeloma. 73-year-old male with progressive, activity-related pain in the thigh. Left radiograph shows radiolucent metastatic lesion with thinning of the cortex. Patient is at significant risk for pathologic fracture. Right radiograph of the femur 3 weeks after prophylactic intramedullary rod fixation. Patient had resolution of pain.

Radiographs courtesy of Dr. Pressley Gilbert

From kidney. Initial symptom was painful mass above knee. Radiograph revealed lytic lesion of femur. Biopsy results indicated adenocarcinoma of kidney, which was confirmed by renal arteriogram and intravenous pyelogram (section below stained with H and E).

Occasionally, breast and prostate metastases are both osteoblastic (causing bone production) and osteolytic in the same patient. Bone necrosis in primary skeletal malignancies is caused by tumor cells. In contrast, bone destruction in metastatic disease results from metastatic tumor cells that produce an *osteoclast-activating factor*. The exact process varies depending on the tumor and is still under investigation. An important part of the process is adherence of the tumor cells to bone and the production of enzymes that facilitate osteoclast-mediated bone destruction.

Patients with skeletal metastases usually seek medical care because of pain or a pathologic fracture. The pain is deep, aching, and often present at rest and at night. Severe pain on walking indicates that bone destruction has progressed to the extent that a pathologic fracture is imminent. Some patients at initial presentation have a bony metastasis but no previous diagnosis of cancer. These patients require a thorough diagnostic evaluation before their skeletal lesions can be treated.

Treatment varies according to the underlying primary disease, the site of skeletal involvement, and the size of the lesion. Chemotherapy may slow growing tumors. Bisphosphonates can markedly slow bone destruction, and are commonly used in metastatic breast carcinoma and multiple myeloma. Radiation therapy decreases pain and controls expansion of the metastasis. Treatment of hypercalcemia of malignancy includes hydration, intravenous bisphosphonate therapy, and effective treatment of the underlying malignancy.

Patients with an existing or impending pathologic fracture often require internal fixation with interlocking intramedullary nails or prosthetic devices. Prophylactic fixation prevents the considerably greater pain and morbidity of a pathologic fracture. The guidelines for intervention, however, are subjective. Factors to consider include the location of the lesion, the amount of cortical bone destruction, the character of the bony involvement, whether stress fracture lines are present, and whether there is pain. The femoral neck, femoral subtrochanteric region, femoral diaphysis, and tibial diaphysis receive greater stress with routine activities, and lesions at these sites are at increased risk for fracture. By comparison, lesions in the pelvis and upper extremity are less likely to fracture. Cortical bone destruction, measured as a percentage of medial, lateral, anterior, and posterior involvement, is an important determinant of fracture risk. The risk of fracture is very high in patients with more than 75% cortical bone destruction and is low in patients with less than 25% cortical destruction; 50% cortical destruction is an indication for prophylactic fixation. Patients with osteoblastic or mixed lesions are less likely to experience fractures than are patients with purely lytic metastases. The presence of an incomplete fracture line on plain radiographs or significant weight-bearing pain strongly suggests an impending fracture. Joint implants are the treatment of choice when the joint surface has been destroyed or an internal fixation device cannot provide rigid fixation.

Before they undergo surgery for internal fixation or joint implants, patients should be tested for anemia, leukopenia, and hypercalcemia. They also should be evaluated for instability of the cervical spine. Some metastatic lesions, particularly renal cell carcinoma, are highly vascular and cause excessive bleeding during skeletal stabilization. Preoperative immobilization may minimize this potential problem.

ADDITIONAL READINGS

Frassica GJ, Frassica DA, Lietman SA, McCarthy EF, Wenz JF. Metastatic bone disease. In: Chapman MW, ed. *Chapman's Orthopaedic Surgery*, 3rd edition. Philadelphia, Pa: Lippincott Williams and Wilkins; 2001:3469–3482.

Simon MA, Springfield DS, Conrad EU, eds. *Surgery for Bone and Soft-Tissue Tumors*. Philadelphia, Pa: Lippincott-Raven; 1998.

Springfield DS, Gebbardt MC. Bone and soft tissue tumors. In: Morrisey RT, Weinstein SL, eds. *Lovell and Winter's Pediatric Orthopaedics*, 5th edition. Philadelphia, Pa: Lippincott Williams and Wilkins; 2001:507–562.

Unni KK. *Dahlin's Bone Tumors: General Aspects and Data on 11,087 Cases*, 5th edition. Baltimore, Md: Lippincott-Raven; 1996.

Fractures and Multitrauma in Adults

Jeffrey O. Anglen, MD, FACS

Trauma is a major public health problem. According to the World Health Organization, traffic accidents kill four times as many people as are killed in wars. Injury is the third leading cause of death in the United States, and in people aged 1 to 44 years, it is the leading cause of death. For each death due to injury, an estimated 180 disabling injuries occur. In the United States, 28.6 million people incur a musculoskeletal injury every year. Approximately half of these injuries result in activity restriction, and the total cost of treatment plus days lost from work is an estimated $41 billion.

As the demographics of industrialized nations shift toward an older population, the incidence of low-impact, *osteoporosis-related fractures* also is increasing. Half of all women and an eighth of all men older than age 50 will have an osteoporosis-related fracture during their lives. In the United States today, 250,000 to 300,000 fractures of the hip are reported in the elderly. A quarter of these patients never return to their prefracture ambulation level. Because the number is expected to double by 2025, this situation is a public health problem of epidemic proportions.

Injury prevention takes several forms. Vehicular modifications such as airbags, seat belts, and crumple zones slow the deceleration of occupants and thus reduce the transfer of kinetic energy, making more accidents survivable. Roadway changes such as improved surfaces, visibility, and traffic control reduce accident occurrence. Injury due to sports participation is reduced by rule modifications and improvements in protective gear. Modification of the environment, such as improved safety mechanisms on machinery or improved lighting in the workplace, and removal of loose throw rugs in the homes of elderly persons, can prevent injuries.

THE PATIENT WITH MULTIPLE TRAUMA

High-energy fractures and multiple sites of injury are in large part a disease of modern times, and most are caused by misuse of motor vehicles, industrial equipment, and cheap handguns. Road traffic accidents are reaching epidemic proportions in the developing nations, and it is estimated that by 2010, they will account for 25% of health care expenditures in those parts of the world.

Fractures contribute significantly to the pathophysiology, morbidity, and mortality of the multiple trauma patient. This is particularly true in patients who have incurred fractures of major long bones or of the pelvis, which can result in substantial blood loss and may cause or worsen hemorrhagic shock. High-energy, markedly displaced fractures create a large amount of devascularized tissue that releases a large quantity of *cytokines*, which, in turn, cause changes in local and systemic hemodynamic regulation, activate the inflammatory system, alter metabolic pathways, and influence endothelial permeability and coagulation. As a result, *adult respiratory distress syndrome* (ARDS; **Figure 9-1**) or even *systemic inflammatory response syndrome* (SIRS), a condition associated with generalized capillary leakage, multiple organ dysfunction, and high metabolic energy consumption, may develop.

Early fracture fixation (within 24 to 48 hours) is beneficial and, for the multitrauma patient, decreases mortality and reduces the risk of pulmonary dysfunction and infectious complications. Furthermore, early fracture stabilization and patient mobilization decrease pain, facilitate nursing care, lower the incidence of skin breakdown, improve gastrointestinal (GI) function, and minimize the psychological effects of trauma. Whether early fracture fixation improves recovery of associated head injuries is controversial. Optimal care of the multiple trauma patient requires prioritization and constant communication and coordination between members of the trauma team. Therefore, patients with multiple injuries are best treated in trauma centers that have the multiple physicians and support staff capable of effectively managing these patients.

Figure 9-1: Adult Respiratory Distress Syndrome (ARDS)

Confusion, disorientation: may progress to coma

Fever

Respiratory distress, tachypnea

Tachycardia

Petechiae

Abnormal blood gasses ($P_{O_2} < 60$ mmHg)

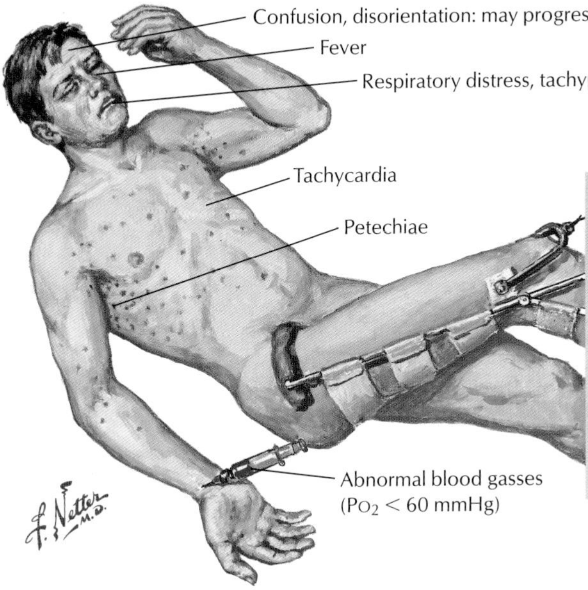

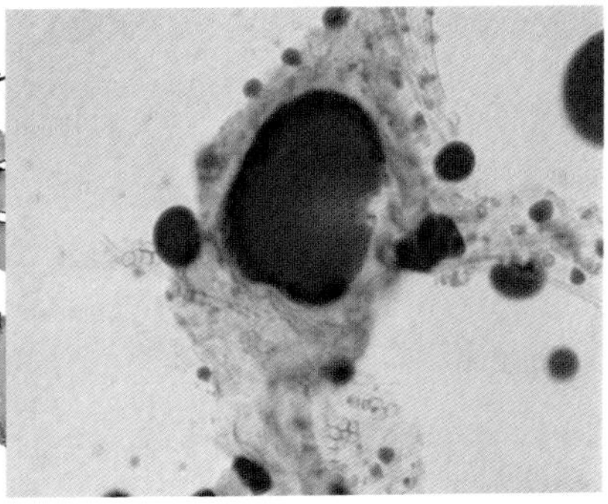

Fat emboli in lung (stained red with Sudan III). Pulmonary edema visible.

Criteria for diagnosis of adult respiratory distress syndrome (ARDS) include an arterial partial pressure of oxygen/fraction of inspired oxygen (PaO_2/FiO_2) ratio less than 200 for 5 or more consecutive days, bilateral diffuse infiltrates on the chest radiograph in the absence of pneumonia, and absence of cardiogenic pulmonary edema. Associated findings of petechiae and confusion merge into systemic inflammatory response syndrome (SIRS).

PHYSIOLOGY OF MUSCULOSKELETAL REPAIR

Bone Fracture and Healing

The ability of any given bone to resist applied forces depends on many factors, including the bone's strength or density, the direction and rate of loading, the type of load applied, and the capability of surrounding muscles and ligaments to absorb part of the injury force. Different loading modes result in different fracture patterns. For example, loading the bone in tension typically results in a transverse fracture, whereas torsional forces produce spiral fractures. Short oblique fractures are caused by axial (compressive) loading, and a long oblique fracture results from a combination of axial and rotational load. A Y-shaped butterfly fracture pattern indicates a bending force (**Figure 9-2**).

Cortical bone and cancellous (trabecular) bone have different mechanical properties; however, both cortical and cancellous bones are stronger when loaded in compression compared with tension. The magnitude of the load required to fracture a bone is reduced in certain disease states that make bone weaker or more brittle, such as osteoporosis, metabolic bone disease, tumor, or infection.

Bone healing is a complex, yet usually reliable, biologic process that has the unique result of complete regeneration of the supporting tissue (bone) rather than healing with scar tissue, as occurs in many other organs. Bone healing requires living tissues with adequate vascularity and involves sequential coordination of a large number of cell types and biologic signals. The process, as we understand it, is summarized in the following section, but the intricate details remain a fascinating mystery and an area of active research.

Fracture repair can be divided into four histologic stages: inflammation, soft callus, hard callus, and remodeling (**Figure 9-3**). The *inflammation stage* begins immediately after injury and is characterized by pain, warmth, tenderness, instability, and, occasionally, fever. Bleeding from the broken bone and

Figure 9-2: Fracture Patterns

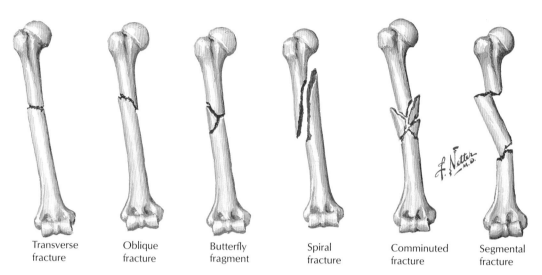

| Transverse fracture | Oblique fracture | Butterfly fragment | Spiral fracture | Comminuted fracture | Segmental fracture |

associated soft tissue injury result in a "fracture hematoma," release of cytokines, clot formation, and migration of acute inflammatory cells into the site of injury. Fibroblasts, mesenchymal cells, and osteoprogenitor cells arrive shortly thereafter. The low pO_2 at the fracture site promotes angiogenesis.

The *soft callus stage* is a period of increased vascularity, resorption of necrotic bone ends, and development of a fibrocartilage callus (collar) that surrounds the fracture. The soft callus progressively widens and stiffens so that at the end of this stage, the bone ends are no longer freely mobile. The *hard callus stage* involves calcification of the fibrocartilage and its conversion into woven bone. During this process, variable amounts of enchondral ossification (conversion of cartilage to bone) and intramembranous bone formation (direct deposition of bone onto surfaces) are noted. The proportions of each depend on the degree of fracture displacement, as well as the type of fracture fixation.

Remodeling, the fourth and final stage of bone healing, may go on for months or years. Remodeling involves the conversion of weaker, woven bone into stronger, lamellar bone by the synchronized function of osteoclasts and osteoblasts organized into "cutting cones" that move through the woven bone, reconstituting the haversian canal system and lamellar bone. Remodeling also responds to biomechanical forces, so that more bone is deposited in areas of greater mechanical stress (Wolff law).

Healing of small, stable defects in bone can proceed by direct, appositional (intramembranous) bone formation. Similarly, fracture lines that can be very well reduced and rendered stable by compression fixation may heal without significant callus formation through a combination of intramembranous bone formation and haversian remodeling across points of stable gap contact (**Figure 9-4**).

Fracture healing at all stages is sensitive to the mechanical environment. The amount of interfragmentary motion or strain that occurs has a significant effect on the differentiation of tissues within the fracture gap, and if strain exceeds the tolerance of the tissue type present, healing may stall. Thus, the theory of "strain tolerance" postulates that only tissues able to tolerate the ambient mechanical strain can differentiate in a fracture gap. As the tissue evolves from loose fibrous tissue to cartilage to bone, the strain tolerance drops; thus, differentiation and progressive healing require progressively less strain or interfragmentary motion. In general, healing bones respond positively to controlled axial loading,

Figure 9-3: Healing of Fracture

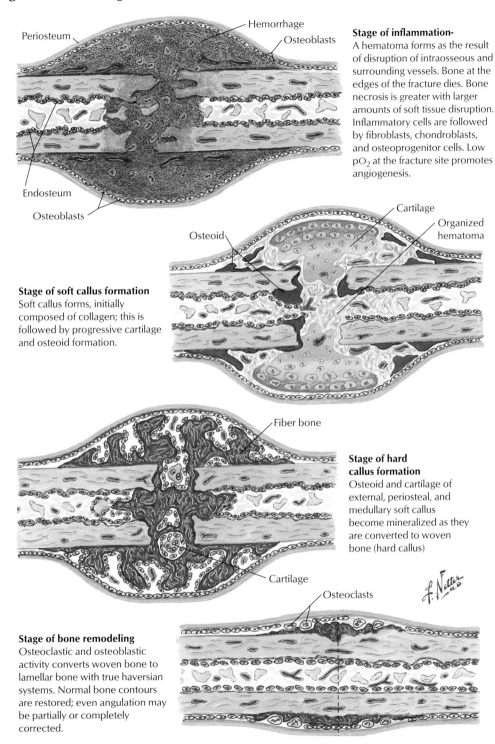

Periosteum
Hemorrhage
Osteoblasts
Endosteum
Osteoblasts

Stage of inflammation-
A hematoma forms as the result of disruption of intraosseous and surrounding vessels. Bone at the edges of the fracture dies. Bone necrosis is greater with larger amounts of soft tissue disruption. Inflammatory cells are followed by fibroblasts, chondroblasts, and osteoprogenitor cells. Low pO_2 at the fracture site promotes angiogenesis.

Cartilage
Organized hematoma
Osteoid

Stage of soft callus formation
Soft callus forms, initially composed of collagen; this is followed by progressive cartilage and osteoid formation.

Fiber bone

Stage of hard callus formation
Osteoid and cartilage of external, periosteal, and medullary soft callus become mineralized as they are converted to woven bone (hard callus)

Cartilage
Osteoclasts

Stage of bone remodeling
Osteoclastic and osteoblastic activity converts woven bone to lamellar bone with true haversian systems. Normal bone contours are restored; even angulation may be partially or completely corrected.

Figure 9-4: Primary Union

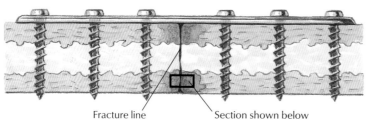

Fracture line   Section shown below

If fractured bone ends are compressed securely so that no motion can take place between them, callus does not form. Dead bone at fracture site not resorbed but revitalized by ingrowth of haversian systems.

Mechanism of healing by primary union

Dead bone Osteoclastic activity Vascular ingrowth Fracture line Osteoid Lamella of new bone Osteoblasts

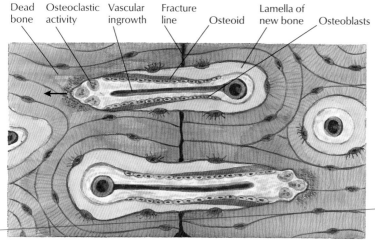

Osteoclasts ream out tunnels through dead bone at fracture edges and across fracture line into opposite bone fragment. Osteoblasts line new tunnels and lay down new lamellae around them to form new osteons, restoring continuity of bone.

a concept that is the principle of functional bracing and early weight bearing. The link between a mechanical stimulus and the biologic response is strain-associated electrical potentials generated when bone is loaded, which leads to an increase in *cytosolic Ca^{++}* and an increase in *activated cytoskeletal calmodulin*, which induces an increase in transforming growth factor-β (TGF-β).

A variety of local and systemic conditions influence fracture healing. Open fractures and high-energy fractures associated with disruption of the surrounding soft tissues and vascular supply have a higher rate of delayed union or nonunion. Other factors that delay bone healing include advanced age, medical illnesses such as diabetes mellitus, malnutrition, poor oxygenation, smoking, long-term corticosteroid use, and deficiencies in vitamin D, vitamin C, retinoic acid,

growth hormone, thyroid hormone, and anabolic steroids.

Soft Tissue Healing

Soft tissue (ie, muscle, ligament, and tendon) healing also proceeds in phases (see Chapter 5). Fracture fixation that allows early motion also has a beneficial effect on ligament and tendon healing, with more rapid reorientation of collagen bundles, as well as increased fibril size and density.

FRACTURE TREATMENT

Although the Hippocratic physicians of ancient Greece left an extensive literature on musculoskeletal injuries, throughout most of human history, treatment of fractures was performed by folk medicine practitioners. These "bone setters" made the diagnosis by examination and history, and their treatments involved local application of poultices, lotions, or ointments; massage; manual traction or manipulation; bandages and splints; and rest, accompanied by the use of charms, incantations, or prayers.

In the 1500s, a shift from the use of classical languages (Greek, Latin, and Arabic) to the use of vernacular in the publication of medical texts allowed a wider dissemination of knowledge. The recorded history of fracture treatment over the following 300 years is interesting and filled with ingenious uses of splints, bandages, traction, and other closed methods. However, the surgical treatment of fractures was very limited and was usually unsuccessful until the introduction of anesthetic and aseptic techniques that lessened pain and the risk of infection. Wilhelm Roentgen's discovery of x-rays in 1895 accelerated the evolution of surgical treatment of fracture. *External fixation* was introduced in 1897 by Clayton Parkhill of Denver, and by Albin Lambotte of Belgium in 1902. By the late 1930s, the use of *intramedullary fixation* was established, largely because of the work of the Rush brothers from Mississippi and Gerhard Küntscher in Germany. In the 1940s, Robert Danis of Belgium designed and used *plates for internal fixation* that enhanced axial compression and stability. In the late 1950s, Maurice Müller of Switzerland, a student of Danis, brought together orthopaedic surgeons and engineers to form the Arbeitsgemeinschaft für Osteosynthesefragen (Association for the Study of Internal Fixation or AO), an organization that continues to study and improve the operative care of fractures.

Fracture care continues to evolve. Implants with new designs and made of newer materials, such as biodegradable polymers, plastics, and ceramics, are constantly being developed. New techniques, such as microvascular free tissue transfer, bone transport and limb lengthening, indirect reduction, and minimally invasive fracture surgery, have extended the possibilities for managing severely injured limbs.

As always, the goal of fracture treatment is to return patients to their preinjury activity level as quickly as possible while minimizing the risk of complications. The care of each patient must be individualized, taking into consideration patient factors such as age, occupation, medical health, and individual risk expectations, as well as injury-related factors such as the nature and number of injuries and concomitant soft tissue trauma.

Evaluation

Assessment of an injured patient begins with a history and physical examination. In the high-energy polytrauma patient, one begins with the "ABC" assessment of airway, breathing, and circulation. Evaluation of the musculoskeletal system is part of the secondary survey, conducted after life-threatening conditions have been ruled out.

The history of the event provides clues to the amount of tissue damage, which is determined by *kinetic energy transfer* (K_E), which in turn is related to *mass* (M) and *velocity* (V) by the equation $K_E = \frac{1}{2}MV^2$. For example, a fall from a curb involves approximately 100 ft-lb of energy; a skiing accident, 300 to 500 ft-lb; a high-velocity gunshot, 2000 ft-lb; and a bumper strike injury, up to 100,000 ft-lb. The mechanism of injury also provides clues about which specific fracture or fractures might be expected. For example, a dashboard injury resulting in an acetabular fracture may also injure the cruciate ligaments in the knee. The time since injury and the setting of the injury (particularly, open fractures) may influence the risk of infection or other complications. Additional complaints of painful areas should be solicited, particularly in the patient who has sustained high-energy trauma. Furthermore, one should seek information about concomitant conditions that may affect treatment decisions, such as diabetes mellitus, infectious disease exposure, heart disease, medication use, allergies, tobacco use, and complications from previous operations and anesthesia.

Physical examination of the high-energy trauma patient should include inspection, palpation, and range-of-motion testing of every bone and joint in a systematic, head-to-toe fashion. Take note of swelling, tenderness, ecchymosis, crepitus, and instability.

Record the presence and any asymmetry of pulses and capillary refill. Palpate soft tissue compartments for possible compartment syndromes. Perform specific motor and sensory examination of nerve roots possibly injured by a spinal fracture, or peripheral nerves possibly injured by an extremity fracture (see **Table 6-1** and **6-2**). Documentation should be specific. For example, "wiggles toes" is not an adequate description or adequate neurologic examination. Open wounds should be noted, and their locations, size, and nature should be described or drawn. After inspection, wounds are covered with a sterile dressing until definitive treatment can be rendered, and fractures are splinted to reduce pain and to protect surrounding soft tissues.

Radiographs of suspected sites of injury should include a good-quality anteroposterior and lateral film that shows the joint above and the joint below the suspected fracture. Additional views are obtained depending on the specific injury. Screening radiographs of the cervical spine and pelvis are obtained in a trauma patient who is obtunded or intubated, or who has multiple painful injuries or unexplained neurologic deficits.

A description of a fracture includes its location, fracture pattern, displacement, and angulation. Location is diaphyseal, metaphyseal, or intra-articular, with diaphyseal fractures further classified as proximal third, middle third, or distal third. Fracture patterns are transverse, short oblique, long oblique, spiral, comminuted, or segmental (see **Figure 9-2**). Displacement and angulation are indicated by reference to the position of the distal portion relative to the proximal portion. Displacement patterns include nondisplacement, minimal displacement, coronal or sagittal translation, rotation, and/or shortening (overlap of fracture fragments). Angulation in the coronal plane is described by *varus,* which means that the distal fragment is angulated toward the midline of the body, or *valgus,* which means that the distal fragment is angled away from the midline (**Figure 9-5**).

Principles of Treatment

Fractures that are nondisplaced or minimally displaced do not require reduction and are mostly immobilized in situ by external devices (eg, casts or splints) for comfort and protection. Internal fixation or external fixation may be required in sites that are difficult to immobilize and that have significant potential risk for displacement (eg, femoral neck fracture).

To reduce a fracture means to realign the fragments, to correct the displacements—in lay terms, to "set the bone." Reduction may be performed by closed means (manipulation of the extremity) or by open techniques (surgical procedures).

Anatomic reduction restores the position of the fragments exactly to their preinjury condition (i.e., the exact shape of the bone is reestablished). This is the goal in treating intra-articular fractures, in which near-perfect alignment of the articular surface is necessary to minimize the risk of traumatic arthropathy. For many fractures, however, anatomic reduction is not necessary and only certain components of the displacement need to be corrected. For example, diaphyseal fractures of a long bone, such as the femur, do not need anatomic reduction but do need to have approximately the correct length, rotation, and reasonable alignment restored so that the hip and knee have the correct relationship to each other.

Once the fracture has been reduced adequately, some form of stabilization is needed for comfort and to prevent re-displacement. After closed reduction has been performed, stabilization is usually provided through a cast, splint, or brace that incorporates the joint above and the joint below the fracture. For example, a displaced fracture of the distal radius treated by closed manipulation and casting typically requires immobilization of the elbow and wrist (a long-arm cast; **Figure 9-6**).

Skeletal traction may provide temporary stabilization, but because of the deleterious effects of prolonged bed rest and the development of better fixation devices, skeletal traction is rarely used today for definitive treatment of fracture in adults.

Figure 9-5: Types of Displacement

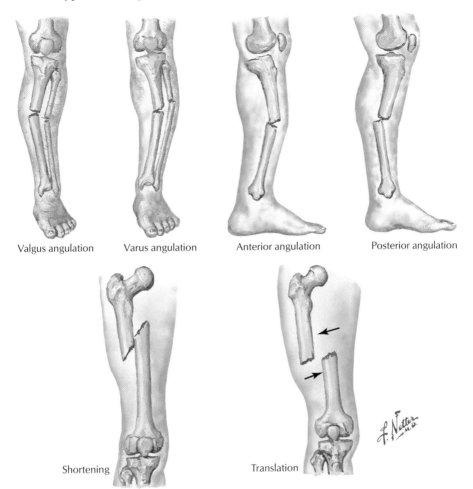

Valgus angulation   Varus angulation   Anterior angulation   Posterior angulation

Shortening   Translation

External fixators have pins or wires that are inserted through or into the bone and connected to external frames (**Figure 9-7**). These are used most commonly when there is damage to the soft tissues, such as occurs with open fractures, burns, or compartment syndromes, or in fractures that do not require internal fixation but require greater fixation than can be obtained with a cast (eg, certain metaphyseal fractures of the distal radius, proximal tibia, and distal tibia).

Implants available for internal fixation include plates and screws, intramedullary nails, pins, wires, staples, and sutures. Screws may be used to attach bone fragments together directly, and when inserted in a manner that compresses the fracture, they are known as *lag screws*. More often, screws are used to attach a plate to the bone, which then functions as an internal splint or a buttress that significantly increases fracture stabilization (**Figure 9-8**).

Intramedullary nails are commonly used for fixation of long-bone diaphyseal fractures, particularly in the femur, tibia, and humerus. Rods are inserted through small incisions distant from the fracture site, thus minimizing disruption of the fracture wound and the risk of infection. Intramedullary rods are biomechanically favorable because of their location near the axis of the long bone. They can be

Figure 9-6: Closed Reduction

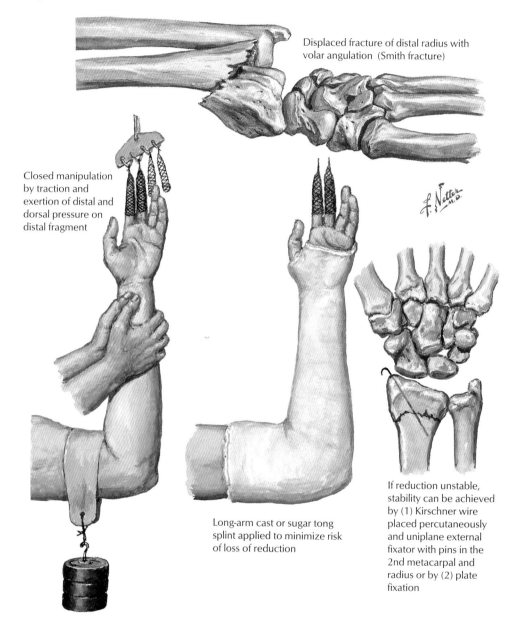

Displaced fracture of distal radius with volar angulation (Smith fracture)

Closed manipulation by traction and exertion of distal and dorsal pressure on distal fragment

Long-arm cast or sugar tong splint applied to minimize risk of loss of reduction

If reduction unstable, stability can be achieved by (1) Kirschner wire placed percutaneously and uniplane external fixator with pins in the 2nd metacarpal and radius or by (2) plate fixation

Figure 9-7: External Fixation

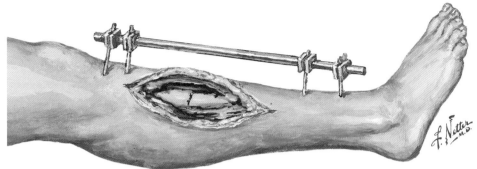

External fixation device stabilizes open fracture and allows access to wound for dressing changes.
Delayed primary closure and placement of intramedullary nail after 3 to 8 days, if wound remains clean

locked proximally and distally to provide stability against rotational or longitudinal displacement (**Figure 9-9**).

A variety of other implants are used in specific locations. Fractures of the patella and olecranon are commonly treated with a technique known as *tension band wiring*. Smooth pin fixation may be used in the hand or foot, or in pediatric fractures, where the forces are weaker, the healing is more prompt, and the size of the bone does not work well with bigger implants.

Figure 9-8: Compression or Buttress Plate

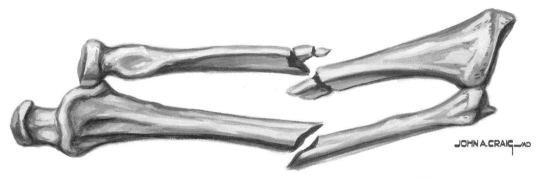

Fractures of radius and ulna with angulation, shortening, and comminution of ulna

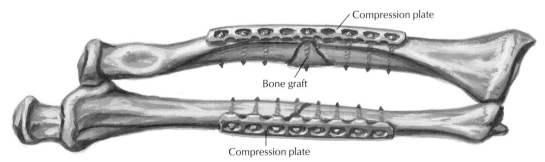

Compression plate

Bone graft

Compression plate

Open reduction and fixation with compression plates and screws through both cortices. Good alignment with restoration of radial bow and interosseous space

Figure 9-9: Interlocked Intramedullary Nail

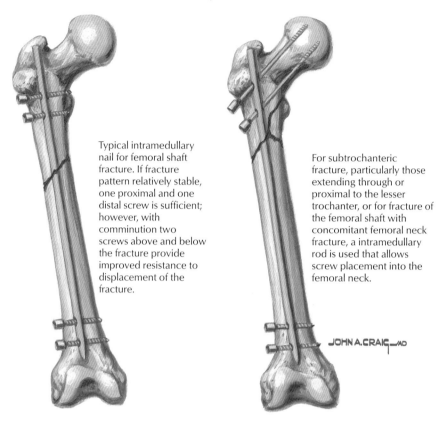

Typical intramedullary nail for femoral shaft fracture. If fracture pattern relatively stable, one proximal and one distal screw is sufficient; however, with comminution two screws above and below the fracture provide improved resistance to displacement of the fracture.

For subtrochanteric fracture, particularly those extending through or proximal to the lesser trochanter, or for fracture of the femoral shaft with concomitant femoral neck fracture, a intramedullary rod is used that allows screw placement into the femoral neck.

JOHN A. CRAIG—AD

Protection and Rehabilitation

The bone must be protected from excessive deformation during healing. *Stable fracture patterns* allow part of the load to be transmitted across the fracture, and they permit early weight bearing in a cast or after internal fixation. *Unstable fracture patterns* do not provide load sharing across the fracture and must be protected by activity restriction or supplemental bracing until adequate healing has occurred.

The *goals of rehabilitation* are to return joints to full range of motion, maintain muscle strength and endurance, and return the patient to as close to full prefracture activity as possible. Joint stiffness and muscle atrophy result from immobilization after injury, and their degree is related to the severity of the injury and the duration of immobilization. Stable fixation facilitates early motion, and early functional weight bearing promotes fracture healing. Early motion is particularly desirable for intra-articular fractures.

Fracture Surgery

The indications for surgery in fracture treatment are as follows, in approximate order of priority:

1. To limit or control life-threatening hemorrhage (as in pelvic fracture reduction).

2. To restore vascularity or nerve function to a limb (as in fractures with vascular injury or vascular embarrassment, such as femoral neck fractures in young adults, neurologic compromise, or compartment syndrome).

3. To prevent infection (as in open fractures).

4. To prevent serious complications of immobilization, such as ARDS or severe joint stiffness (as in a "floating" joint, when there are fractures on both sides of a joint).

5. To achieve and maintain adequate reduction when it cannot be adequately accomplished by closed means (eg, displaced articular fractures, some metaphyseal fractures, and some shaft fractures [femur]).

6. To allow healing in certain fractures that have a high incidence of nonunion when they are treated closed (eg, femoral neck fracture).

7. To facilitate self-care (as in bilateral fractures of the humerus).

8. To allow earlier, better, and less complicated healing (as in some tibial shaft fractures).

The benefits of fracture surgery must always be balanced against the risks of complications, which include infection, wound-healing problems, nerve or vascular injury, delayed union or nonunion, hardware failure, malunion, joint damage, and anesthetic complications. Certain patient characteristics may increase the risk of complications and limit the likelihood of successful achievement of surgical goals. Examples are significant osteoporosis that would compromise fixation; significant medical illness, such as diabetes mellitus, vascular disease, or malnutrition that would impair wound and bone healing; heavy use of tobacco, drugs, or alcohol, which might lead to wound failure or noncompliance; psychiatric disease or personality disor-

der; and a low preinjury functional level that would lower the potential benefits of surgery. The surgeon must evaluate the risks of surgery in each individual patient and balance them against its realistic benefits before discussing treatment options with the patient.

SPECIAL CONDITIONS
Open Fractures

Open fractures are fractures in which a breach in the overlying skin forms, allowing contamination of bone and tissues. Open fractures are at high risk for infection and other complications such as nonunion, delayed union, or malunion. The primary determinant of risk level is severity of the associated soft tissue injury, and for that reason, open fractures are classified according to the size and nature of the soft tissue disruption.

In the Gustilo and Anderson classification (**Figure 9-10**), Type I open fractures have a small (<1 cm) opening in the skin and no significant muscle necrosis or stripping of periosteum from bone. These fractures are usually of relatively low energy without extensive comminution or displacement. Type II open fractures have a larger skin disruption (larger than 1 cm but smaller than 10 cm) but no sig-

Figure 9-10: Gustilo and Anderson Classification of Open Fractures

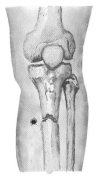 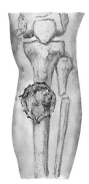 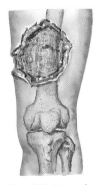 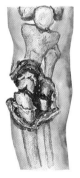 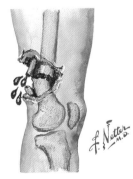

Type I. Wound <1 cm long

Type II. Wound 1 to 10 cm long but without significant soft tissue stripping, gross contamination, or high-energy fracture patterns

Type IIIA. Wound >10 cm long or lesser skin lesions with gross contamination and/or high-energy fracture patterns. Bone coverage adequate

Type IIIB. Extensive soft tissue stripping that typically needs some type of soft tissue flap for coverage

Type IIIC. Large wound with major arterial injury

nificant stripping of periosteum, gross contamination, or high-energy fracture pattern. Type IIIA fractures have extensive lacerations or soft tissue flaps (>10 cm), or lesser skin lesions with gross contamination and/or high-energy fracture patterns. Type IIIB fractures have significant stripping of periosteum and muscle from bone and frequently require some type of soft tissue flap for coverage. Type IIIC fractures have a major vascular injury that requires repair for the limb to be saved.

Open fractures are treated with emergency surgery to minimize the risks of infection and nonunion. Wounds are treated with débridement (removal of all foreign material and devitalized tissue) and irrigation to lower the bacterial load and create a clean, live wound that can repel infection and heal. Stabilizing the fracture promotes vascularization of the wound and is important in preventing infection and promoting bone healing. Stabilization strategies, however, sometimes must be altered in the face of an open fracture. Compared with casts and splints, external fixation provides good access to the wound for dressing changes. External fixation also provides stability without implantation of foreign material at the fracture site. However, external fixation devices are bulky, often interfere with muscle and joint rehabilitation, and, in many situations, do not do as good a job of fixation as plates or intramedullary devices. Therefore, when the wound is adequately cleansed and débrided, fracture fixation with these devices provides better results.

However, if there is doubt about healing, a temporary external fixator may be used until the soft tissue envelope is stabilized, at which time standard plate or intramedullary fixation can be performed with less risk of postoperative wound complications. Patients with open fractures need appropriate tetanus coverage and prophylactic antibiotics. Most protocols include 3 days of cephalosporin administration for grade I and II open fractures, and 5 days of administration of cephalosporin plus an aminoglycoside for grade III open fractures. Gross contamination with soil, injuries in agricultural settings, or aquatic injuries may require additional antibiotics, most commonly anaerobic coverage of bacteria with penicillin. To minimize the risk of abscess formation, open fracture wounds are usually left open and are allowed to heal by themselves, or they are closed in a delayed fashion or covered with flaps or grafts within a week, if conditions permit. A variety of wound care techniques may be used while coverage is awaited, including vacuum-assisted wound closure.

In the treatment of a patient with severely mangled extremities, it is often difficult to decide between attempting limb salvage and performing early amputation. Early amputation is indicated under the following circumstances (refer to Chapter 11 also):

✦ The limb is nonviable (ie, is severely crushed, has had warm ischemia for longer than 8 hours, or has unrepairable vascular injury).

✦ The patient has shock and severe multisystem injuries and thus could not tolerate a prolonged salvage procedure or ongoing blood loss.

✦ The patient has a severe chronic medical illness (eg, vascular disease or diabetes mellitus) that would compromise the success of limb salvage and limb function.

✦ The surgical team believes the time, pain, and ultimate functional results of required reconstruction are not what the patient can, or would want to, withstand.

Treatment of Nonunion

Occasionally, fracture healing fails, and the result is a nonunion, which is defined as a fracture that has failed to unite and that has not demonstrated any progress of healing for 2 to 3 months after the expected time of healing. A related concept is delayed union, in which the healing process has not progressed as expected in the 6 to 9 months after injury. Some delayed unions eventually demonstrate healing; others progress to an obvious nonunion.

A variety of causes lead to nonunion, but, most commonly, it can be attributed to some disturbance in vascularity or inadequate stability. Noncompliance, neuropathy, alcohol abuse, and smoking are contributory causes. It is important to consider, and seek evidence of, a low-grade infection in any nonunion, although bones can and do heal in the presence of infection.

Hypertrophic nonunions have a good blood supply to both fragments, show various degrees of callus formation, and can be treated by enhancing mechanical stability at the fracture site by internal or external fixation and/or by electrical stimulation. *Atrophic or dysvascular nonunions* are associated with necrosis of bone, show no evidence of callus, often have gaps at the fracture site, and require excision of the devitalized bone, as well as implantation of a biologic stimulus (eg, bone graft) and a mechanical stabilizing device (**Figure 9-11**). Large defects may require vascularized bone transplant or local bone transport. Bone stimulators that deliver an electromagnetic signal or a low-intensity ultrasonographic signal may facilitate the healing process.

Fractures With Neurologic or Vascular Compromise

Every injured extremity should undergo detailed neurologic and vascular examination. When deficits are noted, they should be carefully documented before any manipulation is begun, then gentle reduction and splinting should be performed. If function does not return, emergent intervention to restore blood flow may be necessary.

A protocol for the coordinated management of fractures with vascular disruption is helpful. In most cases, arteriography causes an unnecessary delay, and the patient should be taken promptly to the operating room for restoration of blood flow. This treatment may involve a temporary arterial shunt while the fracture wound is treated, or temporary external fixation while the vascular injury is repaired or grafted, then definitive fracture treatment.

Neurologic deficits should be documented and, in most cases, observed in anticipation of eventual recovery. Neurologic deficits that develop during manipulation of a fracture warrant investigation and may require surgical exploration. Fractures that are likely to have an associated nerve injury include the following: radial nerve palsy with fracture of the humeral shaft, median nerve injury with fracture of the distal radius, sciatic nerve injury with hip dislocation or acetabular fracture, and peroneal nerve injury with knee dislocation or tibial plateau fracture (**Figure 9-12**).

Compartment Syndrome

Compartment syndrome is a devastating condition that occurs when the pressure in a closed fascial space rises enough to occlude capillary blood flow, rendering the enclosed muscles and nerves ischemic. It can have a variety of causes such as bleeding into a compartment from arterial injury, infiltration of fluids, overly tight bandages, swelling of the muscle due to injury, reperfusion after ischemia, burns, prolonged pressure, marked and prolonged elevation of the extremity, or overexertion (**Figure 9-13**). Compartment syndrome occurs most commonly in the calf and forearm, but it also may occur in the thigh, buttock, foot, hand, or upper arm.

Early diagnosis is essential because early treatment restores blood flow and prevents irreversible ischemia and resultant muscle and nerve necrosis. When the patient is able to communicate, the earliest, most consistent, and most reliable sign is deep, unrelenting, and somewhat vague but progressive pain that is *out of proportion to the injury* and not responsive to normal doses of pain medication. The pain is exacerbated by passive motion stretch of the involved muscles. For example, plantar flexing the ankle or toes increases pain when the anterior compartment of the leg is involved. The compartment usually feels hard or tense to the touch, especially when compared with the contralateral limb; the skin is tight and shiny and cannot be wrinkled. Other signs (eg, pallor, paresthesia, paralysis, and pulselessness) are late findings or are unreliable.

Treatment of compartment syndrome should be initiated upon clinical diagnosis. In equivocal cases, measuring the pressure in the compartment with a handheld device or adapted manometer can provide useful information. Pressure measurement is also useful in obtunded, intubated, or unreliable patients

Figure 9-11: Nonunion of Fracture

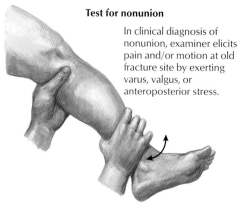

Test for nonunion

In clinical diagnosis of nonunion, examiner elicits pain and/or motion at old fracture site by exerting varus, valgus, or anteroposterior stress.

JOHN A. CRAIG—MD

f. Netter M.D.

Atrophic (dysvacular) nonunion

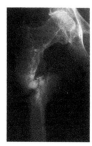 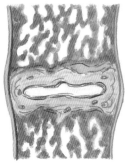

Radiograph shows wide tissue gap and no evidence of callus

Histologic section shows false joint lined with synovial membrane and filled with fluid

Surgical management of atrophic tibial nonunion

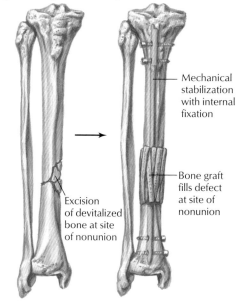

Mechanical stabilization with internal fixation

Bone graft fills defect at site of nonunion

Excision of devitalized bone at site of nonunion

Hypertrophic nonunion

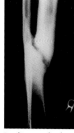 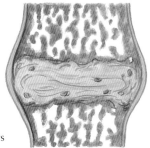

Radiograph shows hypertrophic nonunion of tibia fracture with callus formation

Histologic section shows fracture gap filled with nonossified fibrous cartilage

Devitalized bone excised from site of nonunion. Bone graft implanted and tibia mechanically stabilized via internal fixation

Classification of nonunions

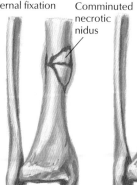 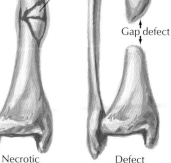 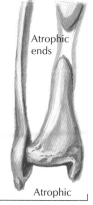

Callus

Comminuted necrotic nidus

Atrophic ends

Gap defect

| Hypertrophic nonunion | Dystrophic | Necrotic | Defect | Atrophic |

Hypertrophic nonunion | Atrophic (dysvascular) nonunions

Figure 9-12: Neurologic Complications of Fractures

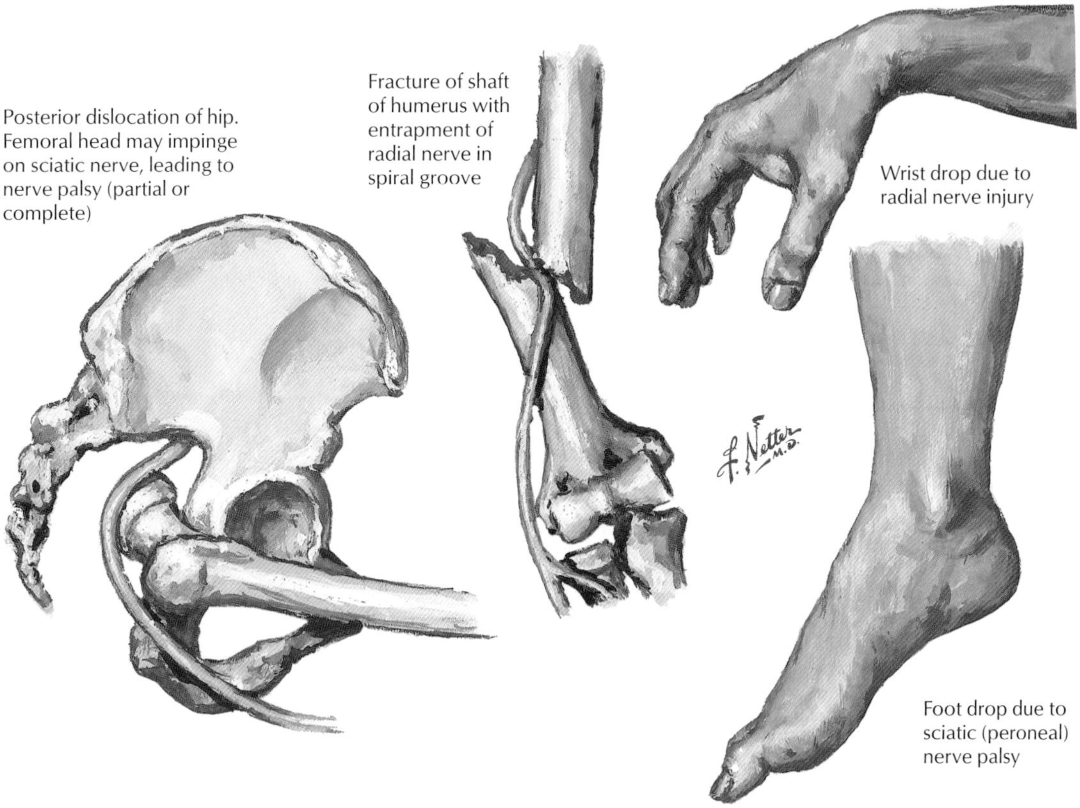

Posterior dislocation of hip. Femoral head may impinge on sciatic nerve, leading to nerve palsy (partial or complete)

Fracture of shaft of humerus with entrapment of radial nerve in spiral groove

Wrist drop due to radial nerve injury

Foot drop due to sciatic (peroneal) nerve palsy

who have a swollen extremity but who otherwise cannot be evaluated. A variety of cutoff pressures have been advocated, but despite numerous studies, there is still disagreement on whether the tissue pressure beyond which capillary circulation ceases and ischemia ensues is an absolute amount or is dependent on the patient's systemic blood pressure. A useful formula is that a compartment syndrome is usually present when the diastolic pressure minus the compartment pressure is less than or equal to 30 mm Hg.

When compartment syndrome is suspected, the limb should be placed at a level equal to the heart, and all casts or dressings should be split to the skin. When the diagnosis is made, the patient should be taken emergently to the operating theater for decompressive *fasciotomy*. All tight compartments must be released. In the calf, all four compart-

ments should be released. Fasciotomy performed through limited skin incisions may compromise results through inadequate release or damage to nerves or blood vessels.

Stress Fracture

Stress fracture, also known as *fatigue fracture*, is a failure of bone that is subjected to multiple repetitive strain cycles, which results in microcracks in the bone. If the repetitive loading continues, these cracks may accumulate faster than the bone can heal them. The result is a complete fracture (**Figure 9-14**). The most common site is the metatarsal, where more than half of stress fractures are found. The calcaneus and tibia account for most of the other half, with the femoral neck and navicular making up less than 5%.

The most common cause of stress fracture is a recent increase in a person's level of load-

Figure 9-13: Compartment Syndrome

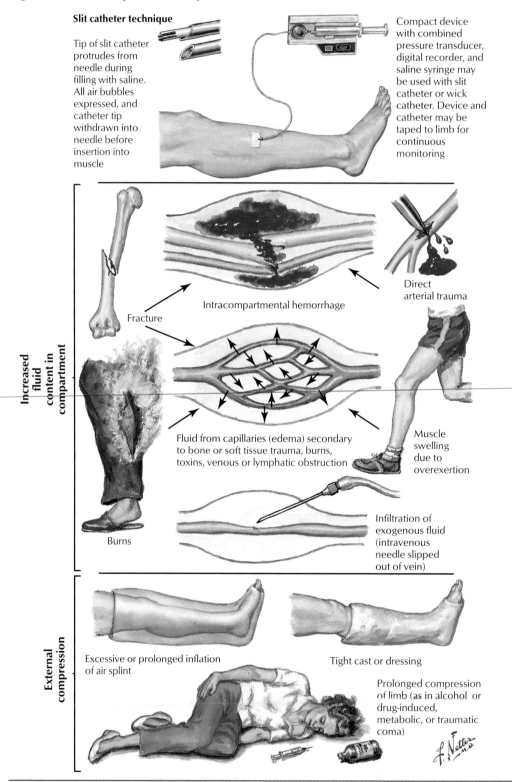

Slit catheter technique

Tip of slit catheter protrudes from needle during filling with saline. All air bubbles expressed, and catheter tip withdrawn into needle before insertion into muscle

Compact device with combined pressure transducer, digital recorder, and saline syringe may be used with slit catheter or wick catheter. Device and catheter may be taped to limb for continuous monitoring

Increased fluid content in compartment

Fracture

Intracompartmental hemorrhage

Direct arterial trauma

Fluid from capillaries (edema) secondary to bone or soft tissue trauma, burns, toxins, venous or lymphatic obstruction

Muscle swelling due to overexertion

Burns

Infiltration of exogenous fluid (intravenous needle slipped out of vein)

External compression

Excessive or prolonged inflation of air splint

Tight cast or dressing

Prolonged compression of limb (as in alcohol or drug-induced, metabolic, or traumatic coma)

Figure 9-13: Compartment Syndrome (continued)

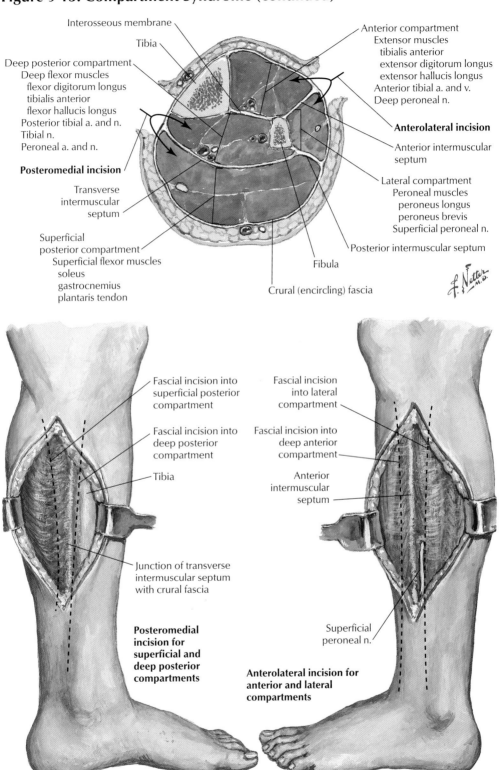

Interosseous membrane

Tibia

Deep posterior compartment
  Deep flexor muscles
    flexor digitorum longus
    tibialis anterior
    flexor hallucis longus
  Posterior tibial a. and n.
  Tibial n.
  Peroneal a. and n.

Posteromedial incision

Transverse
intermuscular
septum

Superficial
posterior compartment
  Superficial flexor muscles
    soleus
    gastrocnemius
    plantaris tendon

Anterior compartment
  Extensor muscles
    tibialis anterior
    extensor digitorum longus
    extensor hallucis longus
  Anterior tibial a. and v.
  Deep peroneal n.

Anterolateral incision

Anterior intermuscular
septum

Lateral compartment
  Peroneal muscles
    peroneus longus
    peroneus brevis
  Superficial peroneal n.

Posterior intermuscular septum

Fibula

Crural (encircling) fascia

Fascial incision into
superficial posterior
compartment

Fascial incision into
deep posterior
compartment

Tibia

Junction of transverse
intermuscular septum
with crural fascia

**Posteromedial
incision for
superficial and
deep posterior
compartments**

Fascial incision
into lateral
compartment

Fascial incision into
deep anterior
compartment

Anterior
intermuscular
septum

Superficial
peroneal n.

**Anterolateral incision for
anterior and lateral
compartments**

Figure 9-14: Stress Fracture

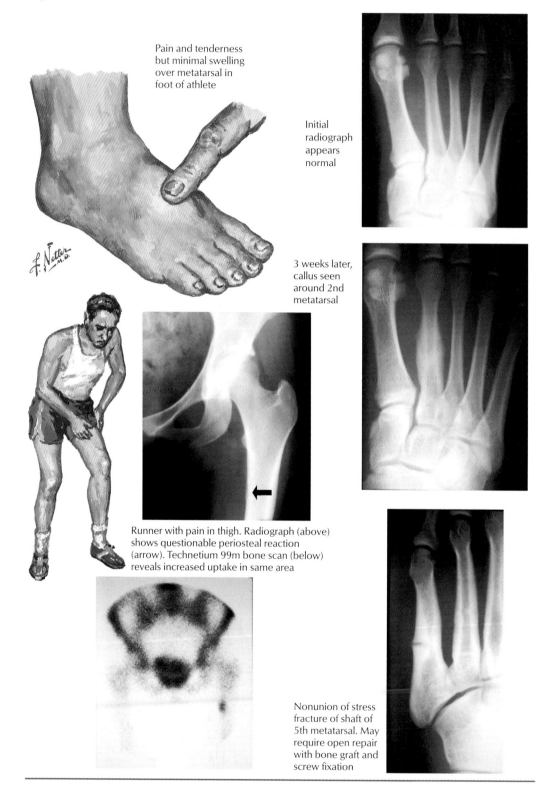

Pain and tenderness but minimal swelling over metatarsal in foot of athlete

Initial radiograph appears normal

3 weeks later, callus seen around 2nd metatarsal

Runner with pain in thigh. Radiograph (above) shows questionable periosteal reaction (arrow). Technetium 99m bone scan (below) reveals increased uptake in same area

Nonunion of stress fracture of shaft of 5th metatarsal. May require open repair with bone graft and screw fixation

ing activity. Classic examples include fracture of the tibia in a military recruit who begins marching and running many hours each day after a previously sedentary existence, or a second metatarsal fracture in a woman who takes a trip and does extended walking and shopping in high-heeled shoes. Stress fractures also occur with normal, unchanged activity levels if the bone is weakened because of osteoporosis or osteomalacia. Stress fractures may be partially due to muscle weakness, because muscles that fatigue easily cannot protect the skeleton from excessive strain.

The clinical presentation includes activity-related pain with an appropriate history. Early radiographs are usually normal, but later ones show periosteal reaction, a sclerotic line, and eventually, callus formation and a line of resorption. Bone scan or magnetic resonance imaging (MRI) shows the lesion at an earlier stage but is not necessary when the history and examination are typical. The diagnosis is most commonly problematic in high-level athletes, who are likely to have musculoskeletal pain from many sources.

Stress fractures are treated with activity modifications to allow healing, and supportive devices (eg, removable walking boots) that reduce pain. The exercise level should be reduced to the level of no or minimal pain. Patients can maintain stretching and strengthening exercises as long as they do not cause pain, and competitive athletes may switch to some type of cross-training activity, for example, runners can use bicycling or rowing to maintain aerobic capacity. Return to the sport should occur when symptoms indicate that this is appropriate; in most cases, athletes are back to full activity in 6 to 8 weeks. Stress fractures of the anterior cortex of the tibial diaphysis, which may occur in jumping athletes, are notorious for requiring a prolonged healing course; surgery may be indicated.

Pathologic Fracture

A fracture through abnormal bone, usually caused by minor, inconsequential trauma, is called a *pathologic fracture*. The cause of the weak bone may be osteoporosis, osteomalacia, a metabolic disorder, or previous infection, surgery, radiation, or tumor (see Chapter 8).

Treatment strategies for pathologic fracture differ from those used in the care of other fractures in the same locations. Preoperative evaluation is needed to identify the underlying cause, and medical treatment is instituted to correct any underlying metabolic disorder or infectious process. To aid healing, patients with metastatic carcinoma usually receive postoperative irradiation to the fracture site. Methyl-methacrylate cement may be used to augment fixation in damaged or porotic bone, but it should be used with care in patients with potential for long-term survival because it will compromise bone healing and is often difficult to remove if further surgery is required. Pathologic fracture of the humeral or femoral head is treated with cemented arthroplasty. Long-bone shaft lesions are usually fixed with intramedullary nails rather than plates because these devices can be inserted with less dissection and provide better stabilization over a longer segment.

Reflex Sympathetic Dystrophy

Also known as *causalgia* or *complex regional pain syndrome*, reflex sympathetic dystrophy (RSD) is an ill-defined and poorly understood syndrome that may develop after fracture or another minor musculoskeletal injury. The pathophysiology is unknown but may involve a self-reinforcing reflex cycle between peripheral sensory nerves and sympathetic neurons in the spinal cord.

Clinical features include *algodynia* (pain and tenderness out of proportion to, and of longer duration than, typical), hyperesthesia, and swelling. Early findings include swelling and warm, red, moist skin that turns purplish at the end of the day. Joint motion is markedly limited. Later on, the skin may be pale, cool, dry, and shiny (**Figure 9-15**). Approximately two thirds of patients will have a diffuse spotty osteopenia on plain radiographs after several weeks. Bone scan typically shows diffuse, increased periarticular uptake on delayed images.

Figure 9-15: Reflex Sympathetic Dystrophy

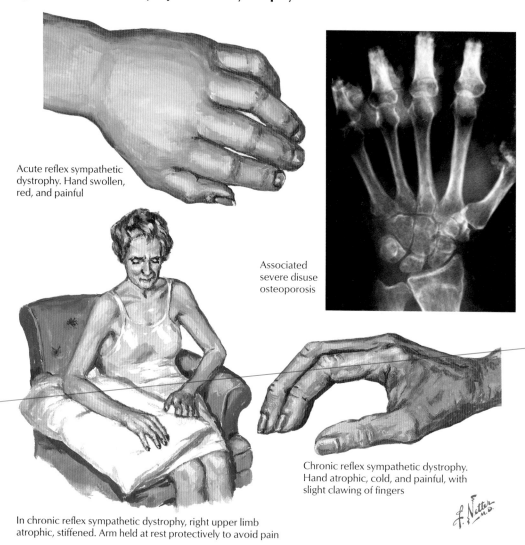

Acute reflex sympathetic dystrophy. Hand swollen, red, and painful

Associated severe disuse osteoporosis

Chronic reflex sympathetic dystrophy. Hand atrophic, cold, and painful, with slight clawing of fingers

In chronic reflex sympathetic dystrophy, right upper limb atrophic, stiffened. Arm held at rest protectively to avoid pain

Treatment is based on breaking the cycle of pain to allow initiation of a functional exercise program. Removal of noxious stimuli, brief immobilization with splints, use of transcutaneous nerve stimulators, biofeedback with thermoregulation, and a variety of medications have been used for this purpose. When these measures fail, serial sympathetic ganglion blocks with local anesthetic may be helpful. Regional intravenous blockade and even surgical sympathectomy are required in refractory cases.

ADDITIONAL READINGS

Bucholz RW, Heckman JD, eds. *Rockwood and Green's Fractures in Adults*, 5th edition. Philadelphia, Pa: Lippincott Williams and Wilkins; 2001.

Chapman MW. Principles of treatment of nonunions and malunions. In: Chapman MW, ed. *Chapman's Orthopaedic Surgery*, 3rd edition. Philadelphia, Pa: Lippincott Williams and Wilkins; 2001:847–885.

Michaud CM, Murray CJL, Bloom BR. Burden of disease—Implications for future research. *JAMA*. 2001;285: 535–539.

Schenk RK. Biology of fracture repair. In: Browner BD, Jupiter JB, Levine AM, Trafton PG, eds. *Skeletal Trauma*, 3rd edition. Philadelphia, Pa: Saunders; 2003:29–73.

ten

Trauma and Osteochondrosis Syndromes in Children

Walter B. Greene, MD

Fractures in children are different from those in adults (**Table 10-1**). The incidence of fracture is higher in children. The strength of bone gradually increases as a child grows, but not until late adolescence does a child's bone become as strong as an adult's. Therefore, bone is the weak link in children, and sprains are uncommon until the later teenage years.

Fractures are uncommon in neonates and toddlers, who are protected by their restrained activity even though their bones are weaker. After 3 years of age, the incidence of fracture in children gradually increases, with peak incidence noted during adolescence. The incidence is also higher in boys and during the summer months.

CHARACTERISTICS OF FRACTURES IN CHILDREN

Unique patterns of injury in children are related to the greater plasticity (modulus of elasticity) of their bone and to the growth plate (physis). Because of its greater plasticity, a child's bone is more likely to bend without completely breaking. The result is much higher incidences of greenstick and torus fractures (**Figure 10-1**). A *torus* fracture is buckling (fracture) of the cortex on only one side of the bone. Torus fractures most commonly occur in children 5 to 10 years old at the metaphysis of the distal radius. These injuries are stable

and require only immobilization for comfort and protection. In a *greenstick fracture*, the cortex is disrupted on the tension side but is intact or only buckled on the compression side. With significant angulation, closed reduction is required. *Physeal fractures* are unique to children and account for 15% to 20% of all pediatric fractures. They are described in greater detail in the following paragraphs.

Ossification (mineralization) of bones is progressive but incomplete in children. A fracture may not be visible or may be difficult to see on initial radiographs when mineralization is incomplete. This characteristic factor causes diagnostic problems, particularly in young children when ossification is immature and when many of the secondary centers of ossification have not developed. These "occult" fractures may be apparent 2 to 3 weeks after injury with the appearance of *periosteal new bone formation*. With a nondisplaced fracture, the periosteum remains intact but may be elevated by the fracture hematoma. New bone formation occurs between the cortex and the elevated periosteum.

Fracture healing is more rapid in children than in adults. For example, a fracture of the femoral shaft in an adult requires 16 to 20 weeks of immobilization if treated in a cast. By comparison, the same fracture needs only 2 weeks of immobilization in an infant and 4 to 6 weeks of casting in a young child. As a corollary to rapid healing, nonunion is uncommon in children.

TREATMENT OF PEDIATRIC FRACTURES

Closed reduction and casting is the primary method of treating pediatric fractures. The thicker periosteum, more rapid healing, and greater potential for remodeling found in children are factors that facilitate closed treatment. Even with a displaced fracture, the

---

Table 10-1
Fractures in Children: Comparison With Adults

More common

Unique patterns:
  Greenstick and torus fractures
  Physeal fractures

Diagnostic problems

More rapid healing

Nonunion uncommon

Treatment:
  Closed treatment is typical
  Internal fixation is often minimal

Greater remodeling potential

Figure 10-1: Greenstick and Torus Fractures in Children

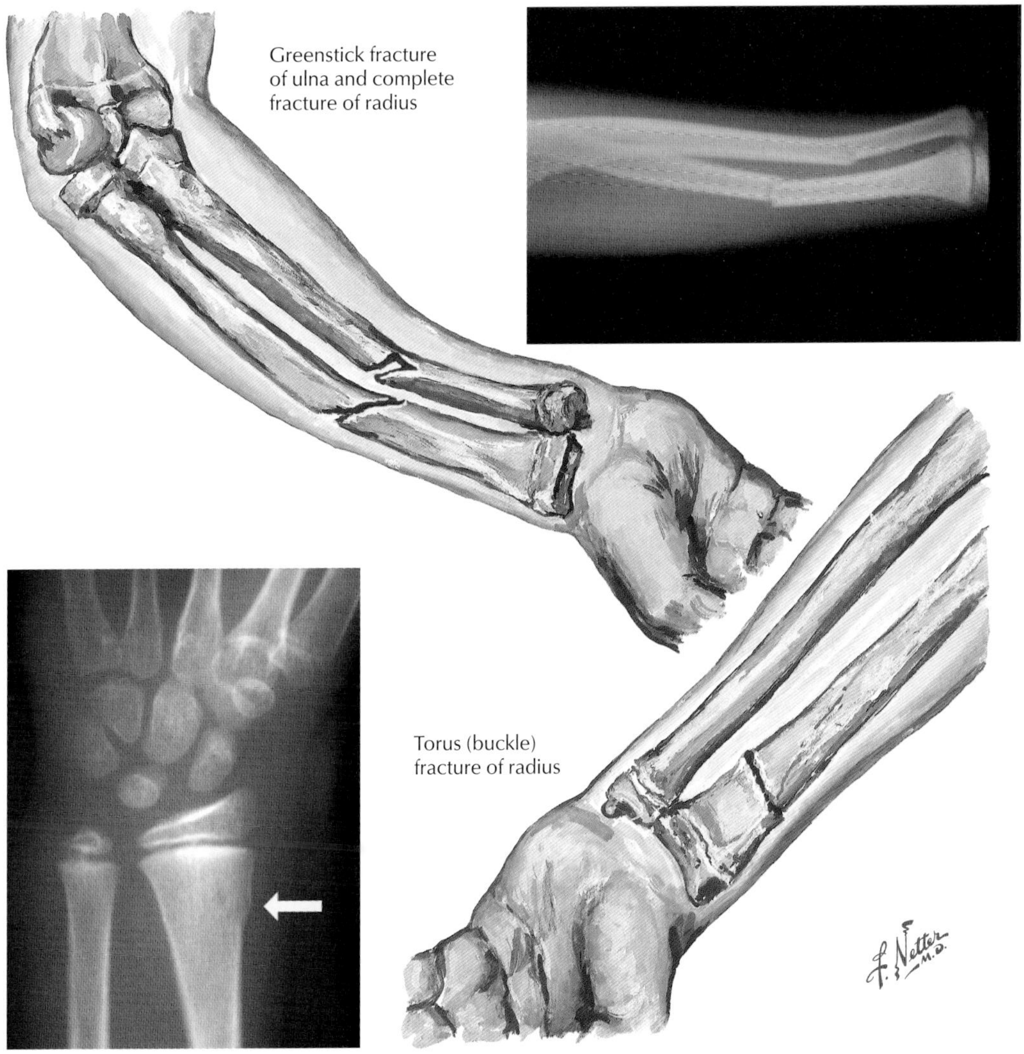

Greenstick fracture of ulna and complete fracture of radius

Torus (buckle) fracture of radius

thick periosteum in children usually remains intact on one side of the fracture. The intact periosteum, combined with appropriate positioning and molding of the cast, helps to maintain closed reduction. The more rapid healing of bone in children reduces the complications associated with prolonged immobilization. Furthermore, complications of prolonged immobilization that are often observed in adults, such as pneumonia and thrombophlebitis, are very uncommon in children. Finally, because remodeling of bone occurs to a greater extent in children, angulation and displacement that

would necessitate open reduction in adults may be acceptable in children without the requirement for open reduction.

Optimal treatment of many fractures in adults requires placement of rigid internal fixation devices to minimize the complications of malunion, nonunion, and prolonged immobilization. Even when operative management of pediatric fractures is required, the best fixation devices typically are small pins or flexible nails, which can be combined with cast immobilization. In children, this combination frequently provides adequate fixation

Figure 10-2: Remodeling of Fracture of Proximal Humerus in a Child

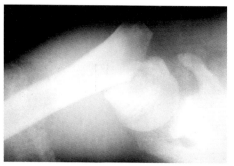

Displaced fracture of proximal humerus

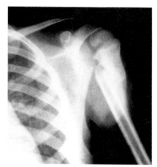

Persistent malalignment despite reduction by traction and manipulation

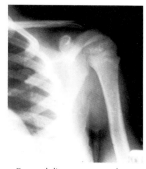

Remodeling over months resulted in relatively normal alignment and unrestricted shoulder motion

while minimizing problems of stress shielding, patient compliance, repeat operation, and pathologic fracture related to the removal of a bulky implant.

Bone remodeling is significantly greater in children, and residual angulation often corrects with subsequent growth (**Figure 10-2**). Remodeling is greater in children who are younger, in fractures close to the physis, and in fractures that are angulated in the plane of motion. For example, a fracture of the distal radius with 35° of volar or dorsal angulation in a 6-year-old child will remodel completely in 1 to 2 years, even if no reduction is performed. In this situation, the primary reason for reduction is to relieve the pressure on adjacent soft tissues. However, remodeling in other planes is less predictable, and rotational deformities are particularly prone to persist. By comparison, in adults, residual angulation in any plane does not remodel to any significant degree.

PHYSEAL FRACTURES

Any fracture that involves the growth plate (the physis) is called a *physeal fracture*. Although supported by the *ring of Lacroix* (a perichondral ring of fibrous tissue), the cartilaginous physis is relatively weak and prone to injury. Physeal fractures may occur at any age until the growth plate closes, but these injuries are more common during the latter part of growth (ie, from 10 to 15 years of age).

Classification of physeal fractures aids in the selection of treatment and provides a prognosis for future complications. Several classifications of physeal fractures have been described. The five-part Salter-Harris classification has been the most commonly used. However, this system does not describe all physeal fractures, and a Salter-Harris type V fracture probably does not occur. The Peterson classification, in contrast, describes six types of physeal fractures; correlates well with anatomic, epidemiologic, and outcome associations; and progresses logically from lesser to greater seriousness of injury, frequency of occurrence, and level of intervention (**Figure 10-3**). Fortunately, the more severe injuries (type IV and type V physeal fractures) are relatively uncommon, and the most severe physeal fracture (type VI) is very uncommon.

As with all fractures, the history of a child with a physeal fracture typically includes a fall, followed by pain, localized tenderness, and swelling. Because the physis is typically outside muscle compartments, vascular and nerve complications are uncommon with fractures of the growth plate. Anteroposterior and lateral radiographs usually identify the fracture; however, oblique views may be necessary.

Physeal fractures heal rapidly. The goals of treatment include reduction (when necessary) by closed manipulation or open techniques, maintenance of reduction during the healing process, and avoidance or minimiza-

Figure 10-3: Peterson Classification of Physeal Fractures

Type I. Metaphyseal fracture with extension to physis is the most common physeal injury. It can be managed by short-term cast immobilization.

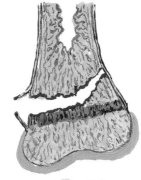

Type II. Line of separation extends partially across deep layer of growth plate and extends through metaphysis, leaving triangular portion of metaphysis attached to epiphyseal fragment. Can be treated by closed reduction and immobilization (Salter-Harris II).

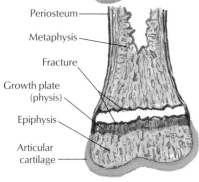

Periosteum
Metaphysis
Fracture
Growth plate (physis)
Epiphysis
Articular cartilage

Type IV. Intra-articular fracture through epiphysis, across deep zone of growth plate to periphery. Open reduction and internal fixation necessary if articular displacement ≥2 mm (Salter-Harris III).

Type III. Complete separation of epiphysis from metaphysis through zone of hypertrophy of the growth plate. No bone actually fractured; periosteum may remain intact. Most common in newborns and young children (Salter-Harris I).

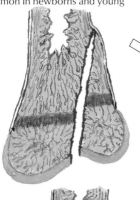
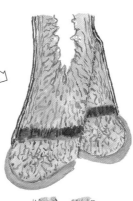

Type V. Fracture line extends from articular surface through epiphysis, growth plate, and metaphysis. Open reduction and internal fixation necessary if articular displacement >2 mm (Salter-Harris IV).

Type VI. Portion of growth plate sheared off. This is always an open fracture and therefore demands immediate surgical attention. Raw surface heals by forming bone bridge across physis. If significant growth remains, angular deformity will develop.

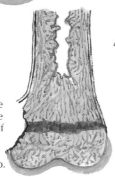
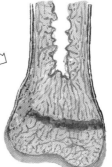

tion of problems of traumatic arthritis and growth arrest.

When fractures are minimally displaced, simple immobilization is sufficient therapy. Type I, II, and III physeal fractures that are displaced are usually treated by closed reduction. Type IV and V physeal fractures with 2 mm or greater displacement at the articular surface require open reduction and internal fixation to prevent joint incongruity and traumatic arthropathy. Type VI fractures are, by definition, open fractures, and they require immediate débridement, irrigation, and appropriate soft tissue closure. Physeal bars always develop after this injury, and reconstructive surgery (ie, excision of the physeal bar, realignment osteotomy, or both) is needed if significant growth remains.

GROWTH ARREST

Premature growth arrest (partial or complete) may occur with any physeal fracture. It is very uncommon with type I, II, and III fractures that occur in the upper extremity; is more common with type II and III fractures that occur in the lower extremity (greater axial load at time of injury); is significantly more common with type IV and V fractures, whatever the site of injury; and is universal with type VI fractures.

If growth arrest involves only one side of the physis, the resultant physeal bar (bony bridge) causes development of an angular deformity (**Figure 10-4**). For example, a *physeal bar* that develops on the medial aspect of the distal femoral physis will result in a progressive genu varum. Genu varum occurs because the medial side is tethered by the physeal bar, while the lateral aspect of the physis continues to grow. If the premature arrest creates a central physeal bar, or if the entire growth plate is prematurely arrested, growth in length stops, and limb-length discrepancy occurs.

If minimal growth remains, the consequences of premature closure of the physis are insignificant. For example, a 13-year-old girl typically has less than 1 cm of growth remaining from the distal tibial physis. Thus, a Peterson type V fracture of the distal tibia will

cause inconsequential angular deformity or leg-length discrepancy, even if the physis closes prematurely. However, younger patients with a similar fracture and significant remaining growth require continued evaluation to detect early growth plate closure.

Excision of a physeal bar with interposition of an inert material may result in resumption of normal growth. If significant angulation has occurred, a corrective osteotomy also will be required. This operation is most successful when the bar makes up less than 50% of the total area of the physis, and when more than 1 year of growth remains at the involved physis.

CHILD ABUSE

Child abuse is far too common. More than 2 million cases are reported annually in the United States. Most involve children younger than 3 years. In addition to physical abuse, child abuse involves starvation, sexual abuse (more common in older children), and emotional neglect.

Parents, larger siblings, or persons outside the family (such as babysitters) may be the abusers. Abuse can occur at any socioeconomic level, but social circumstances associated with abuse include the following:

+ Parents who were abused as children (repeating family history).

+ Social isolation of the parents (no readily accessible grandparent or "good neighbor" support).

+ Drug and alcohol abuse by the parent.

+ Recent family crisis (eg, job loss by parent and no financial reserves).

An isolated fracture may be the initial injury in an abused child. If the abuse is not recognized, the child will be returned to the same environment. In this situation, the risk of death is 5%, and the risk of reinjury is 25%.

All types of fractures occur with child abuse, but certain fracture types are associated with injury from abuse (**Figure 10-5**). The "corner" metaphyseal fracture is most specific. This injury is caused by vigorous pulling on the extremity. A distal traction force may fracture the physis, probably through the zone of hypertrophy. In these relatively low energy injuries, the fracture of the physis may not be

Figure 10-4: Physeal Bar After Fracture of Distal Femur

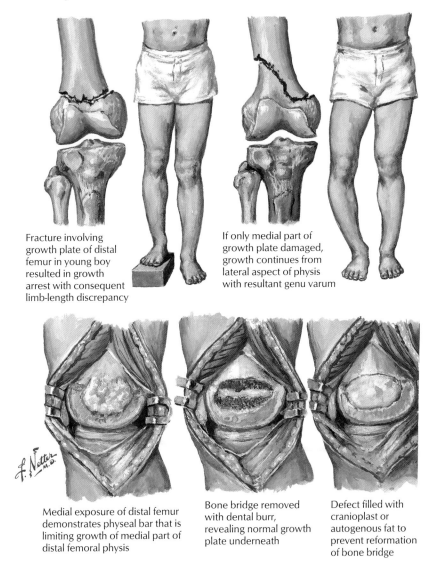

Fracture involving growth plate of distal femur in young boy resulted in growth arrest with consequent limb-length discrepancy

If only medial part of growth plate damaged, growth continues from lateral aspect of physis with resultant genu varum

Medial exposure of distal femur demonstrates physeal bar that is limiting growth of medial part of distal femoral physis

Bone bridge removed with dental burr, revealing normal growth plate underneath

Defect filled with cranioplast or autogenous fat to prevent reformation of bone bridge

evident on plain radiographs, but propagation of the fracture through the corner of the metaphysis can be observed. These metaphyseal avulsion fractures are analogous to the type II physeal fracture, but the metaphyseal chip is often small and may be unilateral or bilateral, involving the medial and lateral metaphysis. Other highly specific injuries for child abuse include posterior rib fractures, fractures of the scapula, and fractures of the sternum that result from compression of the chest.

Multiple fractures at different stages of healing are highly specific for child abuse. The age of the fractures can be approximated with the use of radiographic findings. In a child, callus and periosteal new bone formation may be seen 7 to 14 days after injury. By 14 to 21 days, the initial homogenous callus pattern is transitioning to a more mature trabecular pattern, and the fracture line is less evident. Further organization and greater density of the callus are

Figure 10-5: Fracture in Abused Children

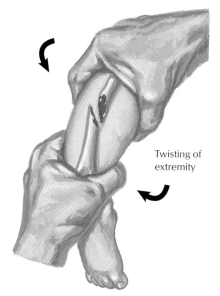

Twisting of extremity

Spiral fractures in young children may occur accidentally but often due to abuse

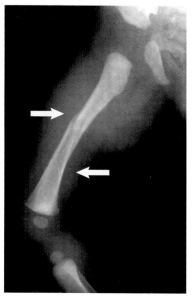

Spiral fracture in infant

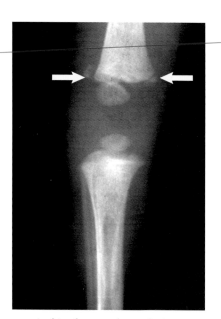

Avulsion fracture of metaphysis

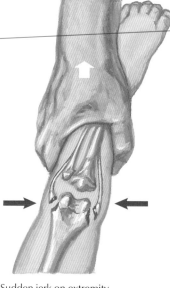

Sudden jerk on extremity avulses metaphyseal tips

JOHN A.CRAIG—AD

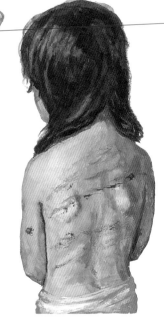

Further examination may reveal bruises, welts, or cigarette burns in various stages of healing on other parts of body

noted 3 to 6 weeks after injury. After 6 weeks, subsequent healing and remodeling will transform the bone so that only spindle-shaped thickening of the cortex is noted at the fracture site. In fractures that are several months old, this thickening is subtle and may be apparent only in comparison with radiographs of the uninvolved side. As with all pediatric fractures, in most cases of child abuse, the bone completely remodels so that no evidence of previous injury is apparent.

Bilateral fractures, complex skull fractures, and fractures of the fingers or spine are highly associated with abuse unless the child has been involved in a motor vehicle or similar accident. Simple linear skull and clavicle fractures that occur in isolation have a low specificity for child abuse.

Isolated long-bone fractures in children younger than 3 years of age are associated with child abuse. For example, approximately 50% of fractures of the femoral shaft in a child younger than 1 year are secondary to child abuse. In one study, all fractures of the humeral shaft in children younger than 3 years (excluding supracondylar fractures) were caused by abuse. Spiral fractures result from a twisting or rotational injury, and this fracture pattern is particularly associated with abuse; however, transverse and oblique fractures caused by a direct blow or bending force are also observed. The "toddler's fracture," a spiral fracture of the distal tibia, is common in 1- to 3-year-old children and, with appropriate history, can be attributed to accidental trauma. It often occurs as a result of a fall with the foot caught and twisted by a chair or some other stationary object.

A thorough history taken in a calm and systematic fashion is particularly important in a possible case of child abuse. It is critical for the clinician to determine whether the history provided by the parents adequately accounts for the injuries. In cases of child abuse, family members frequently provide inconsistent history concerning the injury, particularly when individual persons are questioned in private.

The physical examination must be thorough. Note any areas of skin discoloration and injury. Evaluate the child's mental status. Palpate the chest, abdomen, spine, and limbs for sites of tenderness and swelling. Inspect for signs of sexual abuse.

If abuse is suspected, the child should be admitted to the hospital for further evaluation. Anteroposterior and lateral radiographs of the long bones, hands, feet, spine, chest, and skull are necessary. Coagulation studies are routine, and toxicology screening tests are performed if there is a history of substance abuse. If the mental status or neurologic examination is abnormal, magnetic resonance imaging (MRI) is performed to evaluate the child for the presence of subdural hematomas. If the abdomen is tender, a computed tomography (CT) scan is obtained. If abuse is suspected, the situation should be reported to the appropriate child abuse team and social service agency, which will determine whether the child's constellation of findings meet the criteria for child abuse and, more important, whether the child needs the protection of a foster home.

The differential diagnosis of child abuse includes osteogenesis imperfecta and certain metabolic and genetic diseases. A moderate or mild form of osteogenesis imperfecta and toddler's fracture of the tibia are the two disorders most often confused with child abuse.

SPRAINS, STRAINS, AND OSTEOCHONDROSIS SYNDROMES IN CHILDREN

Sprains and strains occur in children, but this incidence is significantly lower compared to adults until the late adolescent years, when the strength of bone is increasing. Treatment of sprains and strains in adults and children is similar, but the prognosis is better for children.

Various osteochondrosis syndromes may develop in children. These overuse syndromes are associated with the development of secondary ossification or apophyseal centers or

Figure 10-6: Osgood-Schlatter Condition

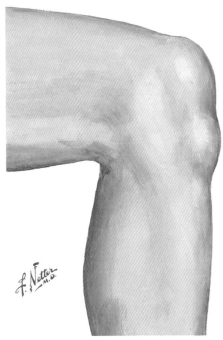

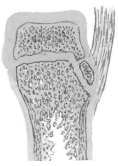

Normal insertion of patellar ligament to ossifying tibial tuberosity

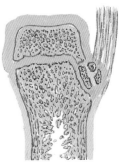

In Osgood-Schlatter lesion, superficial portion of tuberosity pulled away, forming separate bone fragments

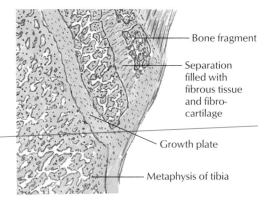

Bone fragment

Separation filled with fibrous tissue and fibro-cartilage

Growth plate

Metaphysis of tibia

High-power magnification of involved area

In Osgood-Schlatter condition, the apophysis of the tibial tuberosity is prominent and has irregular ossification. Fragmentation and separate ossicles may develop

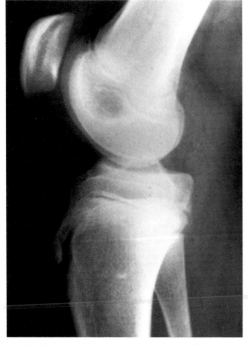

Radiograph shows separation of superficial portion of tibial tuberosity

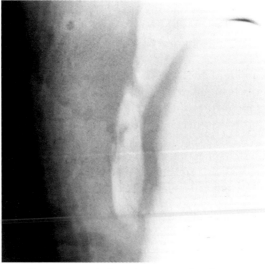

Focal radiograph shows fragment at site of insertion of patellar ligament

Table 10-2
Common Sites of Osteochondrosis in Children

Secondary ossification centers
  Medial epicondylar humerus
    (little leaguer's elbow)
  Ischium (Van Neck syndrome)
  Medial malleolus

Apophysis
  Calcaneus (Sever apophysitis)
  Tibial tubercle (Osgood-Schlatter disease)

Accessory ossification centers
  Bipartite patella (superior lateral pole
    of patella)
  Accessory navicular (medial tuberosity of
    navicula)
  Os trigonum (posterior talus)
  Os subfibulare (distal fibula)
  Os vesalianum (base of fifth metatarsal)

accessory ossification centers (**Table 10-2**). The chief example is Osgood-Schlatter disease, which causes activity-related pain and swelling localized to the tibial tuberosity. The secondary ossification center (apophysis) of the tibial tuberosity develops during early adolescence, a time when body mass and activity have increased. The cartilaginous juncture between the secondary ossification center and the tibia is a weak link. Repetitive contraction of the quadriceps muscles causes repetitive stress at the patellar tendon; traction of the patellar tendon causes injury and microscopic avulsion fractures at the tibial tuberosity and, sometimes, heterotopic ossification or separate bony fragments superficial to the tibial tuberosity (**Figure 10-6**). Osgood-Schlatter disease is more common among males, and a fivefold greater incidence of this condition is seen in children who are active in sports.

Most osteochondrosis syndromes in children can be treated with activity modification. With severe symptoms, short-term immobilization may facilitate healing of the microscopic fractures and resolution of symptoms. With growth, the secondary ossification center coalesces, and the cartilaginous juncture is obliterated. Therefore, long-term symptoms and the need for surgical treatment are very uncommon; surgery is necessary only if the healing response causes residual bony prominence and persistent closure of the tibial tuberosity.

ADDITIONAL READINGS

Beatty JH, Kasser JR, eds. *Rockwood and Wilkins' Fractures in Children*, 6th edition. Philadelphia, Pa: Lippincott Williams and Wilkins; 2005.

Green NE, Swiontkowski MF, eds. *Skeletal Trauma in Children*, 3rd edition. Philadelphia, Pa: WB Saunders; 2003.

Peterson HA: Physeal fractures. Part 3. Classification. *J Pediatr Orthop*. 1994;14:439–448.

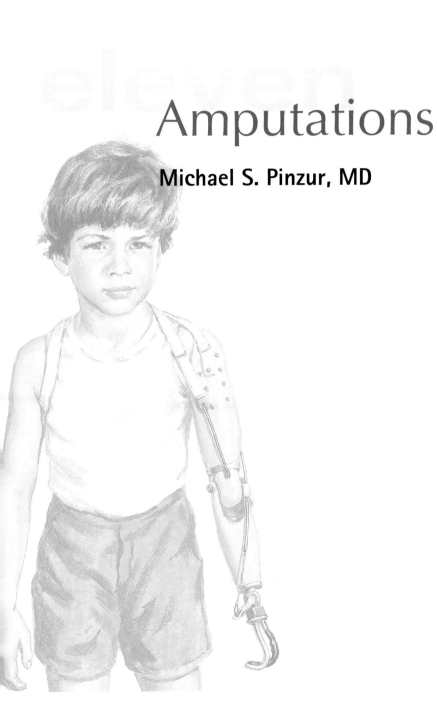

eleven

Amputations

Michael S. Pinzur, MD

A mputation of a limb may be performed as a therapeutic procedure for peripheral vascular insufficiency, chronic infection, irreparable trauma, malignant tumor, or severe congenital deformity. It is performed as an alternative to limb salvage when it has been determined that the patient will be better served by an amputation. For any condition, it should be understood that amputation is a therapeutic procedure that is the first step in a rehabilitation process, as opposed to the last step in a situation of failure.

Persons with lower extremity amputations accomplish weight bearing through load transfer from the residual limb to the prosthesis, which interfaces with the floor. Those with a disarticulation (through-the-joint) amputation accomplish weight bearing and load transfer by end bearing, whereas patients with through-the-bone amputations must accomplish load transfer by total contact. Lower limb prostheses function reasonably well; however, the energy requirements for walking are increased after a lower limb amputation. The increased oxygen consumption is inversely proportional to the level of amputation. A geriatric, dysvascular patient with a transfemoral amputation typically uses maximum energy expenditure during normal walking; therefore, any additional comorbidity may prevent these patients from achieving functional ambulation.

Degree of function after upper extremity amputation also is proportionate to the level of amputation. Prosthetic joints must be controlled individually and sequentially. This factor complicates and compromises function in the more proximal levels of amputation. Because prostheses are insensate, prehension feedback cannot be well regulated, and fine motor activities that are critical to upper extremity function must be performed under visual guidance. This factor also compromises function proportionate to the level of amputation.

AMPUTATION IN CHILDREN

Amputations in children are relatively uncommon, may be congenital (**Figure 11-1**), or as in adults, performed as a therapeutic procedure in the treatment of trauma, tumors, vascular disorders, or infectious complications. Amputations in children are also done to enhance function of a patient with congenital limb deficiency.

Congenital deficiencies are categorized as *transverse* or *longitudinal. Amelia* is the com-

Figure 11-1: Congenital Transmetacarpal Amputation

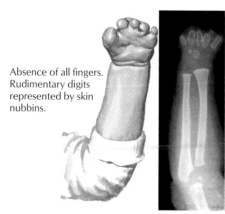

Absence of all fingers. Rudimentary digits represented by skin nubbins.

Radiograph shows absence of phalanges. Metacarpals present but short.

plete absence of a limb; *hemimelia* is the longitudinal absence of a major portion of a limb; and *phocomelia* is the intercalary absence of a section of a limb, with the attachment of a normal or longitudinally deficient terminal limb at or near the trunk. Transverse congenital deficiencies are frequently transdiaphyseal (eg, congenital below-elbow amputation).

Revision or reamputation of an upper limb with congenital deficiency rarely is indicated, as even rudimentary appendages can be functionally useful (**Figures 11-2** and **11-3**). Of note, patients with congenital transverse deficiencies function better than adults who have a similar level of amputation. Indeed, a child with a unilateral congenital below-elbow or more distal amputation will often reject using a prosthesis. However, stability and relative equality of leg length are essential for optimal function of the lower limbs

(see **Figure 17-29**). Fibula and tibia hemimelia frequently cause severe leg-length discrepancy and/or unstable feet. Amputation of an unstable lower limb segment may allow more efficient load transfer and more stable walking.

A disarticulation amputation in a child not only preserves the joint cartilage and permits end-bearing prosthetic function, it also prevents the *recurrent bony overgrowth* often seen with diaphyseal amputations performed in children (**Figure 11-4**). Such bony overgrowth tents the overlying skin, causes pain, compromises prosthetic use, and limits walking. None of the numerous surgical procedures that have been described to manage this recurring problem have been routinely successful. If the joint above the area of damage is functional, a short, nonfunctioning limb segment that is covered by normal skin can

Figure 11-2: Forearm Amputation

Lines of incision

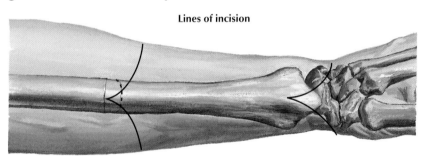

Below-elbow amputation

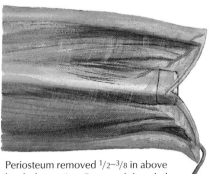

Periosteum removed ¹/₂–³/₈ in above level of resection. Bone ends beveled. Musculotendinous tissues tapered. Skin and fascial flaps formed.

Disarticulation of wrist

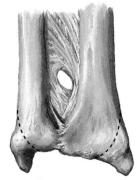

Styloid processes removed (broken lines) to facilitate fitting of prosthesis

Figure 11-3: Body-Powered and Myoelectric Prosthesis

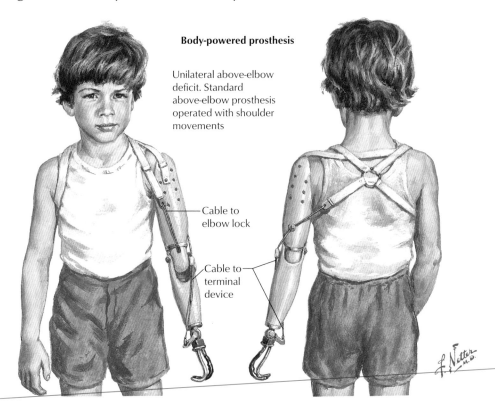

Body-powered prosthesis

Unilateral above-elbow deficit. Standard above-elbow prosthesis operated with shoulder movements

Cable to elbow lock

Cable to terminal device

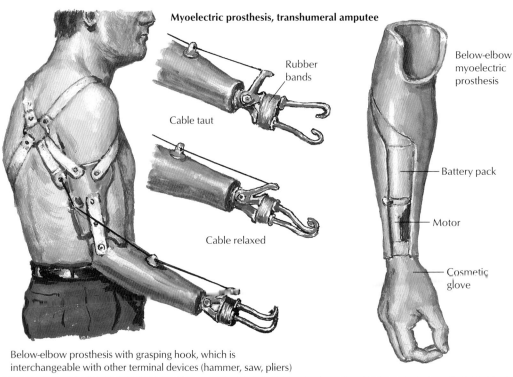

Myoelectric prosthesis, transhumeral amputee

Rubber bands

Cable taut

Cable relaxed

Below-elbow myoelectric prosthesis

Battery pack

Motor

Cosmetic glove

Below-elbow prosthesis with grasping hook, which is interchangeable with other terminal devices (hammer, saw, pliers)

Figure 11-4: Bony Overgrowth

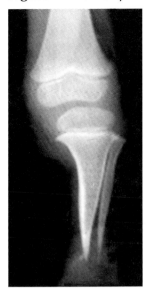

Radiograph of transtibial amputation of a child shows typical "pencil point" overgrowth of tibia and fibula that leads to tenting of the skin and inability to use the prosthesis.

be lengthened to provide improved prosthetic use.

TRAUMATIC AMPUTATION

When a patient sustains a mutilating limb injury, the treating physician often is faced with the dilemma of attempting to reconstruct the limb (ie, limb salvage) or proceeding with amputation. Four questions must be addressed before treatment is initiated (see also Chapter 9, page 206).

First, will limb salvage outperform amputation and prosthetic limb fitting? The surgeon must make a reasonable assessment of the patient's eventual functional outcome after limb salvage and compare it with the projected results of amputation and prosthetic limb fitting. This assessment will vary greatly with the activity level and functional needs of the patient, the potential amputation level, the peripheral nerve and vascular injuries that have occurred, and whether injury has affected the upper or lower extremity.

Second, what is a reasonable outcome expectation? Most traumatic lower extremity amputations occur in young males who earn their living doing physical labor. Based on a reasonable assessment of their functional capacities at the end of treatment, will they be able to re-

cover sufficient strength, agility, and mobility to return to their former work after limb salvage? Will they be able to return to their work after amputation and prosthetic limb fitting?

Third, what are the costs of limb salvage versus amputation? These costs go beyond the financial burden associated with treatment. One must consider the health care system resources that will be necessary to effect treatment. Limb salvage may entail multiple surgeries and hospitalizations, as well as a prolonged time during which the person will be unable to work. During this process, patients may exhaust their financial reserves and experience emotional stress that places a substantial strain on interpersonal relationships.

Fourth, what risks are involved? With multiple surgeries, one also must consider the risks of wound infection and chronic osteomyelitis, as well as the potential systemic complications associated with infection and long-term parenteral antibiotic therapy.

AMPUTATION IN PERIPHERAL VASCULAR DISEASE AND DIABETIC INFECTION

Peripheral vascular disease and diabetic foot infection cause approximately 75% of all lower extremity amputations in adults. Involvement of a single extremity is uncommon in patients with peripheral vascular disease or diabetes mellitus. Patients with vascular disease of one leg are likely to have similar disease in the contralateral limb, heart, carotid arteries, and cerebrovascular system. *Multiple organ systemic disease* also is common in patients with diabetes mellitus. *Cardiopulmonary dysfunction*, coupled with increased energy requirements for walking, may not permit functional prosthetic use in these patients. Furthermore, the *cognitive skills* of memory, attention, concentration, and organization that are necessary for patients to learn to walk with, and care for, a prosthetic limb may be deficient in a geriatric patient. Patients with severe cognitive deficits or psychiatric disease are unlikely to become successful prosthetic users. In patients with lower extremity amputation, one must have realistic goals based on cognitive skills, learning potential, motivation, and the cardiopulmonary reserve necessary to permit functional walking.

Adequate vascular supply, tissue nutrition, and immunocompetence are necessary to achieve successful amputation wound healing. *Adequacy of the vascular supply* can be assessed by Doppler ultrasonographic determination of the ankle-brachial index or ischemic index. Through this method, a blood pressure cuff applied at the level of interest occludes the limb, then pressure on the cuff is slowly released. When the arterial pressure at the affected level can overcome the cuff pressure, the sound of the blood flowing through the partially occluded vessel may be detected with an ultrasonographic Doppler recording device. The *ankle-brachial index* is the ultrasonographic Doppler pressure obtained at the ankle divided by the brachial artery pressure. The ischemic index is the ratio of ultrasonographic Doppler pressure at a level of interest to brachial artery pressure. An ankle-brachial index of 0.5 in patients with diabetes mellitus or 0.45 in patients with peripheral vascular disease indicates sufficient blood supply to support surgical wound healing in the foot or ankle.

Calcified arteries make Doppler ultrasonography an unreliable tool in approximately 15% of patients with peripheral vascular disease. A more reliable prognostic tool is *transcutaneous oximetry*, which measures the oxygen delivery capacity of the patient's cardiovascular system at the surgical level in question. In this method, a probe is applied to the skin at the level of interest. The probe is heated to body temperature to maximize blood flow, and the partial pressure of oxygen is measured. The threshold of transcutaneous oxygen tension needed to support wound healing is between 20 and 30 mm Hg. Because digital arteries seemingly do not become calcified, ultrasound Doppler toe pressures are a good technique if transcutaneous oximetry is not available. Vascular bypass surgery or angioplasty should be considered if blood supply to the level of interest is insufficient.

Patients who are malnourished, immunodeficient, or both have higher rates of wound infection and wound breakdown. Persons are considered *malnourished* if their serum albumin is below 3.5 g/dL. They are considered *immunodeficient* if their total lymphocyte count is below 1500. Dysvascular and diabetic patients with vascular and wound-healing indices above the minimum standards have a 90% successful amputation wound-healing rate. Those with diabetes mellitus who have chronic foot infection, renal failure, or both often have depleted protein stores. Their initial treatment should include removal of infected tissue, followed by open wound management, culture-specific antibiotic therapy, nutritional support, and optimization of renal function. When their wound-healing potential is optimized, amputation can be performed.

TREATMENT OF MUSCULOSKELETAL TUMORS

Advances in the medical management of musculoskeletal neoplasms and in allograft or prosthetic reconstruction have made limb salvage the likely choice of treatment for patients with sarcomas of the extremities. If adequate surgical margins can be obtained, the choice between salvage and amputation should be made after the four questions discussed earlier in the chapter have been addressed.

UPPER EXTREMITY AMPUTATION

The strength of pinch and grasp (prehension) is regulated by tactile sensation; therefore, when even part of a sensate hand that is capable of functional prehension can be retained, the result is frequently greater function than can be attained with an upper extremity amputation. The decision of whether to amputate is based on remaining sensation and ability to achieve functional prehension. Patients who have lost these abilities are often better served by amputation.

Retention of limb length is crucial for retention of function. Prosthetic upper extremity joints are controlled sequentially, and task performance is inversely related to the number of joints that need to be replaced. Suspension of the prosthesis and the ability of the lever arm to manipulate the prosthesis in space vary with the length of the prosthesis within a remaining segment of limb. Patients with wrist disarticulation and distal transradial (below-elbow) amputation achieve the greatest benefit from prosthetic limb fitting, as only one "joint" (ie, the hand) must be replaced. The prosthetic hand will simply need to be opened and closed for tasks to be accomplished.

Patients with elbow disarticulation and transhumeral amputation require sequential control of their prosthetic elbow and hand. This situation leads to less efficient task performance. Shoulder disarticulation necessitates the replacement of three joints. It is unlikely that these patients will achieve meaningful function with a prosthesis, except in special circumstances.

LOWER EXTREMITY AMPUTATION

Walking is relatively simple compared with performance of the fine, coordinated movements of the upper limbs. In contrast to prostheses for the upper extremities, lower extremity prostheses provide good simulation of joint function, and patients with lower extremity amputations often are capable of returning to most of their preamputation activities.

Persons who undergo foot and ankle amputations fare extremely well, as they retain most of the normal weight-bearing tissue (**Figures 11-5** and **11-6**). When the *hallux* is amputated, the proximal aspect of the proximal phalanx should be retained, if possible. This preserves the insertion of the flexor hallucis brevis muscle, keeps the sesamoid bones centralized, and retains the stability of the medial ray of the foot. Loss of the entire great toe leads to lessened stability during the terminal stance phase of gait at the time of push-off, but removal of the lessor toes causes little, if any, disability. *Partial foot amputation* at the transmetatarsal or tarsometatarsal level decreases the lever arm during push-off, but patients can resume walking with simple shoe

modification. Patients with amputations at the hindfoot (talonavicular joint) do not function well. The retained talus and calcaneus are pulled into equinus, and the fit of the prosthesis and walking ability are compromised. In contrast, *ankle disarticulation* allows end bearing on a durable heel pad and adequate space for use of a dynamic elastic-response prosthetic foot that recovers walking propulsion. These persons require minimal training to learn to walk with a prosthesis.

The *transtibial* (below-knee) amputation is performed with a long posterior myofasciocutaneous flap (**Figure 11-7**). This surgery is the most common functional amputation performed. Almost 90% of persons who undergo transtibial amputation recover meaningful walking capability.

Knee disarticulation allows end bearing, but this amputation does not have the walking and running propulsion capacity of the quadriceps–patellar tendon–tibia lever arm that is retained after a transtibial amputation. It also is performed with a long posterior myofasciocutaneous flap (**Figure 11-8**). For individuals who will not become prosthetic users, a knee disarticulation provides a significantly better platform for sitting and a lever arm for transfer from a chair than a transfemoral amputation.

Persons with *transfemoral* (above-knee) amputations do not fare as well as patients with lower-level amputations. The loss of active muscles and dynamic joints, as well as the weight of the prosthesis, greatly limits capabilities (**Figure 11-9**). Because of their limited remaining dynamic motor abilities, patients must "throw" their limbs ahead of them in walking while at the same time achieving knee-joint stability during stance through control of body positioning.

COMPLICATIONS OF AMPUTATION

Wound necrosis, infection, bleeding, and joint contractures are the perioperative complications associated with amputation surgery (**Figure 11-10**). *Wound necrosis* occurs because the amputation is performed at a too distal level through nonviable tissue, or

Figure 11-5: Amputations of the Foot

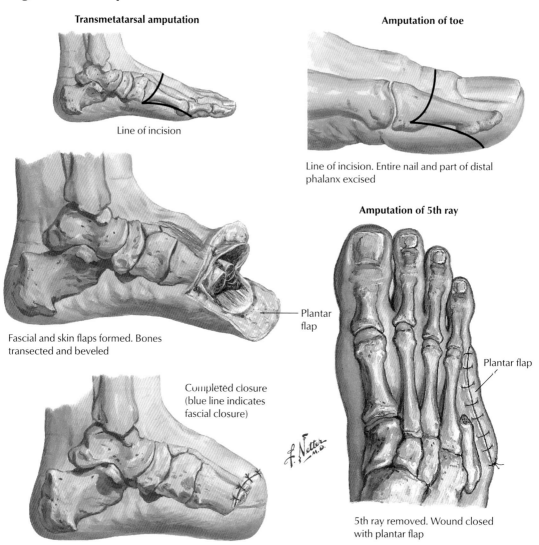

Transmetatarsal amputation

Line of incision

Fascial and skin flaps formed. Bones transected and beveled

Completed closure (blue line indicates fascial closure)

Amputation of toe

Line of incision. Entire nail and part of distal phalanx excised

Amputation of 5th ray

Plantar flap

Plantar flap

5th ray removed. Wound closed with plantar flap

because the wound is closed under too much tension. Treatment of wound necrosis and infection requires debridement of the necrotic or infected tissue, culture-specific antibiotic therapy, and secondary wound closure. Bleeding is controlled via suture ligature of arteries and cautery or ligature of veins. Arteries require suture ligatures for prevention of "pumping" off the suture by arterial pulsations. Joint contractures occur because of surgical muscle imbalance or a rehabilitation program that does not stress mobilization and range-of-motion exercises.

All adults undergoing an amputation experience phantom limb sensation, that is, the perception that the amputated part of the limb is still present. Patients note that their "foot" tingles, itches, or feels like it is receiving electric shocks. After crushing injuries, persons may perceive that the limb remains in the position of injury. Pain in the amputated part—so-called phantom limb pain—usually subsides over time. If these symptoms persist, antiseizure medication, nerve blocks, or transcutaneous electrical nerve stimulation may bring some relief.

Figure 11-6: Ankle Disarticulation (Syme Amputation)

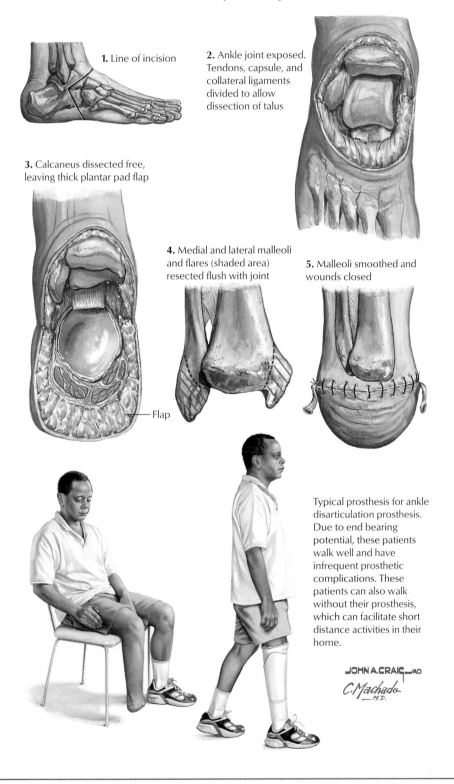

1. Line of incision

2. Ankle joint exposed. Tendons, capsule, and collateral ligaments divided to allow dissection of talus

3. Calcaneus dissected free, leaving thick plantar pad flap

4. Medial and lateral malleoli and flares (shaded area) resected flush with joint

5. Malleoli smoothed and wounds closed

Flap

Typical prosthesis for ankle disarticulation prosthesis. Due to end bearing potential, these patients walk well and have infrequent prosthetic complications. These patients can also walk without their prosthesis, which can facilitate short distance activities in their home.

JOHN A. CRAIG—MD

C. Machado—M.D.

Figure 11-7: Transtibial Amputation

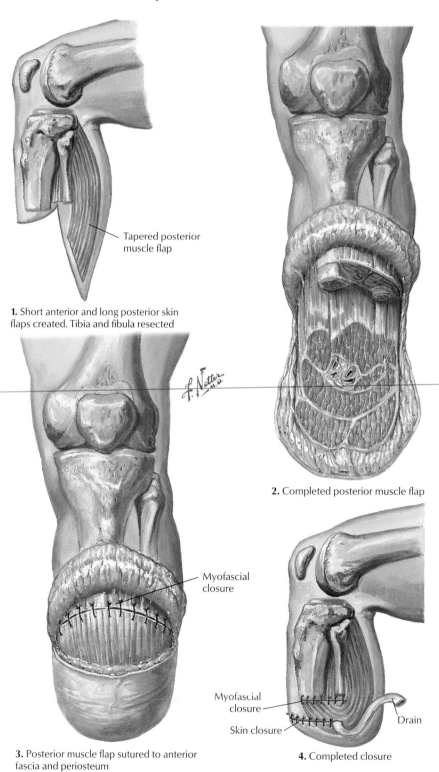

Tapered posterior muscle flap

1. Short anterior and long posterior skin flaps created. Tibia and fibula resected

2. Completed posterior muscle flap

Myofascial closure

3. Posterior muscle flap sutured to anterior fascia and periosteum

Myofascial closure

Skin closure

Drain

4. Completed closure

Figure 11-8: Knee Disarticulation Amputation

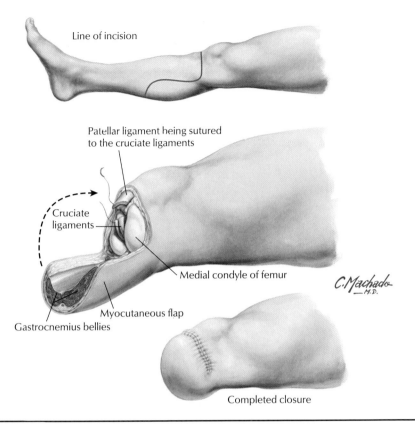

Line of incision

Patellar ligament being sutured to the cruciate ligaments

Cruciate ligaments

Medial condyle of femur

Myocutaneous flap

Gastrocnemius bellies

C. Machado —M.D.

Completed closure

Figure 11-9: Transfemoral Amputation

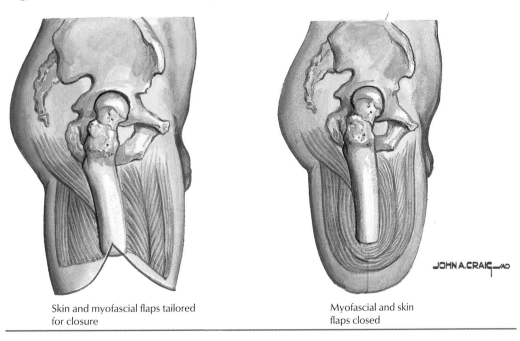

Skin and myofascial flaps tailored for closure

Myofascial and skin flaps closed

JOHN A. CRAIG —MD

Figure 11-10: Complications of Amputation

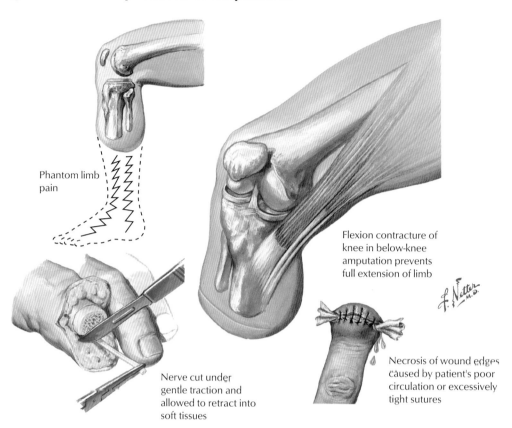

Phantom limb pain

Flexion contracture of knee in below-knee amputation prevents full extension of limb

Nerve cut under gentle traction and allowed to retract into soft tissues

Necrosis of wound edges caused by patient's poor circulation or excessively tight sutures

Pain that develops after amputation is related to the biology of the residual limb or the fit of the prosthetic limb. If prosthetic modification does not resolve the pain, surgical revision may be required for the provision of a more functional residual limb.

ADDITIONAL READINGS

Pinzur MS, Bowker JH, Smith DG, Gottschalk FA. Amputation surgery in peripheral vascular disease. In: Zuckerman JD, ed. *Instructional Course Lectures 48.* Rosemont, Ill: American Academy of Orthopaedic Surgeons; 1999:687–691.

Smith DG, Michael JW, Bowker JH, eds. *Atlas of Amputations and Limb Deficiencies: Surgical, Prosthetic, and Rehabilitation Principles,* 3rd edition. Rosemont, Ill: American Academy of Orthopaedic Surgeons; 2004.

Waters RI, Perry J, Antonelli D, Hislop H. Energy cost of walking of amputees: the influence of level of amputation. *J Bone Joint Surg Am.* 1976;58:42–46.

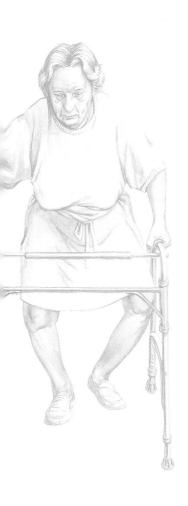

twelve

Rehabilitation

Walter B. Greene, MD

Rehabilitation is an integral part of maximizing the results of treatment after injury or completion of a surgical procedure. The goal is to return the patient to optimal function as quickly as possible. This approach minimizes the profound systemic effects of prolonged immobilization (**Figure 12-1**).

Optimal function may not necessarily be normal function. The return to normal function is impossible with some injuries and disorders. Successful rehabilitation means that the patient has been provided with the physical and psychological means to maximal restoration of function when therapy is curtailed.

Even with modern fracture management, the rehabilitation of musculoskeletal injuries often demands more time and sometimes greater skill than are required for the reduction and fixation. However, for most injuries, rehabilitation does not require complicated equipment or extensive therapy sessions. For most patients, a physician who understands the basic principles usually can outline and monitor an effective program. In contrast, patients with conditions such as paraplegia, multisystem trauma, amputation, chronic arthritis, or intractable low back pain are often best rehabilitated through the coordinated efforts and expertise of a team of physicians and therapists.

This chapter focuses on nonoperative methods of rehabilitation. However, it should be understood that surgical procedures are often an integral part of rehabilitation. For example, tendon transfers may greatly enhance the function and independence of a patient who is paraplegic as the result of a spinal cord injury.

RESTORING JOINT MOTION

Immobilization, whether imposed by a cast or self-imposed by the pain and swelling of an injury, results in muscle weakness and joint stiffness from contracture of the involved ligaments, joint capsules, and muscle-tendon units. Restoration of movement requires stretching of these contracted soft tissues. Regaining motion is more difficult when the fracture was intra-articular, immobilization was prolonged, arthritis was preexistent, or a combination of these factors was present. Fortunately, most sprains, strains, and fractures are not complicated by these factors, and a simple home rehabilitation program usually can be prescribed.

Exercises to regain joint motion may be classified as active, passive, or active-assisted. *Active exercises* involve movements that are under the direct control of the patient. Muscle strengthening is the primary goal of active exercises, but range of motion also may be improved. Active exercise is unlikely to exceed an injury threshold; however, patients with more complex rehabilitation problems or those who are reluctant to initiate movement or muscle contraction require assistance to regain mobility.

In *passive exercises*, a therapist, a family member, or even the patient manually moves the joint (**Figure 12-2**). For example, passive stretching of stiff fingers can be performed easily with the aid of the uninvolved hand. Reinjury may result if the manipulation force exceeds the strength of the healing tissues, but this complication is uncommon if the passive stretch is increased gradually.

Active-assisted exercises combine muscle contraction performed by the patient with assisted movement of the joint. Passive stretch may be applied at the termination of movement. This type of exercise strengthens muscles and stretches ligaments, muscles, and tendons. Active-assisted exercises are particularly useful in the early phase of rehabilitation, when motion is limited and the muscles are too weak for the joint to move through a full arc of motion (**Figure 12-3**).

MEASURING JOINT MOTION

Measuring joint motion allows a simple, objective assessment of disability, as well as

Figure 12-1: Systemic Effects of Immobilization

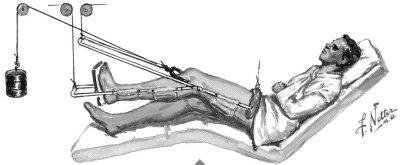

Systemic Effects

Musculoskeletal

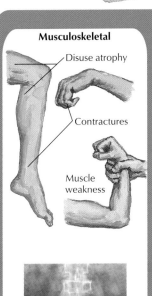

Disuse atrophy

Contractures

Muscle weakness

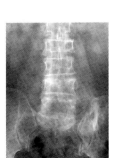

Osteoporosis

Cardiovascular

Increased heart rate, decreased cardiac reserve

Orthostatic hypotension

Altered clotting mechanism, thrombo-phlebitis

Pulmonary embolism

Respiratory

Increased resistance to air flow

Reduced cough and ciliary activity

Atelectasis

Decreased vital capacity

Hypostatic pneumonia

Pulmonary embolism

Neurologic

Confusion, disorientation, anxiety, depression, intellectual deficit

Autonomic lability

Increased dependency

Impaired balance and coordination

Integumentary

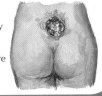

Skin atrophy

Pressure ulcers

Genitourinary

Renal calculi

Hyper-calciuria

Urinary stasis

Urinary tract infection

Gastrointestinal

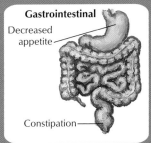

Decreased appetite

Constipation

Mineral-Metabolic

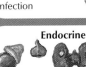

Negative nitrogen, calcium, sulphur, and phosphorus balance. Extracellular fluid shifts

Endocrine

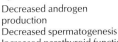

Decreased androgen production
Decreased spermatogenesis
Increased parathyroid function
Reduced insulin binding

Figure 12-2: Passive Exercise

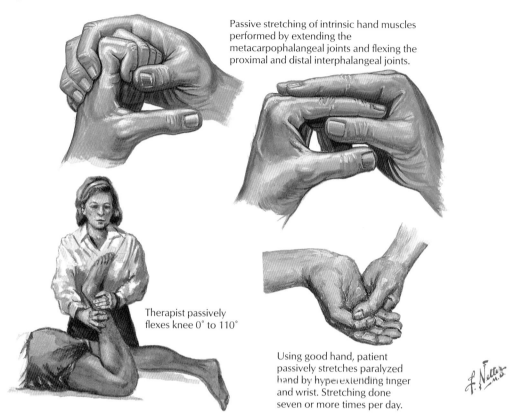

Passive stretching of intrinsic hand muscles performed by extending the metacarpophalangeal joints and flexing the proximal and distal interphalangeal joints.

Therapist passively flexes knee 0° to 110°

Using good hand, patient passively stretches paralyzed hand by hyperextending finger and wrist. Stretching done seven or more times per day.

progress. Standardization of the starting, or zero, position is critical for effective communication. For most joints, the *zero starting position* is the extended, "anatomic" position of the joint. This position is described as 0°

Figure 12-3: Active-Assisted Exercise after Total Knee Replacement

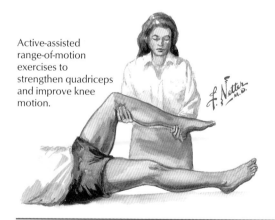

Active-assisted range-of-motion exercises to strengthen quadriceps and improve knee motion.

rather than 180°. Although joint motion may be estimated, a goniometer enhances the accuracy of measurement, is inexpensive, and is easily applied to joints such as the elbow, wrist, finger, knee, and ankle, where bony landmarks allow reproducible alignment of the goniometer (**Figure 12-4**).

MUSCLE STRENGTHENING

Regaining muscle strength is the other primary focus of rehabilitation. Exercises may be classified into three types: isometric, isotonic, and isokinetic. *Isometric strengthening* involves contracting the muscle without moving the joint. This type of exercise is particularly useful in the early rehabilitation process, when joint motion is both painful and limited (**Figure 12-5**). An example of *isotonic strengthening* is lifting of standard barbells. The load placed on the muscle does not change, but the muscular resistance, or force, is continually changing because as the

Figure 12-4: Measurement of Range of Motion

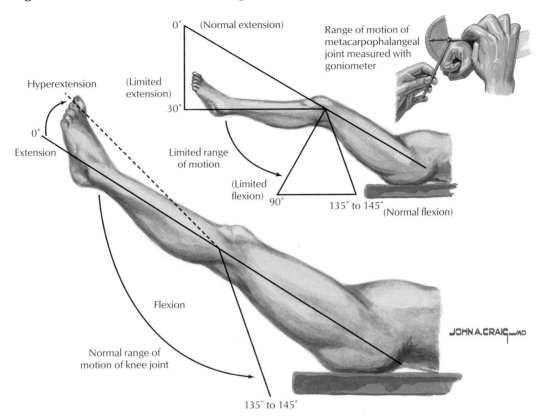

0° (Normal extension)

Range of motion of metacarpophalangeal joint measured with goniometer

Hyperextension

(Limited extension)

30°

0°

Extension

Limited range of motion

(Limited flexion) 90°

135° to 145° (Normal flexion)

JOHN A. CRAIG—MD

Flexion

Normal range of motion of knee joint

135° to 145°

joint moves, the lever arms and efficiency of the muscle are altered. *Isokinetic strengthening* requires special equipment that incorporates a hydraulic system to maintain constant velocity against resistance. Isokinetic exercise allows the muscle to contract maximally throughout its arc of motion and, therefore, should be the most efficient method of strengthening. However, because the ultimate strength achieved by isotonic or isokinetic exercise is similar, it is debatable whether the early difference observed with isokinetic strengthening is great enough to offset the costs of the special equipment.

As a general principle, after injury or surgery, patients should start with isometric and low-resistance isotonic exercises. Vigorous use of isokinetic machines during the early stages of rehabilitation may negatively affect healing and weaken tissues.

MEASURING MUSCLE STRENGTH

Manual grading of muscle strength delineates problem areas, helps in focusing the therapy program, and is useful in assessing progress. Strength is graded on a scale of 0 to 5 (**Table 12-1**). It should be noted that the full range of motion is the *passive* arc of motion, and for a muscle's strength to be graded as fair (grade 3), the muscle must be able to move the joint through that range of motion against gravity. For example, if a patient has a 20° knee flexion contracture and can extend the knee to 20° with some resistance but not with normal strength, then by definition, the quadriceps strength is grade 4, even though the knee does not fully extend.

Figure 12-5: Rehabilitation after Knee Injury or Operation

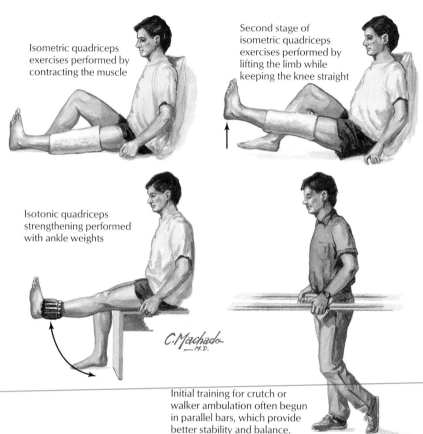

Isometric quadriceps exercises performed by contracting the muscle

Second stage of isometric quadriceps exercises performed by lifting the limb while keeping the knee straight

Isotonic quadriceps strengthening performed with ankle weights

C.Machado M.D.

Initial training for crutch or walker ambulation often begun in parallel bars, which provide better stability and balance.

Likewise, if the patient has full extension of the knee and lacks 20° of active extension of the knee, then that patient has grade 2 quadriceps strength.

When manual muscle testing is performed on specific muscles, the joint should be positioned so as to exclude other muscles that have the same activity. For example, four muscles can dorsiflex the ankle. When the strength of the anterior tibialis muscle is assessed (the best muscle to assess L4 nerve root function), the patient should be instructed to keep the toes flexed. This position inhibits activity of the extensor hallucis longus and the extensor digitorum longus. In addition, the patient should be instructed to pull the foot into dorsiflexion and inversion. This maneuver inhibits the activity of the peroneus tertius.

Instrumented muscle testing provides objective measurement of muscle strength. These techniques provide useful information for research studies, but the cost of such tests does not justify their use in most clinical situations. However, instrumented muscle testing has provided useful information on the limitations of manual muscle testing, which is subjective and dependent on the experience of the observer and on the ability and willingness of the patient to cooperate. The manual classification system also does not correlate in a linear fashion with actual strength (ie, grade 4 strength is typically 40% normal, and grade 3 is 15% normal).

THERAPEUTIC MODALITIES

Physical therapy techniques that use various forms of heat, cold, water, and electrical

Table 12-1
Grading Muscle Strength

Grade	Description
5 (normal)	Complete range of motion against gravity with normal resistance for age and gender
4 (good)	Complete range of motion against gravity, with some resistance
3 (fair)	Complete range of motion against gravity, with no or minimal resistance
2 (poor)	Complete range of motion, with gravity eliminated
1 (trace)	Palpable contraction of the muscle, with no or very limited joint motion
0 (absent)	No contraction of the muscle

modalities are age-old rehabilitation aids. Because such therapies frequently produce a soothing sensation, their psychological effects may be difficult to separate from their physiologic benefits. Regaining motion and strength should be the primary focus of rehabilitation, but physical modalities may enhance the process by decreasing pain and permitting the therapy program to proceed more quickly. Obviously, these techniques are more useful in the initial phases of rehabilitation.

Cryotherapy

Cryotherapy, the use of cold as a treatment modality, is a traditional method for reducing swelling immediately after a sprain or strain. However, cryotherapy also may be a useful modality for reducing pain during the early phases of rehabilitation. Cooling decreases pain, possibly because it acts as a counterstimulant (the gate theory of pain perception), or maybe because it has a direct effect on peripheral nerves.

Techniques of cryotherapy include cold packs, cold compression units, ice massage, cold hydrotherapy, and evaporative cooling sprays. Cold packs and cold compression units are most beneficial immediately after injury or surgery. Ice massage is most frequently used after exercise. Cold hydrotherapy, with water temperatures ranging from 13°C to 18°C for 10 to 20 minutes, has been used to reduce spasticity before physical therapy for patients with upper motor neuron disorders such as cerebral palsy and stroke. Care must be taken to prevent damage to the skin or underlying muscles when cryotherapy is used. Contraindications to cryotherapy include immunologic conditions exacerbated by cold and insensate extremities.

Heat Therapy

Therapeutic heat provides analgesia, hyperemia, local hyperthermia, and reduced muscle tone. Its mechanism of analgesia, similar to that of cold therapy, remains unclear. The application of local heat increases blood flow to skin and subcutaneous tissue; however, penetration of heat to deeper muscular tissues is not only difficult to achieve, it is also unreliable, because control of blood flow to muscle is dependent on metabolic factors within the muscle. If applied before exercise, heat may facilitate stretching of stiff joints that are located superficially.

Contraindications to therapeutic heat treatment include decreased or absent sensation, vascular insufficiency, acute trauma, bleeding disorders, malignancy, and significant cardiac disease.

Hot packs and paraffin baths deliver heat through conduction. Hot packs are warmed to approximately 75°C and are wrapped in towels to protect the skin from thermal injury. The packs are applied for approximately 15 to 20 minutes. Paraffin baths are used most often to transfer heat to arthritic hands. Deeper tissues are not affected by either modality.

Convection therapy circulates a heated substance over a body part and may be administered with the use of moist-air cabinets, hydrotherapy, contrast baths, or fluidotherapy. *Hydrotherapy*, the most frequently used modality, may be carried out in hot tubs, whirlpool baths, and Hubbard tanks. For rehabilitation of minor injuries at home, a warm bath is an excellent way to begin range-of-motion exercises. In therapy centers, hydrotherapy is effectively done in whirlpool tanks that are large enough to enable immersion and exercise of the affected limb in warm (39°C to 45°C) water that is gently agitated. Large tanks and pools that allow walking and running are used to reduce impact loading while providing endurance training, but their effectiveness is controversial.

Fluidotherapy heats and massages tissue by placing the injured part of the body in circulating, heated air that contains suspended particulate matter (cellulose beads). Sensory stimulation from these beads provides additional sedative and analgesic effects. The use of this modality is controversial.

Infrared and visible-light lamps heat only superficial tissues, and their dosage of heat at the tissue level is difficult to calculate. These modalities are rarely used in rehabilitation programs.

Contrast baths alternate cold and heat therapy and thus provide reflex hyperemia and desensitization. This modality is most often used for painful conditions characterized by marked swelling, such as reflex sympathetic dystrophy, but it also may be used at home for symptomatic treatment of painful foot and ankle conditions. Start by placing the affected hand or foot in a cold water bath for 30 seconds. The temperature should be as cold as the patient can tolerate. Immediately switch to a second bucket filled with water that is as warm as can be tolerated. Soak for 30 seconds, then switch back to the bucket of cold water for 30 seconds. Continue to alternate between cold and warm water for a total of 5 minutes. The last soak is performed in cold water.

Diathermy

The two common types of diathermy are ultrasound and shortwave diathermy. *Ultra-sound* involves sound waves above the limit of hearing (approximately 20,000 Hz). Ultrasonography delivers deep heat and also causes nonthermal effects such as cavitation, streaming, and shock waves. Most believe that the benefits of ultrasonography are produced by heat. Because the energy of ultrasonography attenuates rapidly in air, a gel is used as a conduit between the machine and the skin. Continuous movement of the transducer prevents uneven distribution. Because of the practical considerations of penetration, focus, and standardization, most ultrasonography machines use a frequency between 0.8 and 1.0 MHz.

Phonophoresis is an ultrasonographic modality that delivers topical medication (corticosteroids) to deeper structures. However, the effectiveness and depth of penetration of phonophoresis in the clinical situation have not been evaluated conclusively.

Ultrasonography can significantly raise the temperature of tissues that are high in collagen content such as ligaments, joint capsules, and tendons. As the temperature increases within these structures, the collagen elongates, allowing stretching of contracted tissues. Therefore, stretching should begin during the heating of contracted tissue. In muscles, ultrasonography also has an indirect effect in that it increases blood flow. If the treatment damages vessels, blood flow may be adversely affected.

Shortwave diathermy heats deeper tissues through the use of radio waves that produce electrical currents and molecular vibration within the treated tissue. Treatment may be continuous or pulsed. The pulsed approach emphasizes the nonthermal effect and the theoretical resonant effect on cell function.

Although ultrasound and shortwave diathermy are used to treat a great variety of conditions, documentation of their effectiveness compared with simpler modalities is lacking. Contraindications include use in the groin or near the spinal cord after laminectomy. Other relative contraindications include diabetes mellitus, cardiac problems, thrombophlebitis, acute trauma in which bleeding may be exacerbated, and injuries near the physis in children. Additional restrictions on the use of shortwave diathermy are related to its electromagnetic effects.

Electrical Stimulation

Electrical potentials occur in all cells and organs, and therapy that uses electrical stimulation has been prescribed to facilitate healing and reduce pain. Whether this therapy has a significant influence on the healing of soft tissues is inconclusive, but electrical stimulation does seem to be a helpful adjunct in the control of chronic pain.

The use of electrical stimulation for rehabilitation of muscles is probably not justified when voluntary contractions can be generated. However, when immobilization has been prolonged or when voluntary muscle contraction is profoundly inhibited, electrical stimulation is helpful during the initial phases of therapy.

Orthotic Devices

An orthosis may be used for (1) immobilization and protection of an injured part, (2) improvement of function, (3) prevention of deformity, and (4) correction of a deformity. The latter two uses occur primarily in the treatment of pediatric orthopaedic conditions. For example, in conditions that cause muscle imbalance, subsequent growth may lead to progressive contractures. An ankle-foot orthosis frequently is used in the treatment of cerebral palsy to minimize the risk of progressive deformity. Correction of a deformity is illustrated by the use of an abduction harness to reduce and stabilize a hip dislocation in a neonate.

The most common use for an orthosis is protection of an injured part. Although it does not provide as much stability as a circular cast, an orthosis (splint) has the advantage of being removable, thereby allowing bathing and range-of-motion exercises. The decision to use or switch to an orthosis must be individualized; however, most sprains and strains and some fractures can be effectively immobilized with the use of an orthotic device.

Figure 12-6: Orthotics

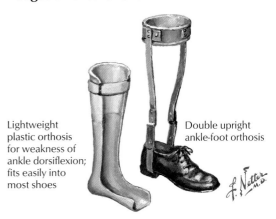

Lightweight plastic orthosis for weakness of ankle dorsiflexion; fits easily into most shoes

Double upright ankle-foot orthosis

An orthosis may improve function. For example, a drop-foot gait caused by peroneal nerve dysfunction may be significantly improved by a below-knee brace made of a lightweight thermoplastic material. A short leg brace made of this material can be worn inside a conventional shoe almost unnoticeably (**Figure 12-6**).

Canes, Crutches, and Walkers

Canes, crutches, and walkers (in that order) reduce weight-bearing stresses on the lower extremities and also improve balance and stability (**Figure 12-7**). The latter may be extremely important in the reduction of falls and fractures in elderly persons and in those who have had strokes.

Canes are light and easily stored. For chronic conditions, a spade handle is easier on the hand than the standard crook handle. To maximize reduction of stress on an arthritic hip, the cane should be used on the contralateral side. A quad cane has four prongs at its base. It is more cumbersome than a single-tipped cane but provides a wider base of support and can be useful after a stroke, when a patient may have only one functional upper limb.

A cane that is too short provides inadequate support. A cane that is too long, in contrast, causes excessive elbow flexion, thus increasing the demand on the triceps muscle,

Figure 12-7: Canes, Crutches, and Walkers

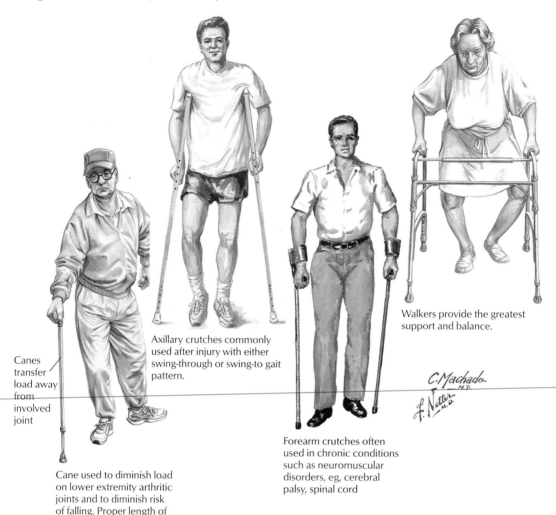

Axillary crutches commonly used after injury with either swing-through or swing-to gait pattern.

Canes transfer load away from involved joint

Cane used to diminish load on lower extremity arthritic joints and to diminish risk of falling. Proper length of cane increases efficiency.

Forearm crutches often used in chronic conditions such as neuromuscular disorders, eg, cerebral palsy, spinal cord

Walkers provide the greatest support and balance.

which is a major stabilizer of the upper extremity when a cane is used. The optimal length of a cane positions the elbow in 20° to 30° of flexion when the tip of the cane is placed approximately 6 inches in front of, and 6 inches lateral to, the little toe.

Crutches offer greater support than a cane but less support than a walker. For short-term use, axillary crutches are satisfactory and economical. Aluminum crutches are more durable than wooden ones, but they cost

more and therefore are prescribed most often for use in chronic conditions. Forearm crutches extend only to the forearm. These crutches are less bulky but require better balance and strength. Platform crutches allow forces through the forearm and are useful for patients with arthritic or traumatic conditions of the hand and wrist.

Crutches that are too long or that are used improperly (with the patient leaning on the top of the crutch) can cause thrombosis or

Table 12-2
Gait Patterns Used With Crutches or Walkers

Type	Description
Swing-through (Variation #1)	Advance both crutches; shift weight, and advance sound leg. No weight on injured limb.
Swing-through (Variation #2)	Advance both crutches; lift the body to advance both feet beyond the crutches.
Swing-to	Advance both crutches; lift the body to advance both feet in line with the crutches.
Four-point	Move one crutch forward; then advance the opposite foot, followed by the ipsilateral crutch, then the contralateral foot. (Three points of contact are always maintained.)
Alternating two-point	Advance one crutch and the contralateral foot at the same time. Shift weight, and advance the other foot and crutch (a progression of the four-point gait).

compression neuropathy. Depending on the height of the patient, the crutch tip should be positioned 4 to 6 inches anterior and lateral to the little toe, and in that position, the length of the crutch should be adjusted to allow 2 inches of clearance between the top of the crutch and the axilla. Adjust the handpiece to permit maximum function of the triceps and latissimus dorsi muscles (i.e., with the elbow flexed 25° to 30°). As a general guideline, the length of the crutch should be approximately 75% of the patient's height.

Walkers have four points of contact and provide the greatest support and balance. The bulkiness of a walker is its major disadvantage. The same principles apply for adjusting the height of a walker and a cane. Elbows should be in approximately 30° of flexion when the patient is in a neutral standing position.

Gait patterns used with crutches or walkers are listed in **Table 12-2**. After an injury, the technique most commonly prescribed is the non–weight-bearing swing-through gait. It is fairly easy to teach patients how to walk on level ground using this method. Ascending or descending steps is more difficult, but the key is to advance the crutches first when going down the stairs and to advance the sound leg first when going up. A training session with a physical therapist is helpful.

ADDITIONAL READINGS

Brotzman SB, Wilk K, eds. *Clinical Orthopaedic Rehabilitation*, 2nd edition. Philadelphia, Pa: Mosby; 2003.

DeLisa JA, Gans BM, Walsh NE, et al, eds. *Physical Medicine and Rehabilitation Medicine: Principles and Practice*, 4th edition. Philadelphia, Pa: Lippincott Williams and Wilkins; 2004.

Greene WB. Principles and techniques of rehabilitation. In: Wilson FC, Lin PP, eds. *General Orthopaedics*. New York, NY: McGraw Hill; 1997:129–139.

Kendall FP, McCreary EK, Provance PG, Rodgers M, Romani W, eds. *Muscles Testing and Function*, 5th edition. Philadelphia, Pa: Lippincott Williams and Wilkins; 2005.

thirteen

Spine

Philip M. Bernini, MD

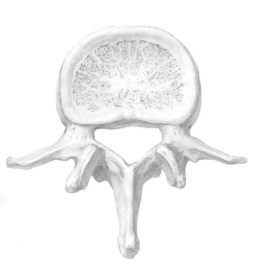

ANATOMY AND BIOMECHANICS
Skeletal and Neural Anatomy

The axial skeleton is composed of 33 vertebrae, including 7 vertebrae in the neck, 12 vertebrae in the thoracic region, 5 vertebrae in the lumbar region, 5 fused vertebrae in the sacrum, and the coccyx that typically includes 4 vertebral bodies, sometimes partially or totally fused together (**Figure 13-1**). Intervertebral discs separate the vertebrae except between the first and second cervical vertebrae (C1 and C2, respectively) and between the sacrum and the coccyx.

The *body* of a vertebra is shaped like a short cylinder and is composed primarily of cancellous, well-vascularized bone covered by a thin layer of cortical bone. With increasing weight-bearing loads, the vertebral body becomes progressively taller and wider from above downward. The *posterior arch* includes right and left *pedicles* that project posteriorly from the posterolateral surface of the vertebral body, and right and left *laminae*

Figure 13-1: Axial Skeleton

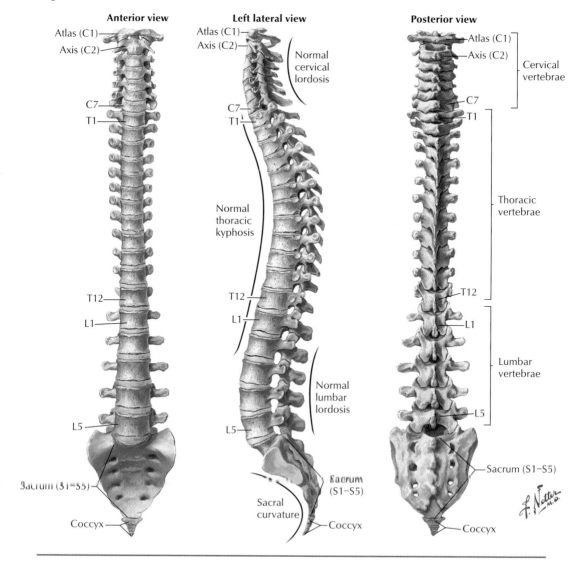

Anterior view

Atlas (C1)
Axis (C2)
C7
T1
T12
L1
L5
Sacrum (S1–S5)
Coccyx

Left lateral view

Atlas (C1)
Axis (C2)
Normal cervical lordosis
C7
T1
Normal thoracic kyphosis
T12
L1
Normal lumbar lordosis
L5
Sacrum (S1–S5)
Sacral curvature
Coccyx

Posterior view

Atlas (C1)
Axis (C2)
Cervical vertebrae
C7
T1
Thoracic vertebrae
T12
L1
Lumbar vertebrae
L5
Sacrum (S1–S5)
Coccyx

that project posteromedially to fuse with the spinous process (**Figure 13-2**). The arch and body enclose and protect the spinal cord and cauda equina and form the vertebral foramen, through which the nerve roots pass.

The *spinous process* projecting posteriorly and the two *transverse processes* that extend laterally from the *pedicle-lamina junction* provide outrigger insertion sites for the multiple muscles and ligaments that move and stabilize the trunk. The *facet joints* provide motion between two vertebrae. The superior articular process and facet joint extend from the pedicle of the vertebra below (caudal) to articulate with the inferior articular process and facet joint that extends from the lamina of the vertebra above.

The vertebral canal extends from the foramen magnum to the sacrum and encloses the spinal cord and its nerve roots. The dura mater is separated from the bones by an epidural space that contains fat and an extensive plexus of epidural veins. The *dural sac* continues inferiorly to approximately the middle of the S2 vertebra. Growth of the spinal cord lags behind longitudinal growth of the axial skeleton. Therefore, the *conus medullaris* (the tapered, inferior end of the spinal cord) extends to the L5 vertebra at the third month of gestation, is opposite the inferior aspect of L2 at birth, and reaches its adult location at the upper border of L2 at 5 years of age. Inferior to

Figure 13-2: Second Lumbar Vertebra

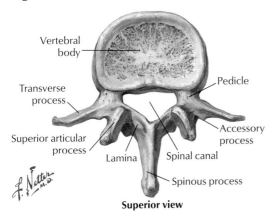

Vertebral body

Transverse process

Pedicle

Superior articular process

Accessory process

Lamina

Spinal canal

Spinous process

Superior view

the conus, the dural sac contains the *cauda equina* (lumbosacral nerve roots) and the *filum terminale*, a cord of tissue that travels inferiorly from the conus to merge with the periosteum on the dorsum of the coccyx (**Figure 13-3**).

The dorsal and ventral nerve roots and the dorsal root ganglion converge to form the *postganglionic spinal nerve* at approximately the level of the respective intervertebral foramen. Because there are eight pairs of cervical nerves and seven cervical vertebrae, cervical nerves are numbered according to the vertebra above which they emerge (eg, the C3 nerve root travels through the foramen above the C3 vertebra, and the eighth cervical nerve emerges through the foramen between C7 and T1). Thereafter, in the thoracic and lumbar regions, spinal nerves are numbered relative to the vertebra below which they emerge; thus, the L3 nerve emerges through the foramen below the L3 vertebra.

The first and second cervical vertebrae are different from the lower five cervical vertebrae (**Figure 13-4**). The *atlas* (C1 vertebra) lacks a spinous process and is essentially an oval ring of bone. The lateral portions of the C1 ring are thickened into a *lateral mass* that articulates with the occipital condyle superiorly and with the lateral mass of C2 inferiorly.

The *axis* (C2 vertebra) has a toothlike protuberance, the dens, that projects upward from the body to provide structural support for the atlas. The C2 superior articular process arises from the body and pedicle rather than from the junction of the pedicle and lamina. The dens provides a pivot point on which the head and atlas can rotate relatively freely on the relatively flat C1-C2 articular facets. From the C2-C3 facet joint and below, the superior facets are oriented primarily in a dorsal and cranial direction, whereas the inferior facets face the opposite direction.

The cervical spine is a mobile platform for the skull and is the most flexible portion of the vertebral column. Motion of the cervical spine includes flexion and extension, right and left lateral bending, and right and left rotation. In young adults, normal neck motion is

Figure 13-3: Spinal Cord and Nerve Root Relationships to Vertebrae

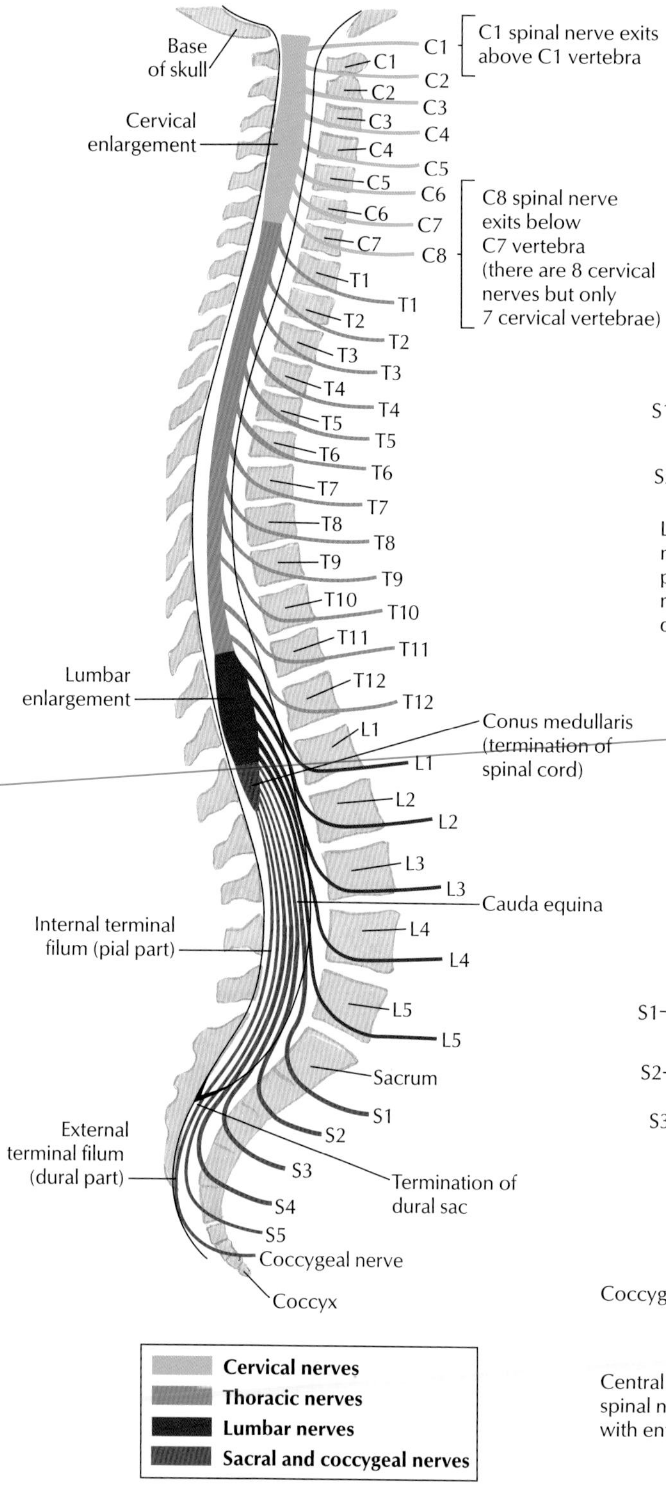
Base of skull
Cervical enlargement
Lumbar enlargement
Internal terminal filum (pial part)
External terminal filum (dural part)
C1
C2
C3
C4
C5
C6
C7
C8
T1
T2
T3
T4
T5
T6
T7
T8
T9
T10
T11
T12
L1
L2
L3
L4
L5
Sacrum
S1
S2
S3
S4
S5
Coccygeal nerve
Coccyx
C1 spinal nerve exits above C1 vertebra
C8 spinal nerve exits below C7 vertebra (there are 8 cervical nerves but only 7 cervical vertebrae)
Conus medullaris (termination of spinal cord)
Cauda equina
Termination of dural sac
Cervical nerves
Thoracic nerves
Lumbar nerves
Sacral and coccygeal nerves

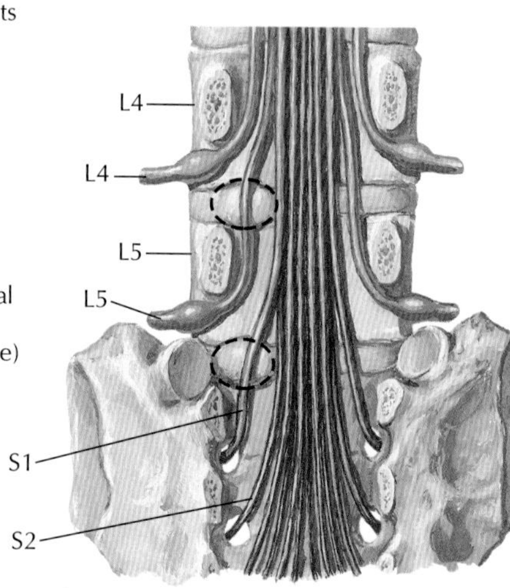
L4
L4
L5
L5
S1
S2

Lumbar disc protusion typically does not affect nerve exiting above disc. Therefore, disc protusion at L4-L5 compresses L5 spinal nerve, not L4 spinal nerve. However, far lateral L4-L5 disc herniation may entrapment L4 nerve root.

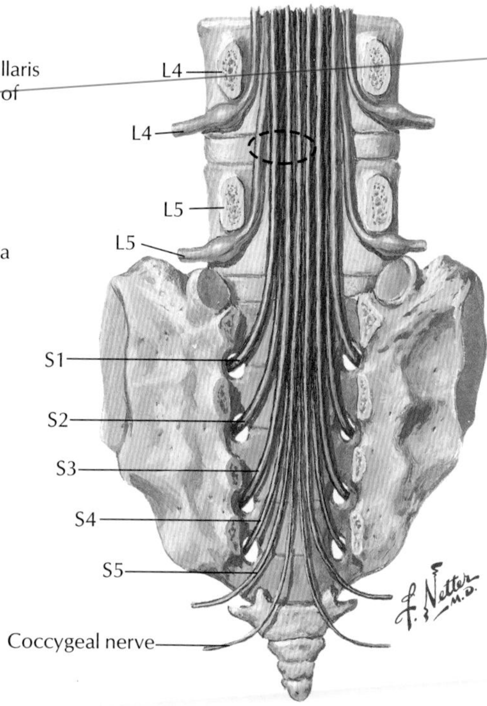
L4
L4
L5
L5
S1
S2
S3
S4
S5
Coccygeal nerve
F. Netter M.D.

Central disc protrusion at L4-L5 uncommonly affects L4 spinal nerve, but may cause cauda equina syndrome with entrapment of L5 and S1-S4 spinal nerves.

Figure 13-4: Cervical Vertebrae

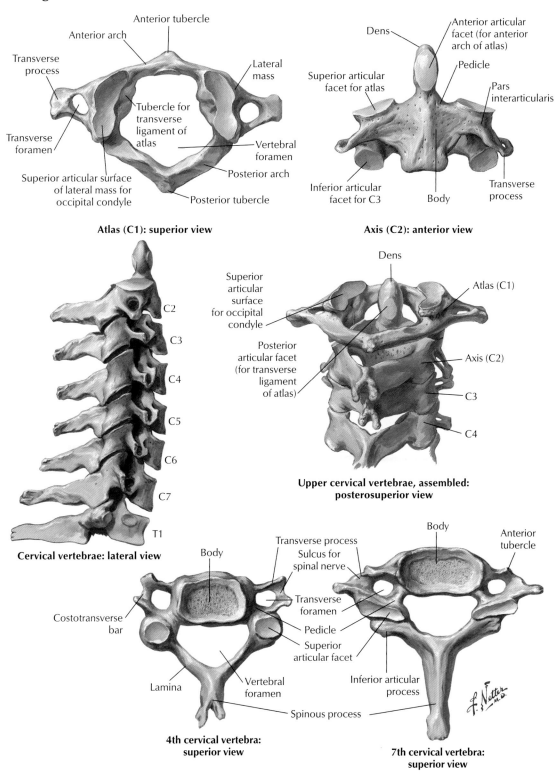

Atlas (C1): superior view

Axis (C2): anterior view

Cervical vertebrae: lateral view

Upper cervical vertebrae, assembled: posterosuperior view

4th cervical vertebra: superior view

7th cervical vertebra: superior view

70° flexion, 70° extension, 50° lateral bending, and 90° rotation to each side.

The degree of motion between two vertebrae is determined primarily by the *orientation of the facets*; therefore, different vertebral segments contribute differing amounts to each plane of motion. This difference is particularly pronounced in rotation of the neck, where approximately 55% to 60% of cervical rotation occurs at the C1-C2 level. Flexion relative to extension is limited at the occiput-C1 joint, but from C1 to C6, the ranges of flexion and extension are approximately equal at each vertebral level. The total arc of flexion-extension, however, is greater in the lower cervical vertebral segments, with peak motion occurring at the C5-C6 level. Motion of the spine is often coupled. For example, lateral bending of the neck is accompanied by rotation, and rotation of the cervical spine is coupled with lateral bending and flexion-extension.

Thoracic vertebrae have costal facets at the upper and lower edges of the junction of the body with the arch on each side. The superior articular facets are directed cranially, dorsally, and laterally, whereas the inferior facets point in the opposite direction. Primary motion in the thoracic spine is lateral bending and rotation, with lateral bending being greater in the lower thoracic segments and rotation being greater in the upper thoracic spine.

Because of the increased axial loads and the lack of surrounding rib support, the horizontal diameter of a lumbar vertebra is greater than its height. Lumbar vertebrae are larger and thicker anteriorly. The superior articular facet of a lumbar vertebra faces mostly medially, and the inferior facet is directed laterally (**Figure 13-5**). Flexion-extension is the primary arc of motion in the lumbar spine, with greater movement occurring in the lower lumbar segments. When the person is leaning forward, flexion occurs first in the lumbar spine, followed by rotation (flexion) of the pelvis at the hip joints. When one goes from flexion to extension, the pattern is reversed, with the pelvis extending first, followed by the lumbar spine.

Motion of the cervical and lumbar spine decreases with age. This decrease occurs sooner and is more severe in males.

Intervertebral Discs

The intervertebral discs contribute approximately 20% of the length of the cervical and thoracic spine and approximately 33% of the length of the lumbar region. In the cervical and lumbar regions, the discs are thicker anteriorly. Cervical lordosis is secondary to the shape of the disc, but lumbar lordosis is a function of the shape of the vertebral body, as well as the disc. Thoracic discs have uniform height. Thoracic kyphosis occurs secondary to the shape of the vertebral bodies.

The intervertebral disc includes the *annulus fibrosus* and the *nucleus pulposus* (**Figure 13-6**). The outer portion of the annulus fibrosus is a ring of highly oriented and densely packed type I collagen fibers that anchor to the vertebral body. The fibrocartilaginous inner portion of the annulus fibrosus is composed mostly of less dense and less organized type II collagen. The central nucleus pulposus is composed of water, type II collagen, and proteoglycan aggregates. This composite structure provides good resistance to repeated loading in both compression and tension. With routine activities, compression pressures on a disc are balanced by hydrostatic pressurization. The negatively charged glycosaminoglycan molecules on the proteoglycan chains attract fluid into the extracellular space. With increased loads, fluid is expressed from the disc. This fluid expression causes an increase in the concentration of negatively charged glycosaminoglycans, with a resultant increase in the imbibition pressure within the disc. As a result, large compressive loads are tolerated. The energy dissipation capability of a healthy intervertebral disc is impressive. The load at the L3-L4 disc ranges from 30 kg while the individual is lying supine to more than 300 kg when the person is lifting a 20-kg weight with the spine flexed and the knees straight. Even with excessive axial loading, the vertebral body and cartilaginous end plate fail before the intervertebral disc does.

Figure 13-5: Anatomy of Lumbosacral Spine

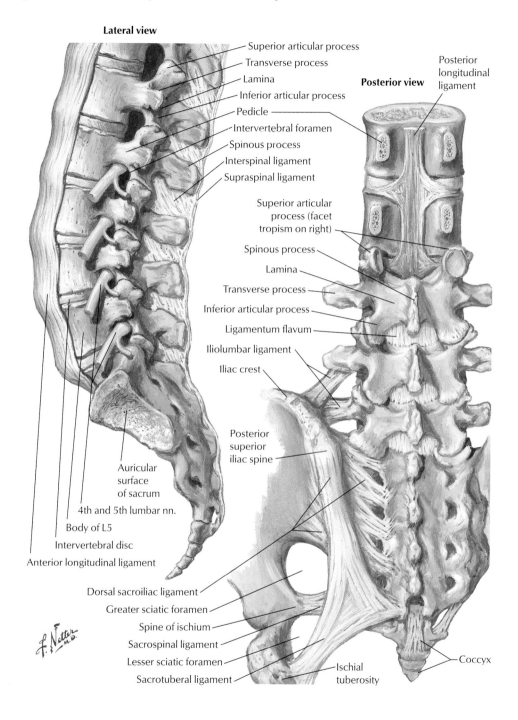

Lateral view

Superior articular process
Transverse process
Lamina
Inferior articular process
Pedicle
Intervertebral foramen
Spinous process
Interspinal ligament
Supraspinal ligament

Auricular surface of sacrum
4th and 5th lumbar nn.
Body of L5
Intervertebral disc
Anterior longitudinal ligament

Dorsal sacroiliac ligament
Greater sciatic foramen
Spine of ischium
Sacrospinal ligament
Lesser sciatic foramen
Sacrotuberal ligament

Posterior view

Posterior longitudinal ligament

Superior articular process (facet tropism on right)
Spinous process
Lamina
Transverse process
Inferior articular process
Ligamentum flavum
Iliolumbar ligament
Iliac crest
Posterior superior iliac spine

Ischial tuberosity
Coccyx

Figure 13-6: Intervertebral Disc

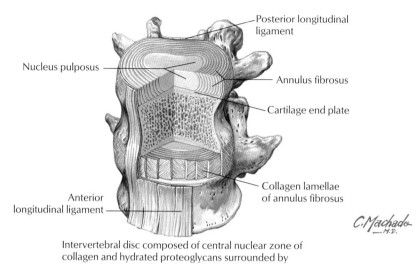

Intervertebral disc composed of central nuclear zone of collagen and hydrated proteoglycans surrounded by concentric lamellae of collagen fibers

Intervertebral discs also have small concentrations of type III, V, and XI fibril-forming collagens and small amounts of type VI, IX, and XII short-helix collagens. Type VI collagen concentration is relatively high in the disc, suggesting that this type contributes to the unique properties of the nucleus pulposus.

During childhood and early adolescence, the nucleus pulposus occupies approximately half of the disc and has a large concentration of water (70% to 80% wet weight) and proteoglycans (approximately 50% dry weight). Age-related changes in the intervertebral disc begin during adolescence. The initiating event appears to be diminished blood flow to the disc as vessels to the annulus and cartilaginous end plate become smaller and less numerous. Proteoglycan aggregates evolve into clusters of short-aggrecan molecules and nonaggregated proteoglycans. During the adult years, the nucleus pulposus becomes progressively smaller and more fibrotic as the proteoglycan and water concentrations decrease. The remaining peripheral blood vessels mostly disappear. Fissures and cracks appear between the lamellae in the outer annulus and progressively extend centrally. In the elderly individual, the disc inside the outer annulus evolves into a stiff fibrocartilage, with few viable cells remaining in the nucleus pulposus.

Spinal Mechanics

The axis of thoracic and lumbar spinal motion is located in the disc, but the center of gravity is anterior to the vertebral body. Therefore, even with erect standing, a bending moment is generated in the spine that must be resisted by the intervertebral discs, spinal ligaments, and spinal extensor muscles. Greatest loads are seen in the lumbar region. The bending moment is markedly increased when an individual is lifting or carrying an object in front of the body. Flexion and torsional movement also greatly increase pressure in the lumbar disc.

PHYSICAL EXAMINATION

Inspect spinal alignment from the back and side. From the posterior view, the spine should be straight. Look for deviations in normal cervical and lumbar lordosis and for thoracic kyphosis. Loss of cervical or lumbar lordosis occurs with painful conditions such as acute sprains, fractures, infections, or neoplastic processes (**Figure 13-7**). The patient who leans to one side may be attempting to alleviate nerve root compression in the cervical or lumbar region.

Figure 13-7: Physical Examination

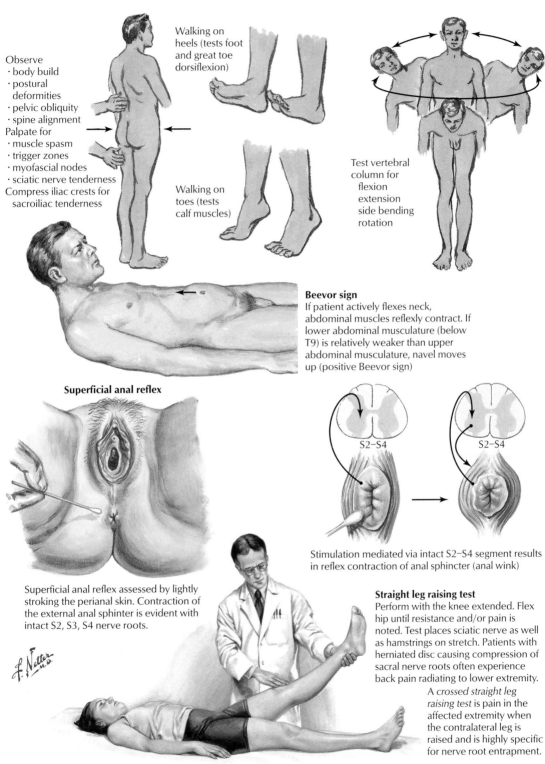

Observe
· body build
· postural deformities
· pelvic obliquity
· spine alignment
Palpate for
· muscle spasm
· trigger zones
· myofascial nodes
· sciatic nerve tenderness
Compress iliac crests for sacroiliac tenderness

Walking on heels (tests foot and great toe dorsiflexion)

Walking on toes (tests calf muscles)

Test vertebral column for
flexion
extension
side bending
rotation

Beevor sign
If patient actively flexes neck, abdominal muscles reflexly contract. If lower abdominal musculature (below T9) is relatively weaker than upper abdominal musculature, navel moves up (positive Beevor sign)

Superficial anal reflex

Superficial anal reflex assessed by lightly stroking the perianal skin. Contraction of the external anal sphinter is evident with intact S2, S3, S4 nerve roots.

S2–S4

S2–S4

Stimulation mediated via intact S2–S4 segment results in reflex contraction of anal sphincter (anal wink)

Straight leg raising test
Perform with the knee extended. Flex hip until resistance and/or pain is noted. Test places sciatic nerve as well as hamstrings on stretch. Patients with herniated disc causing compression of sacral nerve roots often experience back pain radiating to lower extremity.

A *crossed straight leg raising test* is pain in the affected extremity when the contralateral leg is raised and is highly specific for nerve root entrapment.

Palpate the prominent posterior spinous process of C7. The posterior iliac crest is usually at the level of the L4 vertebral body; the posterior superior iliac spine (PSIS), indicated by the dimples of Venus, is on a level with S2.

The Zero Starting Position for assessing spinal motion is with the hip and knees straight and the head and trunk in line with the lower extremities. The neck range of motion should be visually estimated in all six directions. Lumbar flexion is assessed by asking the patient to touch the toes. Normal motion is present if the fingertips extend to at least the distal tibia. A pathologic lumbar condition is more likely if the fingertips are farther than 10 cm from the floor at maximum flexion. Observe the patient as he or she comes from full flexion to extension. Degenerative conditions frequently cause a ratchety-like motion as the spine moves into extension.

Lumbar motion also can be quantified by skin distraction. With the patient in the zero starting position, mark a 15-cm span over the posterior lumbar spine with the distal point on line with the PSIS (dimple of Venus). Then, ask the patient to bend forward as far as possible, and remeasure the distance between these points. With normal lumbar flexion, the distance between the previous 15-cm span typically increases to 20 to 22 cm. With extension of the spine, the distance between the two 15-cm points decreases by 2 to 4 cm.

Evaluate sensory and motor function of each cervical and/or lumbar nerve root that could possibly be affected. This evaluation is most readily accomplished by testing the strength of one muscle and one area of sensation for each nerve root. The muscle selected should exhibit at least good strength if the nerve root being accessed and the nerve roots above it are intact (**Table 13-1**). The clinician can assess thoracic nerve root function by checking sensation in the involved dermatome. The *straight leg raising test* places the L5 and S1 nerve roots on stretch and is done with the patient supine. With the knee

Table 13-1 Evaluation of Cervical and Lumbosacral Nerve Roots			
Nerve	**Muscle**	**Sensory**	**Reflex**
Cervical Nerve Roots			
C5	Deltoid, biceps	Lateral proximal arm	Biceps
C6	Radial wrist extensors	Volar aspect of thumb	Brachioradialis
C7	Triceps, flexor carpi radialis	Volar aspect of long finger	Triceps
C8	Flexor digitorum sublimus to ring finger	Volar aspect of little finger	None
T1	First dorsal interossei	Medial aspect of arm	None
Lumbosacral Nerve Roots			
L1	Hip flexor	Anterior proximal thigh	None
L2	Hip adductor	Middle proximal thigh	None
L3	Quadriceps	Inferior to patella	Patella
L4	Anterior tibialis	Just above medial malleolus	Patella
L5	Extensor hallucis longus	First web space	None
S1	Flexor hallucis longus	Lateral border of foot	Achilles

straight, lift the leg as high as possible, and measure the degree of hip flexion. The *reverse straight leg raising* or *prone rectus femoris test* is performed with the patient prone; it puts the L1-L4 nerve roots under tension. The prone rectus femoris test is easier to perform and is done by flexing the knee with the hip extended.

Special tests to indicate long-track spinal cord involvement include the *Hoffmann sign* and tests to detect superficial abdominal reflexes, Babinski sign, ankle clonus, and increased deep tendon reflexes. The Hoffmann test is performed by flicking the nail of the long finger into flexion. A positive Hoffmann sign is thumb and/or index finger flexion on the ipsilateral side. Superficial abdominal reflexes are assessed by stroking the skin lightly toward the umbilicus. A normal reflex reveals movement of the umbilicus toward the stimulated side. The test is performed in the upper and lower quadrants on both sides. An absent response may indicate cervical or thoracic spinal cord pathology.

DEGENERATIVE DISORDERS

Degenerative axial skeletal syndromes are endemic, with 25% of the adult population reporting neck pain and up to 80% experiencing low back pain. The symptoms cover a continuum from the aches associated with normal, age-related degenerative changes in the disc to disorders that are extremely painful and disabling. Degenerative spinal disorders may begin during late adolescence but occur most frequently in middle-aged and older people.

The clinical presentation varies from neck or back pain with or without radicular symptoms to disconcerting myelopathy with extremity and bowel and bladder dysfunction. Symptoms may coincide with well-defined pain pathways or may be vague and ambiguous. The latter symptoms are especially pronounced when the degenerative process stimulates macrophages and releases various cytokines that adversely stimulate nociceptive nerve endings in and around adjacent spinal structures. Psychological symptoms are aggravated and may become paramount with persistent pain, inability to work at the usual occupation, the need to change jobs with subsequent loss of income, and litigation that may accompany motor vehicle injury or workers' compensation claims.

Cervical Degenerative Syndromes
Neck Pain Alone

Identifying the pathologic nidus is difficult when a patient's only presenting complaint is axial pain, and the only findings are limited range of motion and associated muscle spasm. Imaging studies may demonstrate narrowing and desiccation of the disc and/or the presence of facet osteophytes; however, the meaning of these findings is not clear because, depending on age, 30% to 70% of asymptomatic people may demonstrate these changes. Fortunately, most patients with axial pain can be treated successfully with nonoperative modalities that include pain management, short-term use of supportive orthotics, and therapy to strengthen paraspinal muscles, thereby diminishing stress across the degenerative discs and facet joints.

Cervical Radiculopathy

Cervical radiculopathy is referred neurogenic pain (**Figure 13-8**), usually found in the distribution of a defined nerve root but sometimes associated with *brachialgia* (diffuse, nonspecific pain in the arm). In young adults, the usual cause is a herniated cervical disc that causes compression of the nerve root as it exits the foramen. In older patients, entrapment of the nerve root is more often secondary to narrowing of the disc space, with subsequent arthritic changes at the facet and the *uncinate processes* (a degenerative articulation referred to as Luschka joint) causing narrowing of the foramen.

A typical symptom is pain in the neck or paracervical region that radiates in a dermatomal distribution to the upper extremity. Other possible symptoms include occipital headaches that result from associated compression of upper and midcervical nerve roots or pain radiating to the posterior

Figure 13-8: Cervical Radiculopathy

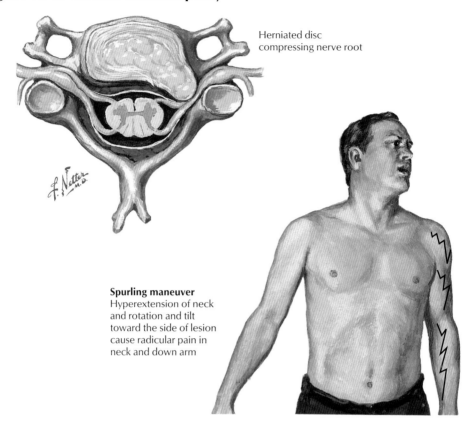

Herniated disc
compressing nerve root

Spurling maneuver
Hyperextension of neck
and rotation and tilt
toward the side of lesion
cause radicular pain in
neck and down arm

shoulder and upper thoracic area with entrapment of lower cervical nerve roots. Weakness, changes in handwriting, dropping of objects from the hand, and difficulty with manipulative tasks that require fine coordination also may be noted. To decrease tension on the involved nerve root, patients often place the ipsilateral forearm over the top of the head.

Examination often shows mild restriction of neck motion. The *Spurling test* is done by having the patient extend the neck while tilting the head to the side of the pain. In this position, the foramen is narrowed, and radicular pain is intensified. Assess motor and sensory function to determine the site of nerve root entrapment. Perform a complete neurologic examination to exclude upper motor neuron involvement and a more complex disorder. Obtain cervical radiographs to rule out other conditions and to identify areas of degenerative disc disease and facet joint changes.

Nonoperative management alleviates symptoms in most patients, but the process can take several weeks. Helpful modalities include adequate pain medication, cervical traction, and physical therapy. Reserve the use of magnetic resonance imaging (MRI) for patients with persistent symptoms who are candidates for operative treatment.

Operative treatment is indicated for persistent and disabling symptoms. Disc excision can be done by an anterior or a posterior approach; however, most patients are treated via the anterior approach with decompression of the disc and concomitant arthrodesis. Spinal fusion prevents the potential problem of cervical instability, and by placing an autograft or allograft of appropriate size, the height of the disc space and foramen can be restored.

Cervical Spondylosis With Myelopathy

Cervical spondylosis with myelopathy can be extremely disabling (**Figure 13-9**). Cervical myelopathy may be caused by a large central disc herniation, but most commonly, it is due to severe spondylitic changes, including stenosis of the canal from ingrowth of bony spurs, as well as thickening and buckling of the ligamentum flavum. The condition is common among older men and persons with conditions that increase spinal instability (eg, rheumatoid arthritis, acute trauma, metastatic spine disease).

Symptoms are variable but classically include stiffness and neck pain that is increased with activity; progressive sensory abnormalities in the upper extremities; and progressive motor weakness, spasticity, and loss of proprioception in the lower extremities. This combination leads to the characteristic *wide-based myelopathic gait.* Tendon reflexes are increased in the lower extremities, but upper extremity reflexes may be decreased or increased, depending on the level of the lesion. The Hoffmann sign, which is indicative of an upper motor neuron disease, is often positive. Abnormalities of bladder function are associated with severe involvement.

Progression of cervical myelopathy is variable. Symptoms most often persist, but significant progression is unlikely if the disability is mild. Even patients with moderate to severe symptoms at presentation have long periods of nonprogressive disability. Indications for surgery include progressive neurologic deficits or a static neurologic deficit associated with radicular pain that does not respond to nonoperative treatment.

Chronic Low Back Pain and Lumbar Degenerative Disc Disease

Low back pain, with or without leg pain, is very common, particularly in middle-aged

Figure 13-9: Cervical Spondylosis with Myelopathy

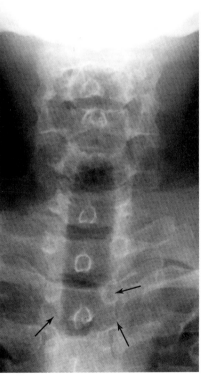

X-ray film showing stenosis secondary to cervical spondylosis and bridging of vertebral bodies by osteophytes

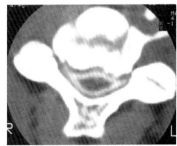

Metrizamide myelogram with CT scan showing spinal cord compression secondary to severe cervical spondylosis

and older adults. Degeneration of the intervertebral disc and some degree of low back pain and stiffness are universal with aging. Degenerated discs have decreased height, increased posterior and lateral bulging, reduced ability to dissipate compression forces, and initially increased mobility. As a result, secondary changes develop and include abnormal loading of the facet joints, greater stress on adjacent ligaments and muscles, subsequent thickening of the ligamentum flavum, and osteophyte formation. The variability of the site and the severity and deep location of the secondary changes make it difficult to isolate the primary source of low back pain.

Chronic low back pain, defined as persistent symptoms for longer than 6 to 8 weeks, is common among people older than 40 to 50 years of age and those working in occupations that require frequent bending and lifting or exposure to repetitive vibrations (truck drivers). Obesity and poor physical fitness are risk factors. Evidence on the association of chronic low back pain with smoking is inconclusive.

A typical complaint is pain that begins in the lower back and radiates to one or both buttocks. Occasionally, the patient notes pain that radiates to the posterior thigh. The pain is increased by lifting and bending activities and is decreased with lying down and after resting at night. As in all chronic pain conditions, depression may aggravate symptoms and complicate treatment.

Examination typically shows mild tenderness in the lower back or sacroiliac region. Flexion of the spine and straight leg raising are mildly affected. With more severe involvement, extension of the spine causes increased discomfort and a dysrhythmic or ratchety-like motion. The neurologic examination is normal. Patients with compounding issues may display nonorganic symptoms such as exaggerated pain behaviors and nonanatomic localization of symptoms. Other conditions should be considered in the evaluation process (**Table 13-2**).

Radiographs and MRI of the spine detect changes that are difficult to differentiate from normal age-related changes. These changes include reduced height of the intervertebral disc, anterior osteophytes, and decreased hydration of the disc. Screening radiographs to rule out tumor, infection, or an inflammatory arthritic process are appropriate for patients with atypical findings or pain lasting longer than 6 weeks. MRI studies should be reserved for patients whose signs and symptoms suggest other conditions, or for preoperative planning in the small proportion of patients who have unremitting symptoms.

Table 13–2
Differential Diagnosis of Chronic Low Back Pain

Intraspinal Source

Degenerative disc changes and herniated disc

Degenerative spondylosis

Lumbar stenosis and intermittent neurogenic claudication

Cauda equina syndrome

Infection
  Osteomyelitis (+/− epidural abscess)
  Discitis

Neoplasm
  Primary
  Metastatic

Inflammatory arthridities

Osteoporosis with compression fracture

Musculotendinous insufficiency

Extraspinal Source

Vascular insufficiency and abdominal aortic aneurysm

Benign gynecologic disorders: ovarian cyst and endometriosis

Intrapelvic or abdominal neoplasm

Sacroiliac arthritis

Arthridities of the hip: osteoarthritis, inflammatory arthritis, osteonecrosis

Trochanteric bursitis and abductor tendinosis

Recurrent episodes of pain are typical, but most can be managed with nonoperative modalities, including intermittent use of nonsteroidal anti-inflammatory drugs (NSAIDs), general conditioning exercises, abdominal and paraspinal strengthening exercises, weight reduction, and cessation of smoking. Unremitting pain necessitates further evaluation. Operative treatment may be indicated, but the results are not always successful. Furthermore, the advantages of, and indications for, the various operative techniques—including posterolateral fusion (with or without instrumentation),

intervertebral disc space arthrodesis with bone graft (with or without metallic implants), and even artificial disc implants—are still unclear.

Lumbar Herniated Disc

The nucleus pulposus may herniate and compress a nerve root, resulting in sciatica (leg pain associated with back pain). The disc may be *protruded* (with the annulus intact), *extruded* (through the annulus but contained by the posterior longitudinal ligament), or *sequestered* (free within the spinal canal) (**Figure 13-10**). Pain results from nerve root

Figure 13-10: Lumbar Disc Herniation

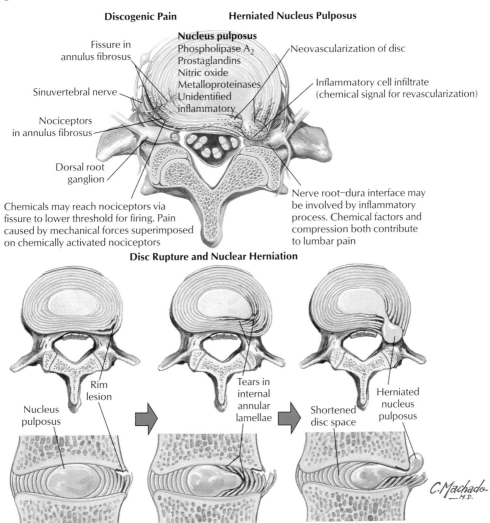

Discogenic Pain

Herniated Nucleus Pulposus

Fissure in annulus fibrosus

Nucleus pulposus
Phospholipase A$_2$
Prostaglandins
Nitric oxide
Metalloproteinases
Unidentified inflammatory

Neovascularization of disc

Sinuvertebral nerve

Inflammatory cell infiltrate (chemical signal for revascularization)

Nociceptors in annulus fibrosus

Dorsal root ganglion

Chemicals may reach nociceptors via fissure to lower threshold for firing. Pain caused by mechanical forces superimposed on chemically activated nociceptors

Nerve root–dura interface may be involved by inflammatory process. Chemical factors and compression both contribute to lumbar pain

Disc Rupture and Nuclear Herniation

Rim lesion

Nucleus pulposus

Tears in internal annular lamellae

Shortened disc space

Herniated nucleus pulposus

C. Machado
—M.D.

Peripheral tear of annulus fibrosus and cartilage end plate (rim lesion) initiates sequence of events that weaken and tear internal annular lamellae, allowing extrusion and herniation of nucleus pulposus

compression and from an inflammatory response initiated by various cytokines released from the nucleus pulposus.

Patients with lumbar disc herniation typically are young and middle-aged adults who have a history of previous low back pain acutely exacerbated by a bending, twisting, or lifting event. The central portion of the posterior longitudinal ligament inhibits direct posterior extrusions. More than 90% of lumbar disc herniations occur posterolaterally at L4-L5 and L5-S1, with subsequent compression of the L5 and S1 nerves, respectively, because lumbar nerve roots emerge from the canal at the superior aspects of the foramina, and a posterolateral herniation compresses the next lower nerve root. However, a far lateral disc herniation at L4-L5 and L5-S1 compresses the L4 and L5 nerves, respectively.

Increasing pressure or stretch on the compressed nerve exacerbates pain. Pain also is increased by sitting, sneezing, and lifting and is decreased by lying down with a pillow under the legs or by lying on the side with the hips and knees flexed. Symptoms are variable, but L5 entrapment typically radiates to the posterolateral aspect of the thigh, the posterior calf, and the medial aspect of the foot. S1 sciatica has a similar distribution in the thigh and calf but radiates to the lateral aspect of the foot.

On examination, look for a list of the spine toward the affected side, a position that decreases tension at the typical site of nerve root entrapement. A positive straight leg raising test (lifting the leg with the knee straight) is the classic sciatic nerve root tension sign, and the test should be performed on both legs. This maneuver may increase symptoms in a variety of spinal conditions, but motion is usually markedly limited on the affected side—ie, less than 50°—with a herniated disc. Reproduction of buttock and/or leg pain on elevation of the contralateral limb (the cross-leg sign) is highly specific for lumbosacral nerve root entrapment. With L4 or higher root compression, pain may be increased by a lying-down position. To put these nerve roots on stretch, a reverse straight leg raising or prone rectus femoris test is performed. Examination should include evaluation of nerve root function (see **Table 13-1**).

Radiographs of the lumbar spine are normal but should be obtained to rule out other conditions. MRI demonstrates changes but is not necessary unless symptoms progress and preoperative planning is undertaken.

Most patients respond to nonoperative treatment. NSAIDs and short-term bed rest are used for the first few days. Muscle relaxants, narcotic medications, or both may be needed for the first 5 to 7 days. To reduce pressure and enhance dissipation of the herniation, patients should lie down frequently, limit initial upright activity to standing, and avoid lifting and prolonged sitting. A short course of steroidal (oral or epidural) medication can ameliorate symptoms but does not change the natural history of the syndrome or alter pain that has persisted for longer than 2 weeks.

Indications for surgery include cauda equina syndrome, urinary retention, progressive neurologic deficit, severe single nerve root paralysis, radicular symptoms that show limited progress for longer than 6 to 12 weeks, and recurrent sciatica that compromises quality of life.

The goal of the operative procedure is to alleviate pressure. The procedure usually involves a small laminotomy and excision of the herniated disc with or without magnification (**Figure 13-11**). Other methods include percutaneous discectomy by suction or endoscopic techniques. Lumbar disc surgery may provide dramatic relief of symptoms and, with proper indications, is generally anticipated to produce good or excellent results in 85% to 90% of patients. Recurrent disc herniation occurs in 5% to 10% of patients. Other possible complications include injury of the neural elements, postoperative septic discitis, bowel perforation, and persistent pain.

Cauda Equina Syndrome

Multiple nerve roots of the cauda equina may be compressed in a relatively short time by central disc herniation or other condition,

Figure 13-11: Discectomy

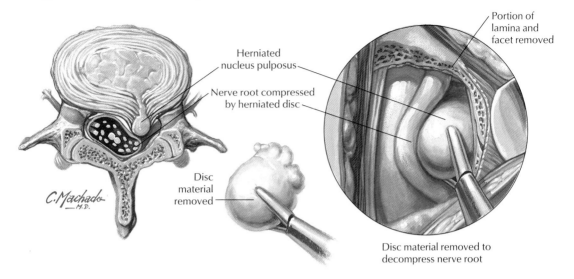

Herniated nucleus pulposus

Nerve root compressed by herniated disc

Portion of lamina and facet removed

Disc material removed

Disc material removed to decompress nerve root

C. Machado
_M.D.

such as epidural abscess, epidural hematoma, or fracture. Midline sacral nerve roots that control bowel and bladder function are particularly vulnerable. Typical symptoms include bilateral lower extremity radicular pain and motor/sensory dysfunction, saddle anesthesia, and difficulty voiding or loss of bladder and anal sphincter control. Lower extremity pain and weakness are typically more severe in one leg.

Patients with cauda equina syndrome usually require urgent surgical decompression. Even with prompt treatment, however, the return of neurologic function is often incomplete.

Lumbar Spinal Stenosis

Lumbar spinal stenosis results from any condition that causes narrowing of the spinal canal and subsequent compression of the nerve roots at one or more levels. The most common cause is degenerative changes, often combined with some degree of spondylolisthesis. Patients with achondroplasia or other conditions that alter growth of the posterior arch may develop stenosis and progressive symptoms in the second or third decade. Other causes of lumbar stenosis are secondary traumatic or postoperative changes.

Approximately 20% to 30% of those older than 60 years have narrowing of the lumbar canal, but most persons are minimally symptomatic. Skeletal changes associated with stenosis in the older population include degenerative changes and osteophyte formation at the facet joints, osteophyte formation at the lamina, narrowing of the disc, and spondylolisthesis. Soft tissue changes associated with stenosis include thickening of the ligamentum flavum and posterior longitudinal ligament, as well as herniation of the disc. Other factors, such as arterial disease, smoking, multiple levels of compression, and duration and severity of compression, cause progression to neurogenic claudication.

Symptomatic lumbar spinal stenosis is common among men older than 60 years who have performed heavy manual labor. Typical symptoms are radicular and progress in a proximal-to-distal direction. Back pain is not prominent and may be absent. Symptoms are often bilateral but more severe in one extremity. Patients note discomfort and progressive weakness with walking, usually beginning in the thighs, then radiating to the calves and feet. Flexion of the spine expands the canal space. Therefore, patients often walk with the hips and knees flexed to keep the spine in flexion. Symptoms may decrease when one is walking up hills or stairs or riding a bike. Patients often note that they "lean on the cart" while grocery shopping.

Vascular claudication should be ruled out but may coexist. Patients with vascular insufficiency have a fixed, as opposed to a variable, claudication distance; have increased pain while using stairs or walking uphill; rarely have back pain or weakness; and typically demonstrate loss of peripheral pulses and calf hair.

Findings on examination are often limited. Lumbar extension may be limited but is often normal for the patient's age. Muscle weakness is often subtle and may be elicited only on treadmill testing. Radiographs often show degenerative listhesis, which is most common of L4-L5 and L3-L4. The differential diagnosis includes arterial insufficiency (vascular claudication), diabetes mellitus with associated neuropathy, abdominal aortic aneurysm, infection, tumor, and vitamin B_{12} and folic acid deficiency.

Nonoperative management includes weight reduction, cessation of smoking, lumbar flexion exercises, bicycling, avoidance of activities that extend the spine, intermittent use of NSAIDs, and empiric use of folic acid. When symptoms are persistent and disabling, operative therapy should be considered after evaluation by MRI or computed tomographic (CT) scanning with contrast has been completed. The principles of operative therapy require adequate decompression of neural structures. When instability is created by complete removal of a single facet joint, removal of more than 50% of both facets, or removal of more than one third of the pars interarticularis bilaterally, a concomitant fusion should be performed (**Figure 13-12**). Surgery is most often successful in patients with persistent and incapacitating neurogenic claudication. Surgery is less successful in patients in whom back pain is the predominant symptom and those with comorbidities such as smoking, obesity, or diabetes mellitus. Recurrent stenosis may occur.

Degenerative Lumbar Spondylolisthesis

Spondylolisthesis is translation (slippage) of one vertebra in relation to an adjacent segment. The superior vertebra typically slips in an anterior or forward direction, but retrolisthesis may occur, particularly in degenerative spondylolisthesis at upper lumbar levels. The causes of spondylolisthesis vary (**Table 13-3**), but most patients have either an isthmic or a degenerative type. Isthmic spondylolisthesis typically begins during adolescence and is discussed later in the chapter.

In degenerative spondylolisthesis, the neural arch is intact, but erosion and narrowing of the disc and facet joints lead to segmental instability. This condition occurs in older adults; is more common in women and blacks; and is most common at the L4-L5 level, probably because of a combination of factors, including degenerative changes and stiffness at all levels, the relative coronal alignment of the facet joint at the L5-S1 level, and resultant force concentration at L4-L5, which is more sagittally aligned. This condition, however, can occur at other levels and may be seen at multiple levels, resulting in a "cascading spine."

Possible symptoms include back pain, radicular pain, and neurogenic claudication. Indications for surgical management are intractable pain, severe myelopathy, and cauda equina syndrome. Because of concomitant instability, decompression usually is combined with arthrodesis. Instrumentation enhances the rate of fusion. Decompression alone or decompression and fusion without instrumentation is indicated in an elderly patient with virtually no disc remaining and no motion detected on flexion-extension lateral radiographs.

Scoliosis in Adults

Scoliosis is a lateral curvature of the spine of more than 10°. In adults, scoliosis either started during the adolescent years or developed during the adult years, usually secondary to degenerative changes in the disc, osteoporosis, or both. Other causes include neuromuscular conditions such as posttraumatic paraplegia.

Figure 13-12: Spinal Stenosis

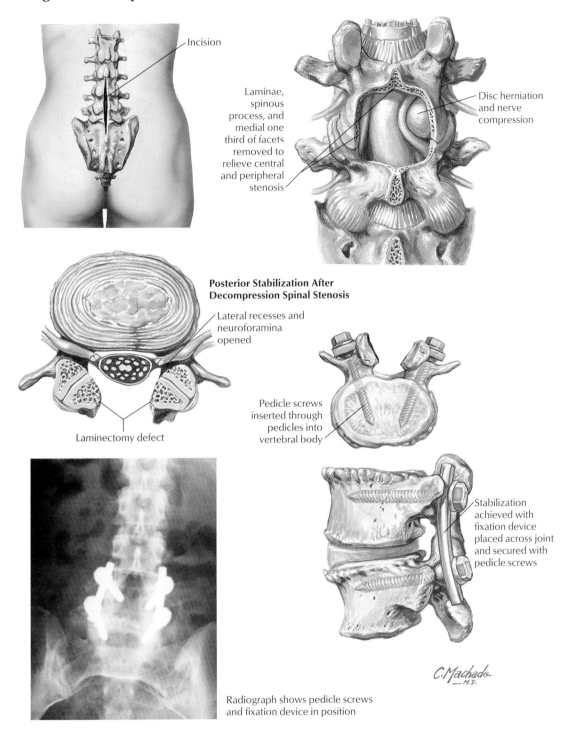

Incision

Laminae, spinous process, and medial one third of facets removed to relieve central and peripheral stenosis

Disc herniation and nerve compression

Posterior Stabilization After Decompression Spinal Stenosis

Lateral recesses and neuroforamina opened

Laminectomy defect

Pedicle screws inserted through pedicles into vertebral body

Stabilization achieved with fixation device placed across joint and secured with pedicle screws

C. Machado M.D.

Radiograph shows pedicle screws and fixation device in position

Table 13-3
Classification of Spondylolisthesis

Type	Description
I: Dysplastic	Congenital incompetency at the lumbosacral junction
II: Isthmic	a. A stress defect in the pars interarticularis b. Attenuation of the pars interarticularis c. An acute fracture of the pars
III: Degenerative	Segmental instability
IV: Traumatic	Acute fracture in the area of the neural arch other than pars interarticularis
V: Pathologic	Metabolic or metastatic disease that causes fracture and instability of the neural arch
VI: Postsurgical	Consequence of surgical decompression (either too much of the facet joint is removed or integrity of the pars interarticularis is compromised)

Curve progression may occur in adults with adolescent idiopathic scoliosis (AIS). Progression is very unlikely when the scoliosis is less than 30° at completion of growth but occurs frequently with 50° to 75° thoracic curves and unbalanced thoracolumbar or lumbar curves of greater than 30°. Older adults with AIS who develop degenerative changes are more likely to have curve progression. Osteoporosis enhances curve progression in patients with degenerative scoliosis.

Pain localized to the area of curvature is the most common symptom. The incidence of back pain may not be different in adults with scoliosis, but the incidence of significant pain is greater. The source of the pain can be difficult to localize, and the pain is often multifactorial. Possible causes include trunk im-

balance with subsequent muscle fatigue or facet/disc/ligament overload, osteoporosis, and spinal stenosis. Symptoms of radiculopathy are more common in patients with degenerative scoliosis. Significant pulmonary dysfunction is unlikely unless the patient has comorbidities such as excessive smoking or preexisting pulmonary disease.

Nonoperative management of painful scoliosis is similar to management of other chronic spine conditions. Indications for surgical management include intractable pain or structurally significant curves with documented progression. Operative management includes stabilization (fusion) with segmental fixation that provides stability for early ambulation. Decompression of spinal stenosis also may be necessary. The rate of major complications is much higher in adults than in adolescents. Possible adverse outcomes include pseudarthrosis, persistent pain, thromboembolism, neurologic injury, infection, and mortality.

SPINAL TRAUMA

Dislocations and fractures of the spine can be devastating injuries. Most such injuries result from motor vehicle accidents or falls. Neurologic injury may occur and may be transient or result in permanent deficits, including quadriplegia or paraplegia. Chronic pain and disability also may occur. Most fractures and dislocations can be classified into one of six mechanisms: compression-flexion, vertical compression, compression-extension, distraction-flexion, distraction-extension, or lateral flexion. Fractures usually result from vertical compression (axial loading) or compression-flexion. Dislocations most often result from distraction-flexion.

Pain, tenderness, and paraspinal spasm are typical symptoms. Radicular symptoms suggest isolated nerve root or cauda equina compression. More global motor and sensory abnormalities suggest spinal cord injury. Palpate the spinous processes for abnormal alignment suggesting significant injury. Examination should include evaluation of all nerve roots distal to the injury. Check perianal sensation and sphincter tone. Sparing of S2-S4 function may be the only early indication of a partial spinal cord injury.

Initial radiographic studies to detect cervical spine injury include anteroposterior, lateral, and odontoid views. Inadequate radiographs may miss upper or lower cervical injuries. The lateral view must include the occiput and the top of T1. Study the radiographs for signs of significant injury, such as more than 7 mm of soft tissue swelling anterior to the C3 vertebra or disruption of the normal lordotic line of the posterior vertebral body. Instability is indicated by more than 3.5 mm of translation or 11° of angulation of adjacent vertebrae on the lateral radiograph, or by malalignment of the spinous processes on the anteroposterior radiograph (**Figure 13-13**). A CT scan should be obtained when plain radiographs show abnormalities or when patients have severe trauma or pain. An MRI study is performed when the injury may be associated with disc extrusion. Lateral flexion-extension radiographs may be helpful but only after muscle spasm has abated.

Initial radiographs for thoracic and lumbar injuries include anteroposterior and cross-table lateral views. As with cervical injuries, CT scans and MRI studies are used for further evaluation.

Initial evaluation includes assessment of the high-energy trauma "ABCs" of airway, breathing, and circulation. To prevent further neurologic injury from an unstable spine, the neck should be immobilized in a hard collar, and all patients with spine injuries should be transported on a backboard. In-line traction of the neck and logroll turning should be used during extrication and transfer maneuvers.

Cervical Fractures

Atlas fractures result from axial compression of the occipital condyles on the C2 lateral masses, leading to fracture of the anterior and posterior ring of C1 (Jefferson fracture) and lateral displacement of the lateral masses of C1 (**Figure 13-14**). Space in the canal is not compromised; therefore, these injuries are not associated with neurologic injury. Radiographic findings include lateral displacement of C1 lateral masses on the odontoid view. Stable injuries can be treated with a hard cervical collar. Unstable injuries should be immobilized in a halo.

Odontoid fractures are of three types: type I is an avulsion fracture of the tip of the odontoid (eg, an injury of the alar ligament); type II, the most common fracture, occurs at the base of the odontoid; and type III fractures extend into the cancellous bone of the vertebral body. Type I injuries are stable and can be treated with a hard collar. Type III injuries are unstable but typically heal with halo cast or vest immobilization. Type II fractures have a higher incidence of nonunion. Halo immobi-

Figure 13-13: Radiographic Signs of Cervical Spine Instability

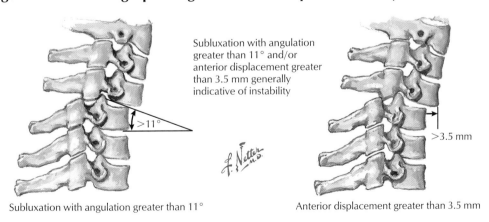

Subluxation with angulation greater than 11° and/or anterior displacement greater than 3.5 mm generally indicative of instability

>11°

>3.5 mm

Subluxation with angulation greater than 11°   Anterior displacement greater than 3.5 mm

Figure 13-14: Cervical Fractures

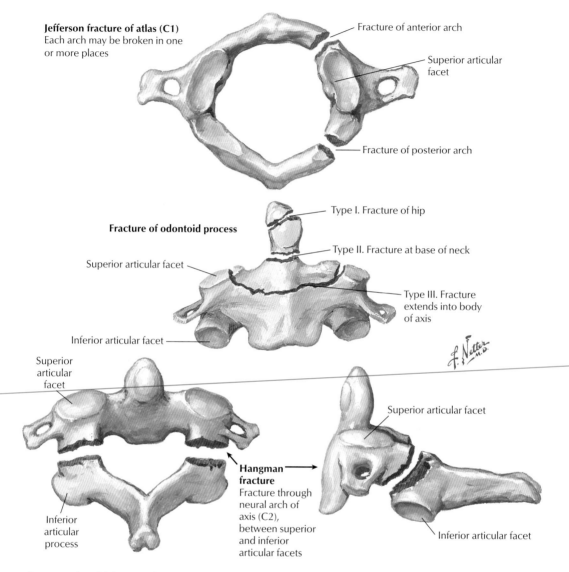

Jefferson fracture of atlas (C1)
Each arch may be broken in one or more places

Fracture of anterior arch

Superior articular facet

Fracture of posterior arch

Fracture of odontoid process

Type I. Fracture of hip

Type II. Fracture at base of neck

Superior articular facet

Type III. Fracture extends into body of axis

Inferior articular facet

Superior articular facet

Superior articular facet

Inferior articular process

Hangman fracture
Fracture through neural arch of axis (C2), between superior and inferior articular facets

Inferior articular facet

lization should be used if less than 5 mm of anterior or posterior displacement or less than 10° of angulation is noted. Otherwise, C1-C2 fusion or anterior odontoid screw fixation should be considered. Nonunion of type II fractures is common in patients older than 40 years.

Traumatic disruption of the C2 pars interarticularis results from extension, axial compression, and subsequent flexion or hyperextension and distraction (hangman fracture). The resultant anterior listhesis of C2 on C3 typically widens the spinal canal; therefore, patients usually do not have neurologic deficits. When displacement measures less than 3 mm, injuries can be treated with the use of a hard collar. Greater displacement is treated with halo immobilization.

Distraction-flexion injuries of C3-C7 include facet subluxation with divergent spinous processes, unilateral facet dislocation with approximately 25% anterior listhesis of the cephalad vertebra, and bilateral facet dislocation with 50% or greater anterior listhesis. Because of the ligamentous disruption, many of these injuries are unstable and require closed reduction by skeletal traction followed by surgical stabilization.

Compression-flexion injuries occur most commonly at the C4-C6 level and range from blunting or fracture of the anterosuperior aspect of the vertebral body (teardrop fracture) to a compression fracture that involves the entire vertebral body. Severe injuries are associated with retropulsion of fragments into the canal and possible disruption of the posterior ligamentous structures. Surgical stabilization is required with posterior ligament disruption or when neurologic decompression is needed. Less severe injuries can be treated with a hard collar or halo immobilization.

Vertical compression injuries occur most commonly at the C6 and C7 vertebrae. The injury pattern ranges from cupping of the superior or inferior vertebral body to severe flattening of the vertebra with retropulsion of the fragments. Surgical decompression and fusion is the treatment for injuries associated with neurologic changes. Otherwise, such injuries can be treated with the use of a brace or halo vest.

Thoracic and Lumbar Fractures

Most thoracic and lumbar fractures result from vertical compression or compression-flexion injuries (**Figure 13-15**). Vertical compression (burst) fractures are most common and typically occur in the thoracolumbar region. In the upper thoracic region (T1-T10), the rib cage provides support and protection. Lower lumbar vertebrae (L3-L5) are larger and more resistant to injury. The thoracolumbar region (T11-L2) is a transitional area between the less mobile thoracic spine and the more flexible lumbar spine.

Figure 13-15: Thoracic and Lumbar Fractures

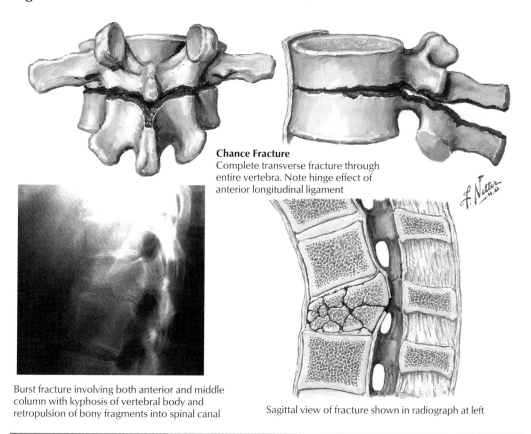

Chance Fracture
Complete transverse fracture through entire vertebra. Note hinge effect of anterior longitudinal ligament

Burst fracture involving both anterior and middle column with kyphosis of vertebral body and retropulsion of bony fragments into spinal canal

Sagittal view of fracture shown in radiograph at left

Treatment is decided after the extent of injury and the presence of neurologic compromise have been discerned. When the thoracolumbar fracture involves only the anterior column (the anterior half of the vertebral body), the injury is stable and can be treated with a supportive orthosis and early ambulation. More extensive injuries also involve the middle column (posterior half of the vertebral body plus the annulus fibrosus and the posterior longitudinal ligament) and the posterior column (all structures posterior to the posterior longitudinal ligament). The injury is stable and can be treated nonoperatively when the fracture involves only the anterior and middle column, no neurologic deficit is noted, and less than 20° of kyphosis and less than 50% canal compromise are observed. Surgical stabilization is usually indicated when a neurologic deficit occurs, when the injury involves all three columns, or when more than 20° of kyphosis or greater than 50% canal compromise is noted.

Minor spine injuries such as transverse process or spinous process fractures can be treated symptomatically. However, such fractures may be associated with more significant injury and require full evaluation.

Fragility fractures of the vertebral body associated with osteopenia and osteoporosis can be very painful, can worsen any premorbid symptoms of back pain associated with degenerative disc disease, and sometimes can be intractable to nonoperative management. Percutaneous vertebroplasty (injection of polymethylmethacrylate into the vertebral body using fluoroscopic control) can be very helpful in decreasing pain by improving the structural integrity of the compromised bone (see **Figure 2-11**). Complications of this procedure include infection, nerve injury, load transfer to other involved vertebrae, and recurrent symptoms.

Injuries of the Spine in Children

Injuries of the spine are uncommon in children but have some unique features, particularly in young children. During the first decade, upper cervical injuries predominate, with fracture of the odontoid being the most common. In adolescents, the injury patterns and treatment principles are similar to adults.

Spinal cord injury without radiographic abnormality (SCIWORA) occurs because a young child's ligaments are more elastic when compared with the spinal cord. MRI often provides useful information concerning the extent of injury. Children with SCIWORA with an unstable ligamentous disruption require spinal fusion. The long-term outcome is largely dependent on the extent of neurologic injury.

Chance fractures are flexion-distraction injuries with the axis of rotation anterior to the vertebral body. The result is that all three columns fail in tension. These injuries can occur in adults but are more frequent in children because children are more likely to wear a lap-type seat belt. Chance fractures may be associated with significant abdominal organ injury. Spinal fusion is indicated with an unstable injury, significant kyphosis, and neurologic injury.

Cervical, Thoracic, and Lumbar Sprains

By strict definition, a cervical, thoracic, or lumbar sprain is a muscle injury in the neck or back. However, because the spine has multiple muscles and ligaments in a deep location, examination and specialized imaging cannot differentiate which soft tissue structure is injured. Therefore, the term *sprain* also is used to describe ligamentous injuries of the spine.

The injury may be trivial (eg, an injury caused by leaning over to pick up a piece of paper) or significant. A typical acute symptom is localized neck or back pain that is increased with motion. The pain, particularly with cervical injuries, may persist for several weeks and may be accompanied by occipital headaches and activity intolerance. Examination typically shows paraspinal tenderness, mild limitation of motion, and pain at extremes of motion. Examination and radiographic studies should exclude neurologic dysfunction and instability.

Treatment includes pain medication, activity modification, and gradual resumption of normal activities. Soft cervical collars or lumbosacral corsets may be helpful. Symptoms typically resolve in 2 to 6 weeks.

Whiplash injuries are rapid flexion-extension neck injuries that result from motor vehicle accidents. The term *whiplash-associated disorders (WADs)* includes perceived neck pain caused by inertial loads applied to the head in motor vehicle accidents. WADs are more common in females and in front-seat passengers who were sitting with an asymmetric posture. Neck pain and stiffness may persist for several months. Neurologic and radiologic abnormalities are typically absent. The cause is probably a relatively severe soft tissue injury combined with the unique motion and load-bearing function of the cervical spine. Persistent pain is often associated with nonorganic amplifiers.

PEDIATRIC SPINAL CONDITIONS
Congenital Muscular Torticollis

Torticollis (wryneck) describes a head positioned with the chin rotated to one side and the head tilted to the other side. Torticollis may be caused by several conditions. Most common is congenital muscular torticollis, which is secondary to a unilateral contracture of the sternocleidomastoid (SCM) muscle. The cause is uncertain, but variable amounts of scar tissue in the muscle suggest that the position of the head in utero or a difficult delivery resulted in a compartment syndrome and eventual fibrosis and contracture of the SCM.

Parents may note a lump or swelling in the SCM when the infant is 3 to 6 weeks of age. The swelling disappears, and the usual reason for concern is the subsequent head tilt and facial asymmetry. Contracture of an SCM tilts the head to the ipsilateral side and rotates the chin to the opposite side (**Figure 13-16**). The face is flattened on the involved side. The differential diagnosis includes Klippel-Feil syndrome, ocular disorders, and congenital anomalies of the base of the skull. The hips should be assessed because approximately 10% of patients have an associated hip dysplasia.

Stretching exercises and positioning of the child to encourage looking away from the affected side are effective in treating many infants. With persistent contracture, surgical release/lengthening is indicated.

Klippel–Feil Syndrome

Patients with Klippel-Feil syndrome have congenital fusion of one or more cervical vertebrae. They frequently have associated problems; more than half of these persons have congenital scoliosis, and a third of them have renal anomalies. Other associated conditions include Sprengel deformity, cardiac anomalies, hearing deficits, and synkinesis.

The typical patient has a short neck, a low posterior neckline, and limited spine motion (**Figure 13-17**). The degree of cervical spine disability depends on the extent and location

Figure 13-16: Congenital Muscular Torticollis

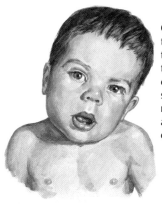

Child with muscular torticollis. Head tilted to left with chin turned to right because of contracture of left sternocleidomastoid muscle. Note facial asymmetry (flattening of left side of face)

Figure 13-17: Klippel-Feil Syndrome

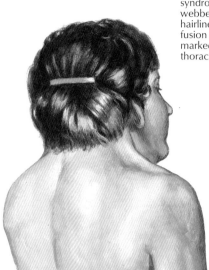

Patient with severe Klippel-Feil syndrome has short, rigid, webbed neck and low posterior hairline. Radiograph reveals fusion of cervical vertebrae and marked deformity of upper thoracic spine.

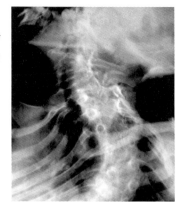

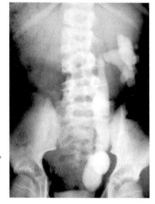

Unilateral absence of kidney with hydronephrosis and hydroureter. Associated anomalies of genitourinary tract or other systems may be less apparent yet more serious than cervical spine fusions.

of the fusion. If only one level is involved, the neck appears normal, and the diagnosis may be made later in life on an incidental radiograph.

Patients should be evaluated for associated problems. Neck problems may develop during the adult years because the fused areas cause increased stress on the surrounding open facet joints.

Atlantoaxial Rotatory Subluxation

Most neck rotation (50%–60%) occurs at the C1-C2 level. Atlantoaxial rotatory subluxation (AARS) may occur in adults but is most common in children between the ages of 2 and 12 years, probably because of the greater ligamentous laxity in children (**Figure 13-18**). AARS most often occurs after a minor trauma or upper respiratory infection.

Children with AARS hold their head in a "cock-robin," or torticollis, position. The posi-

tions of the head and chin are similar to the positions in congenital muscular torticollis, but SCM spasm in AARS is on the opposite, or chin, side. Anteroposterior and lateral cervical spine radiographic findings are normal. The odontoid view shows asymmetry of the space between the odontoid and the C1 lateral

Figure 13-18

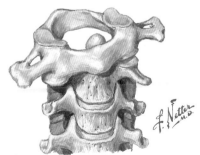

Atlantoaxial rotatory subluxation of C1 on C2

masses; however, this radiographic view is difficult to obtain in AARS. Dynamic CT views with the head maximally rotated to the right, then to the left, may be required for confirmation of AARS.

Symptoms in most patients spontaneously reduce within a week with bed rest and mild analgesics. Longer duration of symptoms requires traction, followed by the use of a hard collar. Rarely, persistent subluxation requires operative treatment.

Congenital Spinal Deformities

Congenital spinal deformities result from abnormal embryonic development of the vertebrae during the first trimester and are caused by failure of formation or by failure of segmentation. Failure of formation causes one or more vertebrae to be hypoplastic, trapezoidal, or wedge-shaped hemivertebra. Depending on the shape and position of the hemivertebrae, subsequent growth may result in scoliosis, kyphoscoliosis, kyphosis, or uncommonly, increased lordosis or lordoscoliosis. Complete failure of segmentation creates two or more blocked vertebrae and slight shortening of the spine, but no abnormal curvature. However, with partial failure of segmentation, growth of the joined portion of the two vertebrae is tethered, and the resultant unbalanced growth causes spinal deformities (**Figure 13-19**). Associated anomalies in patients with congenital scoliosis include genitourinary abnormalities (30%); rib anomalies; and intraspinal deformities such as *diastematomyelia*, *syringomyelia*, and *tethered cord*.

The time to diagnosis varies with the severity of the anomaly. The curvature may be obvious at birth, may become apparent as it grows and progresses, or may be an incidental finding on radiographs obtained for other reasons. At diagnosis, patients should be evaluated for the presence of associated anomalies. The risk of progression depends on the number, position, and type of vertebral anomaly. Bracing is rarely successful in patients with congenital spinal deformities. Surgical options to treat progressive curvatures include in situ fusion, anterior and posterior arthrodesis of the convex side of the curvature, and excision of a hemivertebra with fusion.

Scoliosis

Structural scoliosis is a lateral curvature of greater than 10° (**Figure 13-20**). Scoliosis includes rotation of the vertebrae and is most

Figure 13-19: Congenital Scoliosis

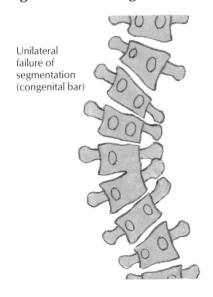

Unilateral failure of segmentation (congenital bar)

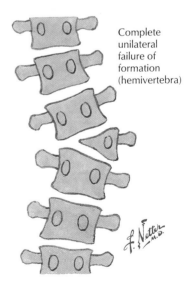

Complete unilateral failure of formation (hemivertebra)

Figure 13-20: Scoliosis

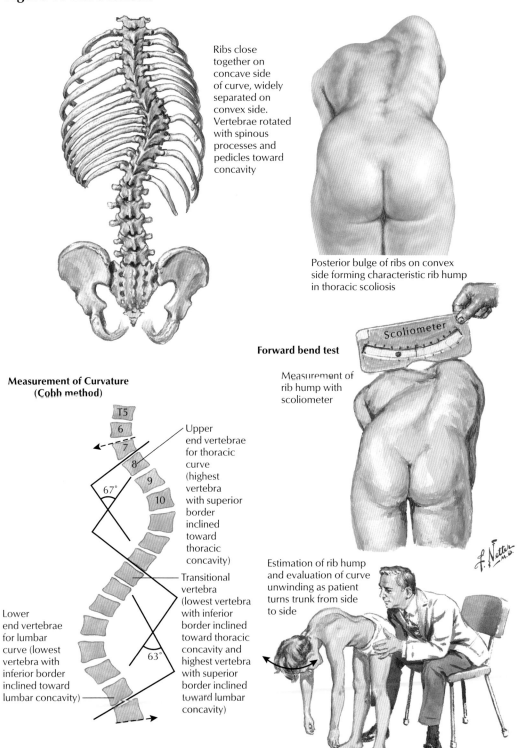

Ribs close together on concave side of curve, widely separated on convex side. Vertebrae rotated with spinous processes and pedicles toward concavity

Posterior bulge of ribs on convex side forming characteristic rib hump in thoracic scoliosis

Forward bend test

Measurement of rib hump with scoliometer

Measurement of Curvature (Cobb method)

T5
6
7
8
9
10

67°

63°

Upper end vertebrae for thoracic curve (highest vertebra with superior border inclined toward thoracic concavity)

Transitional vertebra (lowest vertebra with inferior border inclined toward thoracic concavity and highest vertebra with superior border inclined toward lumbar concavity)

Lower end vertebrae for lumbar curve (lowest vertebra with inferior border inclined toward lumbar concavity)

Estimation of rib hump and evaluation of curve unwinding as patient turns trunk from side to side

often idiopathic but may develop secondary to other conditions (**Table 13-4**). Idiopathic scoliosis is most common and usually develops in early adolescence. The male/female ratio is nearly equal in curves of less than 20°. However, girls are seven to nine times more likely than boys to develop progressive curvature that requires bracing or surgical treatment.

Parents may notice that the child's clothes hang asymmetrically, or the curvature may be noted during a school screening program or routine physical examination. Pain is not characteristic in adolescent idiopathic scoliosis (AIS). Indeed, the presence of significant pain, neurologic abnormality, or both indicates another condition and the need for further evaluation.

Mild degrees of scoliosis may not be apparent when the patient is standing. The *forward bending test* is the most sensitive physical examination test for detecting mild to moderate scoliosis. This procedure exacerbates the rotational deformities of the vertebra and rib. Ask the patient to lean forward with the knees straight and the arms hanging free. Elevation of the rib cage or lumbar paravertebral muscles on one side is a positive finding. An inclination greater than 5° to 7° indicates the need for radiographic evaluation.

Examination should include evaluation for other conditions associated with scoliosis. Left-sided thoracic curvatures have a significant association with syringomelia or other spinal cord anomalies and require detailed evaluation and possible MRI studies. Standing posteroanterior and lateral radiographs and measurements of Cobb angle should be obtained when examination findings are abnormal.

Treatment for AIS involves observation, bracing, or surgical stabilization. Exercise and sports activities do not influence progression. The goal of bracing is to prevent the progression of moderate curvatures during adolescence. Therefore, brace treatment is reserved for patients with growth remaining and progressive curvatures in the range of 20° to 40°. Bracing is not always effective, however, even with a well-made orthosis and a compliant patient.

Surgical fusion is indicated for patients with AIS curves greater than 50° or curves of 40° to 50° that are likely to progress. Scoliosis associated with other conditions is likely to progress and requires surgical stabilization. Possible complications of surgery include infection, neurologic injury, and pseudarthrosis.

Table 13-4
Types of Scoliosis

Type	Possible Cause
Idiopathic	Unknown
	Infantile (before 3 years of age)
	Juvenile (3 to 10 years of age)
	Adolescent (onset after age 10 years)
Congenital	Failure of segmentation
	Failure of formation
Neuromuscular	Cerebral palsy
	Myelomeningocele
	Muscular dystrophy
	Spinal muscular atrophy
	Friedreich ataxia
Vertebral conditions	Benign bony tumors
	Bone infections
	Metabolic bone disease
Spinal cord conditions	Syringomyelia
	Tethered cord syndrome
	Neurofibromatosis type 1
Connective tissue disorders	Marfan syndrome
	Ehlers-Danlos syndrome

Kyphosis

Kyphosis is a sagittal curvature of the spine in which the apex of the curve is posterior. Normal thoracic kyphosis measures 20° to 40° (radiographic measurement from T5 to T12). Kyphosis between 40° and 49° is borderline normal, and curvatures of greater than 50° are abnormal.

Scheuermann disease and *postural kyphosis* are the most common causes of hyperkyphosis in children. Both conditions appear during adolescence. Postural kyphosis is more common in girls, and Scheuermann disease is more common in boys. By definition, Scheuermann disease must demonstrate more than 5° of anterior wedging in at least three successive vertebrae and irregular vertebral end plates (**Figure 13-21**). Kyphosis is typically more severe in Scheuermann kyphosis.

Examine the patient in the forward-bending position. The apex of the kyphosis is found in the mid to lower thoracic spine. When the patient lies in a supine position, the curvature corrects in postural kyphosis but persists in Scheuermann disease. Mild scoliosis may be present in Scheuermann disease.

Figure 13-21: Scheuermann Disease

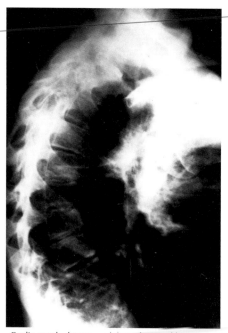

Radiograph shows wedging of several lower thoracic vertebrae, resulting in marked kyphosis. End plates are irregular and narrowed anteriorly

Patients with postural kyphosis usually respond to exercise therapy. Treatment options for Scheuermann disease are similar to options for AIS. Observation is used for patients with curvatures less than 50° to 55°. An orthotic device is prescribed to treat greater degrees of kyphosis if sufficient growth remains. Surgical treatment is anterior and posterior fusion. Indications for operation include refractory thoracic back pain or kyphosis of greater than 75° that has not responded to bracing.

Isthmic Spondylolisthesis

Isthmic spondylolisthesis is caused by a defect in the pars interarticularis, the segment of the posterior arch connecting the pedicle and superior facet to the lamina and inferior facet. The cause is unknown but most cases are probably the result of a stress fracture that fails to unite. This theory is supported by these facts: (1) tension on the pars is greatest in the extended lower lumbar spine, (2) most cases involve the L5 vertebra, and (3) incidence is increased in athletes who repetitively load the extended spine (eg, gymnasts, football players). The condition is more common in males and certain ethnic groups (Eskimo), but the prevalence is low in African Americans. Isthmic spondylolisthesis may be caused by a stress fracture that heals in an elongated position and by acute fractures of the pars.

Most children with isthmic spondylolisthesis present with the insidious onset of low back pain that is aggravated by activity. The pain often radiates to the posterior thigh, and with severe involvement, radicular symptoms may develop. Typical posture includes slight flexion of the hips and knees and decreased lumbar lordosis. Hamstring tightness with concomitant restriction of forward bending and straight leg raising is common. Back pain may begin after an injury but most patients have a preexisting pars defect.

Oblique radiographs demonstrate the pars defect, and lateral views show the degree of

Figure 13-22: Spondylolisthesis

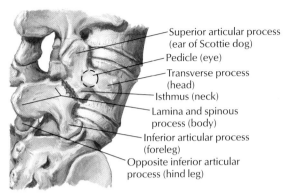
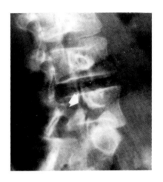

- Superior articular process (ear of Scottie dog)
- Pedicle (eye)
- Transverse process (head)
- Isthmus (neck)
- Lamina and spinous process (body)
- Inferior articular process (foreleg)
- Opposite inferior articular process (hind leg)

Spondylolysis without spondylolisthesis. Posterolateral view demonstrates formation of radiographic Scottie dog. On lateral radiograph, dog appears to be wearing a collar.

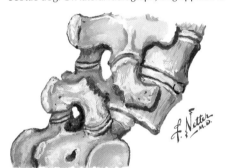
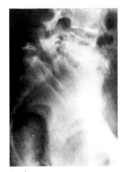

Isthmic-type spondylolisthesis. Anterior listhesis of L5 on S1. Note that the gap in the pars interarticularis is wider.

listhesis (**Figure 13-22**). Most patients respond to stretching and strengthening exercises, short-term activity modifications, and NSAIDs. Periodic radiographs are obtained to assess for the possibility of progressive listhesis with growth. A rigid orthotic device is indicated for the child with severe pain or possible acute injury. Spinal fusion is indicated for patients with intractable pain and those with documented progression and a listhesis greater than 50%.

ADDITIONAL READINGS

Buckwalter JA, Mow VC, Boden SD, Eyre DR, Weidenbaum M. Intervertebral disc structure, composition, and mechanical function. In: Buckwalter JA, Einhorn TA, Simon SR, eds. *Orthopaedic Basic Science: Biology and Biomechanics of the Musculoskeletal System*, 2nd edition. Rosemont, Ill: American Academy of Orthopaedic Surgeons; 2000:547–556.

Frymoyer JW, Wiesel SW, eds. *The Adult and Pediatric Spine*, 3rd edition. Philadelphia, Pa: Lippincott Williams and Wilkins; 2004.

Vaccaro AR, ed. *Fractures of the Cervical, Thoracic, and Lumbar Spine*. New York, NY: Marcel Dekker; 2003.

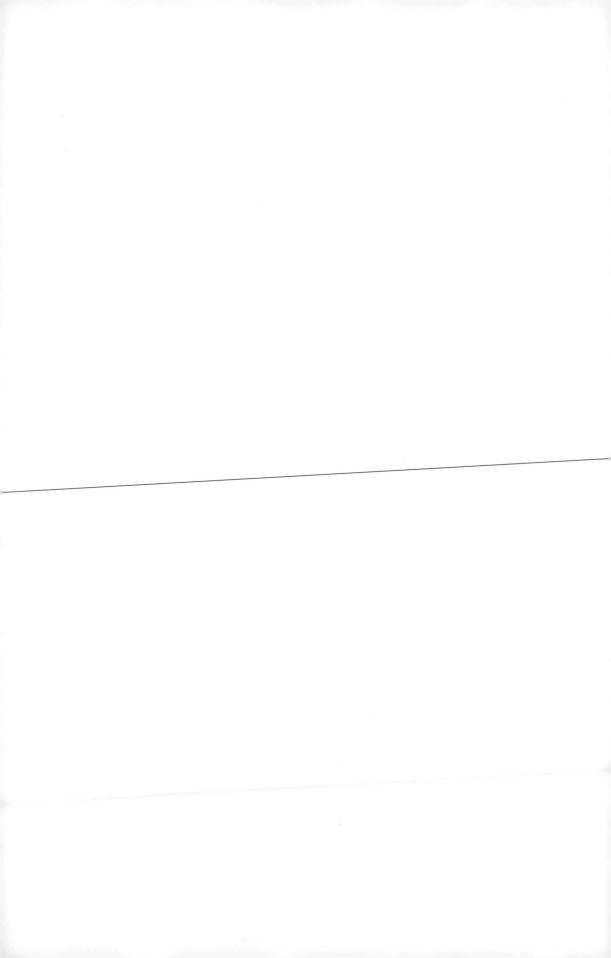

fourteen

The Shoulder and Arm

Keith Kenter, MD

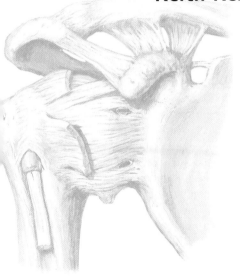

The purpose of this chapter is to review the pertinent basic science of the more common clinical disorders of the shoulder.

ANATOMY AND BIOMECHANICS

The shoulder girdle includes three bones (the scapula, clavicle, and humerus) and three joints (the glenohumeral, acromioclavicular [AC], and sternoclavicular [SC] joints). The scapulothoracic articulation is also considered part of the shoulder girdle. For every 2° of glenohumeral motion, approximately 1° of scapulothoracic motion occurs. The AC and SC joints also participate in this scapulo-humeral rhythm. As a result of this coordinated movement, the shoulder has a greater range of motion than any other joint in the body.

The scapula is a triangular, flat bone that is surrounded by muscle (**Figures 14-1** and **14-2**). Its curved *coracoid process* projects anteriorly from the superior border and is the site of origin for the coracobrachialis and the short head of the biceps muscle. The other notable scapular prominence is the *acromion*, a spinelike process on the posterior aspect. The *coracoacromial ligament* stabilizes the humeral head in the superior direction. The *two coracoclavicular ligaments* prevent the clavicle from riding superiorly. The clavicle is an S-shaped tubular bone that articulates with the acromion laterally and the manubrium medially.

The proximal end of the humerus includes the humeral head, the greater and lesser tuberosities, and the humeral neck. The head of the humerus is retroverted, or posteriorly angled, approximately 30° to match the anterior position of the scapula as it rests on the thoracic cavity. The pear-shaped glenoid fossa articulates with the humerus in a neutral or slightly retroverted position. The *glenoid labrum* is a rim of fibrocartilaginous tissue that increases the surface area of the glenoid fossa and the stability of the shoulder (**Figure 14-3**).

The deltoid is a large, powerful muscle whose primary function is shoulder abduc-tion. The anterior half of the deltoid elevates (flexes) the shoulder, and the posterior half provides extension. Underneath the deltoid are the four rotator cuff muscles: the sub-scapularis, located anteriorly; the supraspina-tus, located superiorly; and the infraspinatus and teres minor muscles, located posteriorly. The deltoid provides most of the power in shoulder motion, whereas the rotator cuff muscles act as a force couple to fine-tune and enhance the efficiency and stability of shoulder motion by compressing, depressing, and thus maintaining the humeral head in the glenoid fossa. Other important shoulder muscles include the trapezius, the latissimus dorsi, the serratus anterior, and the pectoralis major.

The subclavian artery passes under the clavicle and continues as the axillary artery as it traverses the anterior aspect of the shoulder joint. Anastomoses of branches of the axillary artery provide important collateral circulation to the upper extremity (**Figure 14-4**). The main blood supply to the humeral head is the *anterior humeral circumflex artery*. The nerves about the shoulder include the brachial plexus and its terminal branches, the sympathetic nerves, the supraclavicular nerves, and cranial nerve XI.

Important posterior landmarks include the quadrangular space and the triangular interval (**Figure 14-5**). The *quadrangular space* is bordered by the long head of the triceps, the surgical neck of the humerus, the inferior border of the scapula, and the teres major. The axillary nerve and the posterior humeral circumflex artery fill this space. The *triangular interval* houses the radial nerve and the deep brachial artery. Its borders are the teres major superiorly, the long head of the triceps medially, and the lateral head of the triceps laterally.

Figure 14-1: Anterior View Scapula and Proximal Humerus

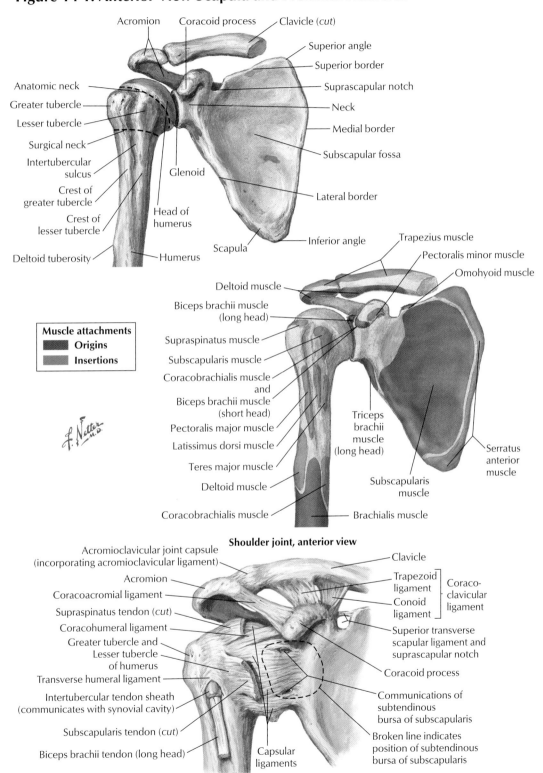

Acromion · Coracoid process · Clavicle (*cut*)

Superior angle

Superior border

Anatomic neck

Greater tubercle

Suprascapular notch

Lesser tubercle

Neck

Surgical neck

Medial border

Intertubercular sulcus

Subscapular fossa

Glenoid

Crest of greater tubercle

Crest of lesser tubercle

Head of humerus

Lateral border

Deltoid tuberosity

Humerus

Scapula

Inferior angle

Trapezius muscle

Pectoralis minor muscle

Omohyoid muscle

Deltoid muscle

Biceps brachii muscle (long head)

Muscle attachments
- Origins
- Insertions

Supraspinatus muscle

Subscapularis muscle

Coracobrachialis muscle and Biceps brachii muscle (short head)

Pectoralis major muscle

Latissimus dorsi muscle

Teres major muscle

Deltoid muscle

Coracobrachialis muscle

Triceps brachii muscle (long head)

Subscapularis muscle

Brachialis muscle

Serratus anterior muscle

Shoulder joint, anterior view

Acromioclavicular joint capsule (incorporating acromioclavicular ligament)

Acromion

Coracoacromial ligament

Supraspinatus tendon (*cut*)

Coracohumeral ligament

Greater tubercle and Lesser tubercle of humerus

Transverse humeral ligament

Intertubercular tendon sheath (communicates with synovial cavity)

Subscapularis tendon (*cut*)

Biceps brachii tendon (long head)

Capsular ligaments

Clavicle

Trapezoid ligament · Conoid ligament — Coraco-clavicular ligament

Superior transverse scapular ligament and suprascapular notch

Coracoid process

Communications of subtendinous bursa of subscapularis

Broken line indicates position of subtendinous bursa of subscapularis

Figure 14-2: Posterior View Scapula and Proximal Humerus

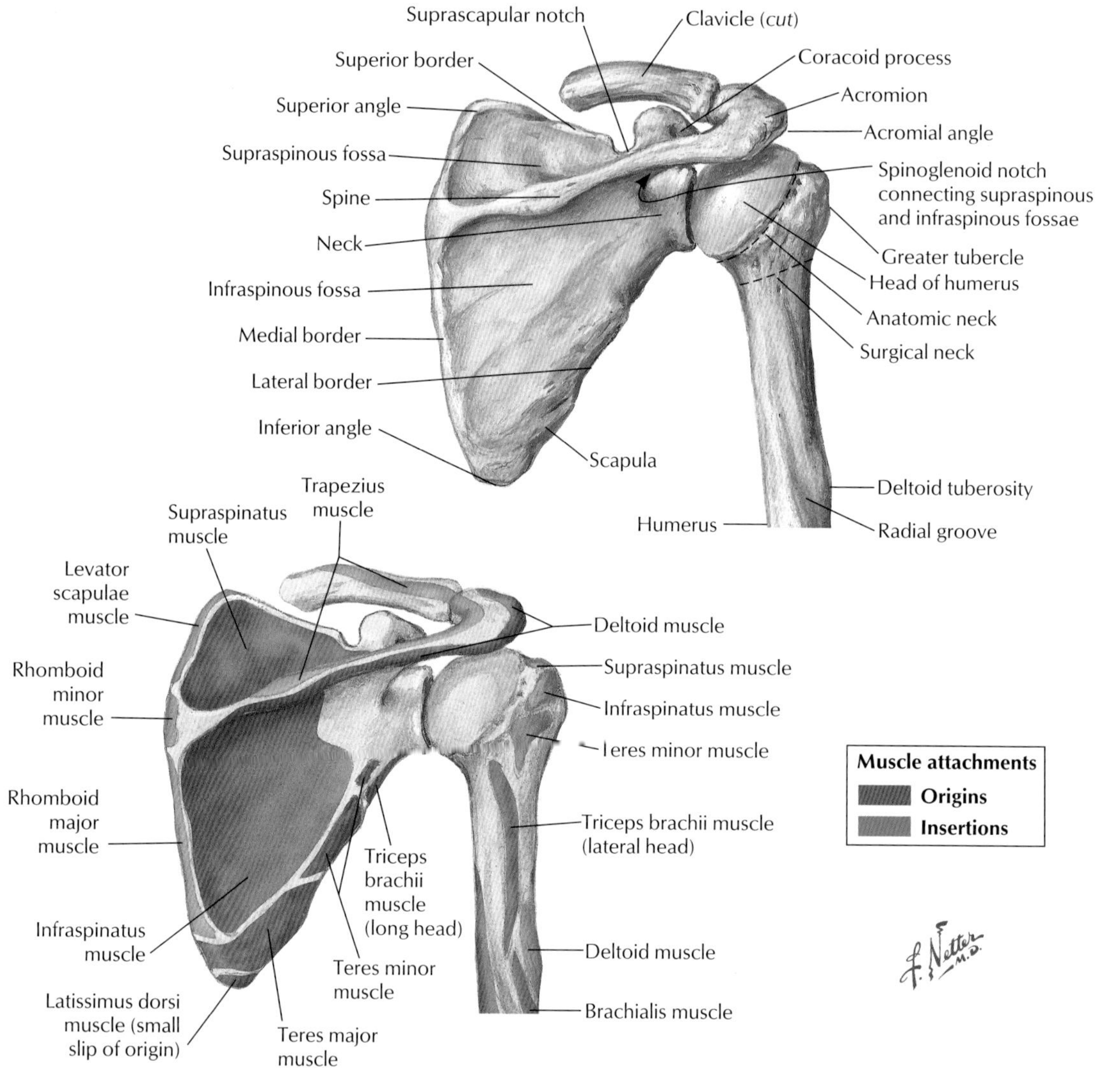

Suprascapular notch
Clavicle (cut)
Superior border
Coracoid process
Superior angle
Acromion
Supraspinous fossa
Acromial angle
Spinoglenoid notch connecting supraspinous and infraspinous fossae
Spine
Neck
Greater tubercle
Head of humerus
Infraspinous fossa
Anatomic neck
Medial border
Surgical neck
Lateral border
Inferior angle
Scapula
Deltoid tuberosity
Trapezius muscle
Humerus
Radial groove
Supraspinatus muscle
Levator scapulae muscle
Deltoid muscle
Rhomboid minor muscle
Supraspinatus muscle
Infraspinatus muscle
Teres minor muscle
Rhomboid major muscle
Triceps brachii muscle (lateral head)
Triceps brachii muscle (long head)
Infraspinatus muscle
Deltoid muscle
Teres minor muscle
Latissimus dorsi muscle (small slip of origin)
Teres major muscle
Brachialis muscle

Muscle attachments	
▨	Origins
▬	Insertions

PHYSICAL EXAMINATION

Begin the physical examination with an inspection of the patient's overall posture and alignment of the shoulder. Look for swelling and ecchymosis, which may indicate recent trauma. Note areas of muscle atrophy suggestive of nerve dysfunction. Injury to cranial nerve XI results in atrophy of the trapezius muscle, which is seen superiorly as a reduced neck-to-shoulder contour. Supraspinatus nerve dysfunction causes loss of the normal posterior shoulder contour and prominence of the scapular spine and acromion.

Next, palpate subcutaneous landmarks to detect deformity or tenderness. For example, with an AC separation, the distal end of the clavicle is prominent. Start at the sternoclavicular joint, and proceed laterally along the clavicle to the acromioclavicular joint. Proceed to the lateral edge of the acromion and the greater tuberosity of the proximal humerus. Also, palpate the long head of the biceps in the bicipital groove of the proximal humerus to detect subluxation or tenderness.

Shoulder range of motion is assessed in four planes (**Figure 14-6**). The zero starting

Figure 14-3: Shoulder Joint Opened (lateral view)

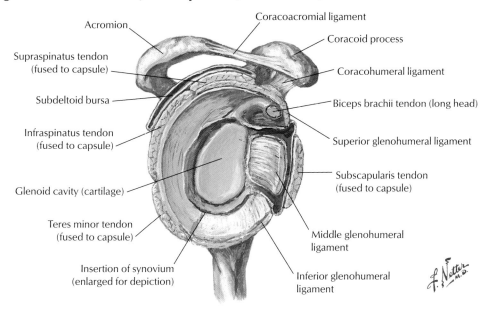

Acromion

Coracoacromial ligament

Coracoid process

Supraspinatus tendon (fused to capsule)

Coracohumeral ligament

Subdeltoid bursa

Biceps brachii tendon (long head)

Infraspinatus tendon (fused to capsule)

Superior glenohumeral ligament

Glenoid cavity (cartilage)

Subscapularis tendon (fused to capsule)

Teres minor tendon (fused to capsule)

Middle glenohumeral ligament

Insertion of synovium (enlarged for depiction)

Inferior glenohumeral ligament

Figure 14-4: Axillary and Brachial Arteries

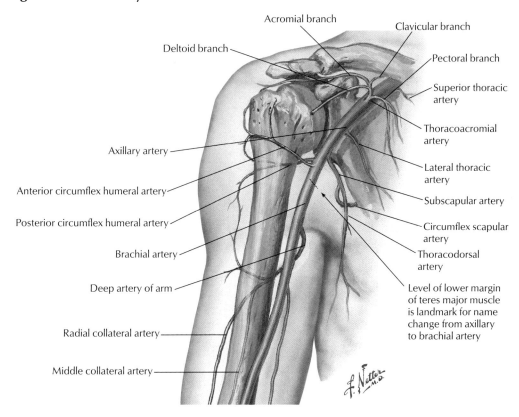

Acromial branch

Clavicular branch

Deltoid branch

Pectoral branch

Superior thoracic artery

Thoracoacromial artery

Axillary artery

Lateral thoracic artery

Anterior circumflex humeral artery

Subscapular artery

Posterior circumflex humeral artery

Circumflex scapular artery

Brachial artery

Thoracodorsal artery

Deep artery of arm

Level of lower margin of teres major muscle is landmark for name change from axillary to brachial artery

Radial collateral artery

Middle collateral artery

Figure 14-5: Posterior View of Shoulder and Arm

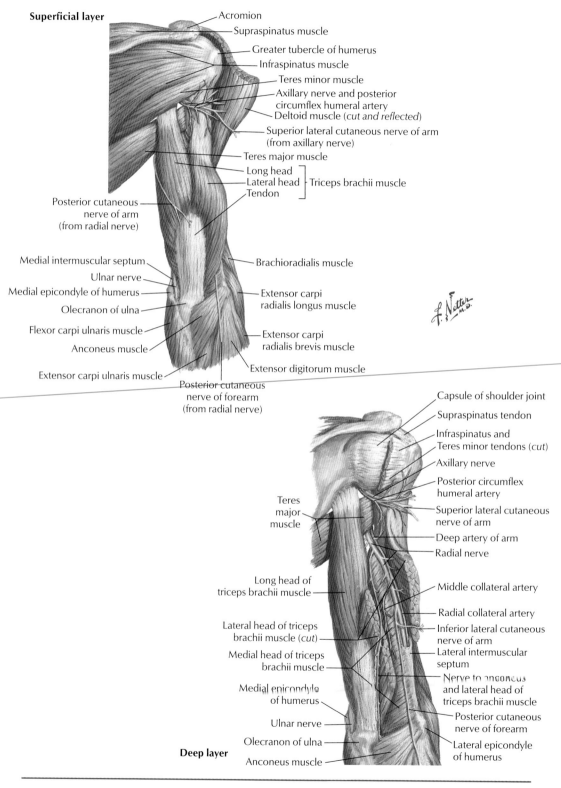

Superficial layer

Acromion
Supraspinatus muscle
Greater tubercle of humerus
Infraspinatus muscle
Teres minor muscle
Axillary nerve and posterior circumflex humeral artery
Deltoid muscle (*cut and reflected*)
Superior lateral cutaneous nerve of arm (from axillary nerve)
Teres major muscle
Long head
Lateral head } Triceps brachii muscle
Tendon
Posterior cutaneous nerve of arm (from radial nerve)
Medial intermuscular septum
Ulnar nerve
Medial epicondyle of humerus
Olecranon of ulna
Flexor carpi ulnaris muscle
Anconeus muscle
Extensor carpi ulnaris muscle
Brachioradialis muscle
Extensor carpi radialis longus muscle
Extensor carpi radialis brevis muscle
Extensor digitorum muscle
Posterior cutaneous nerve of forearm (from radial nerve)

Capsule of shoulder joint
Supraspinatus tendon
Infraspinatus and Teres minor tendons (*cut*)
Axillary nerve
Posterior circumflex humeral artery
Superior lateral cutaneous nerve of arm
Deep artery of arm
Radial nerve
Teres major muscle
Long head of triceps brachii muscle
Middle collateral artery
Radial collateral artery
Lateral head of triceps brachii muscle (*cut*)
Inferior lateral cutaneous nerve of arm
Medial head of triceps brachii muscle
Lateral intermuscular septum
Nerve to anconeus and lateral head of triceps brachii muscle
Medial epicondyle of humerus
Posterior cutaneous nerve of forearm
Ulnar nerve
Olecranon of ulna
Lateral epicondyle of humerus
Deep layer
Anconeus muscle

Figure 14-6: Shoulder Range of Motion

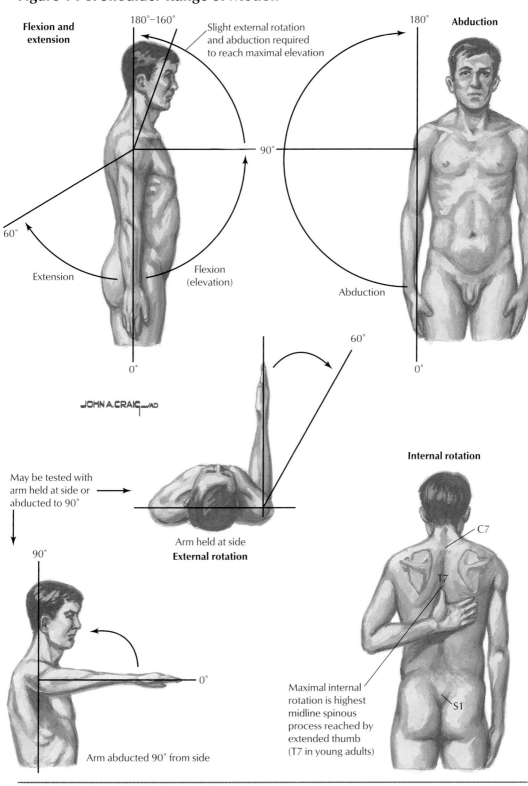

Flexion and extension

180°–160°

Slight external rotation and abduction required to reach maximal elevation

Abduction

180°

90°

60°

Extension

Flexion (elevation)

Abduction

0°

0°

JOHN A.CRAIG_AD

60°

May be tested with arm held at side or abducted to 90°

Arm held at side
External rotation

Internal rotation

C7

T7

90°

0°

Arm abducted 90° from side

Maximal internal rotation is highest midline spinous process reached by extended thumb (T7 in young adults)

S1

position is with the arm at the side of the body. *Flexion*, better described as total *elevation*, is maximum upward movement. Slight external rotation and abduction are required to reach maximum elevation. *Abduction* is maximum movement in the coronal plane. Normal flexion and abduction occur at 160° to 180°. *External rotation* may be measured with the arm at the side or abducted to 90°. The degree of *internal rotation* is the highest midline posterior spinous process reached by the extended thumb. In young adults, internal rotation typically goes beyond the inferior tip of the scapula (approximately the T7 spinous process). Any differences in active versus passive motion, as well as in the quality of movement, should be noted. For example, patients with instability or rotator cuff inflammation may have a dysrhythmic motion. Patients with a rotator cuff tear commonly have a shoulder shrug during abduction. In patients with adhesive capsulitis or arthritis, internal rotation may be limited to the sacrum or the lumbar region.

Assess deltoid muscle strength with the shoulder in 90° abduction. To isolate the anterior deltoid, move the arm forward. Do the reverse to assess the posterior deltoid. The supraspinatus muscle is tested with the shoulder in 90° of flexion and the arm internally rotated and slightly abducted in the plane of the scapula. The external rotation strength of the infraspinatus and the teres minor is tested with the patient's arms at the sides and externally rotated approximately 30°. To test subscapularis strength, internally rotate the arm behind the back to the lumbosacral level, and ask the patient to lift the arm off and away from the back against resistance.

Examination maneuvers that may elicit pain are performed last. Subacromial impingement signs often are present with rotator cuff disease. Keeping the scapula stabilized (depressed) while elevating the arm with the shoulder internally rotated causes the supraspinatus tendon to impinge on the anterior inferior acromion. Another technique is demonstration of pain with the shoulder flexed to 90°, the elbow flexed to 90°, and then moving the

shoulder into internal rotation. Arthritis in the AC joint is suggested when cross-body adduction (ie, flexing the shoulder to 90°, then adducting the arm) elicits pain. Patients with anterior instability may have a positive apprehension test, that is, they express apprehension and a sense of instability when the shoulder is placed in 90° abduction and then maximum external rotation.

Finally, a screening examination of the cervical spine should be performed because some shoulder symptoms may represent cervical spine disease.

DEGENERATIVE DISEASES AND DISORDERS

Rotator Cuff Syndrome

Disorders of the rotator cuff commonly affect patients older than 40 years of age. It represents a spectrum of disorders ranging from subacromial bursitis to rotator cuff tendinopathy to a partial- or full-thickness tear of the rotator cuff. Causes include intrinsic and extrinsic factors. The intrinsic factor is early degenerative changes that are typically observed in the "watershed" region of the supraspinatus tendon (area with diminished blood supply). Extrinsic factors include a thickened coracoacromial ligament, an inflamed subacromial bursa, and a hook-shaped acromion. As the arm is abducted, a degenerative supraspinatus tendon moving under the acromion may be further irritated by these extrinsic factors (**Figure 14-7**). Rotator cuff disease also may be caused by calcium deposited in the tendon as part of the healing response. This calcific tendinopathy may be asymptomatic, or it may aggravate the syndrome and occasionally may cause an acute inflammatory process and severe pain that may be dissipated by spontaneous rupture or needle aspiration.

The typical symptom of rotator cuff disease is dull, aching pain on the lateral side of the shoulder that is worsened by overhead activities and when the patient lies on the affected side. Examination often demonstrates tenderness along the lateral acromion or the lateral aspect of the proximal humerus. Abduction in

Figure 14-7: Rotator Cuff Disease

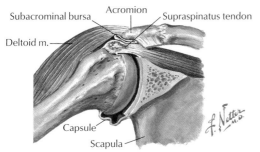

Abduction of arm causes repeated impingement of greater tubercle of humerus on acromion, leading to degeneration and inflammation of supraspinatus tendon, secondary inflammation of bursa, and pain on abduction of arm. Calcific deposits in the supraspinatus tendon may progress to acute calcific tendinitis and sudden onset of severe pain.

the 70° to 120° arc increases pain, which can be decreased by moving the arm into internal rotation. Dysrhythmia of shoulder motion is noted with high-grade tendinopathy. Associated contracture of the posterior glenohumeral capsule results in decreased internal rotation. Weakness of the supraspinatus and external rotators is common and may be caused by pain, a tendon tear, or both. Subacromial impingement signs are often positive.

Most patients with rotator cuff disease can be treated nonoperatively. Activity modifications, ice, and nonsteroidal anti-inflammatory drugs (NSAIDs) are front-line modalities. The focus of physical therapy involves strengthening exercises for the adjacent rotator cuff and parascapular muscles and stretching of the contracted posterior capsule. If the symptoms are severe, a corticosteroid injection into the subacromial bursa may reduce inflammation and pain. With the addition of a local anesthetic, the injection can confirm a diagnosis of rotator cuff disease if pain is relieved on repeat testing of the impingement signs.

If the patient continues to have pain and dysfunction, decompression of the subacromial arch is indicated. This procedure includes a partial acromionectomy that primarily removes the undersurface of the acromion, as well as resection of the inflamed subacromial bursa and coracoacromial ligament (**Figure 14-8**). Rotator cuff tears are also repaired if found at the time of operation. Surgery for rotator cuff disease can be performed as an open or arthroscopic procedure.

Glenohumeral Arthritis

Primary osteoarthritis is the most common type of glenohumeral arthritis. Osteonecrosis and severe rotator cuff tears are the most common causes of secondary osteoarthritis. In addition to pain with activity and pain at the extremes of motion, patients with glenohumeral arthritis complain of inability to comb their hair, touch their contralateral shoulder, or reach behind their back.

Examination reveals reduced motion, particularly in the arc of internal rotation and abduction. On occasion, muscle atrophy

Figure 14-8: Acromioplasty

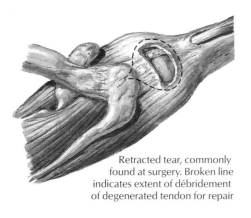

Retracted tear, commonly found at surgery. Broken line indicates extent of débridement of degenerated tendon for repair

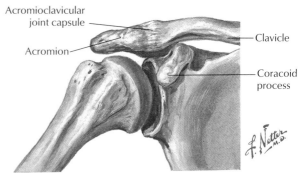

Partial acromionectomy performed with removal of the anterior edge and lateral portion of the acromion. Coracoacromial ligament is also removed. Distal 2.5 cm of distal clavicle resected if acromioclavicular joint is arthritic.

Figure 14-9: Osteoarthritis of the Shoulder

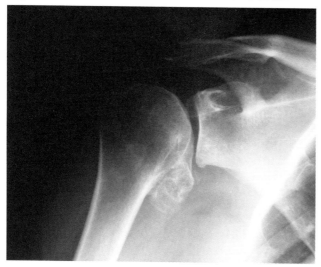

AP radiograph of shoulder demonstrates typical changes of osteoarthritis of the shoulder with narrowing of the joint and prominent osteophyte formation at the inferior aspect of the humeral head.

results from limited use, a large, longstanding tear in the rotator cuff, or both. Radiographs demonstrate decreased joint space, osteophyte formation at the inferior pole of the humeral head, and sclerosis or bony erosion of the glenoid fossa (**Figure 14-9**).

Treatment goals include pain relief and improved function. Nonoperative modalities include activity modification, exercise to improve motion and strengthen muscles in a nonforceful manner, and the judicious use of NSAIDs and intra-articular steroid injections. Surgical alternatives include arthroscopic débridement, arthrodesis, and joint replacement. If arthropathy affects both the humeral head and the glenoid, total shoulder replacement with an unconstrained prosthesis that is combined with soft tissue balancing provides the most predictable outcome (**Figure 14-10**). Possible complications after surgery

Figure 14-10: Prosthetic Replacement of Shoulder Joint

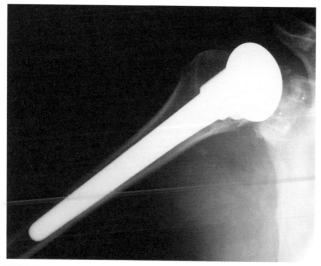

Complete shoulder prosthetic replacement of the humeral head and glenoid can provide good pain relief for patients with degenerative osteoarthritis of the glenohumeral joint.

292

include fracture of the humeral shaft, injury of the axillary or musculocutaneous nerve, infection, glenohumeral instability, and loosening of prosthesis components.

Acromioclavicular Joint Arthritis

Arthropathy of the acromioclavicular joint may be traumatic in origin or may be associated with rotator cuff disease. Typical symptoms include pain at the superior aspect of the shoulder with overhead cross-arm activities and pain exacerbated by bench press and push-up exercises.

Examination demonstrates tenderness at the AC joint and pain with adduction cross-body maneuvers. Associated signs of rotator cuff disease are often present. Radiographs typically reveal osteophyte formation on the undersurface of the distal clavicle. On occasion, periarticular inflammation may cause osteolysis and resorption of the distal clavicle.

Nonoperative treatment includes activity modification, rotator cuff strengthening, and the judicious use of NSAIDs and AC joint corticosteroid injections. The preferred treatment with persistent and disabling symptoms is distal clavicle resection, performed either as an open or arthroscopic procedure.

Adhesive Capsulitis

Adhesive capsulitis, also known as *frozen shoulder,* is a painful disorder characterized by progressive loss of **both** active and passive motion (**Figure 14-11**).The disorder is more common in the 5th to 7th decades, in females, in the nondominant shoulder, and in patients with diabetes mellitus or hypothyroidism. The loss of motion particularly affects overhead activities such as lifting objects off a shelf and activities requiring internal rotation such as fastening a bra.

Adhesive capsulitis is associated with intrinsic shoulder conditions, such as trauma or postsurgical stiffness, and extrinsic disorders that secondarily limit shoulder motion, such as cervical spine disease, acute cardiopulmonary disorders, and breast surgery. The histopathology is characterized by an inflamed synovium with perivascular lymphocytic infiltration.

Over time, the capsule becomes thickened and fibrotic, adhesions develop between the capsule and the cartilage, and the axillary pouch is obliterated.

Examination demonstrates pain at extremes of motion and loss of both active and passive motion. Placing the patient in a supine position and comparing external and internal rotation with the arm at 45° and 90° of abduction to the opposite side is a sensitive test in the early phase of the disease. Radiographs are typically normal. Misdiagnosis of rotator cuff disease may result in improper treatment.

Treatment begins with patient education, pain management, and gentle active and passive range-of-motion exercises. Corticosteroid injections into the glenohumeral joint can help with early pain management and produce a more rapid restoration of motion. Most patients demonstrate gradual recovery of full motion over a few months, but some experience recalcitrant symptoms for years before symptoms abate. In this situation, manipulation of the shoulder under anesthesia should be considered, provided the patient understands that continued physical therapy most likely will be needed. Arthroscopic lysis of adhesions achieved by cutting the thickened capsule near its insertion at the glenoid labrum, then performing a manipulation, can promote rehabilitation. Manipulation must be gentle because forced manipulation may cause intraoperative fracture or tendon tears.

Shoulder Pain in the Overhead Athlete

Glenohumeral joint mobility enhances the performance of the athlete or laborer involved in overhead activities, but repetitive stress also makes the shoulder vulnerable to injury. Most shoulder injuries in overhead athletes are due to poor mechanics and subsequent muscle fatigue. The mechanism of injury is best exemplified in baseball pitchers. The phases of a baseball pitch are (1) windup, (2) early cocking, (3) late cocking, (4) acceleration, (5) deceleration, and (6) follow-through. Phases 3 to 5 put the shoulder at

Figure 14-11: Adhesive Capsulitis

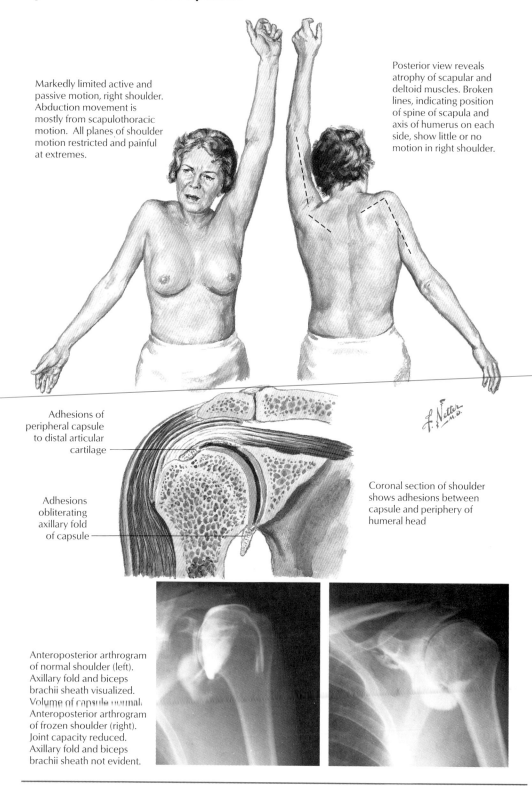

Markedly limited active and passive motion, right shoulder. Abduction movement is mostly from scapulothoracic motion. All planes of shoulder motion restricted and painful at extremes.

Posterior view reveals atrophy of scapular and deltoid muscles. Broken lines, indicating position of spine of scapula and axis of humerus on each side, show little or no motion in right shoulder.

Adhesions of peripheral capsule to distal articular cartilage

Adhesions obliterating axillary fold of capsule

Coronal section of shoulder shows adhesions between capsule and periphery of humeral head

Anteroposterior arthrogram of normal shoulder (left). Axillary fold and biceps brachii sheath visualized. Volume of capsule normal. Anteroposterior arthrogram of frozen shoulder (right). Joint capacity reduced. Axillary fold and biceps brachii sheath not evident.

greater risk for injury. During late cocking, the humerus is moving toward maximum external rotation, a position that places the infraspinatus and teres minor tendons in a more posterior position. In this position, these tendons may impinge on the posterosuperior labrum, a disorder called *internal impingement*. This position also places the humeral head at risk for anterior instability. During the acceleration phase, the humerus internally rotates very rapidly. If the scapular stabilizing muscles have inadequate strength, attrition can develop in the anterior rotator cuff muscles. During the deceleration phase, rapid external rotational forces on the posterior rotator cuff can cause posterior shoulder pain.

Shoulder pain in throwing athletes is typically described as anterior pain that increases as pitching velocity is increased. These patients typically note that they cannot achieve maximum pitching speed. Less common is posterior shoulder pain. In younger patients, such as the high school or collegiate athlete, shoulder pain most often results from glenohumeral instability. The use of improper mechanics during the windup and cocking phases shifts forces typically generated by lower limb and trunk muscles toward greater dependence on shoulder muscles. As rotator cuff muscles fatigue, the humeral head develops abnormal translation at extreme positions of the shoulder. The result is occult instability and secondary impingement. Therefore, treatment is directed toward proper throwing mechanics, stretching of contractures, and strengthening of the rotator cuff and scapular stabilizing muscles.

A tear in the *superior quadrant of the glenoid labrum* is another injury observed in athletes. These SLAP (*superior labrum anteroposterior*) lesions may extend anteriorly or posteriorly and also may violate the attachment of the biceps tendon. A type I SLAP lesion involves degeneration or fraying of the superior labrum but does not affect the attachment of the biceps. Type II tears involve the biceps anchor and are detached from the glenoid fossa. Type III tears are bucket handle–type tears that spare the biceps at-

tachment. Type IV tears are similar to type III tears but involve the biceps anchor. Patients have superior shoulder pain that develops with overhead lifting or throwing activities. If rehabilitation fails, arthroscopic débridement, repair, or both may be helpful.

Nerve Entrapment Syndromes and Injuries

Brachial plexus injuries range from momentary paresthesia to permanent paralysis. The upper plexus (C5, C6, and C7 trunks) is typically stretched and injured when the shoulder is depressed and adducted by a direct blow while the neck is pushed in the opposite direction (**Figure 14-12**). The lower trunks (C8 and T1) are stretched and injured when the arm is forcefully abducted. The entire brachial plexus may be paralyzed by major trauma, causing extreme traction.

Stingers, which are transient stretch injuries to the upper trunk of the brachial plexus, most commonly occur in football players injured by a direct blow to the head, neck, or shoulder. The patient notes sharp shoulder pain that radiates down the arm, is associated with weakness, and lasts a few seconds or minutes. At the other end of the spectrum is high-energy falls or motor vehicle accidents that cause avulsion of the plexus and associated multiple injuries. High-energy falls or motor vehicle accidents are likely to result in axonal disruption and permanent injury.

A detailed neurologic examination is required for determining the extent and location of injury. Preganglionic injuries are more likely with lower plexus injuries. The presence of Horner syndrome, with ipsilateral ptosis, miosis, anhidrosis, and enophthalmos, confirms a preganglionic location and suggests a poor prognosis. With an upper plexus injury, intact function of the serratus anterior and rhomboids (innervated by long thoracic and dorsal scapular nerves) indicates a postganglionic injury and a better prognosis.

The suprascapular nerve travels through the superior notch of the scapula and the spinoglenoid notch to supply the supraspinatus and infraspinatus muscles (see **Figure 14-**

Figure 14-12: Brachial Plexus

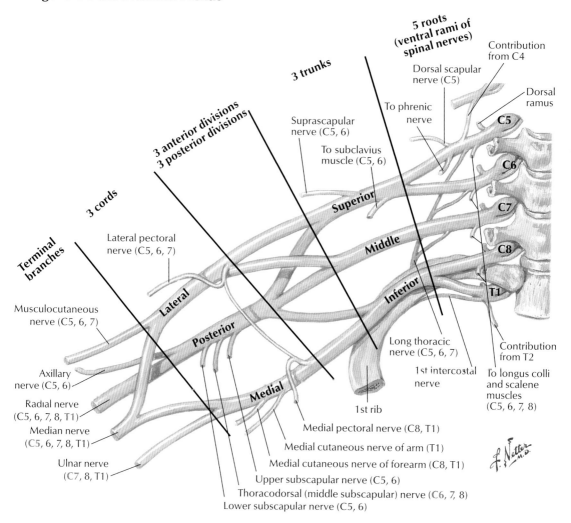

12). In these tight confines, the nerve can become entrapped. Nerve compression at the level of the superior scapular notch affects both *supraspinatus and infraspinatus muscles*. Compression at the *spinoglenoid notch*, which commonly is caused by a ganglion cyst originating from the glenoid labrum, affects only the infraspinatus. Symptoms include a dull ache posterior to the shoulder along the lateral scapula. Examination shows muscle atrophy and weakness.

The musculocutaneous nerve may become compressed within the coracobrachialis muscle. Symptoms include weakness of the el-

bow flexors and hypesthesia of the lateral forearm.

Winging of the scapula can be caused by injury to either of two nerves: the long thoracic nerve or cranial nerve XI. Neuropathy of the long thoracic nerve causes paralysis of the serratus anterior muscle. Patients report the indolent onset of fatigue and aching pain with overhead activities. The strength of the serratus anterior is assessed by asking the patient to keep the arm elevated while applying resistance. Winging and prominence of the vertebral border of the scapula occur with weakness of the serratus anterior, which is an important retractor of the scapula. This neuropathy frequently resolves spontaneously. Injury to cranial nerve XI may result in paralysis of the trapezius muscle and scapular winging. This nerve may be injured during surgery performed in the posterior cervical triangle.

Thoracic outlet syndrome involves entrapment of the brachial plexus, vessels to the upper limb, or both, as they pass through the interval between the scalene muscles and the first rib, then into the axilla. This disorder is described in Chapter 6.

TRAUMA

Fractures in Adults

Fracture of the Proximal Humerus

Fractures of the proximal humerus result from a fall on an outstretched hand or a direct impact. These fractures are particularly common in elderly individuals with osteoporosis. Most of these injuries are minimally displaced fractures through the surgical neck and can be treated by sling immobilization and a progressive rehabilitation program. Displaced fractures may have two, three, or four major fragments consisting of (1) the articular segment, (2) the greater tuberosity with the attached supraspinatus muscle, (3) the lesser tuberosity with the attached subscapularis

muscle, and (4) the humeral shaft (**Figure 14-13**). Fractures are considered displaced if the distance between the fragments is greater than 1 cm or if angulation of the fragments is greater than 45°. The risk of posttraumatic arthritis and osteonecrosis increases with the number of major fragments, the degree of displacement, and associated glenohumeral dislocation.

Treatment options depend on the age of the patient, the activity demands of the patient, the fracture personality, and the quality of the bone stock. Two-part displaced fractures generally require reduction maneuvers with or without internal fixation. Three- and four-part fractures, fortunately, are uncommon and typically require internal fixation or hemiarthroplasty if the blood supply to the humeral head has been disrupted.

Fracture of the Clavicle

The clavicle is the bone that is most frequently fractured. Most clavicle fractures are the result of an indirect force, such as falling on the lateral point of the shoulder or falling on an outstretched hand. The middle third of the clavicle is the most common site of injury; approximately 80% of clavicle fractures occur in this location; 15%, in the lateral third; and 5%, in the medial third (**Figure 14-14**).

Figure 14-13: Fracture of Proximal Humerus

Neer four-part classification of fractures of proximal humerus. 1. Articular fragment (humeral head). 2. Lesser tuberosity. 3. Greater tuberosity. 4. Shaft. If no fragments displaced, fracture considered stable (most common) and treated with minimal external immobilization and early range-of-motion exercise. Displacement of 1 cm or angulation of 45° of one or more fragments necessitates open reduction and internal fixation or prosthetic replacement

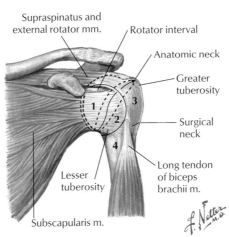

Supraspinatus and external rotator mm.
Rotator interval
Anatomic neck
Greater tuberosity
Surgical neck
Long tendon of biceps brachii m.
Lesser tuberosity
Subscapularis m.

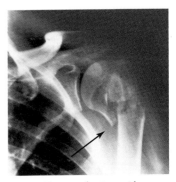

Two-part fracture with some comminution

Figure 14-14: Fracture of the Clavicle

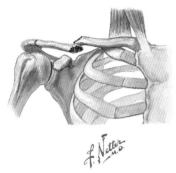

Fracture of middle third of clavicle (most common). Medial fragment displaced upward by pull of sternocleidomastoid muscle; lateral fragment displaced downward by weight of shoulder. Fractures occur most often in children.

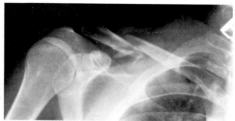

Anteroposterior radiograph. Fracture of middle third of clavicle.

Examination reveals localized tenderness and swelling. An AP radiograph of the clavicle demonstrates most injuries. Most clavicle fractures can be treated nonoperatively with either a sling or a figure-of-eight harness. Injuries with marked displacement in the lateral or middle third of the clavicle have a greater risk of malunion or nonunion and should be evaluated for internal fixation.

Fracture of the Scapula

Most fractures of the scapula result from a high-energy, direct impact to the back. Therefore, concomitant injury to the ribs, lung, thoracic spine, or brachial plexus is common.

Examination shows localized tenderness, swelling, and pain on attempted motion of the arm. Radiographs should include a PA view of the chest, an AP view of the shoulder that includes the scapula, and if possible, an axillary and transscapular view.

Fractures may involve the body of the scapula, the glenoid, the acromion, the coracoid process, or a combination. Because of the surrounding musculature, fractures of the body of the scapula have a good prognosis. They are generally treated nonoperatively with a sling then early range-of-motion exercises as the pain subsides. Displaced intra-articular glenoid fractures (>2 mm), fractures of the neck of the scapula with severe angulation, and displaced fractures of the acromion and coracoid may require internal fixation. A *floating shoulder* is a concomitant fracture of the scapula and ipsilateral clavicle. Whether this injury requires internal fixation of one or both fractures is controversial.

Fracture of the Humeral Shaft

Fractures of the humeral shaft generally are caused by direct trauma. An associated stretch injury of the radial nerve with resultant paralysis of the wrist and finger extensors is relatively common. The nerve injury should be documented and observed, because most resolve in 4 to 6 months.

Nonoperative treatment of humeral shaft fractures is preferred, because the union rate is high, and shoulder and elbow function are excellent even with moderate angulation. The fracture is initially treated with a coaptation splint, followed by prefabricated functional braces that permit shoulder and elbow motion (**Figure 14-15**).

Indications for operative intervention include the following: (1) a segmental fracture that cannot be aligned properly, (2) associated ipsilateral elbow or forearm fractures (floating elbow), (3) open fractures, (4) polytrauma with injuries requiring prolonged bed rest or significant closed head injuries, (5) pathologic fractures, (6) fractures associated with vascular injury, and (7) radial nerve palsy that develops during a closed reduction maneuver (the radial nerve may become entrapped and compressed at the fracture site).

Fractures in Children

The clavicle is the site of most pediatric shoulder injuries and, as in adults, more than 80% involve the middle third. Virtually all do well with nonoperative treatment. The clavicle is the most common site of fracture during delivery with an incidence of approximately

Figure 14-15: Fracture of Shaft of Humerus

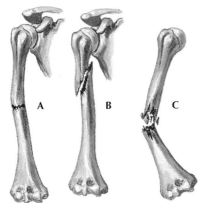

A. Transverse fracture of midshaft
B. Oblique (spiral) fracture
C. Comminuted fracture with marked angulation

After initial swelling subsides, most fractures of shaft of humerus can be treated with functional brace of interlocking anterior and posterior components held together with Velcro straps

3 to 5 per 1000 live births. This injury may cause pseudoparalysis and initial concern of brachial plexus injury.

Fracture of the distal lateral aspect of the clavicle in children occurs by the same mechanism of injury that causes an acromioclavicular separation in adults. These injuries remodel quite well and can be managed with a sling. Fracture of the medial clavicle is the least common site of injury. Medial clavicle fractures in children are commonly physeal injuries, which because the epiphysis of the medial clavicle is the last secondary center to ossify (begins around 18 years of age) may not be apparent on initial radiographs.

Fracture of the proximal humerus in children most commonly is a type II physeal injury (see **Figure 10-3**). Due to large growth potential of the physis of the proximal humerus (provides 80% growth of humerus) and the flexibility of the shoulder joint, these fractures do well with closed management. Moderate angulation of approximately 40° to 50° can be accepted except in the older adolescent (**Figure 14-16**).

Figure 14-16: Fracture of Proximal Humerus in Children

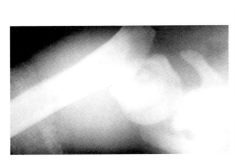

Displaced fracture of proximal humerus

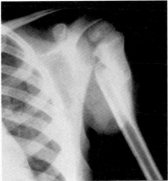

Persistent malalignment despite reduction by traction and manipulation

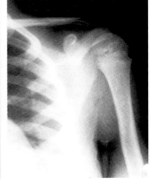

Remodeling over months resulted in relatively normal alignment and full shoulder joint motion

Figure 14-17: Anterior Dislocation, Glenohumeral Joint (Hill-Sachs Lesion)

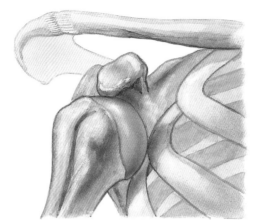

Subcoracoid dislocation (most common)

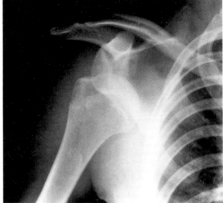

Subcoracoid dislocation. Anteroposterior radiograph.

Acromion prominent

Humeral head prominent

Shoulder flattened

Arm in slight abduction

Elbow flexed

Forearm internally rotated, supported by other hand

Clinical appearance

Stimson maneuver
Patient prone on table with affected limb hanging freely over edge; 10- to15-lb weight suspended from wrist. Gradual traction overcomes muscle spasm and in most cases achieves reduction in 20 to 25 minutes

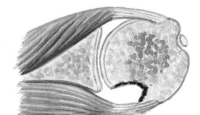

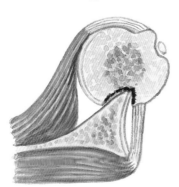

Anterior dislocation. Anterior rim of glenoid indents posterolateral part of humeral head

After reduction. Defect persists, causing instability and predisposing to recurrent dislocation

Dislocations

Dislocation/Instability of the Glenohumeral Joint

Dislocation of the shoulder was described in the Edwin Smith Papyrus (3000 to 2500 BC). Later, Hippocrates described a reduction technique for treatment of acute dislocation and a surgical procedure for treating recurrent instability.

Dislocation of the glenohumeral joint may be anterior, posterior, or multidirectional. Anterior is most common, accounting for approximately 98% of the dislocations. Anterior dislocations may occur at any age but are more common after athletic injuries in adolescents and young adults. The anterior capsule and associated ligaments are stretched or torn with subsequent anterior dislocation of the humeral head when the arm is positioned in abduction, extension, and external rotation. The humeral head usually rests in a subcoracoid position, but it may be positioned inferior to the glenoid or subclavicular.

These patients experience the sudden onset of pain and an inability to use the arm after a fall or forceful throwing movement. Inspection typically shows the patient supporting the arm with the other hand. Examination reveals flattening of the deltoid prominence, prominence of the acromion, fullness of the subcoracoid region, and downward displacement of the axillary fold (**Figure 14-17**). Any attempt at motion elicits pain.

Nerve injury may occur and most commonly affects the axillary or musculocutaneous nerve; however, the median, ulnar, and radial nerves also may be injured and should be examined. Axillary, AP, and scapular Y radiographs should be obtained before reduction so that the type of dislocation and any associated fractures may be documented. Radiographs may show a defect in the posterolateral humeral head, called a *Hill-Sachs lesion*, resulting from impaction of the humeral head on the anterior rim of the glenoid fossa. Avulsion of the anteroinferior glenoid labrum, called a *Bankart lesion,* also may occur. Hill-

Sachs and Bankart lesions are predisposing factors for recurrent instability.

Several methods have been described to reduce an anterior shoulder dislocation. As with any dislocation, the joint should be reduced as soon as possible, and the reduction should not be performed forcefully. Intra-articular injection of local anesthetics and intravenous analgesics and muscle relaxants can significantly reduce the associated muscle spasm. In the traction-countertraction method, a sheet is placed in the axilla and diagonally across the chest. An assistant provides countertraction while the physician applies distal traction to the arm with the biceps relaxed (elbow flexed). Gentle internal rotation may be added. In the Stimson maneuver, the patient is prone, with the arm hanging off the edge of the table. A 10- to 15-lb weight is tied to the wrist for longitudinal traction.

After reduction, AP and axillary radiographs should be obtained to confirm concentric reduction. Hill-Sachs and bony Bankart lesions also may be identified on postreduction radiographs. The arm is immobilized in a sling, and the patient begins circumduction exercises at 1 week and range-of-motion exercises at 3 weeks. The abduction–external rotation position is avoided for 6 weeks. Strengthening exercises are initiated after the patient has regained full range of motion without apprehension.

Surgical intervention rarely is needed for acute glenohumeral joint dislocation but usually is required for a fracture-dislocation and when the glenohumeral joint remains unreduced. Early surgical repair of a Bankart lesion may be indicated for patients with significant predisposing factors to recurrent dislocation. The presence of chronic instability with recurrent dislocation is more likely in females, younger patients, and patients with a Bankart or Hill-Sachs lesion. Surgical reconstruction in cases of chronic instability includes repair of an avulsed glenoid labrum and further tightening of the anterior capsule as needed.

Posterior glenohumeral dislocations are uncommon, and the diagnosis may be missed, particularly if only an AP radiograph is obtained (**Figure 14-18**). Posterior dislocations occur with an internal rotation–adduction force and are more common in patients who have a seizure disorder or who have experienced an electric shock injury. Examination reveals decreased fullness of the deltoid, posterior prominence of the humeral head, and marked restriction of abduction and external rotation. Appropriate radiographs are the same as for an anterior dislocation. Reduction is accomplished by distal traction and the application of manual pressure to the humeral head in an anterior direction.

Patients with chronic anterior shoulder instability may provide a history of recurrent dislocation and/or a history that the shoulder slips or feels unstable when the arm is in a position of abduction and external rotation. The apprehension sign is typically present. Patients whose shoulder instability has a traumatic cause usually have a unidirectional instability and a Bankart lesion, and they often require surgery—thus, the acronym TUBS. The atraumatic type of shoulder instability is usually multidirectional, bilateral, and more likely to respond to a rehabilitation program. However, if surgery is required, an inferior shift of the capsule with closure of the rotator interval is the preferred technique—thus, the acronym AMBRI.

It should be emphasized that treatment for glenohumeral instability should start with muscle-strengthening exercises. Neuromuscular coordination exercises designed to develop proper mechanics are also part of the rehabilitation program. Taping or bracing during athletic activity may minimize recurrence.

Acromioclavicular Joint Dislocation

Acromioclavicular joint dislocation, or shoulder separation, is most commonly caused by a fall on the lateral point of the shoulder. Examination reveals localized tenderness and prominence of the displaced distal clavicle. The severity of the separation is based on the amount of injury to the acromioclavicular (AC) and coracoclavicular (CC) ligaments (**Figure 14-19**). Grade I and II injuries are treated nonoperatively. Most grade III AC joint dislocations may be treated by range-of-motion and strengthening exercises after the

Figure 14-18: Posterior Dislocation, Glenohumeral Joint

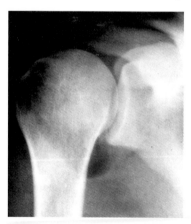 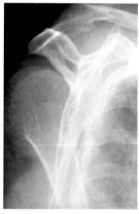

Anteroposterior radiograph. Difficult to determine if humeral head within, anterior to, or posterior to glenoid cavity

Lateral radiograph (parallel to plane of body of scapula). Humeral head clearly seen to be posterior to glenoid cavity

Figure 14-19: Acromioclavicular Dislocation

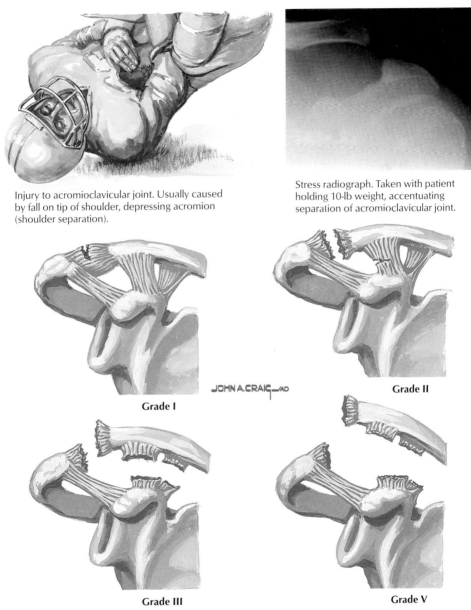

Injury to acromioclavicular joint. Usually caused by fall on tip of shoulder, depressing acromion (shoulder separation).

Stress radiograph. Taken with patient holding 10-lb weight, accentuating separation of acromioclavicular joint.

JOHN A. CRAIG—MD

Grade I

Grade II

Grade III

Grade V

pain subsides. For some athletes in contact sports and workers in jobs that require heavy labor, however, surgical intervention may yield more predictable results. Grade IV–VI AC separations (IV and VI not shown) are uncommon (<1%) and, because of their severity, require open repair.

Sternoclavicular Joint Dislocation

Dislocations of the SC joint are uncommon. Anterior dislocation with the clavicle displaced anterior to the sternum is the most common type. The typical mechanism of injury is an indirect force on the lateral aspect of the shoulder, resulting in anterior translation of the medial clavicle. Examination reveals a prominent bump and tenderness over the SC joint. Reduction can be performed with lateral traction and pressure over the medial clavicle. Redislocation is common, but further treatment is not necessary because most chronic anterior SC dislocations become asymptomatic.

Posterior SC joint dislocations are rare but more serious because of the potential resultant injury to the great vessels that exit the heart and the vital structures of the neck, especially the trachea. Dyspnea, dysphagia, or signs of venous congestion are indicative of a posterior SC dislocation.

Tendon Ruptures

Most tendon ruptures about the shoulder are similar to those in other anatomical areas and are associated with attritional changes, are most common in middle-aged patients, and typically occur at the musculotendinous junction. The most common rupture occurs at the proximal aspect of the long head of the biceps. The rupture may be spontaneous or associated with lifting. A popping sound followed by sharp pain is typical.

Examination shows mild swelling, ecchymosis, and a bulge in the midarm that results from distal retraction of the biceps. The bulge is accentuated when the patient contracts the biceps against resistance with the elbow flexed (**Figure 14-20**).

Figure 14-20: Rupture of Long Head Biceps Brachii Muscle

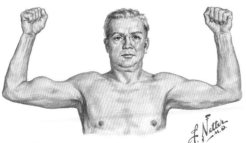

Rupture of tendon of long head of right biceps brachii muscle indicated by active flexion of elbow

Nonoperative treatment is satisfactory for most patients because motion is regained and loss of strength is minimal and not disabling. Operative repair should be considered in young athletes and heavy laborers.

Rupture of the distal biceps tendon is relatively uncommon, is disabling, and should be repaired.

Other tendon ruptures about the shoulder include the pectoralis major, deltoid, subscapularis, and long head of the triceps. These injuries are uncommon, subsequently are more disabling, and frequently require surgical repair.

PEDIATRIC DISORDERS

Neonatal Brachial Plexus Palsy

Neonatal brachial plexus palsy is paralysis of upper extremity muscles noted at birth. The incidence is approximately 1 per 2000 births. Because of improved obstetric care, the neurologic injury is less severe than in the past, but the incidence is approximately the same. This condition typically arises from traction injuries that occur during delivery of large neonates (birth weight >4000 g), pelvic dystocia, or both. An upper plexus injury (Erb palsy) is most common and typically occurs during a cephalic delivery when the head has presented but there is difficulty in delivering the shoulder. A lower plexus injury (Klumpke paralysis) is associated with a breech delivery in which the upper limb is forced into full abduction. Pan plexus palsy is a more severe traction injury that involves the entire brachial plexus.

Examination findings vary according to the pattern and severity of nerve injury. Because of weakness of the deltoid, shoulder external rotators, elbow flexors, and wrist extensors, neonates with Erb palsy keep the shoulder adducted and internally rotated, the elbow extended, the forearm pronated, and the wrist flexed (headwaiter position). Klumpke paralysis, in contrast, primarily affects the wrist and hand. Pan plexus palsy causes the upper extremity to be flail. Horner sign may be present in Klumpke or pan plexus palsy.

Figure 14-21: Sprengel Deformity

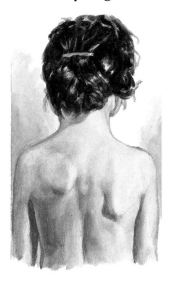
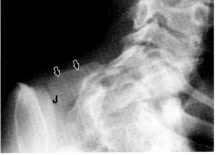

Radiograph shows omovertebral bone (arrows) connecting scapula to spinous processes of cervical vertebrae via osteochondral joint (J)

Initial treatment involves a month of rest in a position that protects the stretched nerves, followed by stretching of contracted muscles while the patient awaits recovery. Most children have significant recovery without surgical treatment. Early plexus surgery should be considered at 4 to 6 months in infants who have not regained palpable elbow flexion or who have pan plexus palsy. Older children (2 to 4 years of age) with significant muscle imbalance can be helped by muscle releases and tendon transfers that improve function and decrease the risk of progressive deformity. Earlier procedures are indicated in children who develop posterior shoulder subluxation or dislocation.

Congenital Elevation of the Scapula (Sprengel Deformity)

Sprengel deformity results from failure of scapular descent during in utero development (**Figure 14-21**). The scapula, in addition to being elevated, is mildly hypoplastic. The affected side of the neck appears fuller and shorter. Patients with Sprengel deformity often have congenital scoliosis, Klippel-Feil syndrome, and renal abnormalities. An omovertebral bone is an osseous or cartilaginous bridge that connects the cervical spine to the superior angle of the scapula and is often associated with Sprengel deformity. This bridge and associated muscle contraction combined with abnormal position of the scapula results in variable loss of shoulder motion.

Surgical intervention is indicated to correct severe deformities. Common surgical techniques include resection of the omovertebral bar and inferior repositioning of the scapula. Clavicular osteotomy may be performed to minimize the risk of brachial plexus injury.

Cleidocranial Dysostosis

Cleidocranial dysostosis is an autosomal dominant condition that affects intramembranous bone formation and results in incomplete formation of the clavicles, skull, and pubis. The entire clavicle may be absent, or only a small segment of the middle or distal third may be missing. The defect is bilateral 80% of the time. The child typically has a large head, a small face, a long neck, drooping shoulders, and a narrow chest. Hypermobility of the shoulder girdles is demonstrated by the patient's inability to position the humeral heads in the anterior midline. Cleidocranial dysostosis usually is not disabling, but parents should make sure the child with open fontanelles wears protective headgear and receives appropriate treatment for abnormal dentition.

Congenital Pseudarthrosis of the Clavicle

Congenital pseudarthrosis of the clavicle is due to pressure from the developing subclavian artery. It usually involves the right side unless *situs inversus* occurs. The affected side has a bony prominence, but functional deficits are mild. For children with pain or cosmetic concerns, internal fixation and bone grafting are usually successful. The appearance of the surgical scar must be considered in the surgical decision.

ADDITIONAL READINGS

DeLee JC, Dres D Jr., Miller MD, eds. *DeLee and Drez's Orthopaedic Sports Medicine: Principles and Practice*, 2nd edition. Philadelphia, Pa: Saunders; 2003.

Matsen FA III, Lippitt SB, eds. *Shoulder Surgery: Principles and Procedures*. Philadelphia, Pa: Saunders; 2004.

Miller MD, Cooper DE, Warner JJP, eds. *Review of Sports Medicine and Arthroscopy*. Philadelphia, Pa: Saunders; 2002.

Elbow and Forearm

Edward D. Wang, MD
Lawrence C. Hurst, MD

ANATOMY

The elbow is a functional link for positioning the hand in space, a fulcrum for the forearm lever, and a load-carrying joint. As such, it requires a combination of mobility and stability. The three articulations of the elbow provide flexion and extension, as well as forearm rotation (**Figure 15-1**). Control and stability of flexion and extension are provided primarily through the *ulnohumeral* (trochlea and olecranon) articulation and secondarily through the *radiohumeral* (capitellum and radial head) articulation. The *trochlea* is shaped like a spool and fits in the wrench-shaped trochlear notch. This anatomic configuration, in conjunction with the collateral ligaments, provides a stable hinge joint that can lift heavy objects. Rotation of the forearm occurs through the proximal and distal radioulnar articulations.

Distal to the radial head, the bone tapers to form the radial neck, then flares at the *radial tuberosity*—the insertion site of the biceps tendon. Between the radius and the ulna is the interosseous membrane—a thickened, ligamentous structure that connects the two

Figure 15-1: Bones of Right Elbow Joint

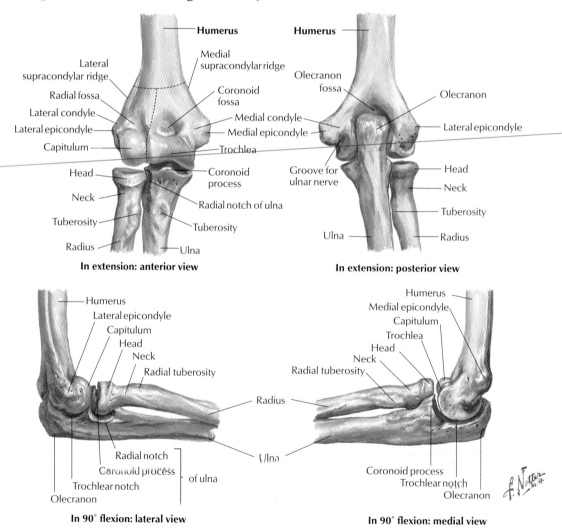

In extension: anterior view

In extension: posterior view

In 90° flexion: lateral view

In 90° flexion: medial view

bones in a manner that provides stability while allowing forearm rotation.

Muscles that cross the elbow anteriorly include the elbow flexors and the flexor-pronator forearm muscles that originate from the medial epicondyle (**Figure 15-2**). In the forearm, the volar muscles are arranged in three layers. The superficial group includes the pronator teres, flexor carpi radialis, palmaris longus, and flexor carpi ulnaris. The middle layer is the flexor digitorum superficialis. The deep layer comprises the supinator, flexor digitorum profundus, flexor pollicis longus, and pronator quadratus. The flexor-pronator muscle group primarily provides wrist flexion and forearm pronation. The biceps is a secondary flexor of the elbow and a strong supinator. Immediately deep to the biceps lies the brachialis muscle—the major flexor of the elbow.

Posterior elbow muscles include elbow extensors, wrist and finger extensors, and the supinator. Posterior forearm muscles are arranged in two layers. The superficial group originates from a common tendon at the lateral epicondyle and includes a lateral component (brachioradialis, extensor carpi radialis longus, and extensor carpi radialis brevis) and a medial subgroup (extensor digitorum, extensor digiti minimi, extensor carpi ulnaris, and anconeus). The deep posterior forearm muscles are the supinator, abductor pollicis longus, extensor pollicis brevis, and extensor pollicis longus (see **Figure 15-2**).

The brachial artery, the main artery of the arm and elbow, travels in the anterior compartment of the arm adjacent to the median nerve. Proximal to the elbow, it gives off collateral arteries that help form a rich plexus of vessels around the elbow. At the level of the radial head, the brachial artery bifurcates into the radial and ulnar arteries. The ulnar artery enters the forearm posterior to the pronator teres, whereas the radial artery travels between the brachioradialis and the supinator muscle.

The median nerve enters the forearm between the humeral and ulnar heads of the pronator teres and travels inferior to the flexor digitorum superficialis muscle (**Figure 15-3**). The *anterior interosseous nerve* branches in-

nervate the index, and sometimes, the long, finger component of the flexor digitorum profundus, the flexor pollicis longus, and the pronator quadratus. Because of the location of its fibers in the median nerve, isolated paralysis of the anterior interosseous nerve may occur with an elbow fracture. The rest of the median nerve innervates all the volar forearm muscles except the ulnar half of the flexor digitorum profundus (fourth and fifth fingers) and the flexor carpi ulnaris, both of which are supplied by the ulnar nerve.

The ulnar nerve exits the anterior compartment of the arm, passing behind the medial epicondyle into the cubital tunnel at the elbow, then enters the forearm between the two heads of the flexor carpi ulnaris (**Figure 15-4**). It innervates the flexor carpi ulnaris muscle, the ulnar half of the flexor digitorum profundus muscle, and, ultimately, the intrinsic muscles of the hand.

In the arm, the radial nerve travels within the posterior compartment, then enters the anterior compartment lateral to the humerus. In the antecubital fossa, the radial nerve innervates the brachioradialis and extensor carpi radialis longus before dividing into superficial (sensory) and deep (mostly motor) branches (**Figure 15-5**). The superficial radial nerve provides sensation to the radial dorsal wrist and hand. The deep branch innervates the remaining extensor muscles of the forearm. It travels deep and through the supinator muscle and exits this muscle as the posterior interosseous nerve. Distal to the radial tuberosity, the deep branch of the radial nerve may lie "on the bone" and, as such, is vulnerable to injury in fractures of the proximal radius or in operations at this site.

PHYSICAL EXAMINATION

Inspect the elbow for swelling and ecchymosis, and determine the carrying angle (the axial alignment of the humerus and the ulna with the elbow extended). The normal carrying angle is 10° to 20°, with most studies observing slightly greater *cubitus valgus* in females. Angular deformities may occur secondary to previous trauma, growth distur-

Figure 15-2: Bony Attachments of Muscles of Forearm

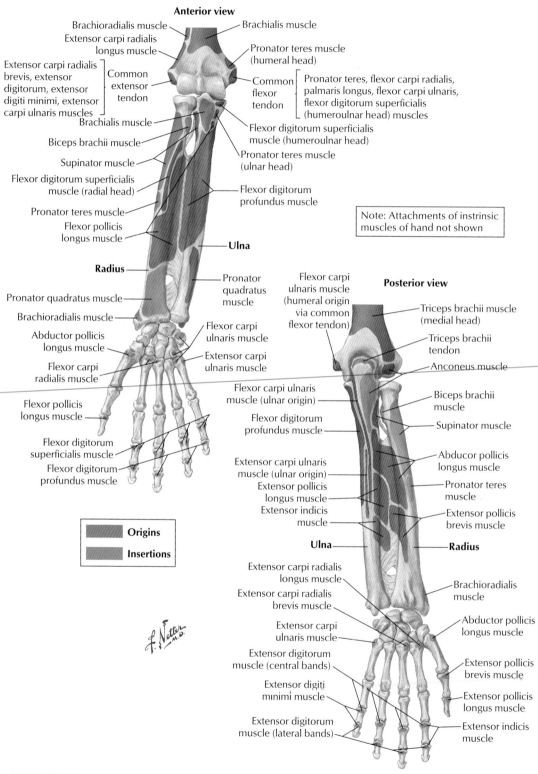

Anterior view

Brachioradialis muscle

Extensor carpi radialis longus muscle

Extensor carpi radialis brevis, extensor digitorum, extensor digiti minimi, extensor carpi ulnaris muscles

Common extensor tendon

Brachialis muscle

Biceps brachii muscle

Supinator muscle

Flexor digitorum superficialis muscle (radial head)

Pronator teres muscle

Flexor pollicis longus muscle

Radius

Pronator quadratus muscle

Brachioradialis muscle

Abductor pollicis longus muscle

Flexor carpi radialis muscle

Flexor pollicis longus muscle

Flexor digitorum superficialis muscle

Flexor digitorum profundus muscle

Brachialis muscle

Pronator teres muscle (humeral head)

Common flexor tendon

Pronator teres, flexor carpi radialis, palmaris longus, flexor carpi ulnaris, flexor digitorum superficialis (humeroulnar head) muscles

Flexor digitorum superficialis muscle (humeroulnar head)

Pronator teres muscle (ulnar head)

Flexor digitorum profundus muscle

Note: Attachments of instrinsic muscles of hand not shown

Ulna

Pronator quadratus muscle

Flexor carpi ulnaris muscle

Extensor carpi ulnaris muscle

Flexor carpi ulnaris muscle (humeral origin via common flexor tendon)

Posterior view

Triceps brachii muscle (medial head)

Triceps brachii tendon

Anconeus muscle

Biceps brachii muscle

Supinator muscle

Abducor pollicis longus muscle

Pronator teres muscle

Extensor pollicis brevis muscle

Flexor carpi ulnaris muscle (ulnar origin)

Flexor digitorum profundus muscle

Extensor carpi ulnaris muscle (ulnar origin)

Extensor pollicis longus muscle

Extensor indicis muscle

Ulna

Radius

Extensor carpi radialis longus muscle

Extensor carpi radialis brevis muscle

Extensor carpi ulnaris muscle

Extensor digitorum muscle (central bands)

Extensor digiti minimi muscle

Extensor digitorum muscle (lateral bands)

Brachioradialis muscle

Abductor pollicis longus muscle

Extensor pollicis brevis muscle

Extensor pollicis longus muscle

Extensor indicis muscle

Origins

Insertions

f. Netter M.D.

Figure 15-3: Median Nerve

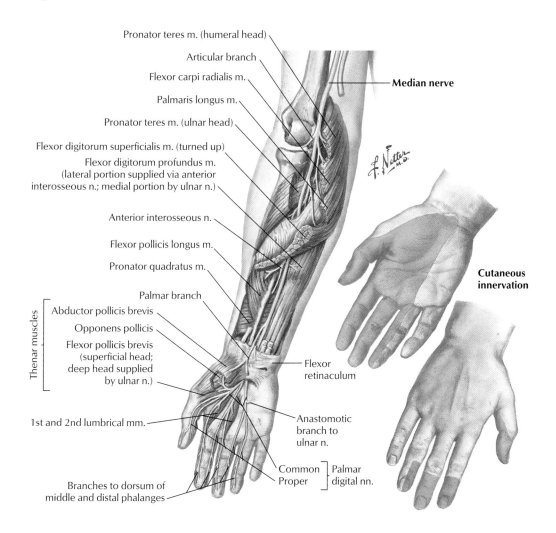

Pronator teres m. (humeral head)

Articular branch

Flexor carpi radialis m.

Median nerve

Palmaris longus m.

Pronator teres m. (ulnar head)

Flexor digitorum superficialis m. (turned up)

Flexor digitorum profundus m.
(lateral portion supplied via anterior
interosseous n.; medial portion by ulnar n.)

Anterior interosseous n.

Flexor pollicis longus m.

Pronator quadratus m.

Cutaneous
innervation

Palmar branch

Thenar muscles

Abductor pollicis brevis

Opponens pollicis

Flexor pollicis brevis
(superficial head;
deep head supplied
by ulnar n.)

Flexor
retinaculum

1st and 2nd lumbrical mm.

Anastomotic
branch to
ulnar n.

Common ⌉ Palmar
Proper ⌋ digital nn.

Branches to dorsum of
middle and distal phalanges

bances, or genetic syndromes. Ecchymosis, swelling, or both about the elbow indicate a muscle or tendon injury, fracture, or elbow sprain or dislocation.

Palpate subcutaneous landmarks for sites of tenderness, deformity, or effusion that indicate the site of occult fracture, tendinosis, ligament sprain, or tendon rupture. From lateral to medial, the structures in the antecubital fossa are the biceps tendon, brachial artery, and median nerve. A palpable defect is key to diagnosing rupture of the distal biceps tendon or disruption of the triceps tendon. Joint effusion is best detected in the "soft spot" between the lateral epicondyle, radial head, and

olecranon. Tenderness over the radial head or humeral condyles may indicate an occult fracture that is not visible on radiographs.

The *zero starting position* for measurement of elbow motion is a straight extremity (**Figure 15-6**). Young children commonly extend the elbow by 10° to 15°, but adults usually cannot extend the elbow past the zero starting position. The normal range of elbow flexion-extension is 0° to 145°. The plane of forearm rotation is pronation-supination. *Pronation* literally means "the state of being prone" or, as it relates to the forearm, "the palm being turned backward." Likewise, *supination* literally means "the state of being supine" (ie, the

Figure 15-4: Ulnar Nerve

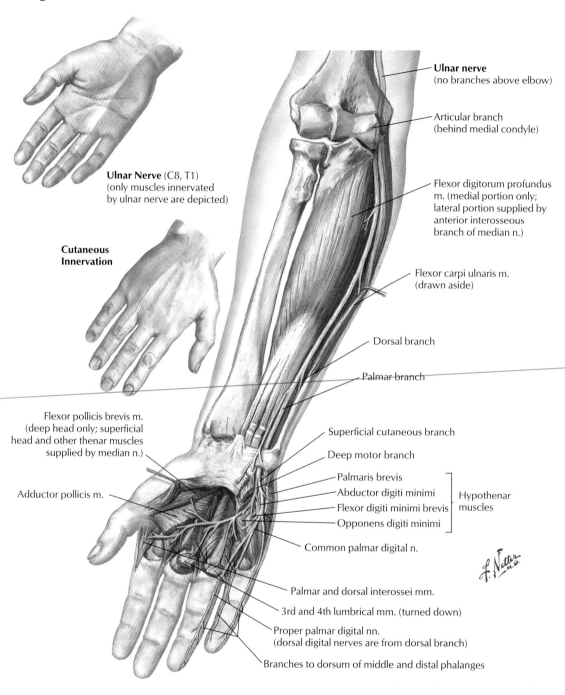

Ulnar nerve
(no branches above elbow)

Articular branch
(behind medial condyle)

Flexor digitorum profundus
m. (medial portion only;
lateral portion supplied by
anterior interosseous
branch of median n.)

Flexor carpi ulnaris m.
(drawn aside)

Dorsal branch

Palmar branch

Superficial cutaneous branch

Deep motor branch

Palmaris brevis

Abductor digiti minimi

Flexor digiti minimi brevis

Opponens digiti minimi

Hypothenar
muscles

Common palmar digital n.

Palmar and dorsal interossei mm.

3rd and 4th lumbrical mm. (turned down)

Proper palmar digital nn.
(dorsal digital nerves are from dorsal branch)

Branches to dorsum of middle and distal phalanges

Ulnar Nerve (C8, T1)
(only muscles innervated
by ulnar nerve are depicted)

**Cutaneous
Innervation**

Flexor pollicis brevis m.
(deep head only; superficial
head and other thenar muscles
supplied by median n.)

Adductor pollicis m.

Figure 15-5: Radial Nerve

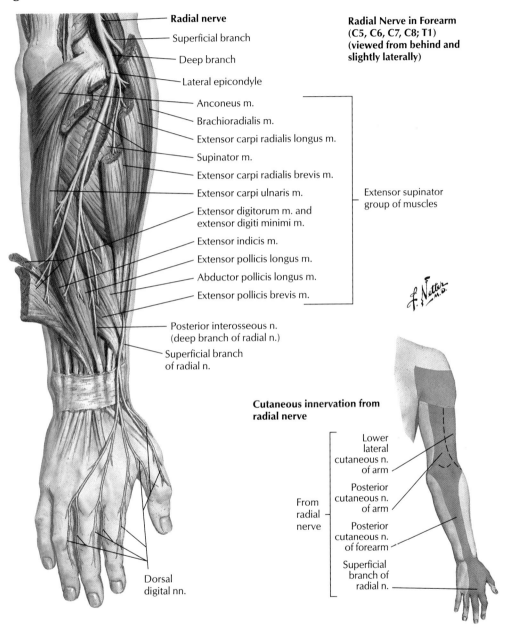

Radial nerve
Superficial branch
Deep branch
Lateral epicondyle
Anconeus m.
Brachioradialis m.
Extensor carpi radialis longus m.
Supinator m.
Extensor carpi radialis brevis m.
Extensor carpi ulnaris m.
Extensor digitorum m. and extensor digiti minimi m.
Extensor indicis m.
Extensor pollicis longus m.
Abductor pollicis longus m.
Extensor pollicis brevis m.
Posterior interosseous n. (deep branch of radial n.)
Superficial branch of radial n.

Radial Nerve in Forearm (C5, C6, C7, C8; T1) (viewed from behind and slightly laterally)

Extensor supinator group of muscles

Dorsal digital nn.

Cutaneous innervation from radial nerve

From radial nerve

Lower lateral cutaneous n. of arm
Posterior cutaneous n. of arm
Posterior cutaneous n. of forearm
Superficial branch of radial n.

Figure 15-6: Measurement of Flexion/Extension

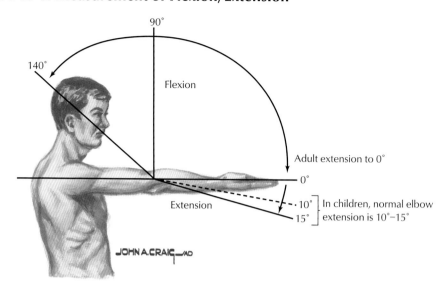

palm turned forward, or anteriorly). In forearm rotation measurement, the patient's arm is stabilized against the chest wall, and the elbow is flexed to 90° (**Figure 15-7**). The zero starting position occurs with the thumb aligned with the humerus. Normal motion in adults is 75° pronation and 85° supination. Mild elbow contractures are of limited functional consequence, as most activities of daily living are accomplished in an arc of motion from 30° to 130° flexion and 50° each of pronation and supination.

DEGENERATIVE DISORDERS OF THE ELBOW

Arthritis

Primary osteoarthritis of the elbow is relatively uncommon and accounts for 2% to 7% of elbow arthritis. These patients often work at a job or hobby that repetitively loads the elbow. Males and the dominant extremity are more commonly affected. Manifestations include stiffness, loss of motion, and pain with activity. Terminal extension typically increases pain. Secondary osteoarthritis of the elbow most often follows intra-articular fractures. Rheumatoid arthritis is by far the most common cause of inflammatory arthritis

of the elbow. Of patients with rheumatoid arthritis, 20% to 50% eventually have elbow involvement.

Most patients with elbow arthritis can be treated with standard nonoperative modalities. Arthrotomy or arthroscopy may be indicated for loose body removal, osteophyte resection and capsular resection, or synovectomy. Elimination of locking and decreased pain are more predictable after removal of a loose body than is increased motion. Injury to neurovascular structures is a potential risk of elbow arthroscopy, but complications are generally minimal, and recovery time is shorter compared with open procedures.

Resection ulnohumeral arthroplasty that includes resection of the tip of the olecranon, débridement of the olecranon fossa, and resection of osteophytes from the coronoid may be used to treat patients with extensive humeral osteophytes and disabling pain at the extremes of motion, but no pain at rest or in the mid arc of motion. Patients should have good elbow stability and normal musculature. Concomitant transposition of the ulnar nerve is indicated for patients with symptoms of entrapment. Increased motion and decreased pain have been reported in 85% of patients who undergo this procedure. Symptoms often

Figure 15-7: Measurement of Pronation-Supination

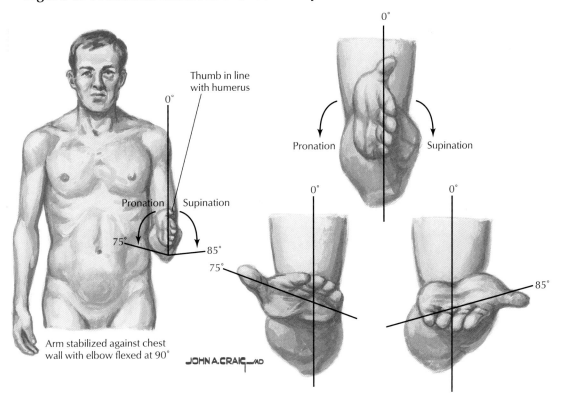

Thumb in line with humerus

0°

Pronation | Supination

75°   85°

Arm stabilized against chest wall with elbow flexed at 90°

JOHN A. CRAIG—MD

0°

Pronation   Supination

0°   0°

75°   85°

return; however, the interval improvement and delay in the need for total joint arthroplasty are helpful. Resection arthroplasty that includes the distal humerus and radial head may be combined with interposition of autogenous fascia or dermis between the bone surfaces for patients with more severe arthritis.

Arthrodesis of the elbow is seldom indicated because no single position provides reasonable function. The rare indications include (1) incurable sepsis or (2) the need for a strong, stable joint in a young manual laborer who has a normal shoulder and contralateral limb.

Total elbow arthroplasty provides consistent short-term results. A semiconstrained prosthesis that depends on both the component and the surrounding soft tissues for joint stability provides the best compromise for function and the highest long-term survival rates (approximately 95% at 7 years) (**Figure 15-8**). Loosening of the implant with resultant instability and recurrent pain is the most com-

mon long-term complication. At the elbow, the rate of loosening is higher and prosthetic revision is less predictable and more complicated than at other sites of joint replacement. In general, total elbow arthroplasty is preferred in the older patient, whereas resection or interposition arthroplasty is preferred in the younger patient. Because of severe erosion and joint instability, total elbow arthroplasty is indicated in nearly all patients with rheumatoid arthritis.

Lateral Epicondylitis

Lateral epicondylitis, commonly known as "tennis elbow," occurs secondary to a tendinosis of the extensor carpi radialis brevis origin immediately distal to the lateral epicondyle. The name is misleading because the lateral epicondyle is not the site of involvement, inflammation is not present, and most patients are not active tennis players. The typical patient is 35 to 50 years of age and expe-

Figure 15-8: Prosthesis for Total Elbow Arthroplasty

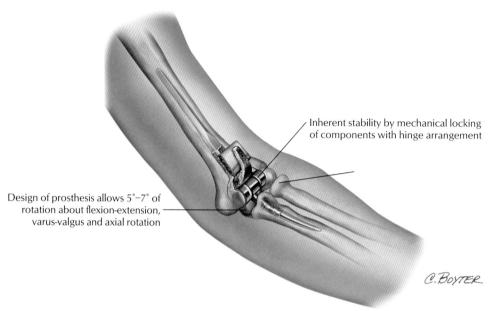

Inherent stability by mechanical locking of components with hinge arrangement

Design of prosthesis allows 5°–7° of rotation about flexion-extension, varus-valgus and axial rotation

C.BOYTER

Three types of total elbow arthroplasty have been used. The constrained design replaced the elbow joint with a hinged prosthesis. All stability of the joint was dependent on the prosthesis which was not built to accommodate the rotational demands of the elbow joint. Due to an unacceptably high failure rate, this prosthesis has been abandoned. Results were better with an unrestrained prosthesis but with 5%–20% incidence of postoperative instability, most patients are now treated with a semi-constrained prosthesis, which has inherent stability by linking of the component usually with a hinge (shown above) or a snap-fit axis arrangement.

riences an insidious or acute lateral elbow pain that is exacerbated by activities that involve forceful wrist extension. Motions such as turning a screwdriver or opening a door can aggravate the symptoms. Over time, the pain can become severe and may interfere with routine activities.

Examination shows pain just distal and posterior to the lateral epicondyle that is exacerbated when the extensor carpi radialis brevis is stressed in an elongated position (wrist extension against resistance with the elbow extended) (**Figure 15-9**). Elbow motion and radiographic findings are normal. The differential diagnosis includes radial nerve (posterior interosseous branch) entrapment, arthritis involving the radiohumeral articulation, lateral elbow instability, and referred pain from cervical radiculopathy.

Nonoperative treatment consists primarily of patience, modification of activities, and progressive strengthening exercises. Patients should be taught to "grasp and lift only in supination." A counterforce strap worn around the proximal forearm may decrease pain during lifting activities. Corticosteroid injections at the site of maximum tenderness should be infrequently used. Operative treatment, which is infrequently required, involves excision of the pathologic area of degenerated tendon. It results in an 85% to 90% return to full activity without pain. Persistent pain usually occurs secondary to an incomplete resection or an incorrect diagnosis.

Medial Epicondylitis

Medial epicondylitis, commonly known as "golfer's elbow," occurs secondary to tendinosis of the flexor-pronator origin. Examination demonstrates tenderness just distal and anterior to the medial epicondyle. Pronation and wrist flexion against resistance exacer-

Figure 15-9: Epicondylitis

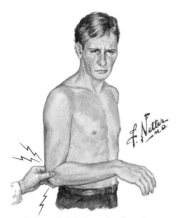

Epicondylitis (tennis elbow)
Exquisite tenderness approximately
1 cm distal to the lateral epicondyle

bate the pain. As in lateral epicondylitis, elbow motion and radiographic findings are usually normal. The differential diagnosis includes ulnar nerve entrapment, medial elbow instability, and cervical radiculopathy. Treatment principles for the noncompetitive athlete are similar to those used for lateral epicondylitis.

NERVE ENTRAPMENT SYNDROMES

Ulnar Nerve Entrapment

Compression of the ulnar nerve at the elbow, or cubital tunnel syndrome, is the most common cause of peripheral nerve entrapment after carpal tunnel syndrome (**Figure 15-10**). The cubital tunnel extends from 8 cm above the medial epicondyle, where the ulnar nerve passes from the anterior to the posterior compartment of the arm, to 5 cm distal to the elbow, where the ulnar nerve enters the anterior compartment of the forearm. Compression of the nerve may occur at any site within this tunnel. A hypermobile or subluxating ulnar nerve also may produce symptoms, and this condition may be aggravated by increased mobility and snapping of the medial triceps.

Symptoms vary with the duration and the severity of compression. Aching on the medial aspect of the elbow and numbness on the dorsal and palmar surfaces of the fingers innervated by the ulnar nerve that is aggravated by elbow flexion are typical (see **Figure 15-4**). Examination shows a positive Tinel sign and altered ulnar nerve sensation in the fingers that typically is exacerbated by flexion of the elbow and pressure on the ulnar nerve. Loss of sensation on the dorsoulnar aspect of the wrist and hand and weakness of the intrinsic muscles causing decreased pinch and grip strength may or may not be present. The differential diagnosis includes ulnar nerve entrapment at the wrist, cervical radiculopathy, thoracic outlet syndrome, and medial epicondylitis.

Nonoperative treatment may include nighttime splinting to keep the elbow in a relatively extended position, as well as avoidance of prolonged leaning on the elbow, use of vibrating tools, or activities that repetitively flex the elbow. Operative treatment is recommended for persistent moderate or severe symptoms. The procedure most commonly used is decompression and transposition of the nerve anterior to the medial epicondyle.

Median Nerve Entrapment

At the elbow, entrapment of the median nerve can occur at several locations, including an anomalous supracondylar process of the humerus and the lacertus fibrosus (**Figure 15-11**). Fibrous constriction arches also may entrap the nerve as it passes beneath the two heads of the pronator teres or flexor digitorum superficialis. The most common location of entrapment is the pronator teres—hence, the alternative name, pronator syndrome.

Typical symptoms include an aching pain in the mid to proximal forearm that is aggravated by repetitive lifting activities. Numbness and weakness in the median nerve distribution are variable and may be absent. Aggravation of symptoms after 90 seconds of resisted pronation or resisted activity of the flexor digitorum superficialis of the long finger suggests median nerve entrapment. Nerve conduction tests are less useful in this syndrome but should be performed. A lidocaine and corticosteroid injection may be beneficial and diagnostic.

Figure 15-10: Cubital Tunnel Syndrome

Clinical signs

Nonsurgical management

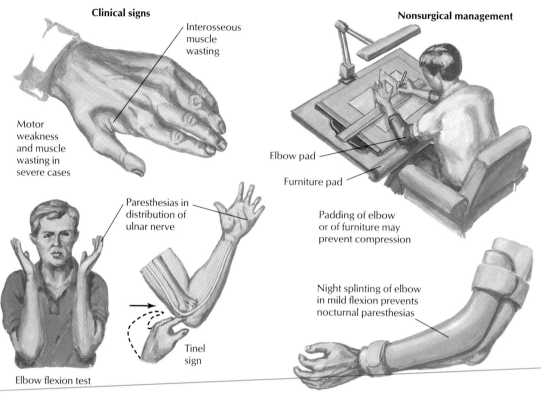

Interosseous muscle wasting

Motor weakness and muscle wasting in severe cases

Paresthesias in distribution of ulnar nerve

Tinel sign

Elbow flexion test

Elbow pad

Furniture pad

Padding of elbow or of furniture may prevent compression

Night splinting of elbow in mild flexion prevents nocturnal paresthesias

Submuscular transposition of ulnar nerve

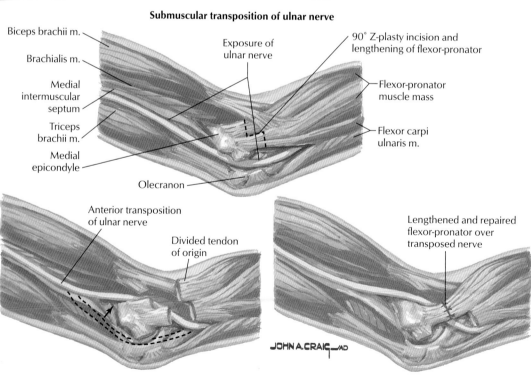

Biceps brachii m.

Brachialis m.

Medial intermuscular septum

Triceps brachii m.

Medial epicondyle

Olecranon

Exposure of ulnar nerve

90° Z-plasty incision and lengthening of flexor-pronator

Flexor-pronator muscle mass

Flexor carpi ulnaris m.

Anterior transposition of ulnar nerve

Divided tendon of origin

Lengthened and repaired flexor-pronator over transposed nerve

JOHN A.CRAIG—AD

318

Figure 15-11: Proximal Compression of Median Nerve

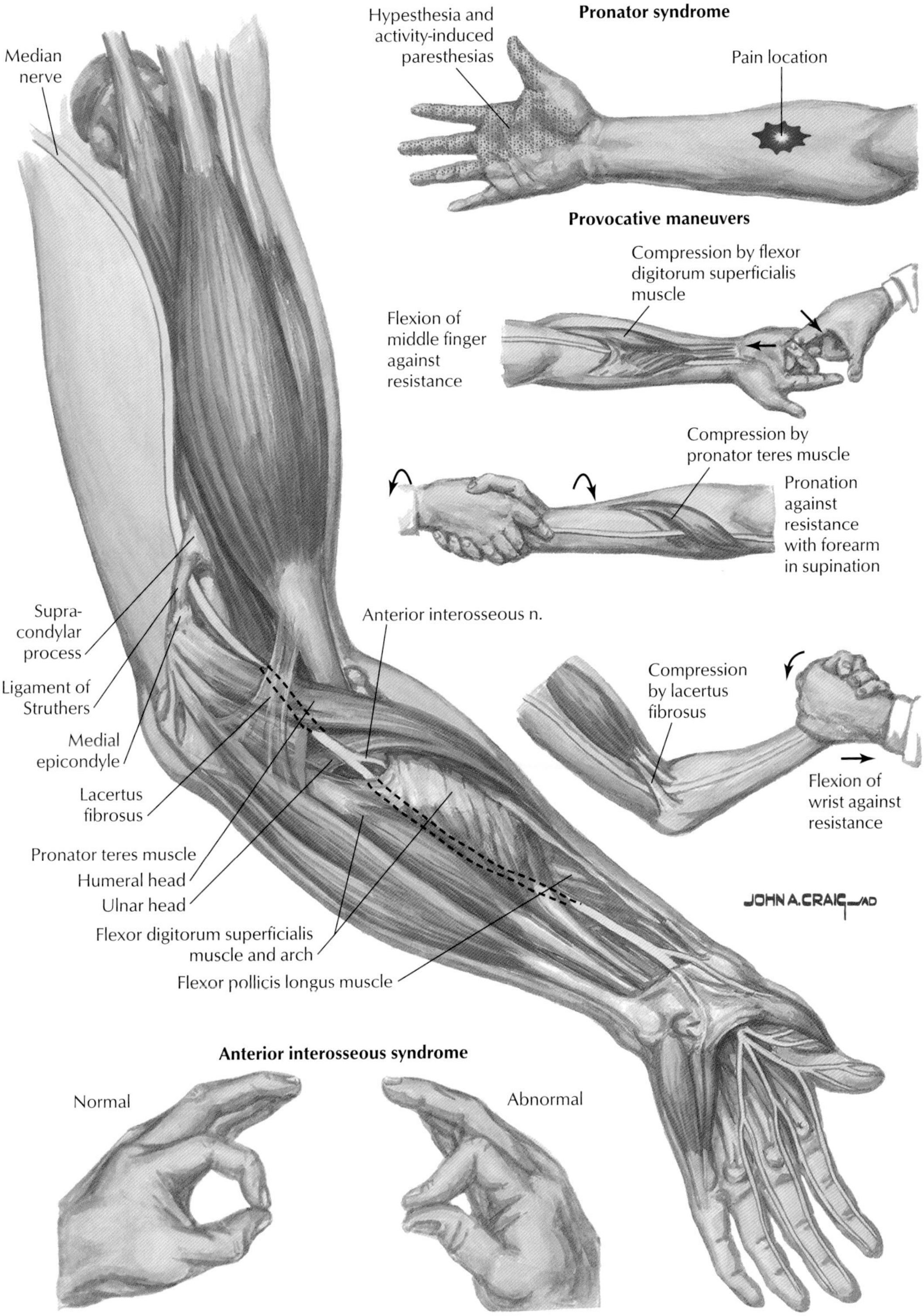

Median nerve

Pronator syndrome

Hypesthesia and activity-induced paresthesias

Pain location

Provocative maneuvers

Compression by flexor digitorum superficialis muscle

Flexion of middle finger against resistance

Compression by pronator teres muscle

Pronation against resistance with forearm in supination

Supra-condylar process

Ligament of Struthers

Medial epicondyle

Lacertus fibrosus

Pronator teres muscle
Humeral head
Ulnar head

Flexor digitorum superficialis muscle and arch

Flexor pollicis longus muscle

Anterior interosseous n.

Compression by lacertus fibrosus

Flexion of wrist against resistance

JOHN A. CRAIG—AD

Anterior interosseous syndrome

Normal

Abnormal

319

The differential diagnosis includes muscle tears in the proximal forearm and carpal tunnel syndrome. Carpal tunnel syndrome can be ruled out if there is loss of sensation at the thenar eminence (supplied by the palmar branch originating proximal to the wrist) or weakness of the flexor pollicis longus. If avoidance of inciting activities does not relieve the symptoms, surgical decompression is indicated. All areas of possible compression should be explored.

Radial Nerve Entrapment

Radial nerve entrapment at the elbow typically involves compression of the posterior interosseous branch of the radial nerve, most commonly as it passes beneath the proximal edge of the supinator muscle at the arcade of Frohse (**Figure 15-12**). Because the posterior interosseous nerve is purely motor, the posterior interosseous syndrome affects only motor function of the thumb, finger extensors, and extensor carpi ulnaris (see **Figure 15-5**). Symptoms and signs of motor weakness are often vague in the early phase of the condition, and radial tunnel syndrome sometimes masquerades as a resistant lateral epicondylitis.

Diagnosis is based on history and an examination that typically shows tenderness over the proximal supinator muscle (approximately 5 cm distal to the lateral epicondyle). Pain is typically exacerbated by extension of the long finger against resistance with the elbow extended.

Surgical decompression with release of the impinging fibrous bands of the supinator muscle is usually helpful if symptoms are severe or do not resolve after a period of observation. The course of the posterior interosseous nerve through the full extent of the supinator muscle should be explored because entrapment also may occur in the midsubstance of the muscle and in its distal margin.

MISCELLANEOUS CONDITIONS

Acute Sprains

The medial collateral ligament (MCL) complex includes the anterior bundle, the poste-rior bundle, and the transverse ligament (**Figure 15-13**). The anterior bundle of the MCL originates at the midportion of the medial epicondyle and inserts onto the coronoid tubercle of the ulna. The anterior bundle is the primary restraint to valgus stress. Its eccentric location provides valgus restraint throughout the full arc of flexion-extension. With the elbow in full extension, stability to valgus stress is conferred equally by the MCL, anterior capsule, and bony articulation. With the elbow in 90° of flexion, the MCL provides 55% of valgus stability. The contribution of the radiocapitellar articulation to valgus stability is secondary and significant only when the anterior bundle is disrupted.

The lateral collateral ligament (LCL) complex includes the radial collateral ligament, the annular ligament, the accessory lateral collateral ligament, and the lateral ulnar collateral ligament. The *lateral ulnar collateral ligament* originates from the anteroinferior portion of the lateral epicondyle, inserts on the supinator crest of the proximal ulna, and is the primary lateral stabilizer. The *annular ligament* serves as a checkrein for the radial head.

Patients with acute sprains report a history of acute pain after a fall or forceful throwing injury. Valgus distraction injuries transmit loads primarily to the MCL complex and the medial flexor-pronator muscular origin. Injuries to the LCL typically occur with a varus stress to the elbow joint when it is in extension and the forearm is in pronation. In acute injuries, the global swelling and tenderness, as well as the unreliability of stress maneuvers, make it virtually impossible for the clinician to determine precisely which ligament components are injured. Avulsion fractures may be seen on radiographs. Short-term immobilization and gradual resumption of activities are successful in treating most acute elbow sprains.

Chronic Medial Elbow Pain and Instability

Medial elbow pain and MCL instability typically develop in athletes involved in repetitive throwing activities. Pain is usually gradual

Figure 15-12: Radial Nerve Compression

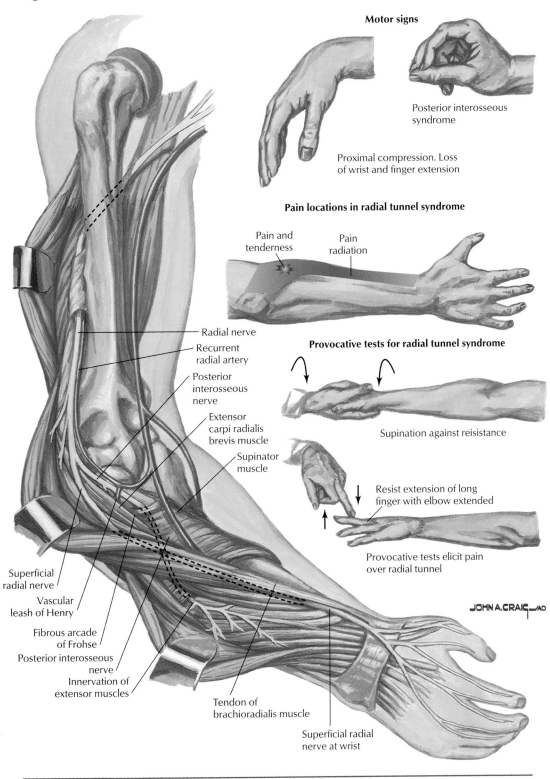

Motor signs

Posterior interosseous syndrome

Proximal compression. Loss of wrist and finger extension

Pain locations in radial tunnel syndrome

Pain and tenderness

Pain radiation

Provocative tests for radial tunnel syndrome

Supination against reisistance

Resist extension of long finger with elbow extended

Provocative tests elicit pain over radial tunnel

JOHN A. CRAIG—AD

Radial nerve

Recurrent radial artery

Posterior interosseous nerve

Extensor carpi radialis brevis muscle

Supinator muscle

Superficial radial nerve

Vascular leash of Henry

Fibrous arcade of Frohse

Posterior interosseous nerve

Innervation of extensor muscles

Tendon of brachioradialis muscle

Superficial radial nerve at wrist

321

Figure 15-13: Ligaments of Right Elbow Joint

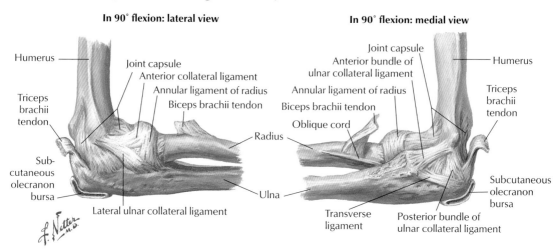

In 90° flexion: lateral view

- Humerus
- Joint capsule
- Anterior collateral ligament
- Annular ligament of radius
- Biceps brachii tendon
- Triceps brachii tendon
- Subcutaneous olecranon bursa
- Lateral ulnar collateral ligament
- Radius
- Ulna

In 90° flexion: medial view

- Joint capsule
- Anterior bundle of ulnar collateral ligament
- Annular ligament of radius
- Biceps brachii tendon
- Oblique cord
- Humerus
- Triceps brachii tendon
- Subcutaneous olecranon bursa
- Transverse ligament
- Posterior bundle of ulnar collateral ligament

f. Netter m.d.

in onset, localized to the medial aspect of the elbow, and most severe during the acceleration phase of pitching (ie, the phase of pitching in which maximum valgus stress is transmitted to the elbow). MCL disruption or attenuation is most often noted at the mid-substance of the anterior bundle. Concomitant symptoms of lateral elbow pain may occur secondary to the valgus overload, causing compression, shear injury, and osteochondral fragments and/or osteochondritis dissecans of the capitellum.

Examination reveals tenderness on the medial aspect of the elbow. Valgus instability is assessed with the elbow in 25° of flexion to relax the ulnohumeral articulation. The patient should be evaluated for the presence of a concomitant ulnar entrapment neuropathy. Radiographs should be inspected for signs of osteochondral loose bodies, medial osteophytes, and osteochondritis dissecans. Magnetic resonance imaging (MRI) can be helpful in preoperative planning.

Nonoperative treatment includes activity modification followed by a gradual rehabilitation program. For persistent symptomatic instability, operative treatment includes reconstruction of the MCL with a tendon graft, removal of any associated osteophytes or loose bodies, and decompression of ulnar neuritis.

Posterolateral Rotatory Elbow Instability

Posterolateral rotatory instability develops after injury to the ulnar collateral component of the LCL. With a lax or attenuated ligament, patients report lateral elbow pain and catching or giving way of the elbow. The lateral pivot test may be difficult to perform except when the patient is completely relaxed under anesthesia. MRI studies often identify the ligament disruption. Reconstruction of the lateral ulnar collateral ligament with a tendon graft is required for treatment of persistent and disabling symptoms.

Rupture of the Distal Biceps Tendon

Rupture of the distal biceps brachii tendon is uncommon; however, timely diagnosis of these injuries is important because failure to recognize and repair the lesion before the onset of irreversible muscle contraction decreases the strength of elbow flexion and forearm supination by 30% to 50%. Predisposing factors include a male older than 40 years and the presence of preexisting degenerative changes in the tendon. Rupture typically occurs at the insertion of the biceps tendon into the radial tuberosity (see **Figure 15-13**).

Injury results from an extension force on a partially flexed and contracting biceps muscle.

Patients frequently report the acute onset of sharp pain in the anterior aspect of the elbow, followed by a chronic, dull ache that is exacerbated by lifting activities. Examination shows tenderness and a defect in the antecubital fossa resulting from absence of the normally prominent bicipital tendon. If the aponeurosis remains intact, the defect is not as obvious. If the tendon rupture is incomplete, no defect is obvious, but the patient experiences pain and weakness on flexion of the elbow against resistance. Radiographs are usually normal. MRI may be helpful in evaluation of equivocal cases.

Partial ruptures can be managed with splinting and activity modifications. Complete ruptures are treated more successfully with operative repair. Injury to the radial nerve is a possible complication of surgical repair.

Olecranon Bursitis

The olecranon bursa is easily irritated because of its superficial location (see **Figure 15-13**) and the tendency for people to lean on their elbows. Precipitating factors include falls or direct blows, an inflammatory arthritis such as rheumatoid arthritis or gout, and occupations and avocations that cause prolonged irritation. Olecranon bursitis also may develop in patients with chronic lung disease who lean on their elbows to aid breathing. Septic bursitis (infection) may occur primarily, but it is more likely to develop as a secondary complication of aseptic olecranon bursitis.

The onset of pain and swelling is relatively rapid when caused by trauma or infection but is indolent when caused by other conditions. Pain is variable, exacerbated by elbow flexion, and more intense with infection. Examination reveals a boggy swelling over the olecranon process. Erythema and increased warmth are common in patients with acute bursitis and universal in individuals with septic bursitis. Tenderness is less marked in chronic, recurrent aseptic bursitis.

If the olecranon bursitis is small and only mildly symptomatic, treatment should include observation, avoidance of direct pressure,

and, occasionally, short-term splinting with the elbow extended. Patients with more symptomatic bursitis should have the bursa aspirated for Gram stain and culture. Patients without infection should have the elbow protected and immobilized in relative extension with a foam or compressive dressing. Patients with septic bursitis require limited surgical drainage or daily aspiration and antibiotic administration that covers penicillin-resistant *Staphylococcus aureus*. Excision of a chronically inflamed olecranon bursa should be avoided if at all possible because recurrence is common and operative treatment may lead to chronic infection.

FRACTURES

General Considerations

When a patient reports an injury to the elbow or forearm, inspect for swelling, ecchymosis, deformity, and open wounds. Palpate the area of maximum tenderness, and assess joint swelling and distal pulses. Assess function of the median, radial, and ulnar nerves. Anteroposterior and lateral radiographs of the elbow are adequate for assessing most elbow injuries, but complicated intra-articular injuries may necessitate oblique views and computed tomographic (CT) scans. The radial head should point to the capitellum in both anteroposterior and lateral views; otherwise, a dislocation or subluxation is present. Look for a fat pad sign if no fracture is obvious. In a normal elbow, the anterior fat pad can be seen on a lateral radiograph, but the posterior fat pad is not visualized. Any process that causes an elbow effusion elevates both anterior and posterior fat pads (**Figure 15-14**). Forearm injuries necessitate anteroposterior and lateral radiographs that visualize bony anatomy from the elbow to the wrist.

Fractures about the Elbow in Adults

Distal Humerus

In adults, fractures of the distal humerus are usually caused by high-speed injuries with the elbow flexed more than 90°. As a result, these fractures are frequently comminuted

Figure 15-14: Fat Pad Locations

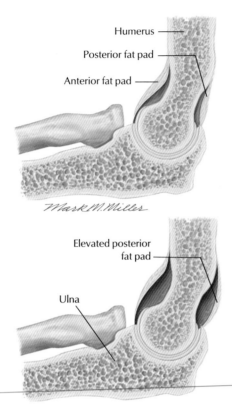

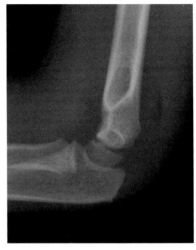

Lateral radiograph of elbow in a 5-year-old female who fell from monkey bars sustaining injury to left elbow. Radiograph shows elevation of anterior and posterior fat pads. No apparent fracture on this view, but subsequent radiographs confirmed presence of a nondisplaced supracondylar humerus fracture.

and intra-articular. Fracture patterns include supracondylar, transcondylar, T or Y intercondylar, and lateral/medial condylar, as well as the rare isolated capitellar or trochlear fracture.

Displaced fractures usually require open reduction. The type of internal fixation used depends on the bony anatomy. The distal end of the humerus is triangular, with medial and lateral columns (condyles). As the distal humerus widens in the medial-lateral plane, it thins in the anterior-posterior plane. Only the columns are thick enough to support plate fixation. Single-condyle fractures may be fixed with screws only, but two plates placed at right angles provide the best fixation for supracondylar, transcondylar, and intercondylar fractures. The lateral column is fixed with a posteriorly positioned plate, and the medial column, with a plate on the medial ridge (**Figure 15-15**). Protection and transposition of

the ulnar nerve is an appropriate adjunct of surgical management.

Radial Head

Fracture of the radial head is the most common elbow fracture in adults. The radial head typically fails under a compressive axial and valgus load when the person falls on an outstretched hand with the forearm pronated and the elbow slightly flexed. Females are twice as likely as males to fracture the radial head. Associated injuries may include fracture of the capitellum, coronoid, or olecranon; disruption of the ulnar collateral ligament; or tear of the interosseous ligament with dislocation of the distal radioulnar joint.

The Mason classification is helpful in determining the appropriate treatment for simple radial head or neck fractures (**Figure 15-16**). Type I fractures are treated with limited immobilization for a few days, followed by early

Figure 15-15: Elbow Fractures

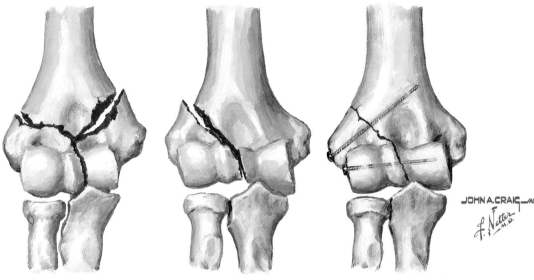

Intercondylar (T or Y) fracture of distal humerus

Fracture of lateral condyle of humerus. Fracture of medial condyle less common

Fractured condyle fixed with one or two compression screws

JOHN A. CRAIG—MD

F. Netter M.D.

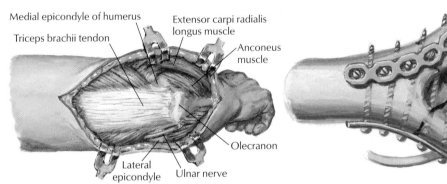

Open (transolecranon) repair. Posterior incision skirts medial margin of olecranon, exposing triceps brachii tendon and olecranon. Ulnar nerve identified on posterior surface of medial epicondyle. Incisions made along each side of olecranon and triceps brachii tendon

Articular surface of distal humerus reconstructed and fixed with transverse screw and buttress plates with screws. Ulnar nerve may be transposed anteriorly to prevent injury. Lateral column fixed with posterior plate and medial column fixed with plate on the medial ridge.

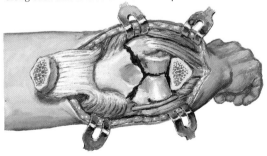

Olecranon osteotomized and reflected proximally with triceps brachii tendon

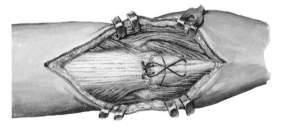

Olecranon reattached with longitudinal Kirschner wires and tension band wire wrapped around them and through hole drilled in ulna

Figure 15-16: Fracture of Head and Neck of Radius

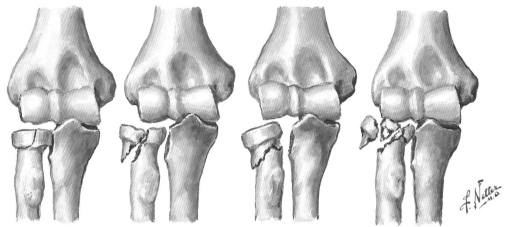

Type I: nondisplaced or minimally displaced.

Type II: displaced single fragment (usually >2 mm) of the head or angulated (usually >30°) of the neck.

Type III: severely comminuted fractures of the radial head and neck.

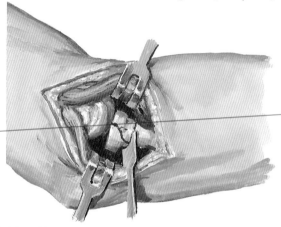

Excision of fragment or entire radial head via posterolateral incision. Radial head should be replaced with a prosthesis in patients with certain complex fractures.

Comminuted fracture of radial head with dislocation of distal radioulnar joint, proximal migration of radius, and tear of interosseous membrane (Essex-Lopresti fracture)

range-of-motion exercises. Type II fractures with acceptable fracture patterns should be treated with open reduction and internal fixation. In equivocal situations, particularly if the patient has a low-demand occupation, type II injuries can be treated nonoperatively, with delayed excision of the radial head if persistent pain or significant limitation of forearm rotation occurs. Uncomplicated type III fractures should be treated with excision of the radial head. When radial head fractures are associated with dislocation of the elbow and severe ligament injury or disruption of the forearm interosseus, the fragments should be removed and the radial head replaced by a prosthesis.

Results of treatment are uniformly good for type I fractures and often satisfactory for simple type II and type III fractures. Potential complications include loss of motion, elbow instability, posttraumatic arthritis, myositis ossificans, and distal radioulnar symptoms.

Olecranon Fractures

Olecranon fractures are caused by a direct blow or an indirect avulsion injury (eg, a fall on an outstretched hand with the elbow

Figure 15-17: Olecranon Fracture

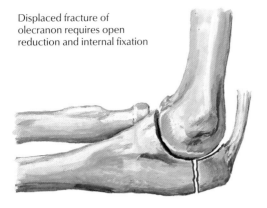

Displaced fracture of olecranon requires open reduction and internal fixation

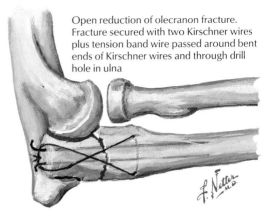

Open reduction of olecranon fracture. Fracture secured with two Kirschner wires plus tension band wire passed around bent ends of Kirschner wires and through drill hole in ulna

slightly flexed while the triceps is contracting). Avulsion injuries create a transverse or slightly oblique fracture pattern. Direct blows typically are associated with some degree of comminution. A palpable defect is present with displaced fractures. The skin should be evaluated carefully for possible open injury. Radiographs should be scrutinized for detection of associated fractures of the radial head or coronoid process.

Nondisplaced fractures can be treated with a splint or cast (**Figure 15-17**). The elbow is positioned in approximately 45° of flexion to relax the pull of the triceps. Displaced fractures require open treatment. Tension band wiring, which transforms distraction forces into compression, is the most common form of fixation. Plate fixation is required for fractures that extend to the coronoid or ulnar shaft. Comminuted fractures can be managed by excision of the fragments and repair of the triceps tendon. If the collateral ligaments are intact, as much as 70% of the proximal olecranon can be excised without resultant instability.

Monteggia Fractures/Dislocations

The Monteggia fracture/dislocation is a fracture of the ulna that is associated with dislocation of the radial head (**Figure 15-18**). Bado classified these injuries into four types. The radial head is dislocated anteriorly in type 1, posteriorly in type 2, and laterally in type 3, and the ulnar fracture is angulated in the direction of the radial head dislocation. In a type 4 injury, the proximal radius and ulna are fractured, and the radial head is dislocated anteriorly. Type 1 and type 2 account for 70% to 90% of Monteggia injuries. Type 1, the most common, may be caused by a direct blow or a fall on the outstretched hand with the forearm in full pronation. Type 2 injuries occur most often in adults. Radial nerve injury, often isolated to the posterior interosseous branch, is relatively common in Monteggia lesions.

These injuries are frequently misdiagnosed, particularly in children, in whom palpation of an anteriorly displaced radial head is more difficult. Another common mistake is to recognize the fracture of the ulna but miss the dislocated radial head, either because the radiograph did not adequately show the elbow or because the evaluator did not understand that on both anteroposterior and lateral radiographs, a line through the axis of the proximal radius and the radial head should pass through the capitellum.

If recognized early, Monteggia injuries in children usually can be treated by closed reduction and cast immobilization. Adults require open reduction and internal fixation of the ulnar fracture. When the ulna is anatomically reduced, the radial head typically reduces and becomes stable without additional surgical intervention.

Figure 15-18: Monteggia Fracture/Dislocation

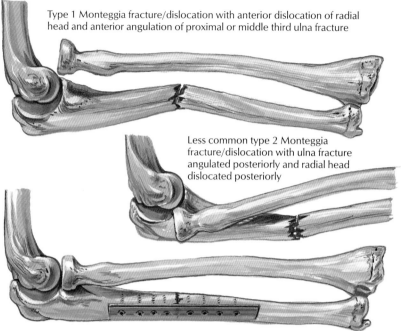

Type 1 Monteggia fracture/dislocation with anterior dislocation of radial head and anterior angulation of proximal or middle third ulna fracture

Less common type 2 Monteggia fracture/dislocation with ulna fracture angulated posteriorly and radial head dislocated posteriorly

Fracture of ulna treated with open reduction and internal fixation using compression plate and screws. After reduction of ulna, radial head spontaneously reduced

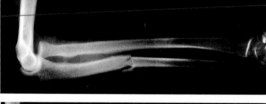

Preoperative radiograph shows Type I Monteggia fracture/dislocation

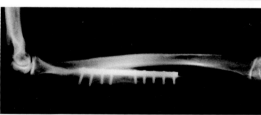

Postoperative radiograph shows compression plate in place

with
C.A. Luce

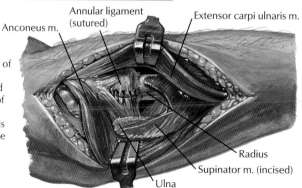

Annular ligament (sutured)

Anconeus m.

Extensor carpi ulnaris m.

If radial head does not reduce after angulation of ulna is corrected, open reduction of radial head dislocation and repair of annular ligament are needed. Typically, this is done through a separate incision between the anconeus and extensor carpi ulnaris muscles

Radius

Supinator m. (incised)

Ulna

Fractures of the Diaphysis of the Radius and Ulna

In adults, motor vehicle accidents or falls from a considerable height usually cause both-bone forearm fractures. Displacement, angulation, and shortening are common when both the radius and the ulna are fractured. A direct blow usually fractures only one bone—typically the ulna, as the forearm is positioned to stop the oncoming injury ("nightstick" fracture). Because only one component of the "structural rectangle" has been disrupted, direct-blow injuries of the ulna or radius are minimally displaced and usually can be treated by nonoperative methods. However, a fall on the outstretched hand with the forearm pronated can cause a fracture at the middle/distal third junction of the radius with associated disruption of the distal radioulnar ligaments (Galeazzi fracture). In this injury, two sides of the structural rectangle are injured; therefore, the fracture of the radius is displaced and unstable.

Displaced forearm fractures in adults are best treated by open reduction and internal fixation. This procedure minimizes the relatively high rates of malunion, nonunion, and loss of forearm rotation associated with management by closed techniques. Bone grafting should be considered with comminution of more than a third of the diameter of the bone or with a segmental fracture.

Fractures About the Elbow in Children

Fractures about the elbow are more common in children than in adults, and treatment in children often differs from treatment of injuries at similar locations in adults. Occult fractures are more common in children, particularly young children, in whom low-impact falls are common. A significant portion of the bone in young children has not ossified, so some fractures are more difficult to visualize on initial radiographs. A child who has a history of injury, tenderness about the elbow, and a positive posterior fat pad sign should be assumed to have an occult fracture and should be immobilized for 3 weeks.

Supracondylar Fractures

Fracture of the supracondylar humerus is the most common elbow fracture in children. The typical age group is 2 to 12 years—a time when a child is able to hyperextend the elbow. The typical mechanism of injury is a fall on the outstretched arm with the elbow in full extension. The distal fragment is displaced posteriorly (**Figure 15-19**). The less common flexion injuries cause anterior displacement of the distal humerus and are more common in the adolescent years.

Supracondylar fractures are associated with a relatively high incidence of neurovascular injury. Usually only one nerve is injured. The median, radial, or ulnar nerve may be

Figure 15-19: Supracondylar Fracture of the Humerus

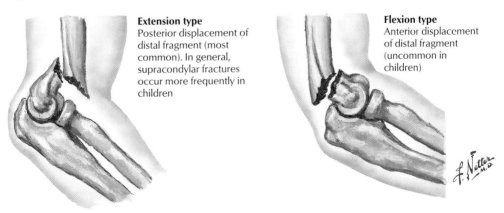

Extension type
Posterior displacement of distal fragment (most common). In general, supracondylar fractures occur more frequently in children

Flexion type
Anterior displacement of distal fragment (uncommon in children)

involved. Median nerve injury, the most common type, may be limited to the anterior interosseous branch. Compartment syndrome of the forearm may occur, and failure to treat this problem in a timely fashion may result in Volkmann ischemic contractures of the wrist and fingers. Malunion with resultant cubitus varus is another potential complication.

To minimize the risk of complications, displaced fractures typically are treated with closed manipulation and percutaneous pinning. If the radial and ulnar pulses are absent, the fracture is reduced. Frequently, the pulse returns after the fracture is reduced and the proximal fragment no longer stretches the brachial vessels. If the pulse does not return but the capillary refill is normal and there are no signs of compartment syndrome, the patient may be treated with observation with careful monitoring. If the pulse does not return after the fracture has been reduced and the fingers or forearm show signs of ischemia, the vessels should be explored.

Cubitus varus, the "gunstock deformity," results from malrotation and the resultant tilt of the distal fragment. The thin, spadelike shape of the distal humerus, in combination with a swollen arm and the small size of a child's bone, is a predisposing factor. The deformity is primarily a cosmetic rather than a functional problem.

Transphyseal Fracture Separation of the Distal Humerus

Transphyseal separations of the distal humerus typically occur in infants and young children as a result of child abuse. Radiographs may be difficult to interpret because the secondary centers of ossification have not developed in children this young. Typically, the proximal forearm is displaced medially and posterior to the humeral shaft. Arthrography, MRI studies, or ultrasonography may be necessary to distinguish this lesion from an elbow dislocation or lateral condylar fracture.

Lateral and Medial Condyle Fractures

Fracture of the lateral condyle of the distal humerus is the second most common elbow injury in children. Lateral condyle fractures result from a fall on a varus, supinated elbow, with the condyle avulsed by attached extensor muscles. Medial condyle fractures are uncommon, but the treatment principles are the same as for lateral condyle fractures. When these fractures cross the articular surface, displacement >1 mm at the joint requires reduction and pinning to minimize associated problems of nonunion, cubitus valgus, tardy ulnar nerve palsy, and traumatic arthritis.

Lateral and Medial Epicondyle Fractures

Lateral epicondyle fractures are uncommon in children, but avulsion of the medial epicondyle by forceful contraction of the flexor-pronator muscles with the elbow in valgus is the third most common pediatric elbow fracture. The injury typically occurs in a 10- to 15-year-old child. A concomitant posterior dislocation of the elbow may occur. In this situation, open reduction should be performed if the medial epicondyle fragment is incarcerated in the joint. Otherwise, medial epicondyle fractures, even when markedly displaced, do not commonly cause residual disability and can be treated with short-term splinting.

Radial Neck Fractures

In children, fracture of the proximal radius typically involves the physis, with extension into the neck of the radius (Peterson II or Salter II). The typical age group is 7 to 12 years. Associated injuries may include fracture of the olecranon or medial epicondyle, as well as dislocation of the elbow. Isolated fractures result from a fall on an extended elbow with valgus stress.

Treatment depends on the age of the child and the degree of angulation. Tilt of more than 30° may result in loss of forearm rotation. With more than 30° angulation, closed reduction with or without percutaneous manipulation of the fracture should be attempted with the goal of reducing angulation to less than 30°. Open reduction may be required but has a greater risk of osteonecrosis of the radial head and synostosis between the radius and ulna. Premature fusion of the physis usually is of little significance, because 80% of the growth of the radius occurs at the distal physis.

Olecranon Fractures and Diaphyseal Fractures of the Radius and Ulna

Olecranon fractures are uncommon in children and are likely to be nondisplaced. Displaced fractures usually require open reduction and tension band wire and pin fixation.

Most diaphyseal forearm fractures in children can be managed by closed techniques. Proximal and middle third forearm fractures account for only 15% to 20% of pediatric forearm fractures, but these injuries are more likely to develop complications such as compartment syndrome, malunion, or synostosis.

Dislocation of the Elbow

The elbow is the most commonly dislocated joint in children and the second most common site of dislocation in adults (**Figure 15-20**). Posterior dislocations are most common. Anterior dislocation is rare because of the shape of the olecranon process. *Divergent dislocation* with separation of the radius and the ulna results from severe disruption of the soft tissues.

Posterior dislocations typically occur in a fall on the outstretched hand with the shoulder abducted. Axial compression at the elbow combined with an external and valgus stress at the elbow (the body internally rotates) results in a continuum of ligamentous injury that typically starts laterally and moves

Figure 15-20: Dislocation of Elbow Joint

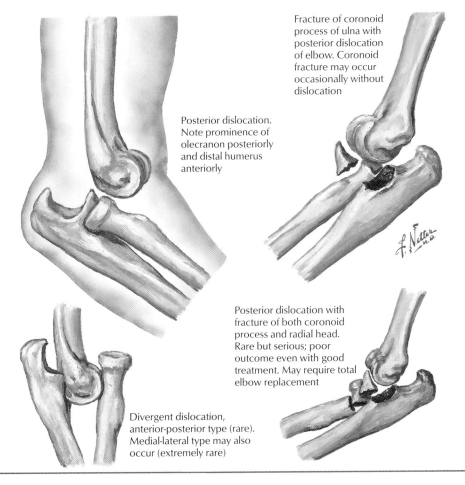

Fracture of coronoid process of ulna with posterior dislocation of elbow. Coronoid fracture may occur occasionally without dislocation

Posterior dislocation. Note prominence of olecranon posteriorly and distal humerus anteriorly

Posterior dislocation with fracture of both coronoid process and radial head. Rare but serious; poor outcome even with good treatment. May require total elbow replacement

Divergent dislocation, anterior-posterior type (rare). Medial-lateral type may also occur (extremely rare)

medially. The first stage tears the ulnar portion of the lateral collateral ligament (LCL), followed by disruption of the entire LCL complex, then the anterior and posterior capsules, then the posterior band of the medial collateral ligament (MCL), and lastly, the anterior band of the MCL. Associated injuries may include avulsion of the medial and lateral epicondyles, radial head and radial neck fractures, and coronoid fractures. These additional injuries increase instability and may necessitate internal fixation.

Isolated dislocation of the elbow is treated by closed reduction. Distal traction is applied with the elbow in extension and the forearm in supination. After reduction, elbow stability is assessed with the forearm in pronation. If ligament disruption involves the anterior band of the medial collateral ligament, instability is noted with the elbow in extension. This injury will need 3 to 6 weeks of protection, starting with the elbow in pronation and 90° of flexion. More stable injuries should be immobilized for a short time (1 to 2 weeks) to prevent the complications of elbow stiffness and loss of extension. Other complications, such as heterotopic ossification, brachial artery injury, ulnar nerve injury, and compartment syndrome, are associated with high-energy injuries and concomitant fractures.

Subluxation of the Radial Head

Subluxation of the radial head, also called a "pulled elbow" or "nursemaid's elbow," is the most common elbow injury in children younger than 5 years. Subluxation occurs with a pull on the forearm when the elbow is extended and the forearm pronated. The annular ligament (see **Figure 15-13**) slips proximally and becomes interposed between the radius and the ulna. This injury is associated with ligamentous laxity, a condition that is almost universal in young children and typically occurs when a young child is "helped along" or lifted by pulling on the forearm.

Immediately after the injury, the child will cry, but the initial pain quickly subsides. Thereafter, the child is reluctant to use the arm but otherwise does not appear to be in great distress. The extremity is held with the elbow slightly flexed and the forearm pronated. Tenderness over the radial head and resistance on attempted supination are the only consistent findings. Radiographic findings are normal.

Reduction is accomplished by applying pressure over the radial head, followed by quick supination. If this maneuver fails to produce the snap of reduction, the elbow should be flexed. Resistance is perceived just before full flexion. As the elbow is pushed through that resistance, the annular ligament will reduce, and a snap will be perceived as the radial head is reseated. If the reduction is successful, the child will resume use of the extremity in a few minutes. In a child who presents for evaluation 1 to 2 days after injury, however, swelling may obscure the snap of reduction and deter the immediate resumption of normal function. If the elbow has full flexion and supination, the radial head has been reduced. Immobilization is ineffective as slings are quickly discarded.

PEDIATRIC DISORDERS

Congenital Dislocation of the Radial Head

Isolated congenital dislocation of the radial head, although present at birth, is usually not diagnosed until a child is 2 to 5 years of age, when the parents note mild limitation of elbow extension and an abnormal prominence (**Figure 15-21**). The dislocation may be bilateral or unilateral. Most dislocations are posterior or posterolateral, but they may be anterior. The limitation of motion is rarely dysfunctional, and most patients are asymptomatic. Excision of the radial head, after completion of growth, is indicated for relief of pain from joint incongruity; however, elbow motion does not improve after the procedure.

Congenital Radioulnar Synostosis

Congenital radioulnar synostosis is an uncommon congenital abnormality caused by failure of separation of the proximal radius and ulna during fetal development. As a result, forearm rotation is lost. The synostosis is frequently an isolated event but may be

Figure 15-21: Congenital Dislocation of Radial Head

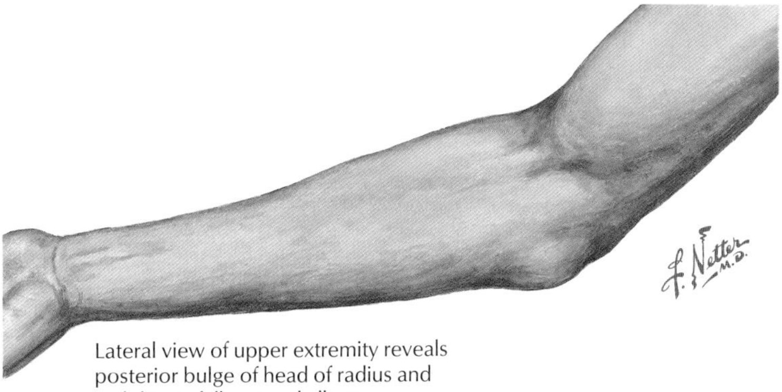

Lateral view of upper extremity reveals posterior bulge of head of radius and inability to fully extend elbow

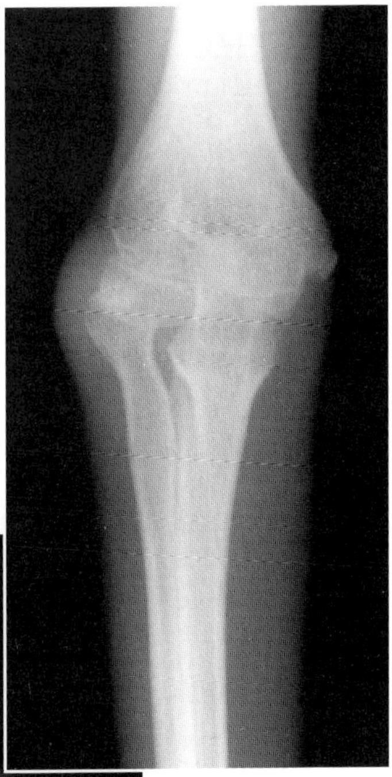

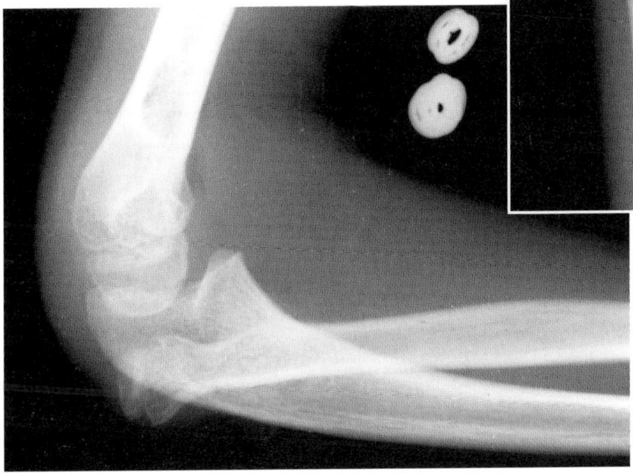

Anteroposterior and lateral radiographs reveal posterior dislocation of radial head, most evident on elbow flexion. Note also hypoplastic capitulum of humerus.

associated with other conditions. Most cases involve some degree of fixed pronation. The degree of disability depends on the amount of fixed pronation and whether the condition is unilateral or bilateral. Patients with bilateral involvement and forearms fixed in greater than 60° of pronation have the greatest difficulty with activities such as holding a fork, dressing, and maintaining good personal hygiene after bowel movements. Patients with less fixed pronation often can substitute shoulder motion.

Surgery to resect the synostosis and restore motion has not been successful. Rotational osteotomy through the synostosis to change the position of the forearm varies according to the amount of functional impairment. Typi-

cally, the dominant forearm is positioned in 0° to 20° of pronation. Compartment syndrome is the most common postoperative complication.

Osteochondrosis of the Elbow

Children involved in repetitive throwing activities or gymnastics repetitively overload the elbow into valgus with tension on the medial epicondyle and compression on the capitellum. Traction apophysitis of the medial epicondyle, better known as "little leaguer's elbow," may develop. The resultant pain responds well to a relatively short period of rest.

Chronic lateral elbow pain in pediatric athletes usually occurs secondary to osteonecrosis of the capitellum and is more problematic.

Figure 15-22: Osteochondrosis of the Capitellum

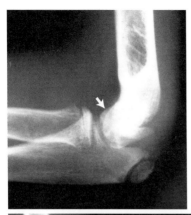

Bone resorption seen as radio-lucent areas and irregular surface of capitulum of humerus

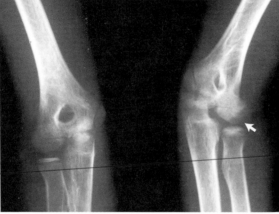

Characteristic changes in capitulum of left humerus (arrow) compared with normal right elbow

When osteonecrosis occurs in children younger than 10 years, the condition is called *Panner disease* and has a good prognosis for healing with a period of rest and, sometimes, immobilization. When the condition occurs during adolescence, it is called *osteochondritis dissecans of the capitellum* and has a more guarded prognosis.

Adolescents with osteonecrosis of the capitellum report the insidious onset of lateral elbow pain that is aggravated by throwing activities. Examination shows tenderness over the lateral elbow, tenderness at the extremes of passive elbow motion, and a flexion contracture of 10° to 30°. Typical radiographic changes include lucency and fragmentation of the anterior central capitellum (**Figure 15-22**). Osteochondral loose bodies may be present. An MRI study often helps define the extent of osteonecrosis. Treatment for patients in this age group includes activity modification, excision of osteochondral fragments, and occasionally, drilling of the defect to stimulate a fibrocartilaginous response.

ADDITIONAL READINGS

Chen FS, Rokito AS, Jobe FW. Medial elbow problems in the overhead-throwing athlete. *J Am Acad Orthop Surg.* 2001; 9:99–113.

Morrey BF, ed. *The Elbow and Its Disorders*, 2nd edition. Philadelphia, Pa: Saunders; 2000.

Staheli LT, ed. *Pediatric Orthopaedic Secrets*, 2nd edition. Philadelphia, Pa: Hanley and Belfus; 2003.

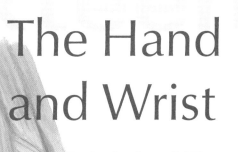

The Hand
and Wrist

John D. Lubahn, MD
D. Patrick Williams, DO

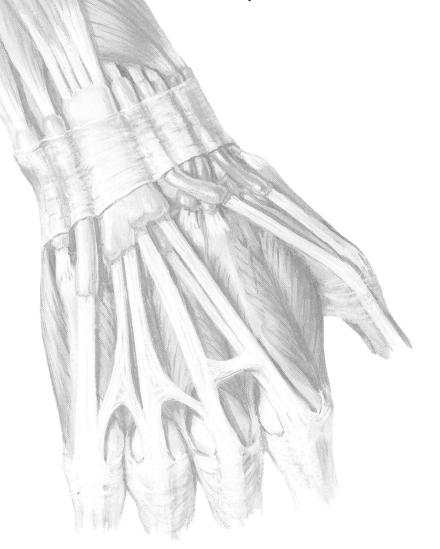

The human hand, as an extension of the brain, allows us to manipulate and interact with our environment and to perform activities as routine as opening a door or as intimate as caressing a loved one. The hand also functions as part of the sensory system, providing tactile sensation for complex hand movements without the necessity of constant visual guidance; this function is epitomized by blind people who read and musicians who entertain. An understanding and careful examination of hand anatomy and function is crucial for the student of medicine.

ANATOMY AND BIOMECHANICS

The carpus, or wrist, is composed of eight carpal bones that link the forearm to the hand (**Figure 16-1**). The proximal carpal row (scaphoid, lunate, and triquetrum) articulates with the distal radius and ulna, as well as the distal carpal row (trapezium, trapezoid, capitate, and hamate). The pisiform, also part of the proximal row, is a sesamoid bone in the flexor carpi ulnaris tendon that articulates only with the triquetrum. The bones of the hand are the metacarpals and phalanges. The carpometacarpal (CMC) joint of the thumb is saddle-shaped, a configuration that permits abduction-adduction, as well as the circumduction that permits opposition of the thumb to the fingers. The metacarpophalangeal (MP), proximal interphalangeal (PIP), and distal interphalangeal (DIP) joints basically are flexion-extension hinge joints.

The skin on the dorsal surface of the hand is thin and flexible to allow full flexion of the fingers, whereas the palmar surface skin is thicker and characterized by creases. The

Figure 16-1: Bones and Joints of Hand

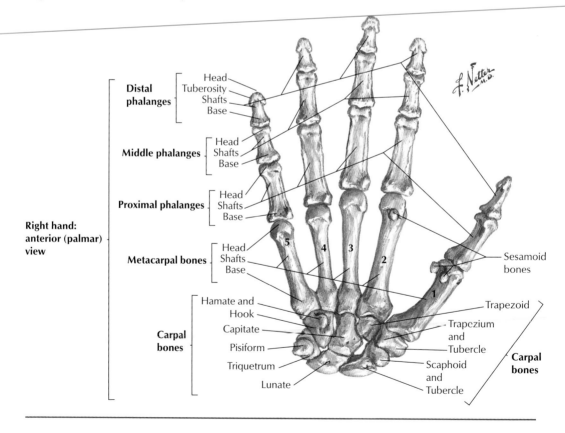

Right hand: anterior (palmar) view

Distal phalanges: Head, Tuberosity, Shafts, Base
Middle phalanges: Head, Shafts, Base
Proximal phalanges: Head, Shafts, Base
Metacarpal bones: Head, Shafts, Base

Carpal bones: Hamate and Hook, Capitate, Pisiform, Triquetrum, Lunate

Sesamoid bones
Trapezoid
Trapezium and Tubercle
Scaphoid and Tubercle
Carpal bones

distal volar crease of the wrist crosses the proximal scaphoid and the pisiform. The distal palmar crease of the hand corresponds to the MP joint, and the proximal finger crease is at the base of the proximal phalanx.

The extrinsic muscles of the wrist and hand originate on the medial and lateral humeral condyles and the proximal radius and ulna (see **Figure 15-2**). The extrinsic extensor tendons cross the wrist and are surrounded by tendon sheaths in *six compartments* bounded by the extensor retinacular ligament (**Figure 16-2**). The extrinsic finger and thumb flexor tendons and the median nerve enter the hand through the carpal canal (**Figure 16-3**). The *transverse carpal ligament*, a thick band extending from the hamate and pisiform to the scaphoid and trapezium, forms the inelastic roof of the carpal canal. A decrease in the size of the canal or an increase in the size of its contents can cause compression of the median nerve (carpal tunnel syndrome).

Intrinsic musculature includes thenar, hypothenar, and interosseous muscles (**Figure 16-4**; see also **Figures 15-4** and **15-5**). The thenar muscles are the abductor pollicis brevis, the opponens pollicis, and the superficial head of the flexor pollicis brevis. The hypothenar muscles are composed of the abductor digiti quinti, the opponens digiti quinti, and the flexor digiti quinti. The dorsal interossei, commonly referred to as *dorsal intrinsics,* abduct the fingers; the palmar interossei (*palmar intrinsics*) adduct the fingers.

The DIP joint of the fingers is flexed by the flexor digitorum profundus (FDP). It has a separate muscle belly for the index finger (which therefore flexes independently) but a common muscle belly for the long, ring, and small fingers (which tend to work as a single unit). The PIP joint of the fingers is primarily flexed by the flexor digitorum superficialis (FDS). It has individual muscle bellies for each finger, thus providing the individual finger flexion at the PIP joint that is necessary for activities such as playing a musical instrument and typing. The FDS separates into two parts before its point of insertion, and the FDP passes through the split (**Figure 16-5**). Both finger flexors are enclosed in a common tendon sheath. The proximity of the FDS and FDP tendon to the surrounding sheath promotes efficient movement, but adhesions from injury or infection can be problematic in this region.

The interossei, along with the lumbrical muscles, flex the MP joints and extend the PIP and DIP joints. The lumbrical muscles are unique in that they originate from the profundus tendons to insert into the dorsal apparatus of the antagonistic extensor mechanism (see **Figure 16-5**). The interossei and the two ulnar lumbricals are innervated by the ulnar nerve, but the two radial lumbricals are innervated by the median nerve.

The MP joints of the fingers are extended by the extensor digitorum longus, extensor indicis proprius, and extensor digiti quinti. When the MP joints are flexed, these muscles also can extend the PIP joints; otherwise, the intrinsic muscles extend the PIP and DIP joints. The complex arrangement of the tendons on the dorsum of the hand provides the necessary synchrony and balance between flexors and extensors during the multiple precise motions of the MP, PIP, and DIP joints working in concert. The main insertion of the extrinsic extensor muscle tendon is through the *central slip* at the base of the middle phalanx. The intrinsic muscles join with the extrinsic extensor through the interdigitating transverse and oblique fibers of the dorsal apparatus to extend the PIP and DIP joints.

Contracture or spasticity of the intrinsic muscles creates increased tension on the dorsal hood. A swan-neck deformity develops, with PIP joint hyperextension and MP and DIP joint flexion (**Figure 16-6**). Laceration of the central extensor tendon proximal to its insertion into the middle phalanx allows the lateral bands to slip volarly and produces the opposite flexion, *boutonnière* (French from "button hole") PIP joint deformity.

The radial artery lies radial to the flexor carpi radialis tendon at the wrist (see **Figure 16-3**). After crossing the snuffbox (see **Figure 16-2**), the radial artery passes through the first intermetacarpal space to the palm as the main contributor to the *deep palmar arch,*

Figure 16-2: Extensor Tendons at the Wrist

Posterior (dorsal) view

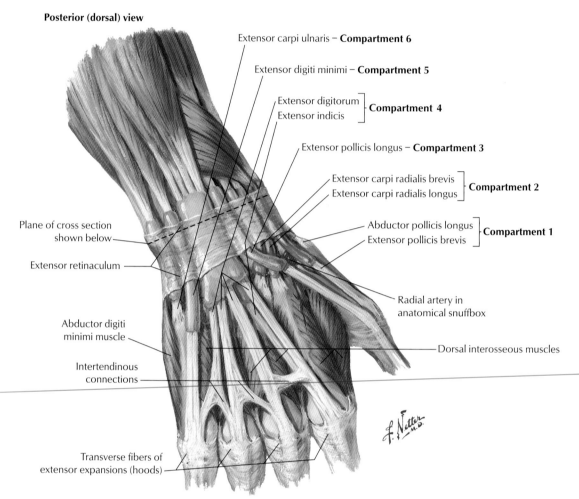

Extensor carpi ulnaris – **Compartment 6**

Extensor digiti minimi – **Compartment 5**

Extensor digitorum
Extensor indicis } **Compartment 4**

Extensor pollicis longus – **Compartment 3**

Extensor carpi radialis brevis
Extensor carpi radialis longus } **Compartment 2**

Abductor pollicis longus
Extensor pollicis brevis } **Compartment 1**

Plane of cross section shown below

Extensor retinaculum

Radial artery in anatomical snuffbox

Abductor digiti minimi muscle

Dorsal interosseous muscles

Intertendinous connections

Transverse fibers of extensor expansions (hoods)

Cross section of most distal portion of forearm

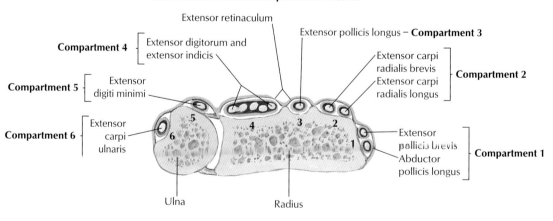

Extensor retinaculum

Extensor pollicis longus – **Compartment 3**

Compartment 4 { Extensor digitorum and extensor indicis

Extensor carpi radialis brevis
Extensor carpi radialis longus } **Compartment 2**

Compartment 5 { Extensor digiti minimi

Compartment 6 { Extensor carpi ulnaris

Extensor pollicis brevis
Abductor pollicis longus } **Compartment 1**

Ulna

Radius

Figure 16-3: Flexor Tendons, Arteries, and Nerves at Wrist

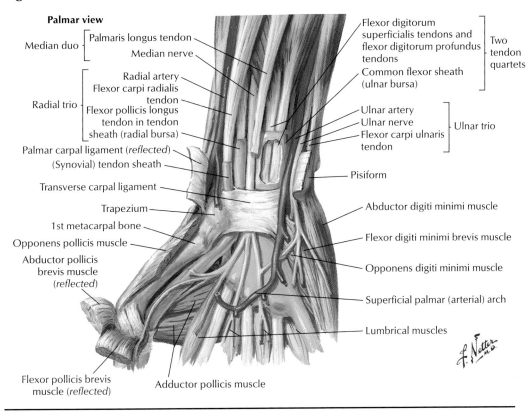

Palmar view

Median duo { Palmaris longus tendon
Median nerve

Radial trio { Radial artery
Flexor carpi radialis tendon
Flexor pollicis longus tendon in tendon sheath (radial bursa)

Palmar carpal ligament (*reflected*)
(Synovial) tendon sheath
Transverse carpal ligament
Trapezium
1st metacarpal bone
Opponens pollicis muscle
Abductor pollicis brevis muscle (*reflected*)

Flexor pollicis brevis muscle (*reflected*)
Adductor pollicis muscle

Flexor digitorum superficialis tendons and flexor digitorum profundus tendons
Common flexor sheath (ulnar bursa) } Two tendon quartets

Ulnar artery
Ulnar nerve
Flexor carpi ulnaris tendon } Ulnar trio

Pisiform
Abductor digiti minimi muscle
Flexor digiti minimi brevis muscle
Opponens digiti minimi muscle
Superficial palmar (arterial) arch
Lumbrical muscles

Figure 16-4: Intrinsic Muscles of Hand

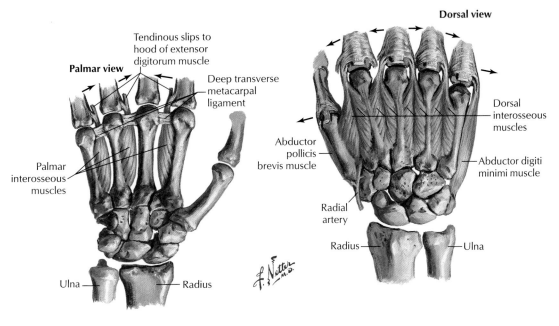

Palmar view

Tendinous slips to hood of extensor digitorum muscle
Deep transverse metacarpal ligament
Palmar interosseous muscles
Ulna
Radius

Dorsal view

Dorsal interosseous muscles
Abductor pollicis brevis muscle
Abductor digiti minimi muscle
Radial artery
Radius
Ulna

Figure 16-5: Flexor and Extensor Tendons in Fingers

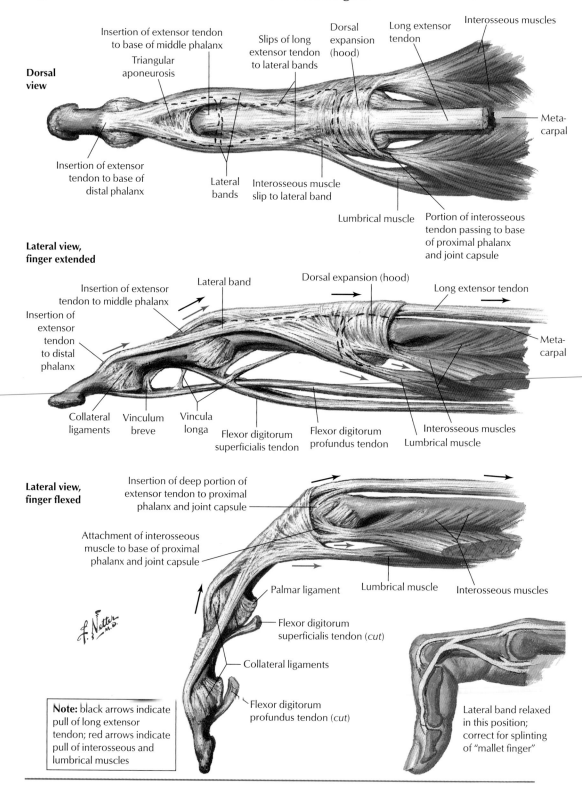

Dorsal view

Insertion of extensor tendon to base of middle phalanx

Triangular aponeurosis

Insertion of extensor tendon to base of distal phalanx

Slips of long extensor tendon to lateral bands

Dorsal expansion (hood)

Long extensor tendon

Interosseous muscles

Meta-carpal

Lateral bands

Interosseous muscle slip to lateral band

Lumbrical muscle

Portion of interosseous tendon passing to base of proximal phalanx and joint capsule

Lateral view, finger extended

Insertion of extensor tendon to middle phalanx

Lateral band

Dorsal expansion (hood)

Long extensor tendon

Insertion of extensor tendon to distal phalanx

Meta-carpal

Collateral ligaments

Vinculum breve

Vincula longa

Flexor digitorum superficialis tendon

Flexor digitorum profundus tendon

Interosseous muscles

Lumbrical muscle

Lateral view, finger flexed

Insertion of deep portion of extensor tendon to proximal phalanx and joint capsule

Attachment of interosseous muscle to base of proximal phalanx and joint capsule

Palmar ligament

Lumbrical muscle

Interosseous muscles

Flexor digitorum superficialis tendon (*cut*)

Collateral ligaments

Flexor digitorum profundus tendon (*cut*)

Note: black arrows indicate pull of long extensor tendon; red arrows indicate pull of interosseous and lumbrical muscles

Lateral band relaxed in this position; correct for splinting of "mallet finger"

Figure 16-6

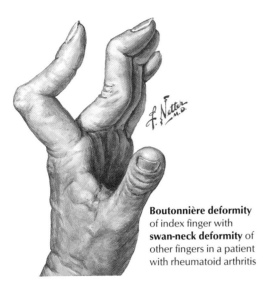

Boutonnière deformity of index finger with **swan-neck deformity** of other fingers in a patient with rheumatoid arthritis

which is completed by the deep palmar branch of the ulnar artery. The ulnar artery and nerve lie radial to the flexor carpi ulnaris and pisiform as they enter Guyon canal and the palm. The ulnar artery is the main contributor to the *superficial palmar arch*, which is completed by a branch of the radial artery.

After traversing Guyon canal, the ulnar nerve branches into a superficial cutaneous branch that provides sensation to the ulnar aspect of the palm and the ulnar one and a half fingers, and a deep motor branch that supplies the hypothenar muscles. The ulnar nerve then travels with the deep palmar arch, supplying all the interossei, the third and fourth lumbricals, the adductor pollicis, and the deep head of the flexor pollicis brevis (see **Figure 15-4**). The median nerve supplies the remaining thenar muscles and the first and second lumbricals, and it provides sensation to the thumb and radial two and a half fingers (see **Figure 15-3**).

PHYSICAL EXAMINATION

Inspect the hand for atrophy of the thenar muscles (innervated by the median nerve) or hypothenar and intrinsic muscles (innervated by the ulnar nerve). Intrinsic muscle weakness causes atrophy between the metacarpals on the dorsum of the hand. Look at the nails for evidence of pitting or signs of other systemic disorders. Palpate bony landmarks and any swelling or osteophytes. At the wrist, the radial and ulnar styloid processes are palpable; the radial styloid is approximately 1 cm distal to the ulnar styloid. The dorsal tubercle at the distal radius, commonly called *Lister tubercle*, is palpable. It functions as a pulley for the extensor pollicis longus and is a marker for surgical approaches. The pisiform on the volar aspect of the wrist is a landmark for the ulnar nerve and artery.

The *zero starting position* for determining wrist motion is the forearm in pronation and the carpus aligned with the plane of the forearm. In young adults, normal wrist motion is approximately 75° of flexion, 75° of extension, 20° of radial deviation, and 35° of ulnar deviation (**Figure 16-7**).

Finger joint motion occurs primarily in the flexion-extension plane, with flexion accounting for most of the motion. The wrist should be in the neutral position when finger or thumb flexion is measured. When the wrist is flexed, the extensor digitorum communis and thumb extensors are under tension, thereby limiting finger and thumb flexion. Flexion and extension can be measured at the MP, PIP, and DIP joints, but from a functional perspective, finger flexion is a composite movement of motion from the three finger joints. Ask the patient to touch the distal palmar crease. In young and middle-aged adults, the fingertip should touch this crease. Lack of full finger flexion can be quantified by measuring the distance from the fingertip to the distal palmar crease (see **Figure 16-7**).

The planes of thumb motion are flexion-extension, abduction-adduction, and opposition. Opposition is a composite motion at the CMC, MP, and interphalangeal (IP) joints that is critical to daily activities. In disability ratings, opposition is valued as 50% to 60% of thumb function. In normal opposition, the tip of the thumb touches the base of the little finger (see **Figure 16-7**). Impaired opposition can be quantified by measuring the distance from

Figure 16-7: Measurement of Wrist Motion and Finger Motion, Lack of Finger Flexion, and Thumb Opposition

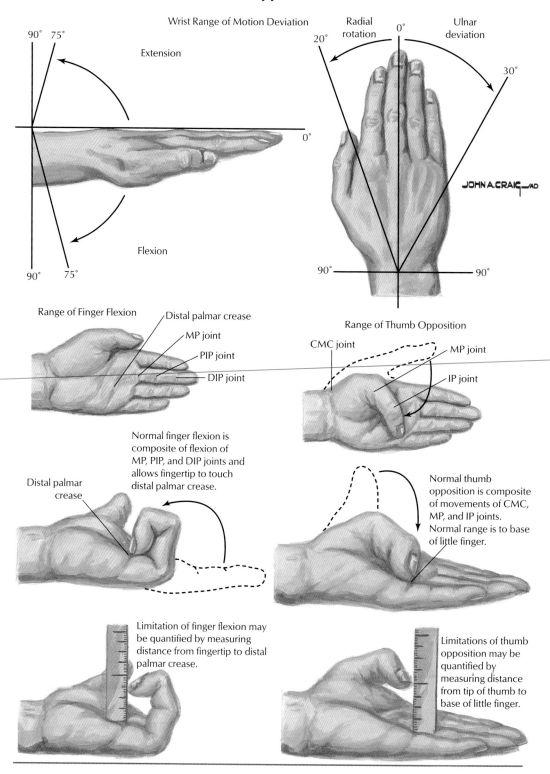

Wrist Range of Motion Deviation

90° 75°

Extension

0°

90° 75°

Flexion

Radial rotation

0°

20°

Ulnar deviation

30°

90°

90°

JOHN A. CRAIG—AD

Range of Finger Flexion

Distal palmar crease

MP joint

PIP joint

DIP joint

Normal finger flexion is composite of flexion of MP, PIP, and DIP joints and allows fingertip to touch distal palmar crease.

Distal palmar crease

Limitation of finger flexion may be quantified by measuring distance from fingertip to distal palmar crease.

Range of Thumb Opposition

CMC joint

MP joint

IP joint

Normal thumb opposition is composite of movements of CMC, MP, and IP joints. Normal range is to base of little finger.

Limitations of thumb opposition may be quantified by measuring distance from tip of thumb to base of little finger.

the tip of the thumb to the base of the little finger.

All thumb joints move in flexion and extension, but this range is difficult to quantify at the CMC joint. Flexion at the thumb MP joint is typically 50° to 60°. Extension is not typically observed at the thumb MP joint. Normal thumb IP motion in young adults is 55° to 75° of flexion and 5° to 10° of extension.

To assess the strength of the wrist flexors, the most powerful of which is the flexor carpi ulnaris, resist the patient's effort to flex the wrist with the elbow flexed to 90° and the thumb and fingers in the extended, neutral position (eliminates action of finger flexors). To test the wrist extensors, the most powerful of which are the extensor carpi ulnaris and the extensor carpi radialis brevis, resist the patient's effort to extend the wrist with the elbow flexed to 90° and the fingers flexed (eliminates action of the finger extensors). To test the integrity of the FDP tendon, hold the PIP joint in extension, and ask the patient to flex the distal phalanx. To assess the flexor digitorum sublimis, neutralize the profundus tendon by holding all the fingers except the one being tested in full extension, and ask the patient to flex the finger.

Median nerve paralysis above the elbow causes weak pronation, wrist flexion, and an "ape hand" with thenar atrophy and weakness of thumb opposition. Thenar muscle strength (motor branch of median nerve) can be evaluated by asking the patient to position the thumb in abduction as you push it into adduction. Assess sensation of the median nerve at the volar tip of the thumb.

Test intrinsic muscle weakness (motor branch of ulnar nerve) by asking the patient to abduct the index finger against resistance while you palpate the first dorsal interosseous muscle. In addition, ask the patient to pinch a piece of paper while you pull on it. Weakness of the adductor pollicis results in flexion of the IP joint of the thumb (positive Froment sign) (**Figure 16-8**). Assess ulnar nerve sensation at the volar tip of the little finger. If ulnar nerve entrapment or laceration occurs above the wrist, sensation may be lost on the dorsum of the hand.

If the ulnar nerve is divided distal to the mid-forearm, all the intrinsic muscles of the hand are paralyzed except for the first and second lumbricals and the thenar muscles. Lack of intrinsic muscle function to the ring and little fingers causes an ulnar claw hand, or *hand of benediction*, with the fourth and fifth fingers hyperextended at the MP joints and flexed at the PIP and DIP joints (**Figure 16-9**). The intact lumbricals to the index and long fingers provide enough intrinsic muscle function to prevent clawing of these digits. However, if the ulnar nerve is lacerated at or proximal to the elbow, clawing of the ring and little fingers does not occur because the FDP to these fingers is also paralyzed. A distal forearm

Figure 16-8: Positive Froment Sign

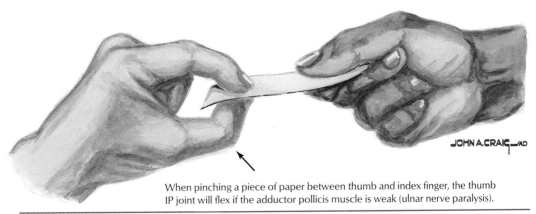

When pinching a piece of paper between thumb and index finger, the thumb IP joint will flex if the adductor pollicis muscle is weak (ulnar nerve paralysis).

Figure 16-9: Hand of Benediction

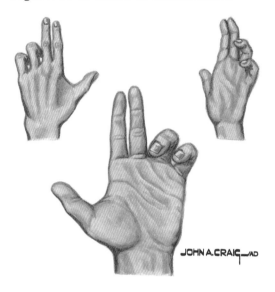

JOHN A.CRAIG—AD

laceration of the median and ulnar nerves results in a complete claw hand because all intrinsic muscles are paralyzed, but the extrinsic flexors and extensors are intact.

DEGENERATIVE DISORDERS
Osteoarthritis

Osteoarthritis may affect any joint of the hand. It is common in the DIP and PIP joints of the fingers with normal aging—a process that usually begins earlier and is more severe in females. Heberden nodes (in the DIP joints) and Bouchard nodes (in the PIP joints) are prominences caused by osteophytes and deformation of the joints (see **Figure 4-7**). A degenerative cystic lesion, referred to as a *mucous cyst,* may be present on the dorsum of the DIP joint. The joints may be painful and stiff early in the process, but the pain usually subsides over time. Although the stiffness and nodules remain, surgical treatment (arthrodesis) of these joints is not commonly required.

Osteoarthritis of the thumb CMC joint is common and affects women more often than men. Predisposing factors are ligamentous laxity and repetitive stress from pinch maneuvers that load the joint (eg, knitting or cutting). Patients report pain with pinch activities. Examination shows swelling and pain over the CMC

joint that are exacerbated by axial pressure of the metacarpal on the trapezium (the grind test). Radiographs show narrowing of the joint and varying degrees of subluxation of the joint (**Figure 16-10**). Nonoperative treatment alternatives include activity modification, nonsteroidal anti-inflammatory drugs (NSAIDs), short-term full-time splinting followed by intermittent bracing, and steroid injections. Reconstructive operations are indicated in patients with persistent, disabling symptoms.

Osteoarthritis of other joints in the hand and wrist is uncommon and usually is secondary to trauma. Predisposing injuries in traumatic wrist arthropathy include intra-articular fractures of the distal radius, unrecognized scaphoid fractures, and ligament disruptions that cause abnormal wrist kinematics.

Kienböck Disease

Osteonecrosis of the lunate, commonly referred to as *Kienböck disease,* can occur at any age but most commonly affects men between the ages of 20 and 40 years. The exact cause is usually not known, but repetitive or single-episode trauma that interrupts the blood supply to a "lunate at risk" is the most accepted theory. Risk factors include a lunate supplied by a single nutrient vessel, which occurs in 7% of the population, and ulnar negative variance (an ulna shorter than the radius). Studies have shown increased contact stress at the radiolunate in patients with negative ulnar variance; however, osteonecrosis of the lunate also occurs in patients with positive ulnar variance.

Patients with Kienböck disease typically present with the insidious onset of wrist pain that is increased with activity. Examination shows variable limitation of wrist motion and mild swelling on the dorsum of the wrist. Routine radiographs are usually diagnostic (**Figure 16-11**). If no changes are apparent in the lunate, a bone scan or magnetic resonance imaging (MRI) may be diagnostic.

Treatment is based on the stage of disease and the degree of disability. Immobilization may be successful if the lunate has not collapsed; however, the effect of immobilization on the natural history of the disease is unclear. Surgical options for patients with no collapse or with some collapse of the lunate but no degenerative changes in the adjacent joints include vascular pedicle transplantation, radial shortening osteotomy, ulna-lengthening osteotomy, and capitate-shortening osteotomy. Surgical options for patients with arthritic changes include limited carpal arthrodesis, resection arthroplasty with interposition of tendon graft or silicone implant, proximal row carpectomy, and wrist arthrodesis.

Figure 16-10: Osteoarthritis of Thumb Carpometacarpal Joint

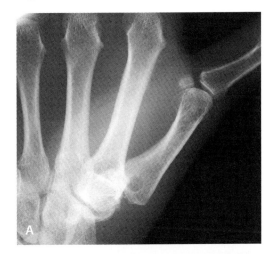
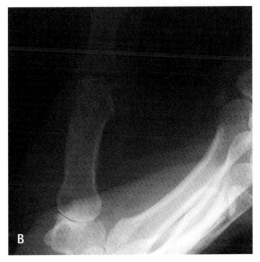
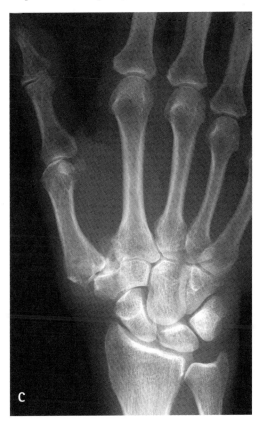

(A) Lateral radiograph and (B) AP radiograph of thumb of 56-year-old male with activity-related pain at base of thumb. Radiographs show early stages of disease with narrowing of thumb CMC and mild subluxation. (C) AP radiograph of hand of 73-year-old female with severe pain at base of thumb. Exam showed swelling and tenderness to palpation at the base of the thumb. Radiographs show subluxation and degenerative changes at the thumb CMC joint with a large osteophyte between the first and second metacarpal. The joint space between the scaphotrapezial was preserved.

Figure 16-11: Radiograph in Kienböck Disease

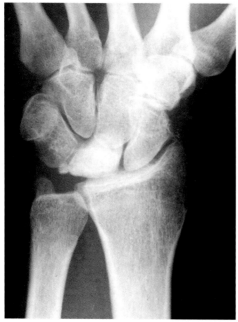

Radiograph of wrist shows characteristic sclerosis of lunate.

Tendinitis of the Hand and Wrist

Tendinitis (tendinosis) of the hand and wrist is common. The most common etiology is predisposing anatomic factors such as a narrow canal for the tendon exacerbated by overuse. Fortunately, most patients respond to nonoperative treatment, including modification of activities, short-term immobilization, NSAIDs, and judicious injections of steroids.

Stenosing tenosynovitis of the finger or thumb flexors, better known as *trigger finger,* is the most common cause of hand tendinitis. Bow stringing of the flexor tendons and its resultant mechanical disadvantage is prevented by five annular and three cruciate pulleys. The first annular pulley may become thickened, causing snapping or locking of the tendon during flexion of the finger or thumb. Predisposing factors include diabetes mellitus, rheumatoid arthritis, and aging.

Patients note pain and catching when moving the finger, as well as a nodule in the distal palm that moves with flexion and extension.

The finger may lock or stick with flexion of the digit (**Figure 16-12**). On awakening, the digit may be locked in the palm and unlocking the digit may require that the finger be pushed into extension. Patients with diabetes mellitus or rheumatoid arthritis may have multiple digit involvement.

Injection of corticosteroid into the tendon sheath is often successful as an initial treatment for trigger finger; however, patients with diabetes mellitus are less likely to improve after an injection. If symptoms persist, release of the A1 pulley is indicated (see **Figure 16-22**).

De Quervain tenosynovitis, the most common cause of tendinitis on the extensor side of the wrist, involves swelling or stenosis of the first dorsal compartment tendon sheath, which surrounds the extensor pollicis brevis and the abductor pollicis longus. It most commonly occurs in patients who have (1) one or more additional anomalous tendons within the compartment, or (2) a septum within the compartment that separates and narrows the space for the extensor pollicis brevis and the abductor pollicis longus. This disorder most commonly occurs in middle-aged women and is frequently brought on by repetitive thumb motion.

Tenosynovitis constricts the tendons as they glide within the sheath. Patients note pain and swelling in the region of the radial styloid that are aggravated by use of the thumb (**Figure 16-13**). Crepitus may be sensed as the compartment is palpated during thumb motion. The *Finkelstein test* is diagnostic with exacerbation of pain when the thumb is flexed and the wrist is then placed in ulnar deviation. Radiographs are typically normal and are used to exclude other possibilities, such as fracture of the scaphoid or arthritis of the wrist or thumb CMC joint.

Treatment begins with immobilization of the thumb in a splint, as well as the use of NSAIDs. If this treatment fails, a corticosteroid injection into the tendon sheath is indicated. Surgical treatment to release the area of stenosis is indicated for relief of persistent symptoms. Anomalous slips of the abductor

Figure 16-12: Trigger Finger

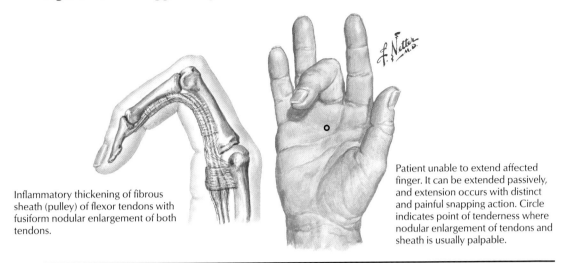

Inflammatory thickening of fibrous sheath (pulley) of flexor tendons with fusiform nodular enlargement of both tendons.

Patient unable to extend affected finger. It can be extended passively, and extension occurs with distinct and painful snapping action. Circle indicates point of tenderness where nodular enlargement of tendons and sheath is usually palpable.

Figure 16-13: De Quervain Tenosynovitis

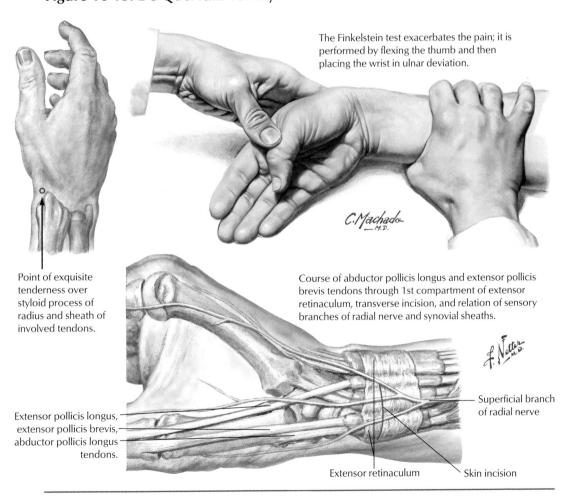

The Finkelstein test exacerbates the pain; it is performed by flexing the thumb and then placing the wrist in ulnar deviation.

Point of exquisite tenderness over styloid process of radius and sheath of involved tendons.

Course of abductor pollicis longus and extensor pollicis brevis tendons through 1st compartment of extensor retinaculum, transverse incision, and relation of sensory branches of radial nerve and synovial sheaths.

Extensor pollicis longus, extensor pollicis brevis, abductor pollicis longus tendons.

Superficial branch of radial nerve

Extensor retinaculum

Skin incision

pollicis longus are commonly noted. The most dorsal tendon of the compartment should be identified as the extensor pollicis brevis; otherwise, a separate septum for this tendon may be overlooked. Complications of surgery include failure to completely decompress all tendons within the sheath, and injury to the superficial radial nerve.

Other potential, but less common, areas of wrist tendinitis include the flexor carpi radialis, extensor pollicis longus (third compartment), extensor digitorum communis (fourth compartment), extensor digiti minimi (fifth compartment), and extensor carpi ulnaris (sixth compartment).

Dupuytren Disease

Dupuytren disease is contracture of the palmar fascia. The pathologic process begins with a proliferation of fibroblasts and type III collagen to produce cords and nodules in the dermis and skin. Predisposing factors include male gender, alcoholism, epilepsy, diabetes mellitus, HIV infection, trauma, and possibly smoking. A genetic, autosomal dominant predisposition has been noted; penetrance is variable, however, as indicated by the fact that the family history is positive in less than 10% of affected patients.

The disease is uncommon before 40 years of age. A typical presentation is a 40- to 65-year-old patient who notices a painless nodule near the distal palmar crease on the ulnar side of the hand. The cords initially may be tender and may occur in other locations. The nodules may remain confined to the palm and cause few symptoms. However, the disease may extend into the fingers, with progressive, albeit variable, flexion contracture of one or more digits at the MP and, in more severe cases, the PIP joints (**Figure 16-14**). The ring finger is most often involved, followed by the little, long, thumb, and index fingers. Concomitant involvement of the plantar fascia, the fascia of the penis, or both occurs in less than 3% of individuals with Dupuytren disease.

Early treatment of a nodule in the palm consists of reassurance that no surgery is needed unless the contracture progresses to functional impairment. Splinting is ineffective. Recent research on collagenase injections has shown promising results. Surgery is indicated for significant contractures that interfere with extension of the fingers and functional activities such as retrieving objects from a pocket. The goals of surgical treatment are to excise the diseased tissue and release the contractures; however, the procedure is technically

Figure 16-14: Dupuytren Disease

Flexion contracture of 4th and 5th fingers (most common). Dimpling and puckering of skin. Palpable fascial nodules near flexion crease of palm at base of involved fingers with cordlike formations extending to proximal palm.

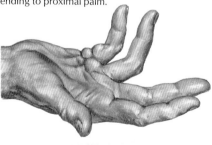
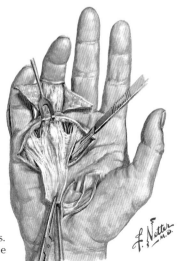

Partial excision of palmar fascia. Proximal portion of fascia divided and freed via thenar incision, then drawn up into palmar incision, where it is further dissected with care to avoid neurovascular bundles. Dissection is then continued into fingers. Buttonholing of skin must be avoided. Nodules and cordlike fascial thickening are apparent.

demanding and may be complicated by nerve injury, skin slough, and recurrent contractures.

Ganglia of the Hand and Wrist

The most common benign tumor of the hand and wrist is a ganglion. These cystic lesions contain a thick, yellowish, mucinous fluid with a composition similar to joint fluid. Ganglia are thought to arise from the degeneration or tearing of a joint capsule or tendon sheath, which creates a one-way valve through which synovial fluid can enter the cyst but cannot easily flow back. The most common age at presentation is 15 to 40 years, but ganglia also develop in children and older adults.

Ganglia may develop at any site. The most common location is the dorsoradial aspect of the wrist over the scapholunate joint (**Figure 16-15**). The lump may be asymptomatic or may cause aching that is aggravated by activities requiring repetitive wrist movements. Examination reveals a firm, cystic mass that transilluminates when a penlight is pressed against its side. The second most common site of ganglia is the volar radial aspect of the wrist between the flexor carpi radialis and the radial styloid. These ganglia originate from the capsule of the scaphotrapezial joint and may wrap around the radial artery.

A volar retinacular ganglion of the flexor tendon sheath typically is just proximal to the MP flexion crease of the finger. This "seed ganglion" is a small, firm nodule that is frequently tender when gripping objects, but does not limit or move with finger flexion/extension. Mucous cysts, a type of ganglion, develop at osteoarthritic DIP joints and most commonly are located on either side of the extensor tendon.

Treatment options include observation, aspiration, and surgical excision. Ganglia may spontaneously recede, and observation is appropriate for patients with minimal symptoms. Aspiration is often successful in the treatment of volar retinacular ganglia, may be useful in the treatment of dorsal wrist ganglia (although recurrence rates are high), and is used with caution in volar wrist ganglia or mucous cysts. Surgical excision includes the joint capsule attachments. The risk of recurrence after surgery is 5% to 10% if the procedure is combined with 2 weeks of immobilization. Mucous cyst excision at the DIP joint requires careful removal of the cyst and any associated osteophytes.

Figure 16-15: Ganglion of Wrist

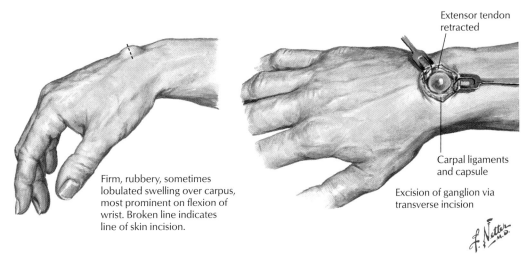

Firm, rubbery, sometimes lobulated swelling over carpus, most prominent on flexion of wrist. Broken line indicates line of skin incision.

Extensor tendon retracted

Carpal ligaments and capsule

Excision of ganglion via transverse incision

NERVE ENTRAPMENT SYNDROMES AT THE WRIST

For signs and symptoms of nerve entrapment syndromes at the wrist, see Chapter 6. Carpal tunnel syndrome is most common in middle-aged or pregnant women. The syndrome is often idiopathic, but predisposing factors that reduce available space in the carpal tunnel or affect peripheral nerve function should be investigated. These factors include tenosynovitis of the adjacent flexor tendons due to rheumatoid arthritis or overuse syndrome; edema resulting from pregnancy or hypothyroidism; and peripheral neuropathy caused by diabetes mellitus, alcoholism, or other conditions. The differential diagnosis includes cervical radiculopathy that affects the C6 nerve root, median nerve entrapment at the elbow, ulnar entrapment at the wrist, and wrist arthritis.

Ulnar nerve entrapment at the wrist in Guyon canal is less common than ulnar entrapment at the elbow. Predisposing factors include a space-occupying lesion (such as a ganglion) or repetitive trauma (such as trauma produced by operating a jackhammer, or that caused by repetitive pressure associated with extended crutch ambulation). The differential diagnosis includes cervical radiculopathy that affects the C8 nerve root, thoracic outlet syndrome, ulnar nerve entrapment at the elbow, carpal tunnel syndrome, and wrist arthritis. More proximal entrapment of the ulnar nerve or C8 nerve root typically causes numbness of the dorsum of the hand.

BITE WOUNDS OF THE HAND

Dog, cat, and human bites account for approximately 1% of all emergency room visits. Dog bites account for approximately 80% to 90% of animal bites, but only 10% of wounds from dog bites become infected. In contrast, approximately 30% to 50% of wounds from cat bites become infected, most likely because the sharp, needlelike teeth of cats inject bacteria deep into the tissues. The causative organisms of dog and cat bite infections are similar. *Pasteurella multocida* is found in 50% of wounds from cat bites and in some dog bite wounds. Other bacteria commonly found in dog and cat bite wounds include α-hemolytic streptococci, *Staphylococcus aureus*, *Bacteroides* species, and *Fusobacterium* species.

Human bite wounds often occur at the fingers (a direct injury) or MP joints (an indirect, clenched fist injury). Because the circumstances of the injury are often embarrassing and the laceration is often small, patients commonly delay evaluation. As a result, many patients with human bite wounds do not present until a well-established infection has developed. Gram-negative, anaerobic organisms—particularly *Eikenella corrodens*—are common in human bite wounds.

Examination should assess location, swelling, erythema, and purulent discharge. Evaluate possible tendon or neurovascular dysfunction. Provide appropriate tetanus prophylaxis, and débride necrotic tissue. Most bite wounds should not be closed primarily. Pending culture results, treat animal bites with oral or intravenous ampicillin-sulbactam. Penicillin and a cephalosporin are the standard initial antibiotic therapy for human bite wounds.

UNIQUE HAND INFECTIONS

The flexor tendons of the fingers and thumb are surrounded by a tenosynovial sheath that extends from the distal palm to the DIP joint (**Figure 16-16**; also **Figure 16-22**). Infections within this sheath usually develop from a puncture wound. Because the sheath is a closed space with limited blood supply, an infection rapidly becomes an abscess. The sheath of the thumb and little finger flexor tendons extends to the radial and ulnar bursae, so infections in these tendon sheaths have the potential for extension into the forearm.

Patients with septic flexor tenosynovitis develop progressive pain and swelling of the digit 24 to 48 hours after injury. Examination reveals diffuse swelling of the finger, maximal tenderness over the tendon, a finger held in a semiflexed position, and marked increased pain on passive extension of the digit. Patients

Figure 16-16: Infections of the Hand

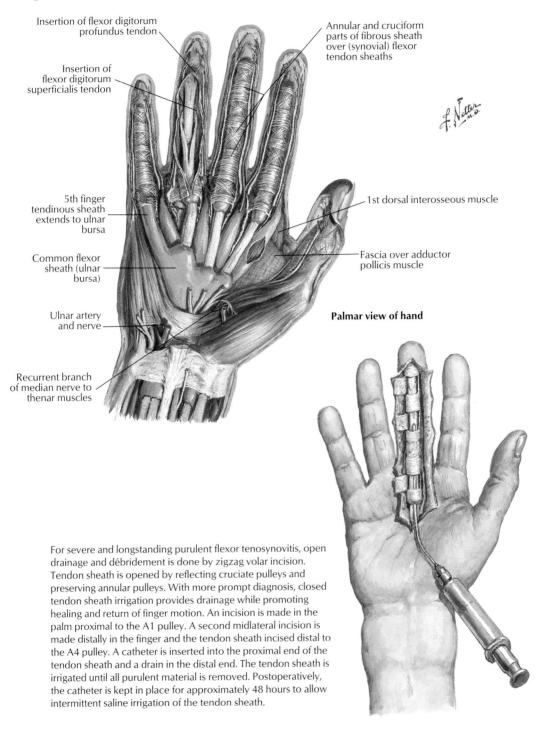

Insertion of flexor digitorum profundus tendon

Insertion of flexor digitorum superficialis tendon

5th finger tendinous sheath extends to ulnar bursa

Common flexor sheath (ulnar bursa)

Ulnar artery and nerve

Recurrent branch of median nerve to thenar muscles

Annular and cruciform parts of fibrous sheath over (synovial) flexor tendon sheaths

1st dorsal interosseous muscle

Fascia over adductor pollicis muscle

Palmar view of hand

For severe and longstanding purulent flexor tenosynovitis, open drainage and débridement is done by zigzag volar incision. Tendon sheath is opened by reflecting cruciate pulleys and preserving annular pulleys. With more prompt diagnosis, closed tendon sheath irrigation provides drainage while promoting healing and return of finger motion. An incision is made in the palm proximal to the A1 pulley. A second midlateral incision is made distally in the finger and the tendon sheath incised distal to the A4 pulley. A catheter is inserted into the proximal end of the tendon sheath and a drain in the distal end. The tendon sheath is irrigated until all purulent material is removed. Postoperatively, the catheter is kept in place for approximately 48 hours to allow intermittent saline irrigation of the tendon sheath.

require prompt treatment for prevention of tendon adhesions and necrosis. If the infection is recognized early, parenteral antibiotic therapy that covers both staphylococci and streptococci may be satisfactory. Most patients, however, require surgical drainage supplemented by closed tendon sheath irrigation and appropriate intravenous antibiotics.

The pulp of the fingertip has fibrous septa that provide support for pinching and grasping activities. These septa create many small compartments in which a felon (pulp space infection) may develop (**Figure 16-17**). A felon typically develops after a puncture wound, most commonly involves the index and long fingers, and is characterized by intense pain and swelling of the palmar tip of the finger. Untreated felons progress to osteomyelitis of the distal phalanx. Surgical drainage can be performed through a central incision that extends from the flexion crease to the fingertip when an abscess collection is identified on the pad side of the finger, or through a midaxial incision when the location of the pus is not visible. "Fish mouth incisions" that extend across the tip of the finger cause painful scars and should be avoided. The wound should be packed open for 24 to 48 hours. The usual infecting organism is *S aureus*.

Herpetic whitlow, a herpes simplex virus infection, can affect the fingertip and may cause swelling that should be differentiated from a felon. Herpetic whitlows have vesicular lesions and typically have less erythema and swelling than occur with felons. Lesions occur in adults and children and are more common in medical personnel, who are frequently exposed to human saliva. The swelling from a herpetic whitlow resolves within 10 to 21 days. Unnecessary surgical drainage predisposes the patient to secondary infection.

Paronychial infections are the most common hand infections. The paronychia is the skinfold radial and ulnar to the fingernail. The eponychium is proximal to the nail. Paronychial infections typically develop from a hangnail, an ingrown nail, or a poorly performed manicure; they also may result from fingernail biting. The infection may involve only one side of the nail or both sides of the nail and the eponychium (see **Figure 16-17**). Early-stage infections may be treated with warm soaks and oral antibiotics that cover *S aureus*. Later-stage infections require elevation of the skinfold or partial or complete removal of the nail.

WRIST AND HAND TRAUMA
Fractures in Adults
Fractures of the Distal Radius

When we fall, the most common protective mechanism involves catching ourselves on an outstretched, hyperextended hand. As a result, Colles fracture of the distal radius is the most common fracture in adults. This injury is more common in women and in older adults; after age 50, the female predominance increases. Colles fracture begins on the volar aspect of the distal radius, which fails in tension. The fracture propagates dorsally, and the bone then is loaded in compression. Therefore, Colles fractures typically reveal dorsal comminution, volar angulation, and dorsal displacement of the distal radius (**Figure 16-18**).

Smith fracture is the opposite of Colles fracture and occurs with a backward fall on a

Figure 16-17: Felon and Paronychia Infections

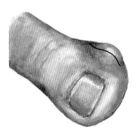

Felon. Line of incision indicated.

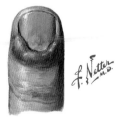

Paronychia

Figure 16-18: Fractures of the Distal Radius

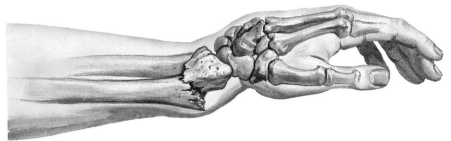

Colles fracture
Lateral view of Colles fracture demonstrates characteristic silver fork deformity with dorsal and proximal displacement of distal fragment. Note dorsal instead of normal volar slope of articular surface of distal radius.

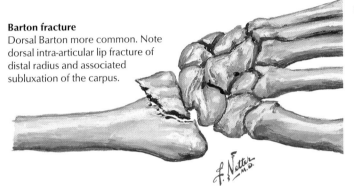

Barton fracture
Dorsal Barton more common. Note dorsal intra-articular lip fracture of distal radius and associated subluxation of the carpus.

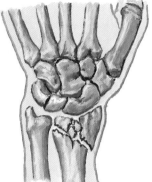

Die-punch, comminuted Colles fracture

flexed wrist. In these injuries, the distal radius is tilted volarly. Barton fracture is a dorsal or palmar lip fracture of the distal radius with associated subluxation of the carpus (see **Figure 16-18**). A die-punch fracture is an intra-articular, depressed fracture of the distal radius that occurs with increased axial compression. A transverse or oblique fracture across the radial styloid (a chauffeur fracture) results from a direct blow to the lateral aspect of the forearm.

Examine the patient to detect swelling and deformity of the distal forearm, and determine the circulatory and neurologic status of the hand. Inspect anteroposterior (AP) and lateral radiographs to determine the direction and magnitude of displacement and whether the fracture is extra-articular or intra-articular. Median nerve dysfunction is the most common associated injury.

The degree of acceptable displacement varies according to the age of the person and whether the fracture is intra-articular or extra-articular. Generally, fractures with 5° to 10° of dorsal angulation, a loss of more than 10° of radial inclination, and more than 2 mm of intra-articular step-off should be reduced and stabilized with the use of sugar tong splints or external or internal immobilization devices. Elderly patients with marked osteopenia and borderline reasons for reduction often function satisfactorily and with fewer complications when treated by short-arm cast or splint immobilization.

Fractures of the Scaphoid

The scaphoid spans the proximal and distal rows of the carpus. Its anatomic location makes it vulnerable to axial loading between the ground and the distal radius when the wrist is hyperflexed (**Figure 16-19**). Therefore, the scaphoid is the most commonly fractured carpal bone. Fractures of the scaphoid are

Figure 16-19: Fracture of Scaphoid

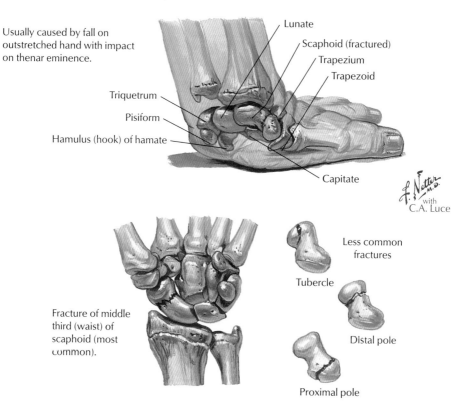

Usually caused by fall on outstretched hand with impact on thenar eminence.

Lunate

Scaphoid (fractured)

Trapezium

Trapezoid

Triquetrum

Pisiform

Hamulus (hook) of hamate

Capitate

F. Netter M.D.
with
C.A. Luce

Fracture of middle third (waist) of scaphoid (most common).

Less common fractures

Tubercle

Distal pole

Proximal pole

more common among males; the age group most often affected is 15 to 40 years, an age at which the distal radius is relatively strong.

Scaphoid fractures have an increased incidence of nonunion and osteonecrosis for two reasons. First, the diagnosis is often delayed or missed. Patients may dismiss the injury as a simple sprain and may not seek medical attention. Furthermore, the radiographic findings of an acute injury are often subtle and may not be apparent unless routine AP and lateral radiographs are supplemented with additional oblique radiographs. The second reason for nonunion and osteonecrosis is a vulnerable blood supply. Articular cartilage covers 80% of the surface of the scaphoid, and the fracture may interrupt the major blood supply, which enters the distal pole at the dorsal ridge.

Tuberosity fractures and incomplete waist (middle third) fractures are stable injuries. Unstable patterns include oblique fractures of the distal pole, complete waist fractures, and proximal pole fractures. Displaced fractures have more than 1 mm of displacement, dorsal angulation, or both. The rate of nonunion markedly increases in displaced fractures. Osteonecrosis is associated with any proximal pole fracture and with displaced waist injuries.

Symptoms include pain and tenderness on the radial aspect of the wrist localized to the anatomic snuffbox, or pain and tenderness on pressure over the scaphoid tubercle on the palmar side of the wrist. In addition to routine posteroanterior and lateral radiographs of the wrist, a posteroanterior view with the wrist in ulnar deviation and an oblique view should be obtained if examination indicates the possibility of a scaphoid fracture.

If the exam suggests a possible scaphoid fracture but radiographs are not diagnostic, treatment should consist of a short-arm cast that includes the thumb for 2 weeks and repeated radiographs. Treatment for acute, stable fractures is a short-arm, thumb-spica cast with the wrist in radial deviation. Nondisplaced, unstable fractures can be treated with either internal fixation or cast immobilization for 12 weeks. Reduction and internal fixation is indicated in patients with displaced fractures or delayed diagnosis.

Fractures of the Metacarpals

Fractures of the base of the thumb metacarpal can be classified as Bennett or Rolando injuries (**Figure 16-20**). These fractures cause functional incompetence of the trapeziometacarpal ligament; therefore, the abductor pollicis longus exerts a subluxating force on the main metacarpal fragment. Displaced fractures require reduction and pinning.

Fractures of the second through fifth metacarpals typically result from axial loading. The most common fracture in the hand is the boxer fracture, a fracture of the fifth metacarpal neck (the distal metaphyseal-diaphyseal junction) that results from a closed fist striking an object (see **Figure 16-20**). Because of the dorsal-palmar mobility of the fifth metacarpal, residual dorsal angulation of 40° to 50° is well tolerated. These fractures usually can be treated with an ulnar gutter splint that positions the fourth and fifth fingers in the "safe, clam-digger" position (MP joints in 80° of flexion, and PIP and DIP joints in extension). The index finger and long metacarpals have less mobility, and only 10° to 15° of angulation is acceptable for metacarpal neck fractures involving these bones.

Displaced fractures of the metacarpal shaft frequently require open reduction and internal fixation to prevent extensor lag at the MP joint (caused by shortening at the fracture) or malrotation of the digit. Rotational malalignment may be difficult to appreciate with the fingers extended but will be evident as the fingers are

Figure 16-20: Base of Thumb Metacarpal and Metacarpal Neck Fractures

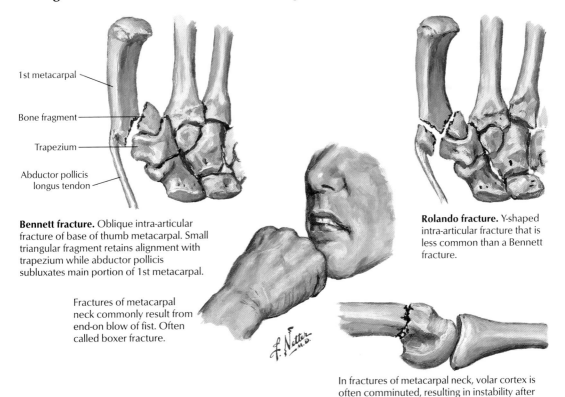

1st metacarpal

Bone fragment

Trapezium

Abductor pollicis longus tendon

Bennett fracture. Oblique intra-articular fracture of base of thumb metacarpal. Small triangular fragment retains alignment with trapezium while abductor pollicis subluxates main portion of 1st metacarpal.

Fractures of metacarpal neck commonly result from end-on blow of fist. Often called boxer fracture.

Rolando fracture. Y-shaped intra-articular fracture that is less common than a Bennett fracture.

In fractures of metacarpal neck, volar cortex is often comminuted, resulting in instability after reduction that may necessitate pinning.

partially flexed. A malrotated metacarpal or phalangeal fracture causes the finger to overlap the adjacent digit. Nondisplaced and minimally displaced fractures are common when only the third or fourth metacarpal is injured. In these injuries, the transverse metacarpal ligament stabilizes and suspends the injured metacarpal between the adjacent ones.

Fractures of the Phalanges

In adults, the distal phalanx is the most commonly injured finger bone, followed by the proximal and middle phalanges. Fractures of the middle and distal phalanges are often nondisplaced and may be managed by splinting or buddy-taping the injured finger to an adjacent digit. Maintenance of reduction is difficult in displaced fractures of the proximal phalanx, so these injuries typically require internal fixation (**Figure 16-21**).

Fractures in Children

The distal third of the forearm is the most common location for fractures in children. Several patterns of injury may occur (**Table 16-1**). These injuries are relatively uncommon before age 4 years and in this age group are mostly torus or greenstick fractures. A torus fracture is the least complicated distal forearm fracture and most commonly involves the dorsal cortex of the radius (see **Figure 10-1**). A metaphyseal fracture isolated to the distal radius is typically minimally displaced.

Most distal forearm fractures in children, including fractures with complete displacement and shortening, can be treated by closed means. Because the distal radial and ulnar physis contribute approximately 80% of forearm length, residual angulation typically remodels completely in 1 to 2 years. Loss of rotational alignment is the only absolute

Figure 16-21: Fracture of Proximal Phalanx

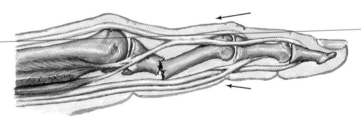

Transverse fractures of proximal phalanx tend to angulate volarly because of pull of interosseous muscles on base of proximal phalanx and collapsing action of long extensor and flexor tendons.

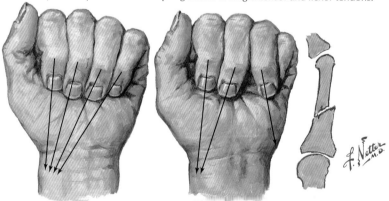

Reduction of fractures of phalanges or metacarpals requires correct rotational as well as longitudinal alignment. In normal hand, tips of flexed fingers point toward tuberosity of scaphoid, as in hand at left. Hand at right shows result of healing of ring finger in rotational malalignment. Rotational malalignment, usually discernible clinically, may also be evidenced on radiographs by discrepancy in cross-sectional diameter of fragments, as shown at extreme right. Discrepancy in diameter is most apparent in true lateral radiograph but is visible to some extent in anteroposterior view.

Table 16-1
Distal Forearm Fracture Patterns in Children (in order of relative severity)
Torus fracture*
Metaphyseal fracture, complete*
Greenstick fracture of the distal radius
Greenstick fracture of the distal radius and ulna
Complete fracture of the distal radius and greenstick fracture of the distal ulna
Complete fracture of the distal radius and ulna
Physeal fracture
Galeazzi fracture
*Typically nondisplaced or minimally displaced.

indication for reduction or remanipulation. The reason for reduction is to relieve pressure on adjacent soft tissues and to facilitate healing. Closed reduction generally is indicated for angulation of 10° to 15°.

Fractures of the wrist and hand are uncommon in children. The most common such injury is a Peterson II (Salter II) physeal fracture of the proximal phalanx. This injury most often involves the little finger and occurs when the finger is caught on an object and is pushed in a lateral direction.

Tendon Injuries

Lacerations cause most tendon injuries in the hand. Examination should carefully assess which tendons are injured, as well as the status of adjacent digital nerves. Flexor tendon injuries in zone II are particularly difficult to treat (**Figure 16-22**). Zone II begins at the ori-

Figure 16-22: Flexor Tendon Anatomy and Injuries

Anatomy of finger flexor tendon sheaths and pulleys

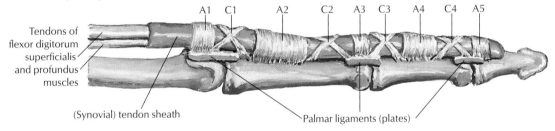

Tendons of flexor digitorum superficialis and profundus muscles

(Synovial) tendon sheath

Palmar ligaments (plates)

A1 C1 A2 C2 A3 C3 A4 C4 A5

Note: Flexor digitorum superficialis and profundus tendons encased in synovial sheaths are bound to phalanges by fibrous digital sheaths made up of alternating strong annular (A) and weaker cruciform (C) pulleys.

Mallet finger

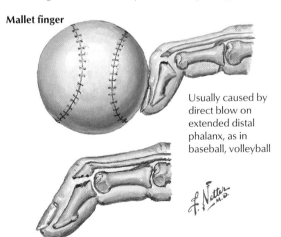

Usually caused by direct blow on extended distal phalanx, as in baseball, volleyball

Jersey finger

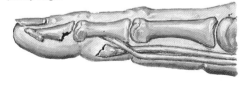

Flexor digitorum profundus tendon may be torn directly from distal phalanx or may avulse small or large bone fragment. Tendon usually retracts to about level of proximal interphalangeal joint, where it is stopped at its passage through flexor digitorum superficialis tendon; occasionally, it retracts into palm. Early open reduction and repair of FDP tendon to insertion site is indicated.

gin of the flexor tendon sheath and extends to the insertion of the FDS. In this zone, both the FDP and the FDS are often lacerated. Laceration may involve the tendons at which the FDS splits to allow passage of the FDP. In addition, injury and repair processes violate the tendon sheath and its associated annular and cruciate pulleys that normally facilitate gliding and nutrition of the tendons. As a result, the site of injury is often complicated by peritendinous adhesions that can seriously compromise function.

Extensor tendon injuries in the distal forearm or wrist often heal well, but lacerations over the metacarpal head and the dorsum of the fingers can be complicated by injury to the sagittal bands and adhesions to surrounding structures that limit flexion. Both flexor and extensor tendon injuries require meticulous operative technique and a postoperative rehabilitation protocol that minimizes adhesions, contracture, and disruption of the repaired tendon. The A2 and A4 pulleys must be repaired or preserved to prevent bow stringing and dysfunction of the flexor tendons.

Avulsion injuries also may disrupt finger tendons. A mallet finger results from forced flexion of the extended finger (eg, when a ball strikes the tip of the finger) and subsequent avulsion of the extensor tendon at the distal phalanx (see **Figure 16-22**). A similar mechanism can result in an intra-articular fracture of the distal phalanx (bony mallet finger). Examination shows a flexion posture of the DIP joint and an inability to actively extend this joint. Splinting the DIP joint in full extension for 6 weeks if the injury is acute, and for 8 weeks if diagnosis is delayed, is often successful.

Avulsion ruptures of the central slip of the extensor tendon insertion into the middle phalanx result in an inability to fully extend the PIP joint. If diagnosis is delayed, lateral bands displace below the axis of rotation, resulting in flexion of the PIP joint and hyperextension of the DIP joint (boutonnière deformity; see **Figure 16-6**). Acute injuries can be treated by splinting of the PIP joint in extension. Chronic injuries may require surgical reconstruction.

Avulsion of the FDP insertion into the distal phalanx usually involves the ring finger (see **Figure 16-22**) and occurs when the flexed finger is caught and is forcefully pulled into extension, as when a sports player is grasping the jersey of another player ("jersey finger"). Examination reveals an inability to flex the DIP joint. Treatment requires operative reinsertion of the FDP to its bony insertion point.

Ligament Injuries and Dislocations of the Hand

Sprains of the hand are common and typically involve a collateral ligament and/or volar plate of the MP, PIP, or DIP joint. Patients note pain and swelling after a jamming type of injury. After obtaining radiographs to rule out a fracture, assess stability by gently stressing the adjacent ligaments. Most sprains of the hand, even those that demonstrate complete disruption, can be treated with splinting. A digit with collateral ligament injury can be buddy-taped to an adjacent digit. Complete ruptures of the volar plate are initially splinted in 30° of flexion for 1 to 3 weeks, with transition to buddy-taping and motion.

Disruption of the ulnar collateral ligament of the thumb MP joint results from forced abduction of the thumb. This injury requires special consideration because this ligament is an important stabilizer of the thumb, and the adductor pollicis tendon may become interposed between bone and torn ligament, thus preventing adequate healing. The term *gamekeeper thumb* is used because English gamekeepers sustained this injury when they killed rabbits by means of a forceful blow from their thumb web space to the back of the hare's neck. The injury is also observed in skiers (from forced abduction of the thumb against the ski pole), in sports players (from the ball's forcing the thumb into abduction), and in persons who have fallen (**Figure 16-23**). Partial injuries can be treated with cast immobilization. Complete disruption requires surgical stabilization.

Finger joint dislocations are typically dorsal and result from hyperextension injuries that disrupt the volar plate. Dislocation of the PIP

Figure 16-23: Gamekeeper Thumb

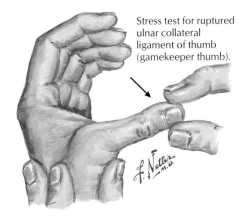

Stress test for ruptured ulnar collateral ligament of thumb (gamekeeper thumb).

joint is the most common. MP dislocations are more common in the thumb and may be simple or complex (interposition of the volar plate between the metacarpal head and the proximal phalanx). Treatment of a PIP or DIP joint dislocation consists of closed reduction after the administration of a digital block anesthetic. Distal traction is followed by appropriate volar and dorsal applied pressure. Stability should be assessed after reduction. Stable injuries can be buddy-taped. When instability is observed with the joint positioned in full extension, the finger should be immobilized with a dorsal extension block splint. Complex dorsal dislocations of the MP joint often benefit from regional block anesthesia. These injuries are reduced by pushing the proximal phalanx over the metacarpal rather than by traction. Complex dislocations of the MP joint may require open reduction.

Nail Injuries

Nail bed and fingertip injuries are common. These include simple lacerations, stellate/crushing lacerations, and avulsion injuries with loss of nail bed tissue. Associated fractures of the distal phalanx are common, as is extension of the laceration through the surrounding skin and pulp. Various levels of fingertip amputation may occur.

The goal of treatment is to prevent hypersensitivity of the fingertip and deformity of the nail such as split, ridged, ingrown, or poorly adherent nails. Assess the extent of injury, including whether the nail bed laceration involves the sterile matrix, germinal matrix, or both. Obtain AP and lateral radiographs of the finger, and note the location and displacement of any fractures.

Simple and stellate/crushing lacerations should be treated by primary repair using digital block anesthesia, a finger tourniquet, loupe magnification, 6-0 chromic suture for the nail bed, and 5-0 nylon suture for any associated skin lacerations. If the germinal matrix is avulsed and lying on top of the nail plate, the nail bed should be repositioned and secured in its anatomic position. Loss of nail bed tissue requires split-thickness or more complicated grafting procedures. Soft tissue loss without exposed bone and with a defect of <1 cm heals well by secondary intention. More complicated injuries with bone exposed require the use of local or regional flaps or shortening of the digit with primary closure. Tuft fractures and nondisplaced fractures of the distal phalanx are treated with symptomatic splinting.

PEDIATRIC CONDITIONS
Syndactyly

Syndactyly is a congenital condition characterized by failure of normal separation of the fingers or toes. At a genetically predetermined time, production of apical ectodermal ridge maintenance factor (AERMF) ceases. If AERMF continues to be produced, apoptosis and disruption of the interdigital space do not occur. The degree of syndactyly can vary from the presence of a thin web of skin to synostosis (bony fusion) of the phalanges. The webbing may extend to the tips of the digits (complete webbing) or may involve only a variable extent of the digit (partial webbing) (**Figure 16-24**). Syndactyly occurs twice as often in males, is 10 times more common in whites than in blacks, and most often involves the long and ring fingers.

Syndactyly may occur in association with other syndromes. Apert syndrome is an auto-

Figure 16-24: Syndactyly

Figure 16-25: Polydactyly

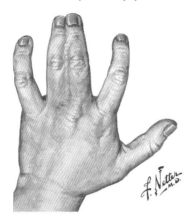

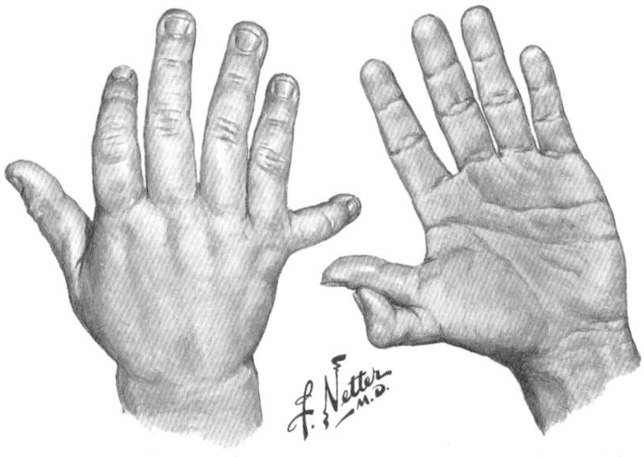

Postaxial   Preaxial

somal dominant condition that results in premature closure of the cranial sutures and complete, complex syndactyly of the hands and feet. Poland syndrome is a sporadic congenital deficiency of the pectoralis major ranging from hypoplasia to absence of the muscle that has a 3:1 male and 3:1 right-sided predominance. Hypoplasia of the distal upper extremity and varying degrees of brachydactyly and syndactyly may be present.

Because fingers differ in length, angular deformity may occur, and release before age 1 year is recommended for index-thumb and ring finger–small finger syndactyly. Long finger–ring finger syndactyly release may be delayed. The results of surgery are improved with a well-designed dorsal commissural flap and liberal use of full-thickness skin grafts. Recurrent web space contracture is the most common long-term complication.

Polydactyly

Polydactyly is the presence of extra digits on the hand or foot (**Figure 16-25**). The condition is usually postaxial (ulnar to the little finger or lateral to the fifth toe) or preaxial (radial to the thumb or medial to the great toe), but it may occur in a central location. Extra digits range from a vestigial digit attached by a narrow bridge of skin to a completely developed digit with its own metacarpal or metatarsal. Polydactyly may occur sporadically or as an autosomal dominant disorder. It is frequently ob-

served in 16 syndromes and is occasionally noted in 31 associated conditions.

Polydactyly of the foot usually causes difficulty with shoe wear. Even when polydactyly of the hand does not create functional difficulties, it causes a significant cosmetic deformity. Vestigial digits can be ablated with the use of a constricting, circumferential suture at the skin bridge. Otherwise, removal of accessory digits should be delayed until the child is 9 to 10 months old.

Camptodactyly

Camptodactyly (bent fingers) usually occurs at the PIP joint of the little finger. The extent of the flexion deformity varies. Approximately 70% of all patients have bilateral involvement. Other fingers may be involved, but incidence decreases toward the radial side of the hand. The natural history of untreated, severe camptodactyly is no improvement or a gradual increase in deformity with growth.

Camptodactyly may occur in isolation or may be associated with syndromes. Almost every conceivable structure has been implicated in the pathogenesis of isolated camptodactyly. Dynamic muscular imbalance is thought to be the primary cause in most cases. No treatment is uniformly successful, probably because it is difficult to differentiate primary and secondary contractures. Treatment begins with splinting. For the young child with persistent PIP joint contractures of 40° or greater and no bony changes, soft tissue releases are useful.

Clinodactyly

Clinodactyly is curvature of the finger in the radial or ulnar plane. The most common deformity is radial angulation of the little finger secondary to a delta-shaped middle phalanx. Clinodactyly is more common in males and is usually bilateral. The disorder is frequently seen in 30 syndromes and is found occasionally in 22 conditions. Isolated clinodactyly is usually simple (no rotation and less than 45° of angulation) and does not require treatment. Surgical realignment is indicated when overlap of the fingers interferes with gripping of objects.

Hypoplasia/Aplasia of the Thumb and Radial Hemimelia

Radial hemimelia and hypoplasia/aplasia of the thumb are part of a spectrum of congenital deletions of the radial portion of the upper limb. Radial hemimelia, also called *radial club hand,* is characterized by partial or complete absence of the radius, variable shortening and bowing of the ulna, radial deviation of the hand, variable defects in the radial carpal bones, and variable presence and stiffness of the thumb and index fingers (**Figure 16-26**). The extent of deficiency is also variable in *congenital hypoplasia/aplasia of the thumb*.

Both conditions may be associated with other disorders, including congenital heart disease (Holt-Oram syndrome), craniofacial abnormalities, vertebral anomalies (VATER association), and Fanconi anemia. TAR syndrome (thrombocytopenia with absent radius) is unique because in this syndrome, the thumb is normal. In other syndromes, if the radius is deficient, the thumb is also hypoplastic or absent.

Operative management is based on the severity of the deficiency. Reconstructive procedures are indicated when the hypoplastic thumb is adequately sized and the CMC joint is stable. Transfer of the index finger to the position of the thumb (index pollicization) is used in the treatment of severe thumb hypoplasia/aplasia. In patients with radial hemimelia, procedures to centralize the hand are performed at approximately 1 year of age, except when a short forearm and limited elbow motion are present.

Figure 16-26: Paraxial Radial Hemimelia

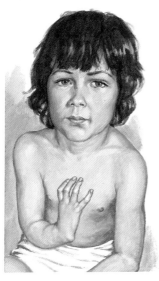 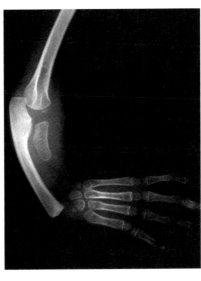

Short, bowed forearm with marked radial deviation of hand. Thumb absent. Radiograph shows partial deficit of radial ray (vestige of radius present). Scaphoid, trapezium, and metacarpal and phalanges of thumb absent.

Ulnar Hemimelia

Children with ulnar hemimelia have a deficiency of bone and soft tissue on the ulnar aspect of the forearm and hand. Deficiency of the ulna ranges from the presence of an ulna that is well formed but short to complete absence of the ulna, which may be associated with radiohumeral synostosis. In contrast to radial defects, ulnar hemimelia is uncommonly associated with abnormalities of other organ systems. However, patients with ulnar hemimelia are more likely to have other skeletal anomalies, including tibial hemimelia and scoliosis. Except to correct the associated digital deformities, surgical reconstruction is not commonly required in ulnar hemimelia.

ADDITIONAL READINGS

Berger RA, Weiss A-PC, eds. *Hand Surgery*. Philadelphia, Pa: Lippincott Williams and Wilkins; 2004.

Green DP, Hotchkiss RN, Pederson WC, Scott WW, eds. *Green's Operative Hand Surgery*, 5th edition. New York, NY: Churchill Livingstone; 2005.

Mackin EJ, Callahan AD, Osterman AL, Skirven TM, Schneider LH, Hunter JM, eds. *Hunter, Mackin, and Callahan's Rehabilitation of the Hand and Upper Extremity*, 5th edition. Philadelphia, Pa: Mosby; 2002.

Smith PJ, Lister G. *Lister's The Hand: Diagnosis and Indications*. Smith P, ed. New York, NY: Churchill Livingstone; 2002.

seventeen

The Pelvis, Hip, and Thigh

Roy K. Aaron, MD

Eric M. Bluman, MD, PhD

Michael G. Ehrlich, MD

Peter G. Trafton, MD, FACS

ANATOMY AND BIOMECHANICS

The pelvis is a basin-shaped structure that supports the spine and joins the axial skeleton to the lower extremities. At maturity, the pelvis includes two innominate bones—the sacrum and the coccyx. Each innominate bone is formed by the fusion of the ilium, ischium, and pubis at the *triradiate cartilage*, a trefoil-shaped growth plate that has an important role in determining the shape of the acetabulum, the congruency of the hip joint, and the propensity to osteoarthritis (**Figure 17-1**).

The ilium is a broad, fan-shaped bone with a concave inner table that tapers inferiorly to form the roof to the acetabulum. The ischium forms the inferior border of the obturator foramen and the posterior wall of the acetabulum. Its thickened tuberous portion bears significant weight when an individual is seated. The pubis forms the anterior wall of the acetabulum and includes the superior and inferior pubic rami, which form the remainder of the obturator foramen before joining together anteriorly at the fibrocartilaginous symphysis pubis.

The sacrum and the coccyx do not contain joints, and they function as a single unit. The posterior sacrum contains five neural foramina to allow passage of the four sacral nerve roots and a single inferior foramen for the filum terminale (**Figure 17-2**). The triangular sacrum is contoured into the two ilia. This interlocking shape, in addition to the very strong anterior and posterior sacroiliac ligaments, transmits the weight of the trunk to the lower extremities. The *sacroiliac joints* are synovial joints, but their interlocking shape permits no significant motion. Stability of the pelvis is enhanced by the sacroiliac, sacrospinous, sacrotuberous, iliolumbar, and symphyseal ligaments.

The ball-and-socket shape of the hip joint provides many degrees of freedom and resultant mobility. The articular surface of the acetabulum includes a broad, horseshoe-shaped outer rim called the *lunate surface*, a central

Figure 17-1: Hemipelvis

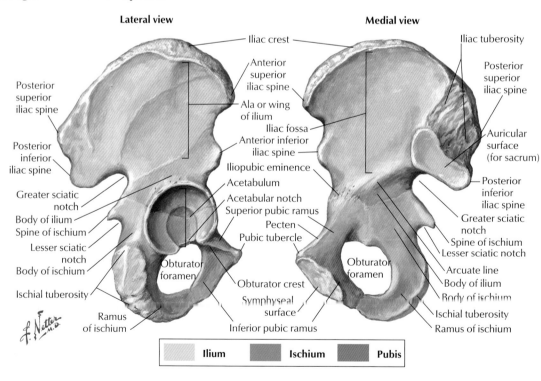

Lateral view   Medial view

Iliac crest

Iliac tuberosity

Anterior superior iliac spine

Posterior superior iliac spine

Posterior superior iliac spine

Ala or wing of ilium

Iliac fossa

Anterior inferior iliac spine

Auricular surface (for sacrum)

Posterior inferior iliac spine

Iliopubic eminence

Acetabulum

Acetabular notch

Superior pubic ramus

Pecten

Pubic tubercle

Posterior inferior iliac spine

Greater sciatic notch

Spine of ischium

Lesser sciatic notch

Arcuate line

Body of ilium

Body of ischium

Ischial tuberosity

Ramus of ischium

Posterior superior iliac spine

Posterior inferior iliac spine

Greater sciatic notch

Body of ilium

Spine of ischium

Lesser sciatic notch

Body of ischium

Ischial tuberosity

Obturator foramen

Obturator foramen

Obturator crest

Symphyseal surface

Inferior pubic ramus

Ramus of ischium

| Ilium | Ischium | Pubis |

Figure 17-2: Sacrum and Coccyx

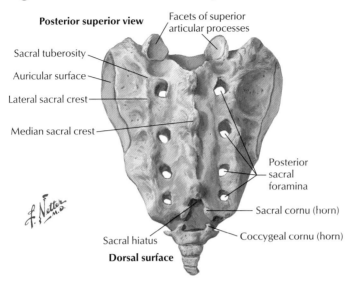

Posterior superior view

Facets of superior articular processes

Sacral tuberosity

Auricular surface

Lateral sacral crest

Median sacral crest

Posterior sacral foramina

Sacral cornu (horn)

Coccygeal cornu (horn)

Sacral hiatus

Dorsal surface

fossa that gives rise to the *ligamentum teres*, and an inferior notch that is bridged by the *transverse acetabular ligament* (**Figure 17-3**). The circumferential fibrocartilaginous acetabular labrum increases the effective surface area of the acetabulum by 40%, thereby reducing stress on the articular cartilage. The shape of the mature hip joint and its strong capsule makes dislocation unlikely without significant trauma.

The femur is the largest bone in the body and provides osseous support for the thigh. The proximal end includes the head, neck, and greater and lesser trochanters at the junction of the neck and femoral shaft. The neck-shaft angle varies somewhat with age and

Figure 17-3: Hip Joint

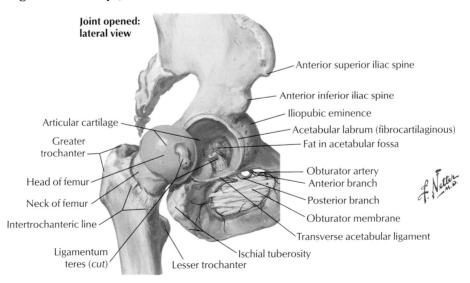

Joint opened: lateral view

Articular cartilage

Greater trochanter

Head of femur

Neck of femur

Intertrochanteric line

Ligamentum teres (*cut*)

Lesser trochanter

Ischial tuberosity

Anterior superior iliac spine

Anterior inferior iliac spine

Iliopubic eminence

Acetabular labrum (fibrocartilaginous)

Fat in acetabular fossa

Obturator artery

Anterior branch

Posterior branch

Obturator membrane

Transverse acetabular ligament

gender but is approximately 125° in adults—a position that places the center of the head at the level of the tip of the greater trochanter. *Coxa valga* is a neck-shaft angle greater than 135°; this condition places the femoral head above the trochanter and predisposes the patient to subluxation. *Coxa vara* is a neck-shaft angle less than 115°—a condition that decreases effective abductor muscle function and effectively shortens the thigh. The neck of the femur is anteverted, or anteriorly angled, in relationship to the femoral condyles, by about 15°. Blood to the femoral head is primarily supplied by the *medial circumflex femoral artery* through its subsynovial retinacular vessels (**Figure 17-4**). The lateral circumflex and ligamentum teres arteries provide minor contributions to the femoral head.

Almost the entire surface of the pelvis and thigh is covered by muscle (**Figure 17-5**). As a result, the pelvis and femur have a very good vascular supply that results in consistent fracture healing (femoral neck fractures are the exception). The chief flexor of the hip is the *iliopsoas,* which in reality comprises two muscles that come together at the iliopsoas ten-

don. Other significant flexors are the *tensor fascia lata, sartorius, rectus femoris, pectineus, adductor longus,* and *adductor brevis.* The chief extensor is the *gluteus maximus.* Other hip extensors are the hamstrings. The hip abductors are the *gluteus medius* and *gluteus minimus.* The hip adductors are the *adductor longus, adductor brevis, adductor magnus,* and *gracilis.* External rotators are the gluteus maximus and several small muscles that insert on or about the posterior edge of the greater trochanter. The primary internal rotators are the gluteus minimus and the tensor fascia lata.

The muscles of the thigh are arranged into three compartments: anterior (quadriceps), medial (adductors), and posterior (hamstrings) (**Figure 17-6**). Several muscles about the hip also cross the knee. Examples include the hamstrings, rectus femoris, sartorius, tensor fascia lata, and gracilis. These *two-joint muscles* are important in fine-tuning movement of the two joints, particularly during forceful activities, such as running. Furthermore, the span of these muscles across two joints must be understood if they are to be accurately examined for strength and possible contracture or strain.

Figure 17-4: Blood Supply to Femoral Head

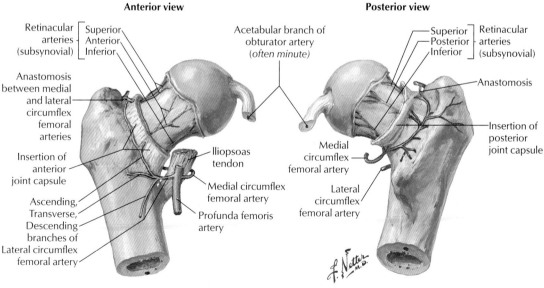

Figure 17-5: Bony Attachments of Buttock and Thigh Muscles

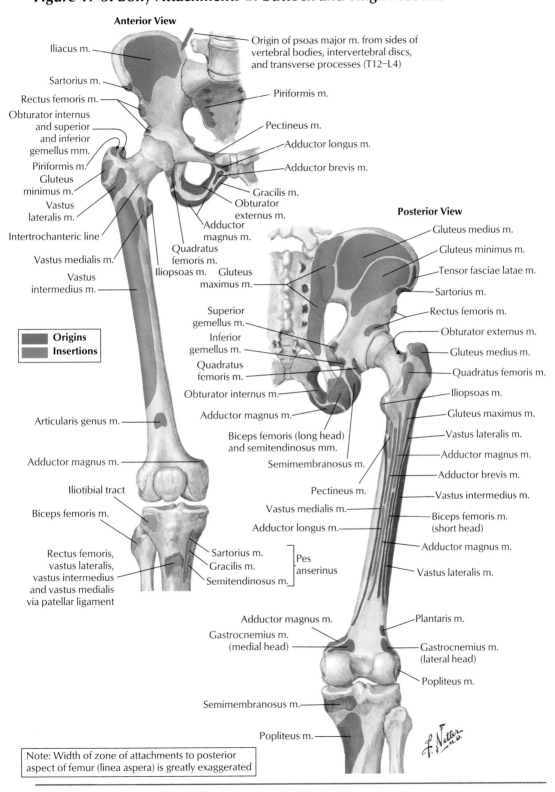

Anterior View

Iliacus m.

Sartorius m.

Rectus femoris m.

Obturator internus and superior and inferior gemellus mm.

Piriformis m.

Gluteus minimus m.

Vastus lateralis m.

Intertrochanteric line

Vastus medialis m.

Vastus intermedius m.

Origin of psoas major m. from sides of vertebral bodies, intervertebral discs, and transverse processes (T12–L4)

Piriformis m.

Pectineus m.

Adductor longus m.

Adductor brevis m.

Gracilis m.

Obturator externus m.

Adductor magnus m.

Quadratus femoris m.

Iliopsoas m.

Gluteus maximus m.

Origins
Insertions

Articularis genus m.

Adductor magnus m.

Iliotibial tract

Biceps femoris m.

Rectus femoris, vastus lateralis, vastus intermedius and vastus medialis via patellar ligament

Superior gemellus m.

Inferior gemellus m.

Quadratus femoris m.

Obturator internus m.

Adductor magnus m.

Biceps femoris (long head) and semitendinosus mm.

Semimembranosus m.

Pectineus m.

Vastus medialis m.

Adductor longus m.

Sartorius m.

Gracilis m.

Semitendinosus m.

Pes anserinus

Posterior View

Gluteus medius m.

Gluteus minimus m.

Tensor fasciae latae m.

Sartorius m.

Rectus femoris m.

Obturator externus m.

Gluteus medius m.

Quadratus femoris m.

Iliopsoas m.

Gluteus maximus m.

Vastus lateralis m.

Adductor magnus m.

Adductor brevis m.

Vastus intermedius m.

Biceps femoris m. (short head)

Adductor magnus m.

Vastus lateralis m.

Adductor magnus m.

Gastrocnemius m. (medial head)

Semimembranosus m.

Popliteus m.

Plantaris m.

Gastrocnemius m. (lateral head)

Popliteus m.

Note: Width of zone of attachments to posterior aspect of femur (linea aspera) is greatly exaggerated

Figure 17-6: Muscles of Hip and Thigh

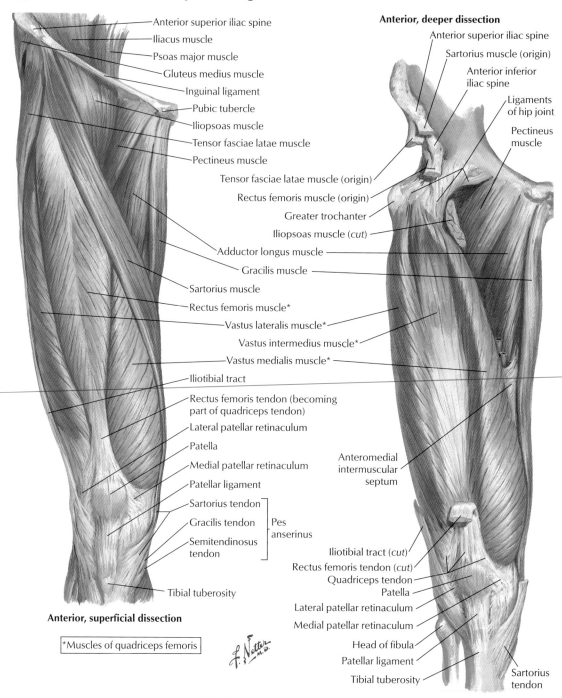

Anterior superior iliac spine
Iliacus muscle
Psoas major muscle
Gluteus medius muscle
Inguinal ligament
Pubic tubercle
Iliopsoas muscle
Tensor fasciae latae muscle
Pectineus muscle
Tensor fasciae latae muscle (origin)
Rectus femoris muscle (origin)
Greater trochanter
Iliopsoas muscle (*cut*)
Adductor longus muscle
Gracilis muscle
Sartorius muscle
Rectus femoris muscle*
Vastus lateralis muscle*
Vastus intermedius muscle*
Vastus medialis muscle*
Iliotibial tract
Rectus femoris tendon (becoming part of quadriceps tendon)
Lateral patellar retinaculum
Patella
Medial patellar retinaculum
Patellar ligament
Sartorius tendon
Gracilis tendon
Semitendinosus tendon
Tibial tuberosity

Anterior, superficial dissection

*Muscles of quadriceps femoris

Anterior, deeper dissection

Anterior superior iliac spine
Sartorius muscle (origin)
Anterior inferior iliac spine
Ligaments of hip joint
Pectineus muscle
Anteromedial intermuscular septum
Iliotibial tract (*cut*)
Rectus femoris tendon (*cut*)
Quadriceps tendon
Patella
Lateral patellar retinaculum
Medial patellar retinaculum
Head of fibula
Patellar ligament
Tibial tuberosity
Sartorius tendon

Pes anserinus

Figure 17-6: Muscles of Hip and Thigh (*continued*)

Posterior, superficial dissection

Posterior, deeper dissection

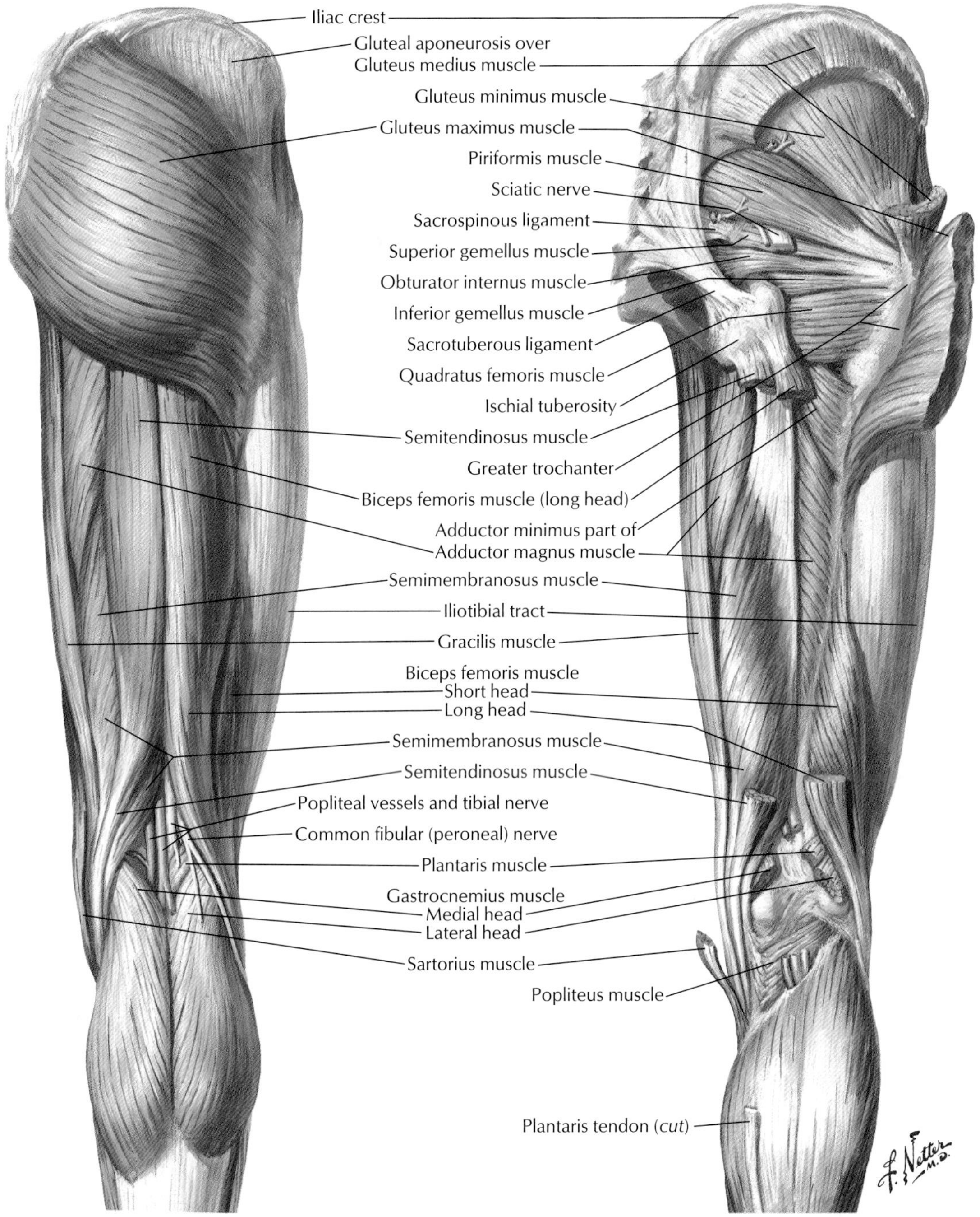

Iliac crest

Gluteal aponeurosis over Gluteus medius muscle

Gluteus minimus muscle

Gluteus maximus muscle

Piriformis muscle

Sciatic nerve

Sacrospinous ligament

Superior gemellus muscle

Obturator internus muscle

Inferior gemellus muscle

Sacrotuberous ligament

Quadratus femoris muscle

Ischial tuberosity

Semitendinosus muscle

Greater trochanter

Biceps femoris muscle (long head)

Adductor minimus part of Adductor magnus muscle

Semimembranosus muscle

Iliotibial tract

Gracilis muscle

Biceps femoris muscle
Short head
Long head

Semimembranosus muscle

Semitendinosus muscle

Popliteal vessels and tibial nerve

Common fibular (peroneal) nerve

Plantaris muscle

Gastrocnemius muscle
Medial head
Lateral head

Sartorius muscle

Popliteus muscle

Plantaris tendon (*cut*)

Figure 17-7: Lumbar Plexus

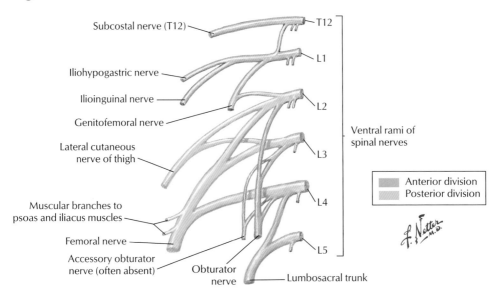

Subcostal nerve (T12)

Iliohypogastric nerve

Ilioinguinal nerve

Genitofemoral nerve

Lateral cutaneous nerve of thigh

Muscular branches to psoas and iliacus muscles

Femoral nerve

Accessory obturator nerve (often absent)

Obturator nerve

T12

L1

L2

L3

L4

L5

Ventral rami of spinal nerves

Anterior division
Posterior division

Lumbosacral trunk

The lumbar plexus is formed by L1–L4 ventral rami (**Figure 17-7**). The *femoral nerve* (posterior branches of L2–L4) enters the thigh lateral to the femoral artery. After supplying motor branches to the sartorius and quadriceps and cutaneous branches to the anterior thigh, the femoral nerve continues as the *saphenous nerve*, supplying sensation to the medial calf and ankle. The *obturator nerve* (anterior branches of L2–L4) supplies the adductor muscles and provides sensation in the medial thigh.

The sacral plexus is formed by the L4–S4 ventral rami (**Figure 17-8**). The nerves from the sacral plexus exit the pelvis posterior to the hip joint. The *superior gluteal nerve* (posterior branches L4–S1) innervates the primary hip abductors (gluteus medius and gluteus minimus). The *inferior gluteal nerve* (posterior branches L5–S2) innervates the primary hip extensor (gluteus maximus). The *sciatic nerve* includes the *tibial nerve* (anterior branches L4–S3) and the *common peroneal nerve* (posterior branches L4–S2). The tibial segment of the sciatic nerve innervates the posterior muscles of the thigh (except for the short head of the biceps femoris). The tibial segment of the sciatic nerve innervates the posterior muscles of the thigh except for the

short head of the biceps femoris, which is innervated by the peroneal component of the sciatic nerve.

The vessels, similar to the nerves, leave the pelvis anterior and posterior to the hip joint. The buttocks are supplied primarily by the *superior and inferior gluteal arteries*, which are branches of the internal iliac artery. The *femoral artery*, a continuation of the external iliac artery, supplies most of the remainder of the lower extremity. The femoral artery exits the pelvis between the femoral vein medially and the femoral nerve laterally and thereafter gives off the *profunda femoris* and the *medial* and *lateral circumflex femoral arteries* before continuing down the leg with the saphenous nerve deep to the sartorius. In the distal thigh, it passes to the posterior thigh through an opening in the adductor magnus, at which time its name is changed to the *popliteal artery* (**Figure 17-9**).

In quiet, two-legged standing, very minimal hip muscle force is necessary to maintain erect stance. However, during the midportion of the stance phase of gait, all the body weight is on one leg while the opposite limb is swinging through. At this time, a force of approximately 3 times body weight must be developed through the abductor muscles

Figure 17-8: Sacral Plexus

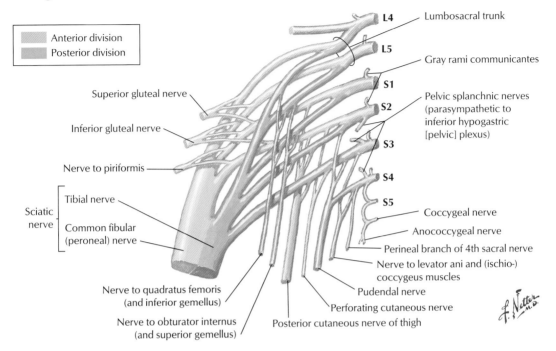

Anterior division
Posterior division

L4 — Lumbosacral trunk
L5
Gray rami communicantes
S1
S2 — Pelvic splanchnic nerves (parasympathetic to inferior hypogastric [pelvic] plexus)
S3
S4
S5

Superior gluteal nerve
Inferior gluteal nerve
Nerve to piriformis
Sciatic nerve
Tibial nerve
Common fibular (peroneal) nerve
Coccygeal nerve
Anococcygeal nerve
Perineal branch of 4th sacral nerve
Nerve to levator ani and (ischio-) coccygeus muscles
Pudendal nerve
Nerve to quadratus femoris (and inferior gemellus)
Perforating cutaneous nerve
Nerve to obturator internus (and superior gemellus)
Posterior cutaneous nerve of thigh

to counteract gravity and keep the pelvis from dropping down on the non–weight-bearing side. Weakness or paralysis of the hip abductor muscles from coxa vara or neuromuscular disorders may require compensatory gait mechanics. The patient leans over the affected hip during the stance phase (abductor or *Trendelenburg* lurch) to decrease the moment arm of the contralateral side. Likewise, an arthritic hip may increase friction at the joint surface, which results in greater abductor force required to balance the moment of body weight and compensation by Trendelenburg lurch. Using a cane in the opposite hand counteracts some of the stance limb weight-bearing forces and can be quite helpful in relieving pain and allowing patients with osteoarthritis or hip abductor weakness to walk more efficiently (see Chapter 12).

PHYSICAL EXAMINATION

With the patient standing, inspect the anterior thigh for quadriceps atrophy and overall alignment of the hip, knee, and ankle. From the posterior aspect, palpate the iliac crests.

Note any pelvic obliquity (one iliac crest lower than the other). A leg-length discrepancy causes an apparent obliquity that can be corrected by placing blocks under the shorter limb, but fixed obliquity from a spinal deformity or hip abduction contracture cannot be corrected by this maneuver. Other palpable landmarks are the greater trochanter; the *anterior superior iliac spine* (ASIS); and, deep to the dimples of Venus, the *posterior superior iliac spine* (PSIS).

Observe the patient walking. If the problem is primarily pain without significant deformity, the patient will shorten the stance phase on the affected side (coxalgic gait). If the problem is abductor muscle weakness or severe arthritis, the patient will compensate by means of Trendelenburg lurch.

The hip joint allows motion in all planes. With the pelvis stabilized (preventing pelvic-vertebral motion), the average range of hip flexion in adults is 120°, and extension is 15°. Abduction averages 40°, adduction averages 30°, and internal and external rotation (with the hip in extension) are both

Figure 17-9: Arteries and Nerves of Thigh

Superficial dissection

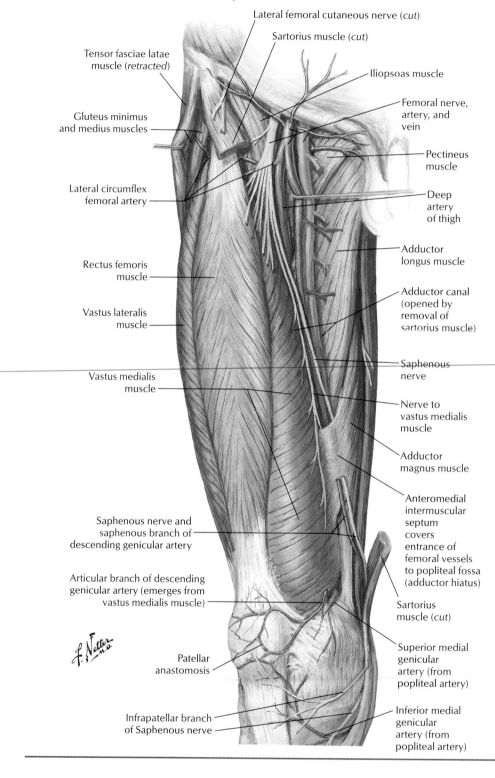

Lateral femoral cutaneous nerve (*cut*)

Sartorius muscle (*cut*)

Tensor fasciae latae muscle (*retracted*)

Iliopsoas muscle

Femoral nerve, artery, and vein

Gluteus minimus and medius muscles

Pectineus muscle

Lateral circumflex femoral artery

Deep artery of thigh

Adductor longus muscle

Rectus femoris muscle

Adductor canal (opened by removal of sartorius muscle)

Vastus lateralis muscle

Saphenous nerve

Vastus medialis muscle

Nerve to vastus medialis muscle

Adductor magnus muscle

Anteromedial intermuscular septum covers entrance of femoral vessels to popliteal fossa (adductor hiatus)

Saphenous nerve and saphenous branch of descending genicular artery

Sartorius muscle (*cut*)

Articular branch of descending genicular artery (emerges from vastus medialis muscle)

Superior medial genicular artery (from popliteal artery)

Patellar anastomosis

Infrapatellar branch of Saphenous nerve

Inferior medial genicular artery (from popliteal artery)

approximately 30° to 40°. Greater degrees of rotation, particularly external rotation, are observed if the measurements are made with the hip flexed.

The *zero starting position* for measuring hip motion is with the thigh in line with the trunk. In measuring flexion and extension, the opposite hip is held in enough flexion to prevent pelvic-vertebral motion. Avoid positioning the opposite hip in excessive flexion because this position will rock the pelvis into abnormal inclination, thereby creating a false-positive

hip flexion contracture. Instead, flex the opposite hip to a position where the lumbar spine just starts to flatten or, more precisely, to a position in which the inclination of the pelvis is similar to a normal standing posture (ASIS inferior to PSIS by approximately 3°). Maximum flexion is the point at which the pelvis begins to rotate. Now, allow the hip to extend. If the patient has a hip flexion contracture, the pelvis will start to rock before the leg reaches the examination table (positive Thomas sign) (**Figure 17-10**).

Figure 17-10: Measurement of Hip Flexion/Extension and Thomas Test

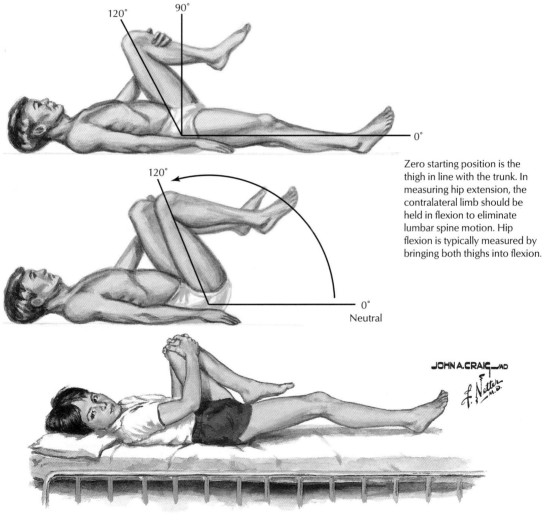

Zero starting position is the thigh in line with the trunk. In measuring hip extension, the contralateral limb should be held in flexion to eliminate lumbar spine motion. Hip flexion is typically measured by bringing both thighs into flexion.

Positive Thomas test indicates a hip flexion contracture, ie, the affected hip cannot be extended to the neutral position.

Measure abduction and adduction with the pelvis level (limbs 90° to a transverse line across the ASISs). Maximum abduction is reached when the pelvis begins to tilt—a movement that you can detect by keeping one hand on the opposite ASIS while moving the leg. For adults, it is more practical to measure rotation with the hips in flexion. However, this approach should not be used in children or when femoral torsion is assessed (see Chapter 3).

Assess hip flexors with the patient seated. To quantify strength, ask the patient to flex the hip, and then resist the effort. Test the gluteus maximus with the patient prone and the knee flexed 90° (to minimize concurrent hamstring activity). Hip abductor strength is measured with the patient lying on the unaffected side; ask the patient to abduct the hip while you resist the effort. *Trendelenburg test* is a useful maneuver for assessing hip abductor function (**Figure 17-11**). Place your hands on both iliac crests, and ask the patient to stand on one leg. A positive test is dropping of the pelvis on the opposite side and results from either abductor weakness or hip dysplasia and resultant abnormal abductor mechanics.

FABER (*flexion*, *abduction*, and external *rotation*) is a stress maneuver that chiefly detects sacroiliac pathology. Place the hip in 90° of flexion and maximum abduction and external rotation. Apply a posteriorly directed force to the knee. A positive test is increased pain. A positive FABER sign, however, is not specific for sacroiliac pathology, as it may be found with hip joint pathology or may be a nonorganic finding.

DEGENERATIVE DISEASES AND DISORDERS

Osteoarthritis

Osteoarthritis of the hip may be primary (idiopathic) or secondary to an underlying hip disorder (eg, pediatric hip disease, osteonecrosis, previous infection, or previous trauma). Typical presenting symptoms are indolent onset of anterior thigh or groin pain that is deep and activity related. Occasionally,

Figure 17-11: Trendelenburg Test

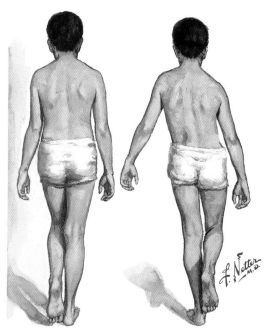

Trendelenburg test
Left: Patient demonstrates negative Trendelenburg test of normal right hip. **Right:** positive test of involved left hip. When patient is standing on the affected side, the pelvis on the opposite side drops, indicating either actual weakness of the gluteus medius muscle, functional weakness of the hip abductors secondary to altered alignment of the hip joint, or a painful arthritic hip joint that cannot tolerate the normal force of hip abductor contraction during single-legged stance. The trunk shifts to the left as patient attempts to decrease biomechanical stresses across involved hip and thereby maintain balance.

the pain is referred to the buttocks or distal thigh. As degeneration of the articular cartilage progresses, the duration and the frequency of the pain intensify. Pain at rest or pain that wakens the patient at night is associated with severe arthritis.

The most sensitive sign of early osteoarthritis of the hip is loss of internal rotation (**Figure 17-12**). As the disease and joint contractures progress, decreased abduction, flexion, and extension are observed. A coxalgic limp, with or without Trendelenburg lurch, is often present.

Anteroposterior (AP) and lateral radiographs show joint space narrowing in the early stages and osteophytes, cyst formation, and sclerosis as the disease progresses (**Figure 17-13**). Osteophytes can occur in the

Figure 17-12: Osteoarthritis of the Hip

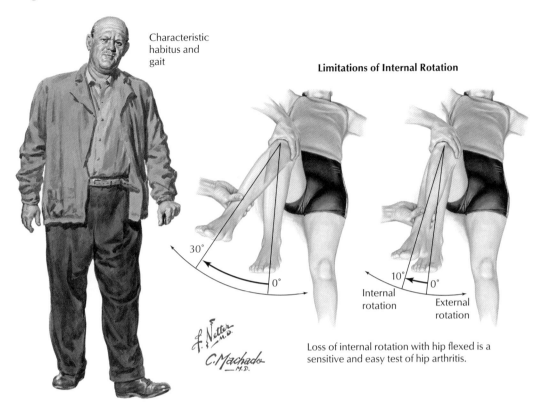

Characteristic habitus and gait

Limitations of Internal Rotation

30°

0°

10°

0°

Internal rotation

External rotation

Loss of internal rotation with hip flexed is a sensitive and easy test of hip arthritis.

floor of the acetabulum and around the periphery of the femoral head and may cause lateralization and proximal migration of the femoral head.

Figure 17-13: Osteoarthritis of the Hip

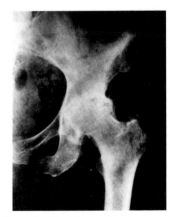

AP radiograph of the hip showing degeneration of cartilage and osteophytes at margins of acetabulum

The differential diagnosis includes:
+ Osteonecrosis of the femoral head (evident on radiographs)
+ Trochanteric bursitis (localized tenderness, normal radiographs)
+ Lateral femoral nerve entrapment (burning pain, sensory changes, normal motion)
+ Lumbar disc herniation or degenerative disc disease (buttock pain, distal motor and sensory changes, no restriction of hip motion)
+ Tumors of the lumbar spine, pelvis, or upper thigh (back pain, night pain, normal motion)

Nonoperative treatment includes education of the patient, activity modification, optimization of any leg-length discrepancies (often with a small heel lift), and judicious use of nonsteroidal anti-inflammatory drugs (NSAIDs). Physiotherapy to improve range of motion is often unsuccessful because this type of exercise provokes joint pain. Low-impact exercises, particularly swimming, may improve muscle strength. As the disease progresses, the patient will benefit from the use of a cane in the opposite hand.

Adolescents and young adults who have malalignment of the acetabulum, proximal femur, or both, may benefit from realignment osteotomies of the pelvis, proximal femur, or both. Arthrodesis should be considered for adolescents or young adults with unilateral end-stage arthritis and no other significant limb dysfunction. In other patients who have severe pain and joint erosions, a total hip replacement arthroplasty is indicated (see **Figure 4-8**). These procedures can dramatically reduce pain and improve function, but the decision for surgery should be made with an understanding of potential complications, including infection (0.5% to 1.0%), dislocation (8% to 10%), and deep venous thrombosis (40% to 60% if no prophylaxis is used).

The long-term concern of total joint arthroplasty is aseptic loosening. When a joint implant is loose and has to be revised, less bone stock is available and the rates of all complications are higher, particularly the rate of recurrent loosening. The risk of needing to replace a hip arthroplasty is very low in a patient older than 65 years, who typically places moderate demands on the joint and who has a limited life expectancy, but it is virtually universal in a young adult who is in good health and places more strenuous demands on the joint. Appropriate preoperative planning and better implants have improved the results of both primary and revision arthroplasty.

Osteonecrosis

The femoral head, with its vulnerable circulation (see **Figure 17-4**), is the most common site of osteonecrosis. The true incidence is difficult to establish, but osteonecrosis accounts for 5% to 10% of the total hip replacements done in the United States. The cause and pathophysiology of osteonecrosis are discussed in Chapter 2; in brief, some disturbance of circulation causes death of osteocytes in a variably sized segment of the femoral head. Subsequent secondary structural changes lead to femoral head collapse and, ultimately, end-stage arthritis.

Common causes of femoral head osteonecrosis include trauma (hip dislocations and femoral neck fractures), corticosteroid use, sickle cell disease, systemic lupus erythematosus, and alcohol abuse. The male-to-female ratio is approximately 4:1. Osteonecrosis is bilateral in approximately 50% of patients, but the onset of disease and symptoms is typically earlier on one side.

Indolent onset of dull, activity-related pain is the usual presenting symptom, with the pain most often located in the groin or buttock. However, the onset of pain may begin suddenly if an acute collapse or shear fracture involves the articular surface. Early signs include decreased internal rotation and abduction. As incongruity of the joint progresses, the pain increases, the gait becomes antalgic, and range of motion decreases.

Good-quality AP and lateral radiographs are important in making the diagnosis. Sclerosis is a typical radiographic finding early in the disease process; however, in the early stage of osteonecrosis, the radiographs may be normal, but magnetic resonance imaging (MRI) will be positive (see **Figure 2-14**). MRI also is useful in defining the extent of osteonecrosis and identifying early osteonecrosis in patients who are susceptible to bilateral involvement and who have normal radiographs of the contralateral hip.

Treatment and prognosis depend on the extent of osteonecrosis and the degree of joint congruity. Observation is indicated if the area of osteonecrosis is small and unlikely to cause collapse of the articular surface. The optimal procedure if the area of osteonecrosis is large but the joint has not collapsed is highly debatable at this time. Options include vascularized or nonvascularized structural bone grafts, osteoinductive grafts, osteotomies, and electrical stimulation. For hips that have progressed to significant segmental collapse, total hip arthroplasty is the best salvage procedure. Because many patients are young, subsequent revision arthroplasty, with its attendant problems, is common.

MISCELLANEOUS AND SPECIAL CONDITIONS

Trochanteric Bursitis

Inflammation of the greater trochanteric bursae, known as *trochanteric bursitis,* is the most common cause of bursitis about the hip. This problem is more common in females and middle-aged to older patients. The problem may be isolated or associated with lumbar spine disorders, hip conditions, leg-length discrepancy, rheumatoid arthritis, previous surgery about the hip, and ipsilateral quadriceps weakness and knee conditions. Sometimes, it is difficult to distinguish whether the pain over the greater trochanter is referred pain or a concomitant bursitis. Tendinosis of the gluteus medius and minimus tendons is also difficult to distinguish.

Typical symptoms include pain and tenderness in the region of the greater trochanter that may radiate to the lateral thigh. Symptoms may be increased in the morning on initiation of walking, after extended walking, or on rising after sitting for a period of time. Patients note discomfort when lying on the affected side. Examination demonstrates tenderness over the lateral aspect of the greater trochanter that is exacerbated at the extremes of adduction and internal rotation.

Treatment includes activity modifications, use of a cane, and NSAIDs. Injection of the bursa with corticosteroids and a local anesthetic can be diagnostic and therapeutic. Surgery is rarely needed.

Snapping Hip

Snapping or popping sensations about the hip are usually caused by tendons sliding over bony prominences, but occasionally may be symptoms of uncommon problems such as acetabular labral tears or intra-articular loose bodies. In most patients, the snapping is mild clicking that is not painful and resolves without treatment. A few patients have pain that is persistent and limiting.

The iliotibial band moving over the greater trochanter is the most common site of snapping. If symptoms are severe, the patient feels that "the joint is coming out of the socket." Snapping and pain are commonly noted when climbing stairs, when rising from a seated position, or when lying with the affected side up and rotating the leg. Examination typically shows no restriction of motion or abnormal gait. Snapping of the iliotibial band can be provoked if the patient stands with the leg adducted, then rotates the hip. A snap or subluxation will be perceived over the greater trochanter.

Snapping of the iliopsoas tendon is caused by subluxation of the tendon over the iliopectineal eminence as the hip goes from flexion to extension. Patients perceive pain in the groin.

AP and lateral radiographs of the hip are obtained to exclude other conditions such as osteoarthritis, osteonecrosis, and intra-articular loose bodies. Treatment in most patients constitutes explanation of the condition and observation. Patients with pain are managed with activity modification, judicious use of NSAIDs, and stretching exercises for associated iliotibial band contractures. Corticosteroid injections may be helpful for more resistant cases. Surgery is infrequently needed and is reserved for cases that do not respond to nonoperative management.

Meralgia Paresthetica

Meralgia paresthetica is entrapment of the *lateral femoral cutaneous nerve,* usually between the inguinal ligament and the medial edge of the sartorius. This syndrome is associated with obesity, direct compression from tight clothing or straps around the waist (eg, tool belts or backpacks), scar tissue from previous operations, or repetitive trauma over the nerve. Infrequently, an intrapelvic mass causes compression of the nerve.

Typical symptoms include pain and dysesthesia that radiate to the lateral aspect of the thigh. Examination typically shows decreased sensation in the distribution of the lateral femoral cutaneous nerve and positive Tinel sign medial to the ASIS. Muscle strength, hip motion, and the abdominal examination are normal unless a concomitant disorder is present.

Treatment includes avoidance of clothes or activities that compress the nerve. Weight reduction can alleviate symptoms in obese patients. A corticosteroid and local anesthetic injection can be diagnostic and occasionally therapeutic. Surgical release is indicated for persistent and severe symptoms.

TRAUMATIC DISORDERS

Fractures of the Pelvis

Although the acetabulum is part of the pelvis, the term *pelvic fractures* is typically restricted to fractures of the pelvic ring. These fractures range from low-impact injuries that are simple to treat to high-impact injuries that cause hemodynamic instability, may be life threatening, and result in a very unstable pelvis.

Pelvic ring injuries can be classified as stable or unstable. Stable injuries involve only one side of the ring. Examples include direct-impact fracture of the sacrum, coccyx, or iliac wing and isolated pubic ramus fractures associated with low-energy falls in osteoporotic elderly individuals (**Figure 17-14**). Stable injuries can be treated symptomatically with crutch- or walker-assisted ambulation.

Unstable pelvic fractures include fracture and/or ligamentous disruption in two parts of the ring. Examples include *straddle injuries* with bilateral superior and inferior pubic rami fractures, *lateral compression injuries* with overlapping pelvis, *open book fractures* with disruption of symphysis pubis and anterior sacroiliac ligaments, and *vertical shear fractures* with ipsilateral disruption of the anterior and posterior ring (**Figures 17-15** and **17-16**). Some unstable pelvic fractures can be treated nonoperatively with a period of bed rest to

Figure 17-14: Stable Pelvic Ring Fractures

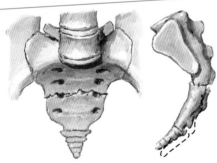
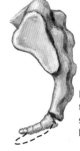

Transverse fracture of the sacrum that is minimally displaced

Fracture usually requires no treatment other than care in sitting; inflatable ring helpful. Pain may persist for a long time.

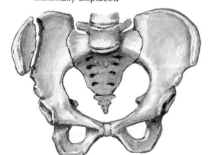

Fracture of iliac wing from direct blow

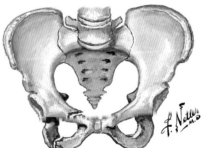

Fracture of ipsilateral pubic and ischial ramus requires only symptomatic treatment with short-term bed rest and limited activity with walker- or crutch-assisted ambulation for 4 to 6 weeks.

Figure 17-15: Unstable Pelvic Fractures

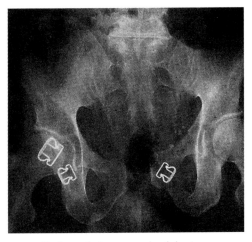

Radiograph shows open book fracture.

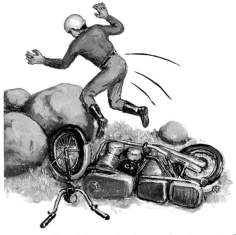

Caused by forceful impact to knee or foot transmitted to pelvis or by direct blow to pelvis.

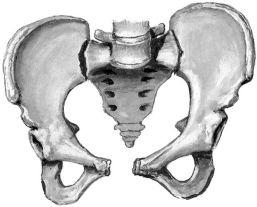

Open book fracture. Disruption of symphysis pubis with wide anterior separation of pelvic ring. Anterior sacroiliac ligaments are torn, with slight opening of sacroiliac joints. Intact posterior sacroiliac ligaments prevent vertical migration of the pelvis.

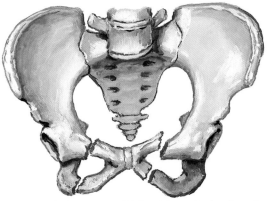

Straddle fracture. Double break in continuity of anterior pelvic ring causes instability but usually little displacement. Visceral (especially genitourinary) injury likely.

Vertical shear fracture.
Upward and posterior dislocation of sacroiliac joint and fracture of both pubic rami on same side result in upward shift of hemipelvis. Note also fracture of transverse process of 5th lumbar vertebra (L5), avulsion of ischial spine, and stretching of sacral nerves.

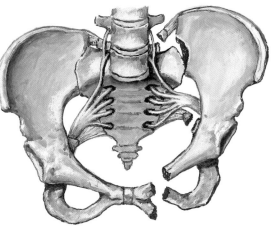

Figure 17-16: Internal Fixation for Type of Vertical Shear Fracture

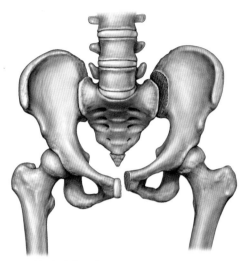

Vertical shear fracture with disruption of symphysis pubis and sacroiliac joint

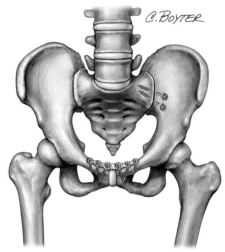

Reduction and internal fixation with percutaneous screw fixation of the sacroiliac joint and open reduction and plate fixation of the symphysis pubis disruption

allow initial healing, followed by progression to assisted ambulation. Other injuries require reduction and internal fixation of one or both sides of the ring to avoid or minimize the risk of pelvic deformity and associated pain and dysfunction.

Examination shows tenderness on compression and possible instability of the pelvis. Evaluation should include assessment for all potential associated injuries. Most injuries are obvious on an AP radiograph of the pelvis; however, special views and computed tomographic (CT) scans are frequently required to delineate the full extent of injury.

Acetabular Fractures

Acetabular fractures often result from high-impact falls or motor vehicle accidents that transmit force most commonly from an impact to the greater trochanter or the flexed knee. These intra-articular fractures may result in a disabling, traumatic arthropathy. Associated injuries such as posterior dislocation of the hip and fracture of the femoral head complicate treatment and results.

Examination should include assessment of sciatic, femoral, and obturator nerve function.

The peroneal segment of the sciatic nerve is at greatest risk. Radiographic evaluation includes AP radiographs of the pelvis, and internal and external Judet views (AP radiographs centered on the hip with the pelvis rotated 45° internally and externally). A CT scan further characterizes the injury.

The Judet and Letournel classification of acetabular fractures is most commonly used (**Figure 17-17**). If the injury involves a significant portion of the weight-bearing dome and the articular surface is displaced more than 2 mm, open reduction and internal fixation are required to minimize the risk of traumatic arthritis (**Figure 17-18**).

Hip Dislocation

Approximately 90% of hip dislocations are posterior and are caused by a high-energy impact on the knee of a person sitting with the hip flexed and adducted (**Figure 17-19**). Less adduction of the hip at injury makes an associated posterior acetabular wall fracture more likely. These injuries typically occur to unbelted automobile occupants and would be rare if seat belt use were more prevalent. Fracture of the acetabulum,

Figure 17-17: Acetabular Fractures

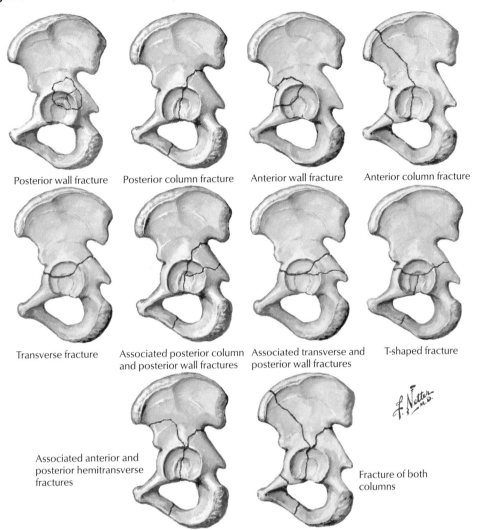

Posterior wall fracture

Posterior column fracture

Anterior wall fracture

Anterior column fracture

Transverse fracture

Associated posterior column and posterior wall fractures

Associated transverse and posterior wall fractures

T-shaped fracture

Associated anterior and posterior hemitransverse fractures

Fracture of both columns

shear fracture of the medial femoral head, or both, may be present. The vascular supply to the femoral head and the sciatic nerve are vulnerable.

Anterior dislocations often occur in sporting events. A forceful abduction and external rotation movement ruptures the stout anterior capsule, with the femoral head typically displaced to an inferior obturator position (**Figure 17-20**). Impaction fractures of the posterior femoral head may occur. The femoral nerve and artery are vulnerable.

Patients with posterior dislocations present with the hip held in flexion, adduction, and internal rotation and have apparent shortening of the limb. Persons with anterior dislocations present with the leg in marked abduction and external rotation. An AP radiograph of the pelvis and a cross-table lateral view confirm the diagnosis.

Prompt treatment of posterior dislocations is mandated because the incidence of osteonecrosis of the femoral head progressively increases when reduction is delayed. Most

Figure 17-18: Acetabular Fracture Fixation

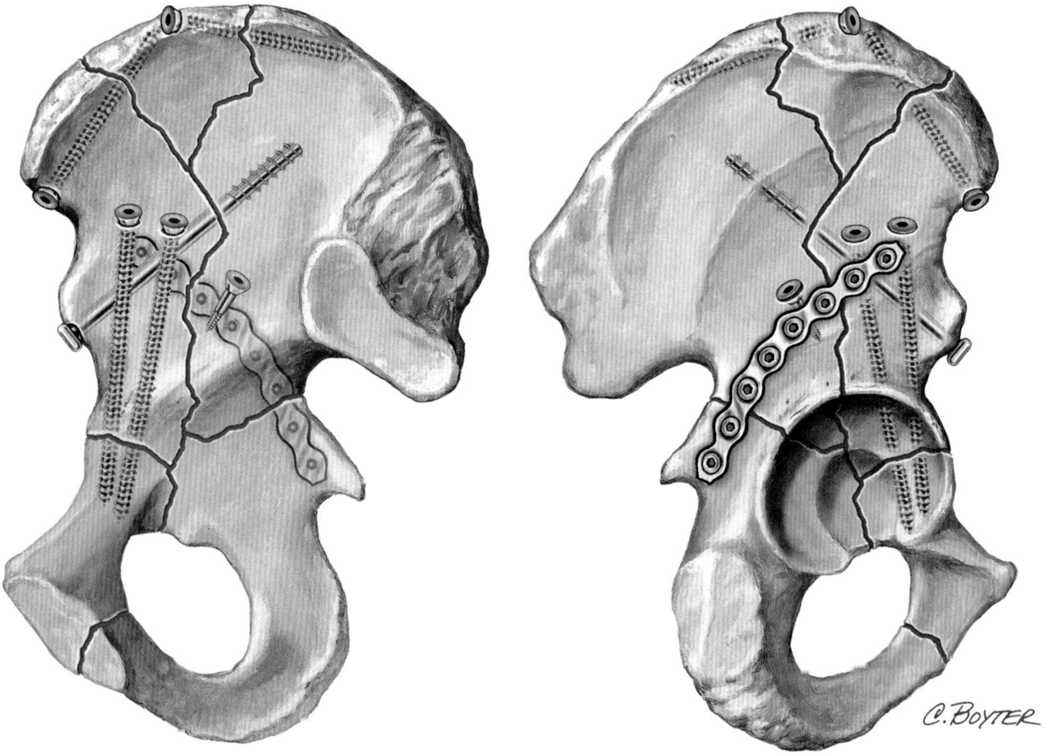

Representative fixation for both-column fracture with associated iliac wing fractures

hip dislocations can be reduced by closed means using either conscious sedation or general anesthesia. Principles of reducing a posterior dislocation include traction with the hip in a position of 90° flexion and slight adduction. As the femoral head reenters the acetabulum, there is a palpable clunk. Post-reduction radiographs are critically assessed to confirm a congruent reduction and no evidence of osteochondral fragments in the joint. Subsequent management depends on associated injuries and stability of the joint. Uncomplicated dislocations can be managed with activity modifications and crutch-assisted ambulation.

Fractures of the Proximal Femur

Fractures of the proximal femur, often called *hip fractures,* are very common in the elderly population. After the age of 50 years, the incidence of hip fractures doubles for every 6 years of age. Factors that increase the risk of fracture are those that exacerbate osteoporosis and those that increase the likelihood of a fall. Therefore, associated risk factors include age, gender, race, alcoholism, rheumatoid arthritis, sedentary lifestyle, cerebral dysfunction, dementia, cerebrovascular disease, use of psychotropic medications, and peripheral neuropathies.

The goals of treatment are to reduce mortality (10% to 30% in elderly patients at 6 months after hip fracture) and return patients to their preoperative functional status. Increased mortality is associated with male gender, advanced age, poorly controlled systemic disease, cerebral dysfunction, institutionalization, internal fixation before optimization or correction of medical problems, and postoperative complications. Factors associated with return to independent function include absence of mental impairment,

Figure 17-19: Posterior Dislocation of Hip

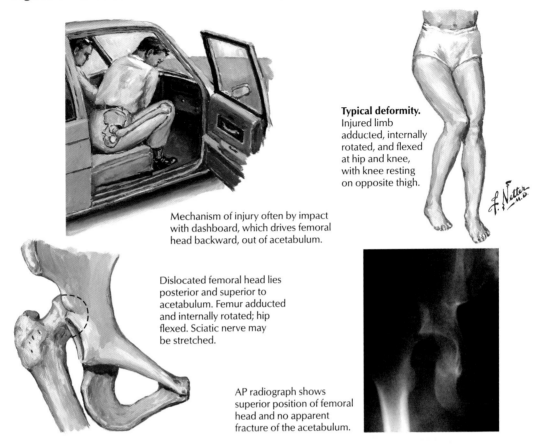

Mechanism of injury often by impact with dashboard, which drives femoral head backward, out of acetabulum.

Typical deformity. Injured limb adducted, internally rotated, and flexed at hip and knee, with knee resting on opposite thigh.

Dislocated femoral head lies posterior and superior to acetabulum. Femur adducted and internally rotated; hip flexed. Sciatic nerve may be stretched.

AP radiograph shows superior position of femoral head and no apparent fracture of the acetabulum.

Figure 17-20: Anterior Dislocation of Hip, Obturator Type

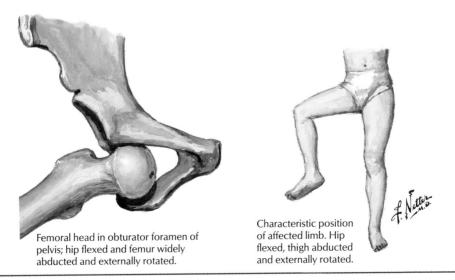

Femoral head in obturator foramen of pelvis; hip flexed and femur widely abducted and externally rotated.

Characteristic position of affected limb. Hip flexed, thigh abducted and externally rotated.

independent community ambulation prior to injury (as opposed to walking only in therapy sessions or around the house), the presence of another person in the home, and interdisciplinary management.

Most hip fractures are caused by a fall from a standing position with a direct blow over the greater trochanter. The two patterns of injury are femoral neck and intertrochanteric fractures (**Figures 17-21** and **17-22**). Osteonecrosis of the femoral head and nonunion may complicate femoral neck fractures; however, patients with intertrochanteric fractures have an overall poorer prognosis because, on average, they are older and typically have more limited preoperative ambulation function.

Presenting symptoms include an inability to walk after a fall and pain in the groin or buttock. Patients with a displaced fracture lie with the extremity shortened and with the hip in external rotation and slight abduction. Patients with nondisplaced fracture may have no obvious deformity but a positive *log-roll test* (pain on internal and external rotation of the limb).

AP and cross-table lateral radiographs of the hip demonstrate most fractures. MRI is the most sensitive test for identifying an occult fracture.

Treatment and complications are determined by whether the fracture is in the femoral neck or the intertrochanteric region. *Femoral neck fractures* that are impacted or nondisplaced have a low rate of nonunion (<5%) and avascular necrosis (<10%); however, in displaced femoral neck fractures, the incidence of avascular necrosis (AVN) is approximately 40%, and the nonunion rate is 10% or greater. Nondisplaced femoral neck fractures are best treated by multiple-screw fixation. Displaced femoral neck fractures in active, healthy elderly patients are best treated by reduction and screw fixation, but this injury in older, sedentary individuals is better managed by a hemiarthroplasty prosthetic replacement.

Fractures of the femoral neck occurring in young adults are usually secondary to high-impact motor vehicle accidents. The degree of soft tissue damage is greater, and therefore, the incidence of AVN is much higher (approximately 80% in persons 20–40 years of age). This is a "vascular emergency," and urgent reduction is required. In the elderly population, the timing of surgery is less urgent; however, unless there are comorbidities that must be corrected, patients do better if the hip fracture is reduced and fixed within 24 to 48 hours.

Although technically a femoral neck injury, a cervicotrochanteric fracture, or fracture at the base of the femoral neck, has a low

Figure 17-21: Fracture of Femoral Neck and Intertrochanteric Fracture of Femur

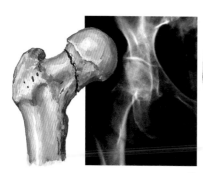

Nondisplaced femoral neck fracture

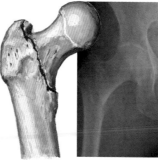

Two-part, minimally displaced intertrochanteric femur fracture

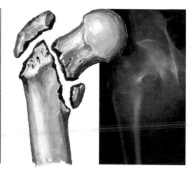

Comminuted four-part intertrochanteric femur fracture

incidence of osteonecrosis. Furthermore, these fractures cannot be adequately fixed with multiple pins and should be managed with techniques used for intertrochanteric fractures.

Intertrochanteric fractures of the femur occur in a region of ample blood supply. Therefore, fracture hemorrhage may be a problem, but the incidences of osteonecrosis and nonunion are low. Stable intertrochanteric fractures are two-part fractures without significant posteromedial comminution in the posterior medial aspect of the region. Unstable fractures have posteromedial comminution and frequently are three- or four-part injuries with separate fractures of the lesser trochanter, greater trochanter, or both.

Intertrochanteric fractures of the femur are best managed by reduction and internal fixation with the use of a device that stabilizes the head and neck to the shaft while the intertrochanteric fracture heals. The development of compression sliding hip screws has significantly reduced the complication of the fixation device cutting out of the osteopenic femoral head during the healing process (**Figure 17-22**).

Fractures of the Femoral Shaft

Femoral shaft fractures in adults are usually the result of high-energy trauma in younger patients with normal bone. Consequently, these fractures usually are displaced and have obvious swelling and pain. AP and lateral radiographs confirm the diagnosis. Over the past 30 years, treatment of femoral shaft fractures has evolved from several weeks of skeletal traction followed by several weeks of cast immobilization to early reduction and intramedullary rod fixation (**Figure 17-23**). This change has greatly reduced the morbidity associated with prolonged immobilization, as well as the incidences of malunion, limb shortening, and nonunion. Furthermore, in multiply injured patients, early stabilization of femoral shaft fractures greatly reduces the risks of pulmonary and other systemic complications.

Figure 17-22: Intertrochanteric Fracture of Femur

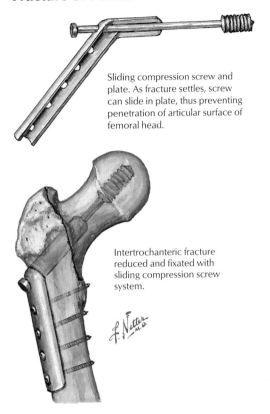

Sliding compression screw and plate. As fracture settles, screw can slide in plate, thus preventing penetration of articular surface of femoral head.

Intertrochanteric fracture reduced and fixated with sliding compression screw system.

Fractures of the Femur in Children

As in adults, fractures of the femur in children may occur anywhere (femoral neck, intertrochanteric, femoral shaft, etc.), but in children, most injuries involve the femoral shaft. In young children, child abuse should be considered. The incidence of abuse is particularly high in children younger than 1 year; at this age it is approximately 50% in those who present with an apparent isolated fracture of the femur.

Treatment of femoral fractures in children varies according to fracture location, age of the child, and degree of displacement. Nondisplaced femoral neck and intertrochanteric fractures can be treated in a spica cast. Displaced fractures in these locations should be treated with reduction and internal fixation, often supplemented by spica casting in a young child.

Femoral shaft fractures in children up to 6 years of age are most often treated by immediate reduction and spica cast immobilization. If the fracture is significantly displaced, children are placed in skeletal traction until enough callus has formed to allow maintenance of alignment in a cast. Older children may be candidates for fixation of femoral shaft fractures. Flexible intramedullary rods are often used in the 6- to 12-year-old child. Older adolescents and younger obese children often require intramedullary rod fixation, but the insertion point should be through the greater trochanter to diminish the risk of osteonecrosis that has a small but greater prevalence when the proximal femoral physis is still open and the standard entry site is used (slightly posterior to the pyriformis fossa).

Strains and Contusions of the Pelvis and Thigh

Strains of thigh muscles typically occur in a sporting event or fall when a muscle forcefully contracts while it is in a relatively lengthened position (on stretch). In addition to the history, the key to diagnosis is location of the pain and exacerbation of the pain on muscle contraction against resistance and on passive stretch of the muscle. The latter is a more sensitive test. For example, a strain of the hip adductors is indicated by groin pain that is increased by contraction of the adductors and by movement of the hip into abduction. The position of the knee and hip must be controlled when two-joint muscles are assessed. For example, a strain of the semitendinous muscle is indicated by pain in the posteromedial thigh that is exacerbated by flexing the hip to 90°, then extending the knee.

For most patients, modification of activities, followed by simple home exercises and progressive resumption to full activity, is adequate. Rehabilitation of elite athletes usually includes a more aggressive and costly regimen.

A direct blow to the anterior thigh can cause a painful and disabling hemorrhage into the quadriceps. Examination should exclude evaluation for a compartment syndrome, and radiographs may be required to exclude a femoral fracture. To enhance rehabilitation and minimize the risk of myositis ossificans, the treatment of a quadriceps contusion should include immobilization of the knee for the first 48 hours, followed by exercises that decrease thigh atrophy and increase knee flexion.

Myositis ossificans may complicate a direct blow to the thigh (see **Figure 8-16**). The incidence correlates with the severity of the associated contusion. The development of this complication is probably related to concomitant injury of the periosteum and the subsequent reparative process, which initiates a metaplastic chondroid and osseous response. The firm mass interferes with knee flexion and may be confused with a neoplastic process. Function can usually be regained with range-of-motion and strengthening exercises, but occasionally, excision of a persistently large mass is necessary once osteogenesis has ceased and the bone is mature.

PEDIATRIC HIP DISORDERS

Developmental Dysplasia of the Hip

Developmental dysplasia of the hip (DDH) includes the typical dislocatable hips present at birth; rigid dislocations at the time of birth from conditions such as arthrogryposis; and hip dysplasia that develops during early childhood, usually from conditions that cause severe ligamentous laxity or neuromuscular dysfunction. Typical DDH usually is detectable at birth. Associated factors in these patients include an increased incidence in females (5:1 ratio), breech presentation (20% for frank breech position), left hip predominance (3:1 ratio), and greater incidence in individuals of northern European and American Indian ancestry. In addition to normal perinatal laxity, additional ligamentous laxity is the cause for the greater incidence in females and the greater incidence in some families.

The acetabulum is relatively shallow in all babies, and breech presentation probably increases the likelihood of DDH by altering the shape of the acetabulum. In the center of the

Figure 17-23: Femoral Shaft Fracture

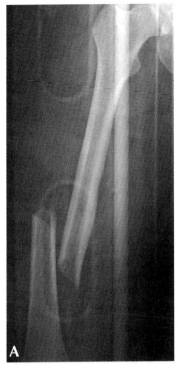
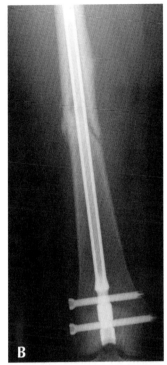
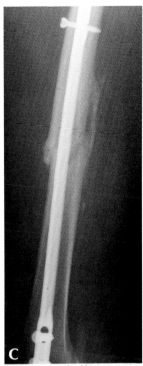

AP radiograph of femur on date of injury

AP radiograph of femur 2 months after retrograde intramedullary nailing

Lateral radiograph of femur 2 months after retrograde intramedullary nailing

20-year-old female who was unrestrained passenger in a motor vehicle accident. The patient sustained multiple fractures including a closed fracture of the right femoral shaft (A), an open grade IIIA comminuted fracture of the junction of the middle third-distal third right tibia and fibula (see Figure 18-19), a closed, comminuted fracture of the middle third of the left tibia and fibula, and comminuted fracture of the right calcaneus (Figure 18-19). On the date of injury, the patient underwent débridement of the right tibia with application of an external fixator, retrograde nailing of the right femur, and intramedullary nailing of the left tibia. Radiographs of the femur 2 months after injury (B and C) show good alignment and interval healing of the fracture.

acetabulum is a growth plate, the triradiate cartilage. Like all growth plates, it responds to pressure. If the femoral head is hyperflexed and adducted (i.e., in a breech position), the pressure will flatten the outer rim of the socket, and the resultant insufficient acetabulum predisposes the hip to dislocate or become dislocatable.

Physical examination is the key to early diagnosis. The examination should be done on a firm surface, with the infant calm and relaxed. Hip instability may not be detected when the infant is upset.

Two provocative maneuvers should be performed during the newborn examination (**Fig-ure 17-24**). The *Barlow test*, a "sign of exit," is done first. A positive test is a clunk as the dislocatable femoral head slides over the posterior rim of the acetabulum. The *Ortolani maneuver* is a "sign of relocation" as the dislocated femoral head is manipulated back into the acetabulum. Again, a clunk and sudden give are perceived as the femoral head slides over the posterior lip of the acetabulum into the socket. If the acetabulum is very shallow, the sense of relocation may be soft compared with the typical clunk, making the diagnosis questionable. To increase the sensitivity of this test, push the femoral head toward the acetabulum when performing this maneuver.

Figure 17-24: Developmental Dysplasia of the Hip

Ortolani (reduction) test

With baby relaxed and content on firm surface, hips and knees fixed to 90˚. Hips examined one at a time. Examiner grasps baby's thigh with middle finger over greater trochanter and lifts thigh to bring femoral head from its dislocated posterior position to opposite the acetabulum. Simultaneously, thigh gently abducted, reducing femoral head into acetabulum. In positive finding, examiner senses reduction by palpable, nearly audible "clunk."

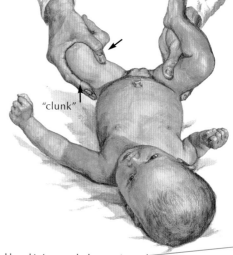

"clunk"

Barlow (dislocatable) test

Reverse of Ortolani test. If femoral head is in acetabulum at time of examination, Barlow test is performed to discover any hip instability. Baby's thigh grasped as in image to the left and adducted with gentle downward pressure. Dislocation is palpable as femoral head slips out of acetabulum. Diagnosis confirmed with Ortolani test

After the neonatal period, perinatal laxity wears off, and with the femoral head in a dislocated position, the joint capsule and hip adductors contract. As a result, by 2 weeks to 3 months of age or older, the hip cannot be relocated by the Ortolani maneuver. Other signs, however, are present. A unilateral dislocation is more obvious because the affected thigh appears shortened (positive *Galeazzi sign*), and decreased abduction of the affected hip causes obvious asymmetry when both hips are abducted (**Figure 17-25**). Furthermore, a toddler with one hip dislocated will stand bending the knee on the normal limb and will walk up on the toes on the affected side to make the leg longer.

Bilateral DDH is more difficult to diagnose. Thigh lengths are equal, and abduction is symmetric. Bilateral DDH is suggested by hip abduction of less than 45˚ to 50˚.

Radiographs are not very useful until the femoral head ossifies (3 to 5 months of age in girls and 5 to 7 months of age in boys). When the newborn examination is equivocal, ultrasonographic examination can be helpful. This study also can help confirm reduction as treatment proceeds. AP radiographs of the pelvis are helpful in older children.

Treatment of DDH should begin as soon as possible. The longer a hip is dislocated, the less likely it is that closed reduction will be possible. Untreated DDH causes a dysfunctional gait and a secondary osteoarthritis that may become painful in the adolescent or young adult years.

The goals of treatment are to concentrically reduce the femoral head into the acetabulum without causing excessive tension on the contracted vascular supply to the femoral head, and to maintain the reduction until the hip

Figure 17-25: Clinical Signs in Older Infant with Developmental Dysplasia of the Hip

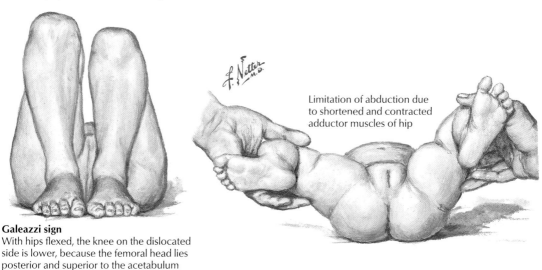

Limitation of abduction due to shortened and contracted adductor muscles of hip

Galeazzi sign
With hips flexed, the knee on the dislocated side is lower, because the femoral head lies posterior and superior to the acetabulum

joint stabilizes. For a dislocatable hip, the treatment of choice in a child up to 6 months of age is a Pavlik harness, a dynamic positioning splint that holds the hips in flexion and abduction, thus promoting normal growth of the acetabulum and stabilization of the somewhat lax and stretched-out hip capsule (**Figure 17-26**). Consistent, full-time wearing of the splint for 2 to 3 months is necessary for treatment of an unstable hip. If reduction does not occur in the harness, or if the child is older than 6 months at diagnosis, an examination and arthrogram under anesthesia, along with a closed or open reduction with application of a spica cast, will be necessary.

Legg–Calvé–Perthes Disease

Legg-Calvé-Perthes (LCP) disease is idiopathic osteonecrosis of the femoral head in children. LCP typically affects children between the ages of 4 and 8 years, but it can occur anytime between 2 and 12 years of age. It is unilateral in 90% of cases, more frequent in boys (4:1 ratio), and uncommon in blacks. The prognosis is worse in older children and in those with severe involvement (osteonecrosis of all or most of the femoral head).

Typical symptoms include the indolent onset of a limp that is activity related (i.e., the limp is usually more noticeable at the end of the day). Pain is often insignificant or mild; therefore, the limp has usually been present for 4 to 8 weeks before the initial visit.

Examination reveals limitation of hip motion, mostly in abduction and internal rotation. Abduction is particularly restricted and usually measures 30° to 40° less on the involved side (60° to 70° abduction normally is present at this age). Good-quality AP and frog-leg lateral radiographs of the pelvis should be obtained. Increased density of the femoral head is an early sign of LCP. The *crescent sign* indicates that a shear collapse has occurred in the subchondral bone (**Figure 17-27**). In the early stages of LCP, plain radiographs may be normal, and MRI may be necessary to document the osteonecrosis. In a child with bilateral LCP, AP radiographs of the hand and knee should be obtained to screen for a possible epiphyseal dysplasia or hypothyroidism.

The healing process in LCP involves revascularization of the femoral head, removal of necrotic bone, replacement with viable bone that is initially weak (woven bone), and remodeling of woven bone to normal lamellar bone. Although this physiologic process occurs more rapidly and with greater consis-

Figure 17-26: Pavlik Harness

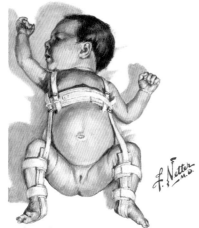

Harness adjusted to allow comfortable *abduction* within safe zone. Forced abduction beyond this limit may lead to avascular necrosis of femoral head.

tency in children, it still requires many (24 to 84) months, and no current interventions accelerate reossification. Furthermore, no treatment modality consistently produces good outcomes or prevents the deformity of the femoral head that occurs when the bone structure is relatively weak (i.e., during revascularization and woven bone formation).

The goal of treatment is to minimize deformity and lateralization of the femoral head. Before any treatment is initiated, motion must be regained. A short period of bed rest and traction is commonly required. Observation is acceptable for children who are unlikely to develop significant deformity. Therefore, observation may be used for children younger than 6 years who do not have significant subluxation of the femoral head and who maintain satisfactory abduction (approximately 40° to 45°). To facilitate early healing, a short period (6 to 8 weeks) of abduction casting may be used at the start of observation.

The principle of active intervention is to "contain" the femoral head within the depth of the acetabulum and thereby maintain, as well as possible, the spherical shape of the femoral head. Options include an abduction brace that extends below the knees or an osteotomy of the femoral head or pelvis. Of note, none of these treatment modalities completely contains the femoral head during all phases of gait. As a general rule, osteotomy is reserved for older children. The abduction brace is used until the lateral portion of the femoral head has reossified, a process that generally takes 12 to 24 months. With a lateral buttress present, the remaining portion of the femoral head is shielded from weight-bearing stresses during the remainder of the reossification process.

Slipped Capital Femoral Epiphysis

Slipped capital femoral epiphysis (SCFE) is displacement of the femoral head (epiphysis) through the physis, which typically occurs during the adolescent growth spurt. During adolescence, the physis of the proximal femur becomes more vertical. That orientation, coupled with increased body size and activity, may cause intolerable shear at the relatively weak physis. The result is microscopic fractures and gradual slippage of the femoral head posteriorly, and usually also medially. Occasionally, an acute event causes sudden displacement of the femoral head—in essence, a fracture or unstable slip.

Obesity, male gender, and heavy involvement with sports activities are predisposing factors. A high degree of femoral retroversion also is a risk factor, which probably explains the greater incidence of SCFE in blacks. Bilateral involvement is eventually found in 40% to 50% of cases.

A small percentage of patients with SCFE have an endocrine disorder that alters the strength or growth of the physis. Hypothyroidism and growth hormone deficiency are most common. In children with hypothyroidism, SCFE often occurs before the endocrine abnormality has been diagnosed.

The mean age at presentation is 12 years for girls (typical range, 10 to 14 years) and 13 years for boys (typical range, 11 to 16 years). Onset before or after the typical range is associated with an increased incidence of some type of endocrine disorder.

Proximal thigh pain exacerbated by activity is the most common presenting symptom.

Figure 17-27: Legg-Calvé-Perthes Disease

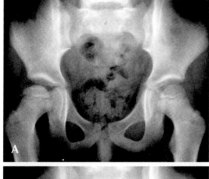

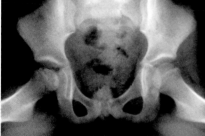

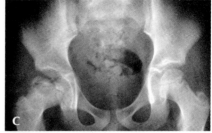

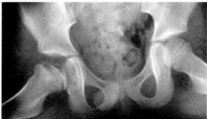

C. Fourteen months later, radiographs show lateral and medial buttress maintained on AP radiographs. Areas of radiolucency are indicative of resorption of the osteonecrotic segments and new woven bone formation.

A. At initial evaluation radiographs demonstrate crescent sign and flattening/mild sclerosis of the right femoral head.

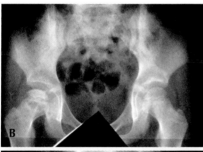

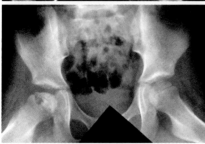

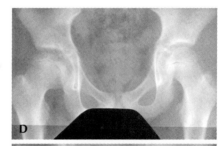

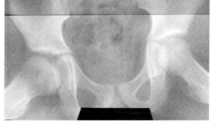

D. Five years after onset of presentation, bone formation is almost complete. Right femoral head shows mild coax magna. Hip function minimally impaired.

B. Three months later, increased sclerosis is evident as woven bone formation is deposited on necrotic trabeculae.

In each group, top image is an AP radiograph and bottom is a "frog leg" position.

Parents may note that the child walks with the foot turned out. In one third of patients, pain is referred to the distal thigh and may be mistaken for a knee problem.

Clinical examination is easy and virtually diagnostic. Loss of hip internal rotation is the most sensitive finding on examination. This limitation is more severe when the hip is flexed and is readily apparent even with minimal displacement of the femoral head (**Figure 17-28**). Furthermore, SCFE is the only pediatric hip disorder that causes greater loss of internal rotation when the hip is flexed. Assessment of internal rotation with the hip flexed to 90° is a useful screening maneuver for all adolescents who have lower extremity pain.

Other findings on clinical examination include mild limitation of hip abduction and extension. Patients typically walk with the leg externally rotated. The affected extremity is 1 to 3 cm shorter, with the degree of shortening dependent on the severity of the slip.

AP and frog-leg lateral radiographs of the pelvis confirm the diagnosis. No displacement is evident in a few patients, but in this pre-slip phase, the physis is widened. The severity of displacement is measured by the degree of posterior displacement as mild (less than 30° displacement), moderate (30° to 50°), and severe (more than 50°). Severe displacement is more likely with long duration of symptoms or an acute, unstable slip. The severity of the slip correlates with the subsequent development of osteoarthritis. Most patients with mild or moderate SCFE remain asymptomatic or do not develop significant arthritis until the older adult years.

The goals of treatment are to prevent further slippage of the femoral head and to promote closure of the physis, an event that

Figure 17-28: Slipped Capital Femoral Epiphysis

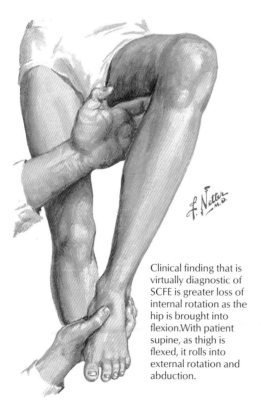

Clinical finding that is virtually diagnostic of SCFE is greater loss of internal rotation as the hip is brought into flexion. With patient supine, as thigh is flexed, it rolls into external rotation and abduction.

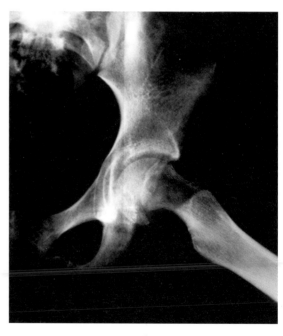

Frog-leg radiograph demonstrating posterior displacement of the epiphysis.

Figure 17-29: Proximal Femoral Focal Deficiency

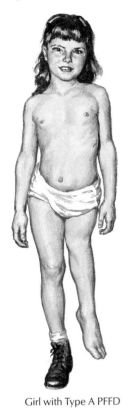

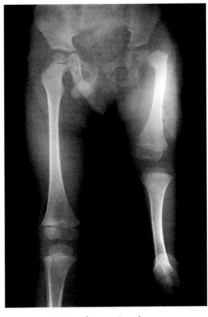

Type A PFFD with associated coxa vara

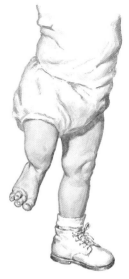

Type B PFFD with associated fibular hemimelia. Foot lies opposite contralateral knee.

Girl with Type A PFFD

Type C PFFD. Femoral head absent or not ossified; acetabulum dysplastic. Femoral shaft very short and displaced laterally and superiorly

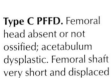

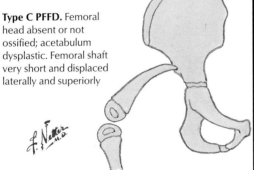

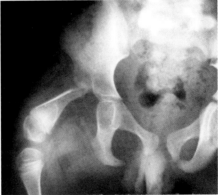

ensures that no further displacement will occur. Most patients are treated by in situ stabilization with a single cannulated screw. This procedure is associated with the lowest risks of osteonecrosis and chondrolysis. A patient with severe deformity may require a realignment osteotomy. Patients with an unstable SCFE experience severe pain after a fall, are unable to walk, and have severe displacement of the femoral head. They are at increased risk for AVN and require urgent reduction and stabilization.

Transient Synovitis

Transient synovitis of the hip is an aseptic effusion that is a common cause of limping or refusal to walk. Children 2 to 5 years of age are most commonly affected, and the incidence is 2 to 3 times greater in boys. The cause is unknown, but mild trauma or overuse at an age when the acetabulum is not fully developed seems to be the best explanation. Numerous studies have failed to identify a bacterial or viral origin.

Typically, the child awakens with a limp or refusal to walk. Later, the limp may improve but will again worsen toward the end of the day. Children old enough to communicate typically localize their pain to the anterior proximal thigh.

Examination reveals mild restriction of hip motion. Abduction is most sensitive and typically is 20° to 40° on the affected side.

Transient synovitis is a diagnosis of exclusion. How much evaluation is performed varies according to the degree and duration of symptoms. Septic arthritis of the hip is the primary disorder to exclude. If the child has very limited motion and a temperature higher than 37.5°C, diagnostic studies should include complete blood count (CBC), erythrocyte sedimentation rate, blood cultures, radiographs, and sometimes aspiration of the hip joint under anesthesia.

Transient synovitis resolves without therapy or sequelae. With a short period of bed rest, symptoms and limping typically resolve within 3 to 14 days.

Proximal Femoral Focal Deficiency

Proximal femoral focal deficiency (PFFD) is an uncommon, sporadic congenital deformity characterized by dysgenesis of the proximal femur. Shortening of the femur is marked. Coxa vara is common, and pseudarthrosis of the femoral neck may be present. Associated abnormalities in the extremity include hip dysplasia, absence of the anterior cruciate ligament, and mild fibular hemimelia. Other organ systems are uncommonly involved in PFFD.

The classification system described by Torode and Gillespie is most useful. In type A, the foot lies opposite the midpoint of the contralateral tibia. These children can be treated by limb equalization procedures and correction of associated coxa vara. In type B, the foot lies opposite the contralateral knee, and the femoral head and neck are absent or have a pseudarthrosis. In type C, the foot lies proximal to the knee joint. Both types B and C require some type of amputation to equalize the limb-length discrepancy (**Figure 17-29**).

ADDITIONAL READINGS

Callaghan JJ, Rosenberg AG, Rubash HE, eds. *The Adult Hip*. Philadelphia, Pa: Lippincott, Williams and Wilkins; 1997.

Chapman MW, ed. *Chapman's Orthopaedic Surgery*, 3rd edition. Philadelphia, Pa: Lippincott Williams and Wilkins; 2001.

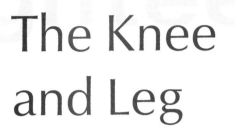

The Knee and Leg

Derrick J. Fluhme, MD
Lee D. Kaplan, MD
Freddie H. Fu, MD

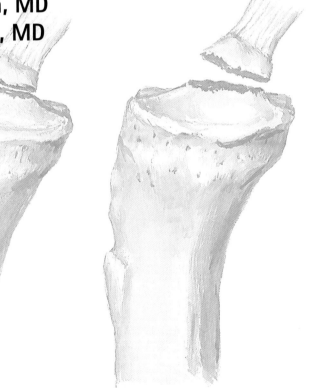

ANATOMY

Compared to the hip and ankle, the intrinsic bony configuration of the knee provides limited support for the weight-bearing demands of walking and running (**Figure 18-1**). Knee stability is created primarily through a complex interplay of passive (collateral ligaments, cruciate ligaments, menisci, and joint capsule) and active stabilizers (quadriceps, hamstrings, and popliteus muscles).

The distal femoral metaphysis expands into a medial and a lateral condyle, each of which is convex and articulates with the corresponding, slightly concave medial and lateral tibial plateaus. The medial condyle is narrower in the anteroposterior (AP) plane and extends farther distally. The articular surfaces of the femoral condyles join anteriorly to articulate with the patella. Posteriorly, they remain separate to form the intercondylar notch.

The proximal tibia is composed of medial and lateral condyles (often called medial and lateral plateaus), which are separated by an intercondylar eminence that has medial and lateral intercondylar tubercles (spines). The intercondylar eminence has no ligament attachments, but the anterior and posterior areas receive the cruciate ligaments and horns

Figure 18-1

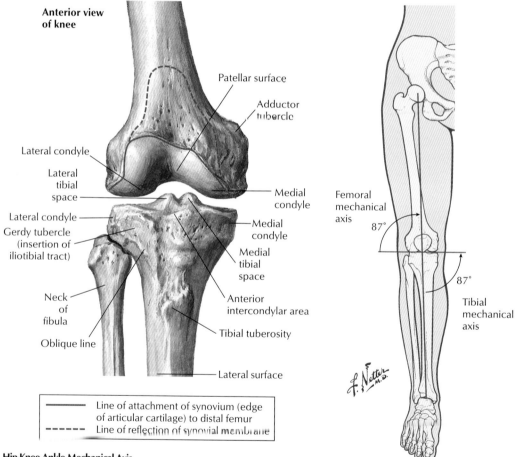

Anterior view of knee

Patellar surface

Adductor tubercle

Lateral condyle

Lateral tibial space

Lateral condyle

Gerdy tubercle (insertion of iliotibial tract)

Neck of fibula

Oblique line

Medial condyle

Medial condyle

Medial tibial space

Anterior intercondylar area

Tibial tuberosity

Lateral surface

Femoral mechanical axis 87°

Tibial mechanical axis

87°

——— Line of attachment of synovium (edge of articular cartilage) to distal femur
- - - - Line of reflection of synovial membrane

Hip-Knee-Ankle Mechanical Axis
Mechanical axis of the lower extremity is the angle from the center of the femoral head to the center of the knee (usually, anterior tubercle of the tibia) to the center of the ankle. Normal is 1° of varus. Femoral mechanical axis is the femoral mechanical axis and a line tangential to the joint line. Normal is 87°. Tibial mechanical axis is tibial mechanical axis line and line tangential to the joint. Normal is 87°.

of the menisci. Palpable insertion sites are the tibial tubercle (patellar tendon) and Gerdy tubercle (iliotibial band).

Abnormal alignment predisposes the joint to osteoarthritis. Normal alignment parameters include the following: both femoral condyles form a horizontal plane parallel to the ground, the plane of the femoral condyles relative to the femoral shaft (the anatomic axis) is 5° to 7° valgus, the mechanical hip-knee-ankle axis (center of the femoral head–center of the knee–center of the distal tibia) is approximately 1° varus, and the tibial articular surface is sloped posteriorly 7° to 10° (see **Figure 18-1**).

The patella, the largest sesamoid bone in the body, lies within the substance of the quadriceps tendon (**Figure 18-2**). The proxi-

Figure 18-2: Medial and Lateral Views of the Knee

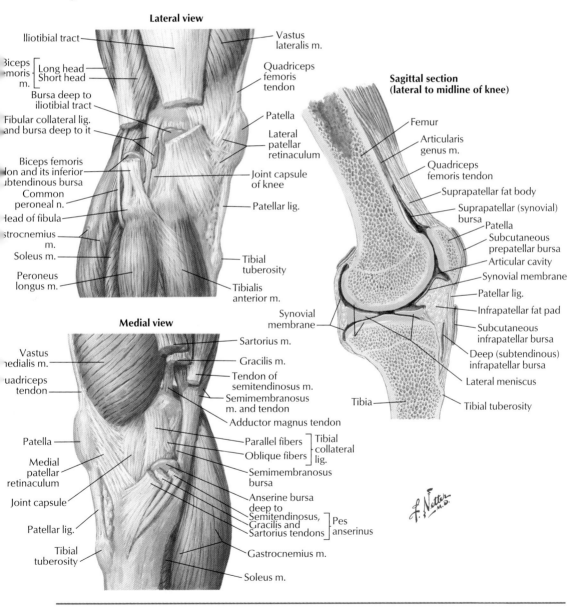

Lateral view

Iliotibial tract
Biceps femoris m. — Long head / Short head
Bursa deep to iliotibial tract
Fibular collateral lig. and bursa deep to it
Biceps femoris tendon and its inferior subtendinous bursa
Common peroneal n.
Head of fibula
Gastrocnemius m.
Soleus m.
Peroneus longus m.

Vastus lateralis m.
Quadriceps femoris tendon
Patella
Lateral patellar retinaculum
Joint capsule of knee
Patellar lig.
Tibial tuberosity
Tibialis anterior m.

Sagittal section (lateral to midline of knee)

Femur
Articularis genus m.
Quadriceps femoris tendon
Suprapatellar fat body
Suprapatellar (synovial) bursa
Patella
Subcutaneous prepatellar bursa
Articular cavity
Synovial membrane
Patellar lig.
Infrapatellar fat pad
Subcutaneous infrapatellar bursa
Deep (subtendinous) infrapatellar bursa
Lateral meniscus
Tibial tuberosity

Synovial membrane
Tibia

Medial view

Vastus medialis m.
Quadriceps tendon
Patella
Medial patellar retinaculum
Joint capsule
Patellar lig.
Tibial tuberosity

Sartorius m.
Gracilis m.
Tendon of semitendinosus m.
Semimembranosus m. and tendon
Adductor magnus tendon
Parallel fibers / Oblique fibers — Tibial collateral lig.
Semimembranosus bursa
Anserine bursa deep to Semitendinosus, Gracilis and Sartorius tendons — Pes anserinus
Gastrocnemius m.
Soleus m.

Figure 18-3: Axial View of Meniscus

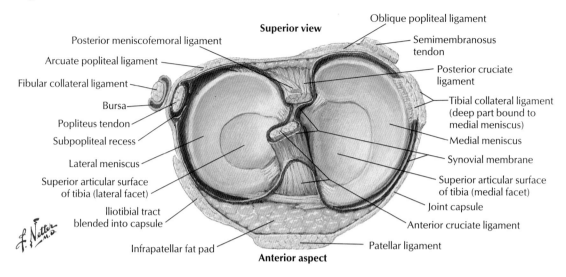

Superior view

Oblique popliteal ligament

Posterior meniscofemoral ligament

Semimembranosus tendon

Arcuate popliteal ligament

Posterior cruciate ligament

Fibular collateral ligament

Tibial collateral ligament (deep part bound to medial meniscus)

Bursa

Popliteus tendon

Subpopliteal recess

Medial meniscus

Lateral meniscus

Synovial membrane

Superior articular surface of tibia (lateral facet)

Superior articular surface of tibia (medial facet)

Iliotibial tract blended into capsule

Joint capsule

Anterior cruciate ligament

Infrapatellar fat pad

Patellar ligament

Anterior aspect

mal two thirds of the patella's undersurface articulates with the anterior surface of the femoral condyles and is divided by a longitudinal ridge into medial and lateral facets. The distal third provides attachment for the patellar tendon; this tendon is more precisely called the *patellar ligament* because it extends from bone to bone (from the patella to the tibial tuberosity). The quadriceps tendon inserts into the superior border of the patella, and retinacular expansions of the vastus medialis and vastus lateralis occupy the corresponding border of the patella.

The medial and lateral menisci are triangular wedge–shaped rims of fibrocartilaginous tissue that line the periphery of the tibial plateaus (see **Figures 18-2** and **18-3**). The menisci aid in load transmission, reduce articular surface stresses, deepen articular surfaces of the tibial plateau, and contribute to joint stability. The medial meniscus is C-shaped, whereas the lateral meniscus forms an incomplete circle. The collagen fibers of the menisci are arranged radially and circumferentially. The circumferential (longitudinal) fibers dissipate "hoop" stresses and allow meniscal expansion under compressive loads.

The broad, flat medial collateral ligament (MCL) is the primary restraint to valgus stress (**Figure 18-4**). The superficial portion of the MCL originates at the medial femoral epicondyle and inserts distally into the proximal tibia, deep to the pes anserinus tendons. The deep portion of the MCL is a thickening of the knee capsule that blends with the fibers of the superficial MCL at its insertion on the tibia. The lateral (fibular) collateral ligament (LCL) is the primary restraint to varus stress. It originates on the lateral femoral condyle, posterior and superior to the popliteus tendon, and inserts on the lateral aspect of the fibular head.

The anterior cruciate ligament (ACL) is the primary restraint (85%) to anterior translation of the tibia relative to the femur. It originates on the posteromedial aspect of the lateral femoral condyle and inserts at the anterior intercondylar area of the tibia. The ACL includes two functional bundles: the anteromedial bundle, which tightens in flexion, and the posterolateral bundle, which tightens in extension. Thus, the ACL maintains some tension throughout the full arc of knee motion. Mechanoreceptors in the ACL provide protective proprioception against abnormal joint translations.

The posterior cruciate ligament (PCL) is the primary restraint (95%) against posterior translation. It originates on the posterolateral aspect of the medial femoral condyle and in-

Figure 18-4: Collateral and Cruciate Ligaments of the Knee

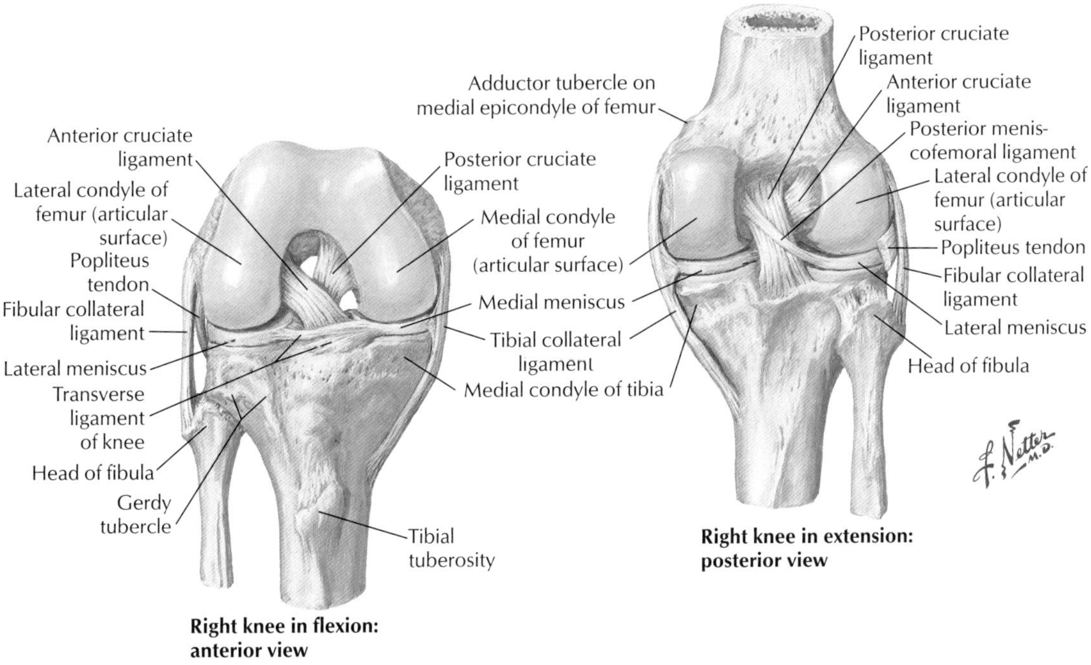

Right knee in flexion: anterior view

Right knee in extension: posterior view

serts in the posterior intercondylar area of the tibia. The PCL also is made up of two functional bundles. The anterior meniscofemoral (ligament of Humphrey) and the posterior meniscofemoral ligament (ligament of Wrisberg) originate from the posterior horn of the lateral meniscus and contribute to the function of the PCL.

The extensors of the knee are the five components of the quadriceps muscle. Knee flexors include the three hamstrings, as well as the sartorius, gracilis, and popliteus muscles. The pes anserinus (goose foot) is the convergence of the sartorius, gracilis, and semitendinosus tendons where they insert on the anteromedial aspect of the proximal tibia (see **Figure 18-2**).

The tibia and the fibula are connected by an interosseous membrane. The slender fibula has limited weight-bearing function. The muscles of the legs are separated into four compartments (**Figure 18-5**). Anterior compartment muscles (tibialis anterior, extensor hallucis longus, extensor digitorum longus, and peroneus tertius) dorsiflex the ankle and

extend the toes. Lateral compartment muscles (peroneus longus and peroneus brevis) originate from the fibula and primarily function as evertors of the foot. Posterior compartment muscles are separated into superficial (gastrocnemius and soleus) and deep posterior compartments (tibialis posterior, flexor hallucis longus, and flexor digitorum longus).

The two components of the sciatic nerve separate within the proximal aspect of the popliteal fossa (**Figure 18-6**). The common peroneal nerve travels across the lateral gastrocnemius; becomes subcutaneous and vulnerable to injury as it goes around the neck of the fibula; and, after penetrating the posterior intermuscular septum, divides into the superficial and deep peroneal nerves. The deep peroneal nerve supplies the anterior compartment muscles, and the superficial peroneal nerve provides motor branches to the lateral compartment. The tibial nerve continues its posterior course and innervates the posterior compartment muscles.

Proximal to the knee, the femoral artery separates from the saphenous nerve, passing

Figure 18-5: Fascial Compartments of the Leg

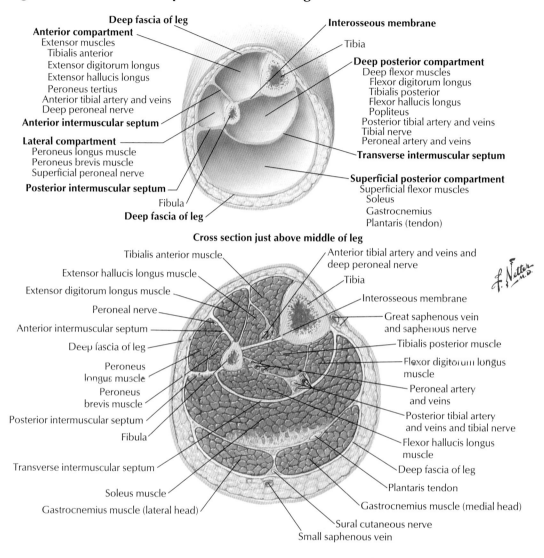

Deep fascia of leg

Anterior compartment
Extensor muscles
Tibialis anterior
Extensor digitorum longus
Extensor hallucis longus
Peroneus tertius
Anterior tibial artery and veins
Deep peroneal nerve
Anterior intermuscular septum

Lateral compartment
Peroneus longus muscle
Peroneus brevis muscle
Superficial peroneal nerve
Posterior intermuscular septum
Fibula
Deep fascia of leg

Interosseous membrane
Tibia
Deep posterior compartment
Deep flexor muscles
Flexor digitorum longus
Tibialis posterior
Flexor hallucis longus
Popliteus
Posterior tibial artery and veins
Tibial nerve
Peroneal artery and veins
Transverse intermuscular septum

Superficial posterior compartment
Superficial flexor muscles
Soleus
Gastrocnemius
Plantaris (tendon)

Cross section just above middle of leg

Tibialis anterior muscle
Extensor hallucis longus muscle
Extensor digitorum longus muscle
Peroneal nerve
Anterior intermuscular septum
Deep fascia of leg
Peroneus longus muscle
Peroneus brevis muscle
Posterior intermuscular septum
Fibula
Transverse intermuscular septum
Soleus muscle
Gastrocnemius muscle (lateral head)

Anterior tibial artery and veins and deep peroneal nerve
Tibia
Interosseous membrane
Great saphenous vein and saphenous nerve
Tibialis posterior muscle
Flexor digitorum longus muscle
Peroneal artery and veins
Posterior tibial artery and veins and tibial nerve
Flexor hallucis longus muscle
Deep fascia of leg
Plantaris tendon
Gastrocnemius muscle (medial head)
Sural cutaneous nerve
Small saphenous vein

from the anterior compartment of the thigh through an opening in the adductor magnus tendon to enter the popliteal space as the popliteal artery. The popliteal artery provides five geniculate and two sural branches before it divides into the anterior and posterior tibial arteries. The anterior tibial artery passes directly forward above the upper end of the interosseous membrane to enter the anterior compartment. The posterior tibial artery continues down the leg, accompanied by the tibial nerve. Its largest branch, the peroneal artery, supplies the muscles of the lateral side of the leg and arises 2 to 3 cm distal to the origin of the posterior tibial artery.

BIOMECHANICS

The primary plane of knee motion is flexion and extension, but small degrees of rotation, adduction/abduction, and anterior/posterior translation occur as well. Maximum stability is needed when the limb is in the midstance phase of walking or running, and several factors enhance stability in this phase (refer to

Figure 18-6: Tibial Nerve and Cutaneous Innervation of Sole

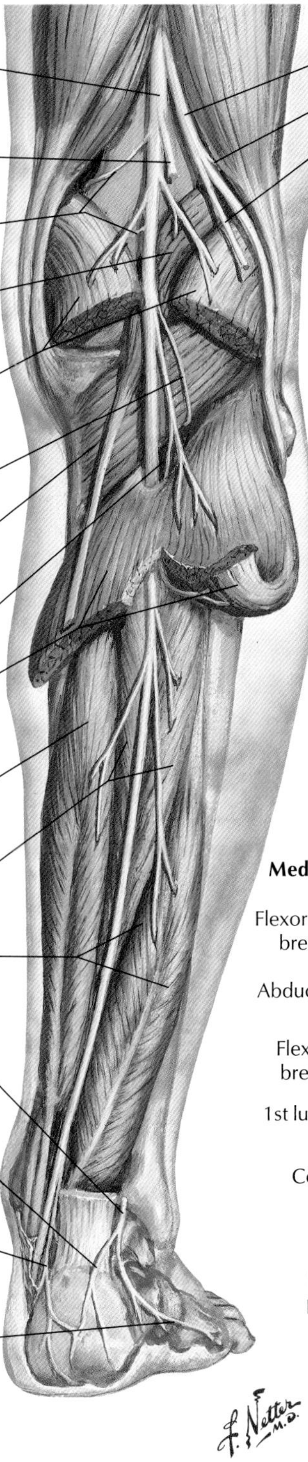

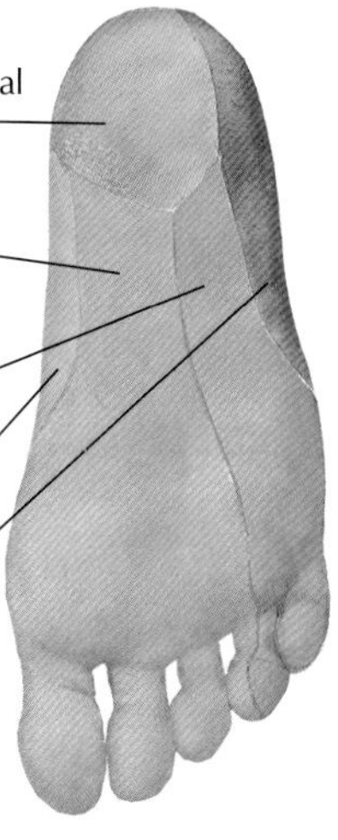

Tibial nerve
(L4, 5, S1, 2, 3)

Medial sural
cutaneous
nerve (cut)

Articular branches

Plantaris muscle

Gastrocnemius
muscle (cut)

Nerve to
popliteus muscle

Popliteus muscle

Interosseous
nerve of leg

Soleus muscle
(cut and partly
retracted)

Flexor digitorum
longus muscle

Tibialis posterior
muscle

Flexor hallucis
longus muscle

Sural nerve (cut)

Lateral calcaneal
branch
sural nerve

Medial
calcaneal branch
tibial nerve

Lateral dorsal
cutaneous nerve

Common fibular (peroneal) nerve
Articular branch
Lateral sural cutaneous nerve (cut)

Medial calcaneal
branches
(S1, 2)

Medial
plantar nerve
(L4, 5)

Lateral
plantar nerve
(S1, 2)

From
tibial nerve

Saphenous nerve
(L3, 4)

Sural nerve
(S1, 2) via
lateral calcaneal
and lateral dorsal
cutaneous
branches

Cutaneous innervation of sole

Tibial
nerve

Medial
calcaneal
branch

**Medial plantar
nerve**

Flexor digitorum
brevis muscle
and nerve

Abductor hallucis
muscle

Flexor hallucis
brevis muscle

1st lumbrical
muscle

Common
plantar
digital
nerves

Proper
plantar
digital
nerves

Lateral calcaneal
branch of sural nerve

**Lateral plantar
nerve**

Nerve to abductor
digiti minimi muscle

Quadratus plantae
muscle

Abductor digiti
minimi muscle

Deep branch
to interosseous
muscles,
2nd, 3rd, and 4th
lumbrical muscles
and Adductor hallucis
muscle

**Superficial
branch** to
4th interosseous
muscle
and
Flexor digiti minimi
brevis muscle

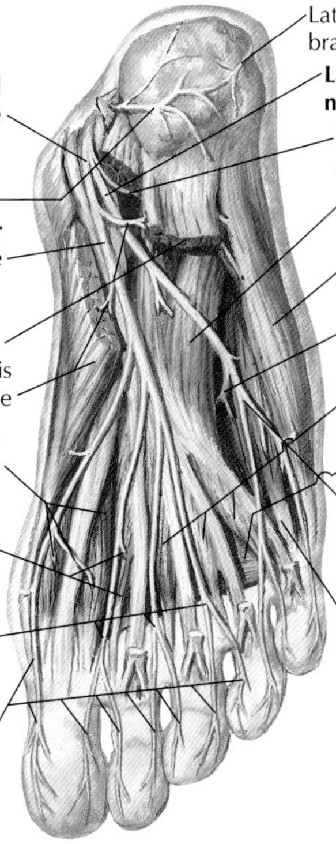

Note: Articular branches not shown

Chapter 19, section on phases of gait). Especially important is that the knee is in almost full extension during midstance. In extension, medial rotation of the femur achieves the close-packed, stable position. The femoral condyles have larger articular surfaces than the tibial condyles. Therefore, knee movement has a component of rolling and gliding of the femoral condyles. As the knee is extended, the shorter, more highly curved lateral condyle reaches its limit sooner. The lateral meniscus is displaced forward on the tibia and becomes firmly seated in a position that blocks further motion of the lateral femoral condyle. However, the medial femoral condyle continues to glide backward, thus bringing its flatter, anterior surface into full contact with the tibia. Medial rotation of the femur also brings the cruciate and collateral ligaments into maximum tension. The tension of the ligaments and the close approximation of the flatter parts of the condyles also make standing in the erect position relatively easy to maintain.

Flexion of the extended knee is initiated by lateral rotation of the femur, a process facilitated by contraction of the popliteus muscle. Lateral rotation relaxes the taut ligaments enough to allow flexion.

An important function of the patella is to reduce the force requirements of the quadriceps muscle by use of a variable-lever arm. As the knee goes into extension, the patella rides up in the femoral notch, thereby increasing the moment arm and extension torque. Less torque is required when the knee is flexed, and the patella sinks into the femoral notch, thereby reducing the quadriceps lever arm. Patellectomy reduces the lever arm and increases, by 15% to 20%, the force required by the quadriceps to bring the knee into full extension.

HISTORY AND PHYSICAL EXAMINATION

A history of acute knee pain typically indicates an injury to ligamentous, meniscal, or bony tissue or a combination of these injuries. Chronic pain without specific cause usually is due to overuse or degenerative problems. Contact injuries may involve single or multiple knee ligaments; in noncontact injuries, often the ACL is the only ligament torn. The sensation of feeling or hearing a pop is associated with ACL tears. An effusion that develops within hours suggests an ACL injury, whereas an effusion that develops overnight suggests a meniscal injury.

Buckling of the knee, a transient sensation of the knee's giving way, may arise from meniscal tears, ligamentous instability, patellar instability (subluxation/dislocation), or weakness of the quadriceps. Locking of the knee, a transient or sometimes longer lasting sensation of the knee being stuck in a semi-flexed position, is associated with displacement of a meniscal tear into and out of its normal alignment. Difficulty with cutting maneuvers suggests ACL or patellar instability. Difficulty climbing or descending stairs is associated with patellofemoral problems.

Observe the patient as he or she walks, to detect antalgic movements. Inspect the knee for swelling, ecchymosis, and malalignment. Examine the knee with the patient first in the supine position, then seated.

With the patient supine, inspect, then palpate the knee for effusion by placing one hand above and one hand below the patella. Any fluid in the knee can then be displaced and palpated proximally and distally. Have the patient point to, then palpate, the site of maximum tenderness. Tenderness at the medial joint line suggests a tear of the medial meniscus or medial compartment arthritis. A history of an acute valgus injury and tenderness anywhere over the MCL suggests MCL sprain. Pain at the medial aspect of the proximal tibia suggests pes anserinus bursitis. Lateral joint line tenderness is associated with a tear of the lateral meniscus, sprain of the LCL, or tendinitis of the popliteal tendon or iliotibial band. Tenderness at the medial-superior border of the patella suggests acute patellar subluxation/dislocation.

When the patient is seated, observe the patella while the patient moves the knee. Note abnormal crepitation and excessive lateral movement. With the quadriceps relaxed and the knee in extension, push the patella laterally, then flex the knee. In a patient who has patellar instability, this test displaces the patella to an abnormal position that creates pain and apprehension as the knee is flexed.

Knee motion is primarily flexion and extension. The zero starting position is a straight knee. Normal knee flexion is 135° to 145° (**Figure 18-7**). Extension beyond the zero starting position is seen more often in young children; adults commonly have a 5° knee flexion contracture.

Test the strength of the quadriceps with the patient seated. Ask the patient to keep the knee extended while you resist the effort by pushing against the tibia. Measure hamstring strength with the patient prone and the knee in 90° of flexion. Ask the patient to extend the hip as you resist the effort by pushing against the thigh.

DEGENERATIVE DISORDERS

Osteoarthritis of the Knee

Osteoarthritis of the knee may be primary but often is secondary to predisposing conditions. Presenting symptoms include activity-related pain and stiffness that characteristically improve as the knee "warms up" (see **Figure 4-6**). Swelling caused by an effusion and mild synovitis may be present. A knee flexion contracture of 10° to 20° and limitation of knee flexion are common. Catching or locking of the incongruent joint may be noted as the knee moves. In addition to displaying the typical shortened stance phase of an antalgic gait, a patient with varus malalignment and resultant stretching of the LCL may demonstrate a lateral thrust during midstance. Similarly, a patient with a valgus knee may demonstrate a varus thrust caused by weight-bearing forces and instability of the MCL.

AP and lateral weight-bearing radiographs show narrowing of the joint space, as well as osteophyte formation, cortical sclerosis, and subchondral cysts. With varus malalignment, the medial aspect of the joint becomes more involved. With valgus deformities, greater narrowing is noted on the lateral side of the joint. Radiographs also should be inspected for concomitant patellofemoral arthritis. An AP standing radiograph with the knee flexed 45° is required if only the posterior aspect of the joint is involved.

Nonoperative management of knee osteoarthritis includes observation, weight re-

Figure 18-7: Zero Starting Position and Arc of Flexion

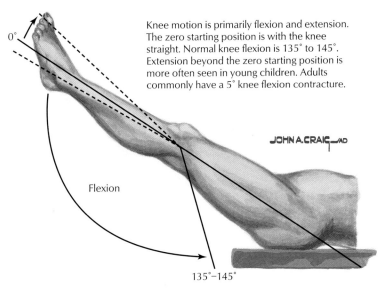

0°

Knee motion is primarily flexion and extension. The zero starting position is with the knee straight. Normal knee flexion is 135° to 145°. Extension beyond the zero starting position is more often seen in young children. Adults commonly have a 5° knee flexion contracture.

JOHN A.CRAIG—AD

Flexion

135°–145°

duction, activity modification, and low-impact exercises such as swimming or cycling, and isometric or closed-chain strengthening exercises. NSAIDs, intra-articular steroid or viscosupplement injections, and force reduction devices such as a cane or unloader braces also may be helpful.

Surgical options for treating disabling arthritis are based on the age and activity of the patient, as well as the type of deformity. Arthrodesis can provide excellent pain relief and allows the patient to withstand the demands of heavy labor; however, it is uncommonly desired because sitting is compromised. It remains the best choice for a young, active adult with unilateral arthritis. Fusion in 15° of flexion is the optimal position for both walking and sitting.

Varus deformity and medial compartment arthritis in a patient younger than 60 years may be treated with a valgus osteotomy of the proximal tibia by the removal of a triangular wedge of bone (a lateral closing wedge) or the medial insertion of a triangular wedge of bone (a medial opening wedge). The goal is to normalize weight-bearing forces so that pain is decreased, activity is maintained, and progression of arthritis is slowed. Results are better with correction to ≥8° valgus. Contraindications include grossly obese patients or those who have either >10° varus, <75° flexion, >15° flexion contracture, and/or gross instability.

The indications for a unicompartmental knee arthroplasty (UKA) are less clear. This procedure, which replaces only the medial or lateral side of the joint, is associated with less postoperative morbidity than a total knee arthroplasty (TKA); however, the long-term functional outcome of UKA is unclear. Most experts agree that both osteotomy and UKA delay the need for TKA. At present, the guidelines for UKA include isolated medial or lateral compartment arthritis, patients >60 years of age who are relatively sedentary, no significant varus/valgus malalignment, and no significant instability or restriction of motion (**Figure 18-8**).

TKA is preferred for older patients with end-stage arthritis because the procedure produces more predictable pain relief and durability (**Figure 18-9**). This procedure is also indicated for younger patients with bicondylar or tricompartmental disease (medial, lateral, and patellofemoral). A young or middle-aged active adult who undergoes TKA will require future revision surgery. To prevent or delay the complications that incrementally increase with each revision replacement, TKA should be delayed as long as possible in these patients by the use of nonoperative or alternative operative methods.

The goals of TKA include restoring normal hip-knee-ankle alignment, preserving (or restoring) a normal joint line, and balancing the collateral ligaments (joint stability). Possible complications include loosening (aseptic and septic), infection, osteolysis with subsequent aseptic loosening resulting from a macro-phage response to particulate metal and polyethylene wear debris, settling of the prosthesis into the cancellous bone and subsequent accelerated wear, peroneal nerve palsy (more likely in a patient with a preoperative valgus deformity and flexion contracture), abnormal patellar tracking, and stress fracture of the patella.

Loosening and settling can be corrected by revision TKA. Infection is particularly difficult to treat because the implants act as foreign bodies in the knee, making antibiotic treatment and drainage alone unpredictable and riddled with failure. The infection can be treated definitively by removal of the prosthesis and cement with complete débridement of all infected tissue, implantation of an antibiotic-coated cement spacer, and a 6-week course of intravenous antibiotics followed by reimplantation of a new TKA.

Osteochondritis Dissecans

Osteochondritis dissecans (OCD) is focal osteonecrosis at an articular surface. In the knee, OCD typically begins during the adolescent years, although symptoms may not occur until the young adult years. The cause is unclear, but the condition most likely occurs secondary to repetitive shear trauma that disrupts the blood supply to surrounding bone.

Figure 18-8: Unicondylar Knee Arthroplasty

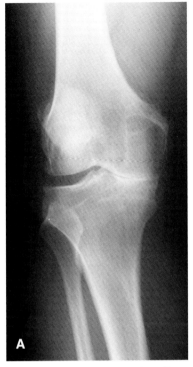 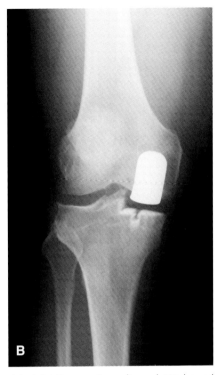

58-year-old male with severe bilateral knee pain on the medial aspect of the joint. Preoperative radiograph (A) showed similar findings in both knees with marked degenerative changes on the medial aspect of the knee and maintenance of joint cartilage on the lateral aspect of the joint. Patient underwent unicompartmental arthroplasty with good relief of pain. (B) Postoperative standing AP radiograph.

The most common location is the lateral aspect of the medial femoral condyle, but any area of the medial or lateral femoral condyle may be involved.

Gradual buckling of the articular surface causes the indolent onset of activity-related pain. With buckling or disruption (dissecans) of the articular surface, patients note effusions and catching or locking symptoms. Eventually, the osteonecrotic fragment may become a loose body (**Figure 18-10**).

Examination may demonstrate tenderness on the involved site. Assess the medial femoral condyle by flexing the patient's knee to 90° and applying pressure just medial to the inferior pole of the patella. Perform the Wilson test with the patient's hip and knee flexed to 90° and the tibia internally rotated.

Positive findings are increased pain as the knee is extended to approximately 30° and reduced pain when the maneuver is repeated with the tibia externally rotated (the abutting tibial spine is now rotated away from the medial condyle). Small lesions may be missed on standard AP and lateral radiographs but may be seen on an AP tunnel view (knee held in 30° flexion).

The prognosis for OCD varies according to the size of the lesion and the age of the patient. If the distal femoral physis has closed, the OCD lesion is unlikely to heal. Younger children have greater potential for osteonecrotic bone repair before the cartilage starts to separate. Activity modification to a level that diminishes shear stresses and eliminates symptoms is paramount. Lesions smaller than 1 cm in diameter

Figure 18-9: Total Knee Arthroplasty

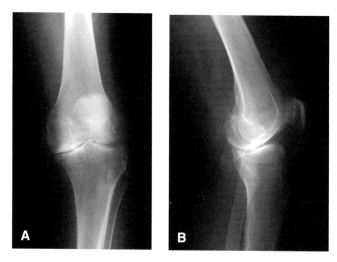

77-year-old male with progressive pain and difficulty walking despite intra-articular injections, NSAIDs, and using a cane. Gait antalgic with varus thrust. AP (A) and lateral (B) standing preoperative radiographs show varus malalignment, marked narrowing of the joint space, and patellofemoral involvement.

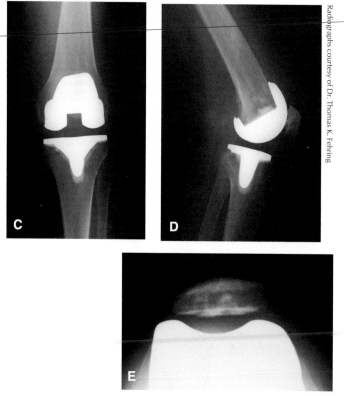

Radiographs courtesy of Dr. Thomas K. Fehring

Postoperative radiographs demonstrating total knee arthroplasty with resurfacing of patella. Alignment of limb improved. Patient walking without pain and without a cane. AP (C) and lateral (D) standing and Merchant view (E).

Figure 18-10: Progression of Osteochondritis Dissecans

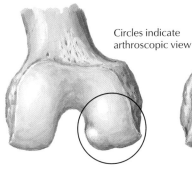

Circles indicate
arthroscopic view

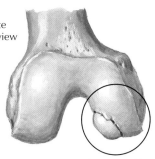

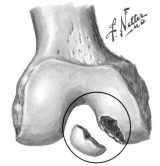

Stage 1. Bulge on medial femoral condyle due to partial separation of bone fragment. Articular cartilage intact, but defect evident on radiographs.

Stage 2. Fragment demarcated by separation of articular cartilage

Stage 3. Fragment of cartilage and bone completely separated as loose body. This often migrates to medial or lateral gutter.

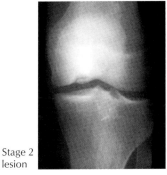

Stage 2 lesion

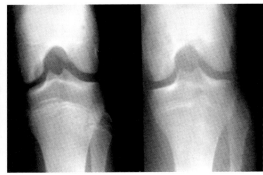

Tunnel view radiographs of small OCD lesion involving medial femoral condyle treated with activity modification. Complete healing occurred

do well, whereas lesions larger than 2 cm carry a poor prognosis for healing without operative intervention (see **Figure 18-10**).

Indications for surgical intervention include a loose body, an unstable lesion, or persistent symptoms despite nonoperative therapy. Drilling the lesion may promote revascularization. However, when partial separation of the articular surface has occurred, treatment should include not only drilling the base of the lesion but also stabilizing the fragment through temporary internal fixation. Surgical options for lesions that have completely separated and are not reparable include removal of loose bodies, drilling the defect to promote fibrocartilate replacement, grafting of the defect by osteochondral autograft (osteochondral autograft transfer system, or OATS, procedure), allograft transplantation and autologous chondrocyte implantation.

Osteonecrosis

Osteonecrosis is similar to OCD, but in the knee, the diagnosis of osteonecrosis indicates a large lesion that typically occurs in a female patient older than 60 years (the female-to-male ratio is 3:1), occasionally in a younger patient with predisposing factors, such as long-term steroid therapy or sickle cell anemia. These patients often present with acute onset of pain secondary to a subchondral fracture and collapse of the articular surface. The medial femoral condyle is most commonly involved, but osteonecrosis also may occur in the lateral femoral condyle and the tibial plateau (usually medial). Initial radiographs may be normal, but eventually show flattening of the articular surface, subchondral radiolucency, and sclerosis of surrounding bone.

Smaller lesions (less than 5 cm^2) typically have a better clinical prognosis, and may be satisfactorily treated with activity modification and assistive devices (ie, cane). Progressive symptoms necessitate drilling of the lesion, realignment osteotomy, or total knee replacement.

Meniscal Tears

The function of knee menisci is to dissipate stress; therefore, they are susceptible to injury from abnormal strain. The common age for traumatic tears is from late adolescence to the late forties. These injuries often occur with a twisting injury while the knee is under stress, that is, the foot planted. Degenerative tears are observed in older patients. These patients uncommonly associate onset of symptoms with significant injury.

The medial meniscus is less mobile and therefore is torn approximately 4 to 5 times more frequently than the lateral meniscus. Tears may be isolated or associated with other knee injuries; lateral meniscus tears are more frequent with acute ACL injuries, whereas medial meniscus injuries are more common with chronic ACL tears.

The torn portion may be unstable and intermittently displaces and interferes with the normal gliding motion of the knee. Symptoms of a torn meniscus include pain and intermittent catching, buckling, or locking. Examination frequently shows tenderness at the medial or lateral joint line. Positive McMurray test results indicate a tear of the posterior horn of the meniscus (most common site of tearing). To assess the medial meniscus, position the knee in maximum flexion and external rotation. Gradually extend the knee while keeping the leg in external rotation. Positive test findings include pain and a popping sensation. Use a similar maneuver with the knee internally rotated to assess the posterior horn of the lateral meniscus.

Small tears that are causing only limited symptoms do not require treatment. Meniscal tears causing persistent symptoms should be treated by excision of the torn portion or repair of the meniscus. The goals include (1) prevent progression of arthritis from erosion of adjacent articular cartilage from repet-

itive buckling and locking; and (2) retain as much of the meniscus as possible. Tears involving the avascular inner two thirds of the meniscus are treated with arthroscopic débridement and partial meniscectomy. The peripheral third of the meniscus has sufficient vascularity that repair should be attempted for all peripheral longitudinal tears in young patients. Meniscal repair is enhanced by placement of a fibrin clot in the tear before the sutures are tightened. The fibrin clot provides a scaffold that facilitates healing. The saphenous nerve is vulnerable in medial meniscus repairs, and the peroneal nerve, in lateral meniscus repairs (**Figure 18-11**).

Discoid Meniscus

A discoid meniscus is a congenital anomaly in which the meniscus is enlarged and shaped like a disc. The lateral meniscus is mostly involved. The three types are *complete*, which covers the lateral tibial plateau; *incomplete*, and the *Wrisberg* variant with absence of posterior meniscotibial attachment (**Figure 18-12**).

Patients typically present during childhood or adolescence with symptoms of pain and popping. Examination may show a palpable clunk as the knee is moved into extension. MRI can be helpful in showing the abnormal meniscus and any associated meniscal tears. Treatment options include observation, partial meniscectomy, and meniscal repair.

Bursitis

The prepatellar bursa is anterior to the patella and may become inflamed by prolonged kneeling (see **Figure 18-2**). In bursitis, the overlying skin is erythematous. The joint appears swollen, but close inspection demonstrates the absence of a knee effusion. Pain is increased by flexing the knee. The primary differential diagnosis is cellulitis.

Treatment includes aspiration and culture, short-term splinting of the knee in extension, activity modification, and other modalities that reduce inflammation. If culture is negative, a steroid injection may be considered. Excision of the bursa is seldom necessary and

Figure 18-11: Types of Meniscal Tears

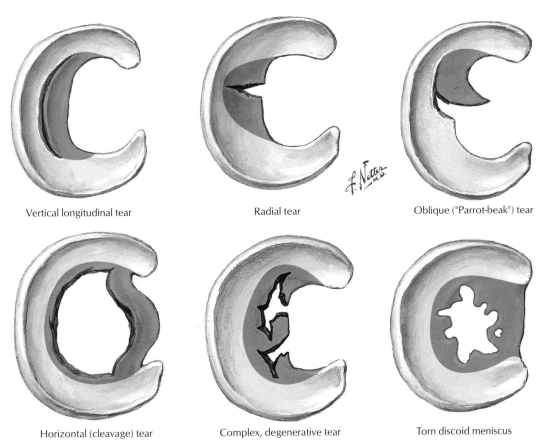

Vertical longitudinal tear   Radial tear   Oblique ("Parrot-beak") tear

Horizontal (cleavage) tear   Complex, degenerative tear   Torn discoid meniscus

Oblique tears are most commonly seen and are best treated by arthroscopic partial meniscectomy (APM). Vertical-longitudinal tears involving the peripheral third are best managed by repair. Radial split tears are usually secondary to trauma, and when the split extends to the capsular rim, repair should be attempted in young people if at all possible. Bucket-handle tears are more likely to cause locking of the knee. Horizontal (cleavage) and symptomatic degenerative tears are best treated by APM.

Figure 18-12: Discoid Meniscus Variations

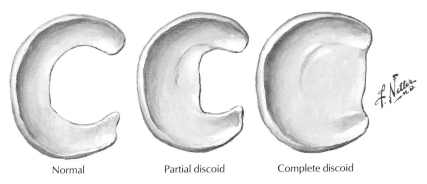

Normal   Partial discoid   Complete discoid

should be avoided due to its subcutaneous position.

The pes anserinus bursa is located between the insertion of the pes anserinus tendon and the underlying medial flare of the tibia (see **Figure 18-2**). Pes anserinus bursitis may be secondary to overuse or may be an early manifestation of medial compartment osteoarthritis. Examination shows mild swelling and tenderness over the bursa. Patients with osteoarthritis may have decreased motion and an antalgic gait. A torn medial meniscus should be excluded. Treatment modalities such as ultrasonography and phonophoresis are often required for patients with this overuse bursitis.

Patellofemoral Pain Syndrome

Anterior knee pain is a common complaint in adolescents, especially females and athletes, particularly runners. The cause is often difficult to identify but probably is a combination of instability/malalignment and overuse. The former is usually more pertinent in adolescents, and the latter makes a greater contribution in athletes.

These patients note peripatellar aching that is increased by extended walking or running activities. Pain is often increased when ascending or descending stairs or sitting with the knee flexed for a prolonged time (theater sign). The knee may give way during running or climbing—activities that create forces of several times the body weight across the patellofemoral joint.

Constraint of the patella in the femoral sulcus and forces acting across the patellofemoral joint are increased in the 20° to 60° arc of flexion (**Figure 18-13**). Factors that decrease constraint include generalized ligamentous laxity, a high-riding patella, a shallow angle/depth of the femoral sulcus, and an increased Q angle (angle formed by the quadriceps/patellar tendon alignment) that is increased with genu valgum or increased femoral anteversion and external tibial torsion. Decreased constraint of the patella causes instability and abnormal lateral translation of the patella during knee flexion/extension. Abnormal stress across the patella can occur with a low-riding patella and other unknown factors. The result is anterior knee pain that may progress to recurrent patellar subluxation/dislocation or patellofemoral arthritis.

Swelling is seldom noted. With instability, increased lateral translation of the patella and a positive apprehension sign (displacing the patella laterally, then flexing the knee with resultant pain and anxiety). Symptoms may be reproduced when the knee is flexed to 40° (patella now constrained) and then moving the patella proximally and distally. Tracking of the patella should be observed as the knee is flexed and extended. Patellar crepitation may be noted with flexion and extension.

Radiographs that include Merchant views should be examined to determine the position of the patella, abnormal subluxation or tilt, and arthritic changes. Most patients respond to nonoperative management that emphasizes strengthening of the quadriceps, particularly the vastus medialis, and stretching of any tightness of the hamstrings, iliotibial band, or gastrocnemius. With persistent symptoms and instability, patients may benefit from procedures that alter the alignment of the patellofemoral joint.

Bipartite Patella

A bipartite patella results from incomplete fusion of secondary centers of ossification. The superolateral corner is involved more than 75% of the time (**Figure 18-14**). These lesions rarely cause symptoms and are typically incidental findings on radiographs. However, a bipartite patella may become painful with overuse or injury. Examination shows localized tenderness that may be increased on maximum flexion. Symptoms typically resolve with rest and short-term immobilization.

Plica Injury

A plica is a normal fold in the synovium. The knee joint has three distinct plicae (**Figure 18-15**). The suprapatellar plica extends from the posterior surface of the quadriceps tendon to the medial or lateral capsule of the knee. The medial plica extends from the medial joint capsule to the infrapatellar fat pad. The infrapatel-

Figure 18-13: Subluxation and Dislocation of Patella

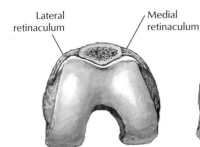

Lateral retinaculum | Medial retinaculum

Skyline view. Normally, patella rides in groove between medial and lateral femoral condyles

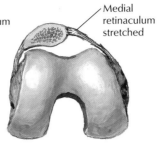

Medial retinaculum stretched

In subluxation, patella deviates laterally because of weakness of vastus medialis muscle, tightness of lateral retinaculum, and high Q angle

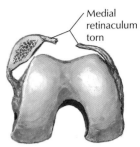

Medial retinaculum torn

In dislocation, patella displaced completely out of intercondylar groove

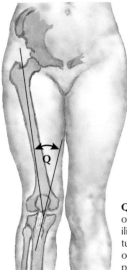

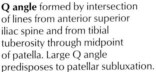

Apprehension test
Displace patella laterally and move the knee into flexion. Unstable patella will displace laterally and pain (apprehension) is noted at approximately 20° to 40° of flexion when the patella is compressed against the edge of the lateral condyle.

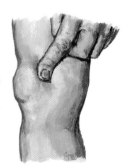

Q angle formed by intersection of lines from anterior superior iliac spine and from tibial tuberosity through midpoint of patella. Large Q angle predisposes to patellar subluxation.

Surgical procedures for recurrent patellar subluxation or dislocation

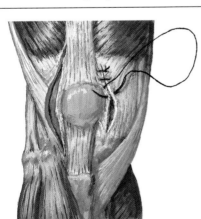

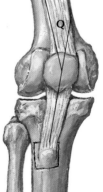

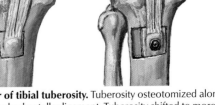

Lateral release. Lateral retinaculum incised, decreasing lateral pull on patella. Torn medial retinaculum sutured or tightened by plication.

Transfer of tibial tuberosity. Tuberosity osteotomized along with attached patellar ligament. Tuberosity shifted to more medial position and fixed with screw, reducing Q angle.

Figure 18-14: Bipartite Patella

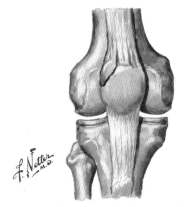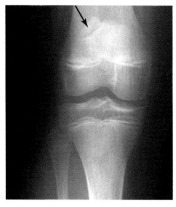

AP radiograph of knee in a 13-year-old boy who presented with pain at superolateral aspect of patella after a fall. Radiographs show bipartite patella. Patient treated with 4 weeks of immobilization for suspected quadriceps strain/slight avulsion of bipartite fragment. Symptoms resolved and patient resumed full activity.

lar plica, also called the *ligamentum mucosa,* can overlap the ACL as it extends from the intercondylar notch to the infrapatellar fat pad.

The medial plica is most likely to become symptomatic. Direct trauma to the anterior-medial aspect of the knee, often combined with repetitive flexion-extension sports, may cause inflammation and subsequent fibrosis and thickening of the plica. The thickened plica snaps across the medial femoral condyle. Patients report activity-related anterior-medial aching pain and occasionally note mild buckling of the knee. Examination shows tenderness on the medial aspect of the patella. The thickened plica may be palpated with the knee flexed. A snap is noted at 60° to 70° as the knee moves from flexion into extension.

Nonoperative management includes activity modification and NSAIDs. Injection of steroids into the plica may reduce inflammation and resolve symptoms. If pain persists and there is no evidence of other disorders, resection of the plica should be considered.

Popliteal Cyst

A popliteal (Baker) cyst is typically located between the semimembranosus tendon and the medial head of the gastrocnemius.

Popliteal cyst in children typically presents with a painless swelling without an apparent precipitating event. Spontaneous resolution is common.

A popliteal cyst in an adult is nearly always secondary to pathologic conditions within the knee, such as a tear of the medial meniscus or synovitis secondary to an inflammatory arthritis. Symptoms in adults include activity-related posterior knee pain and the presence of a mass. Large cysts may rupture, spilling synovial fluid into the surrounding tissues with a resultant acute pain and swelling that simulates deep venous thrombosis in the calf.

Initial treatment is directed at the underlying pathologic condition. The popliteal cyst commonly resolves after excision of a torn medial meniscus.

Chronic Exertional Compartment Syndrome of the Leg

Chronic compartment syndrome most often occurs in the leg. These patients have a thicker, less compliant fascia that does not accommodate the increased blood and muscle volume that develops during exertion and exercise. As a result there is abnormally in-

Figure 18-15: Synovial Plica

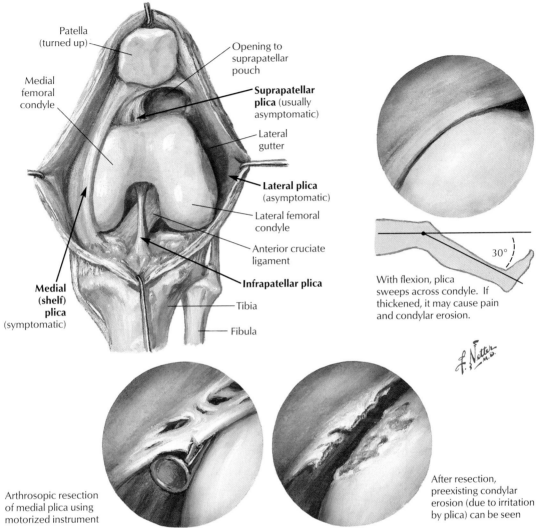

Patella (turned up)

Medial femoral condyle

Opening to suprapatellar pouch

Suprapatellar plica (usually asymptomatic)

Lateral gutter

Lateral plica (asymptomatic)

Lateral femoral condyle

Anterior cruciate ligament

Infrapatellar plica

Medial (shelf) plica (symptomatic)

Tibia

Fibula

With flexion, plica sweeps across condyle. If thickened, it may cause pain and condylar erosion.

30°

Arthroscopic resection of medial plica using motorized instrument

After resection, preexisting condylar erosion (due to irritation by plica) can be seen

creased tissue pressure in one or more of the four leg compartments (see **Figure 18-5**). Patients complain of achy leg pain and sometimes paresthesia radiating into the foot after running or other exercise activities that resolves with rest. The anterior compartment is most often involved.

The examination may be normal or there may be mild discomfort over the involved compartment. A fascial defect allowing muscle herniation during exertion may be pre-

sent. After exercise, the involved compartment is tender, and muscle weakness and paresthesia may be present. The diagnosis is confirmed through measurement of compartment pressures before and after exercise. These patients develop pressures >40 mm Hg with exercise, and the pressure typically remains elevated for a prolonged period (30 minutes or longer).

Nonoperative management includes a period of exercise cessation and sometimes a

Figure 18-16: Fracture of Distal Femur

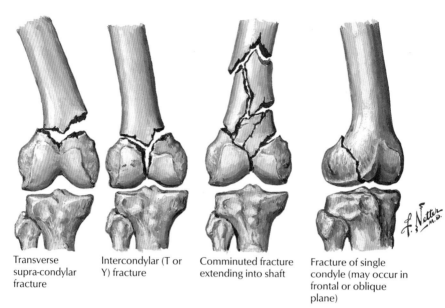

Transverse
supra-condylar
fracture

Intercondylar (T or
Y) fracture

Comminuted fracture
extending into shaft

Fracture of single
condyle (may occur in
frontal or oblique
plane)

continued reduction in exercise intensity. Fasciotomy is indicated for the management of persistent symptoms.

Shin Splints

Shin splints are a common, but poorly understood, condition. The primary symptom is the indolent onset of posteromedial pain in the middle to distal third of the leg, most often after running. The best explanation is inflammation of the periosteum caused by repetitive muscle contraction. Stress fracture of the tibia should be excluded.

TRAUMATIC CONDITIONS
Fractures in Adults

Distal femur fractures may be classified as *supracondylar fractures, supracondylar fractures with intra-articular extension,* or *isolated fractures of the medial or lateral condyle* (**Figure 18-16**). In young adults, these injuries typically result from high-energy axial loading of the flexed knee (eg, dashboard impact in a car crash). Concomitant injuries are common. In the elderly, the trauma that causes the injury may be trivial. Most fractures are displaced and require open reduction.

Fractures of the tibial plateau in young adults may occur with sports play or motor vehicle accidents (**Figure 18-17**). The lateral plateau is injured from a valgus, axial-loading force. More than 2 mm displacement of the articular surface necessitates operative reduction and internal fixation. Larger amounts of displacement can be accepted in a patient with osteoporosis and reduced activity.

Fractures of the patella usually are caused by a direct blow, but a powerful quadriceps contraction with the knee partially flexed can cause a transverse avulsion fracture. Direct trauma typically causes variable degrees of comminution. Displaced fractures require open reduction to restore articular congruity and the extensor mechanism (**Figure 18-18**). Markedly comminuted fractures may require partial or complete patellectomy, although the latter should be avoided if at all possible

Fractures of the tibial shaft are common in adults, and open fractures are more common in the tibia than in any other long bone. Fractures of the tibial shaft also are more likely to be complicated by nonunion, malunion, and infection. Closed treatment is primarily used in closed, minimally displaced, and axially stable injuries.

Figure 18-17: Tibial Plateau Fractures

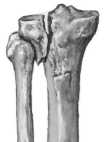
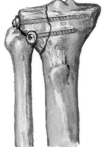

Split fracture of lateral tibial plateau. Repair with long cancellous screws

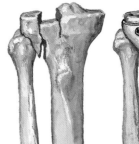
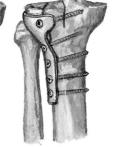

Split fracture of lateral condyle plus depression of tibial plateau. Repair by elevation of depressed segment plus bone graft and buttress plate

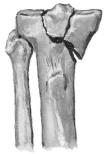

Comminuted split fracture of medial tibial plateau and tibial spine. Repair with buttress plate

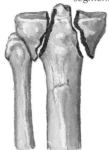

Bicondylar fracture involving both tibial plateaus with widening. Repair with two buttress plates and lag screws or with single locking plate

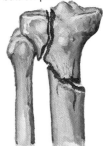

Fracture of lateral tibial plateau and tibial shaft at the metaphyseal-diaphyseal junction. Repair with locking plate

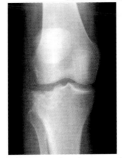

Split depression fracture of lateral tibial plateau

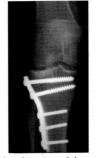

Repair by elevation of depressed segment plus bone graft and buttress plate

Intramedullary nailing is preferred for most open and unstable closed tibial shaft fractures.

Fractures in Children

Displaced distal femoral supracondylar and growth plate fractures can be difficult to reduce or to maintain reduction in casts. Open treatment with pin fixation and supplemental cast immobilization is commonly used for these injuries. Patellar fractures are uncommon in children and are treated similar to adult injuries.

Proximal tibia fractures in children occur in the adolescent years. The exception is a *metaphyseal* fracture, which is typically seen in the 2- to 8-year-old child. These fractures may cause genu valgum secondary to overgrowth of the medial aspect of the proximal tibial physis.

Fractures of the tibial tubercle occur during adolescence (**Figure 18-19**). Type I injuries

Figure 18-18: Fracture of the Patella

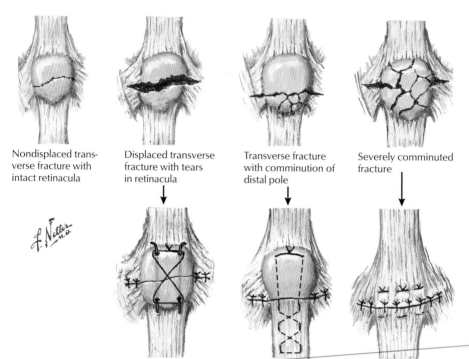

Nondisplaced transverse fracture with intact retinacula

Displaced transverse fracture with tears in retinacula

Transverse fracture with comminution of distal pole

Severely comminuted fracture

Displaced transverse or slightly comminuted fractures fixed with Steinmann pins through vertical drill holes plus figure-of-8 tension band wire and suture of retinacula.

Complete excision of lower pole plus re-attachment of patellar ligament to remainder of patella with wire through drill holes. Retinacula repaired.

In badly comminuted fractures, patella removed, quadriceps femoris tendon sutured to patellar ligament with nonabsorbable sutures, and retinacula repaired.

may be treated by casting in extension, while type II and type III injuries require open re-duction and screw fixation. Tibial spine frac-tures affect the attachment of the ACL. Type I and type II injuries can be treated by casting in extension. Type III injuries require open or arthroscopic reduction with suture or screw fixation.

Tibial shaft fractures in children can usually be treated by closed methods. A *toddler's fracture* occurs in a 1- to 3-year-old whose foot catches on an object while running or falling. The result is a rotational injury of the distal tibia that may be difficult to visualize on initial radiographs (occult fracture). The goal of reduction for displaced fractures is coronal angulation <10° in children and 5° in adoles-cents, <10° of sagittal angulation, and <1.5 cm of shortening. Grade III open fractures usually are treated with external fixation.

Dislocation/Subluxation of the Patella

Lateral subluxation/dislocation of the patella can result from a direct blow but most often occurs with the foot planted, the knee flexed 20° to 40°, and a valgus external rotation stress on the knee. These traumatic injuries merge with and have similar predisposing fac-tors as observed in patients with instability and the patellofemoral pain syndrome.

Patients report severe pain and that their knee popped out of place. The patella fre-quently reduces spontaneously, but closed re-duction may be required. Dislocation of the patella causes tearing of the medial retinacular tissues. Examination shows swelling, decreased

Figure 18-19

Fracture of Tibial Tubercle and Tibial Spine
Tibial spine (eminence) fracture

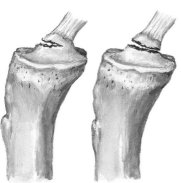
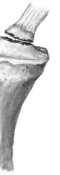
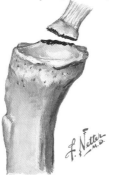

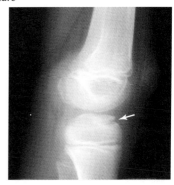

Type I. Incomplete
fracture of tibial
spine

Type II. Complete
fracture,
nondisplaced

Type IIIA. Complete
fracture, displaced

Type I tibial spine fracture

The terms tibial spine, tibial
eminence, and intercondylar
eminence are used
interchangeably to designate
the nonarticular portion of the
adjacent medial and lateral
tibial plateaus to which the
anterior cruciate ligament is
attached anteriorly. Injuries
that typically cause ruptures of
the anterior cruciate ligament in
adults often cause a fracture of
the tibial spine in children 7 to
14 years of age

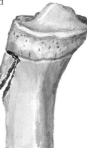
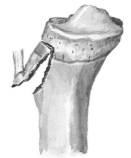
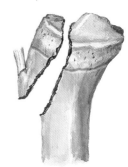

Type I

Type II

Type III

Fracture of the Tibial Shaft

20-year-old female who was
unrestrained passenger in a motor
vehicle accident. The patient sustained
multiple fractures including a closed
fracture of the right femoral shaft (A),
an open grade IIIA comminuted
fracture at the junction of the middle
third-distal third right tibia and a closed,
comminuted fracture of the middle
third of the left tibia and fibula, and a
comminuted fracture of the right
calcaneus. On the date of injury, the
patient underwent débridement of the
right tibia with application of an
external fixator, and retrograde nailing
of the right femur, and intramedullary
nailing of the left tibia. Nine days after
injury, intramedullary nailing of the
right tibia and open reduction and
plating of the right calcaneus were
done.

AP (B) and lateral (C) radiographs of
the tibia 2 months after intramedullary
nailing show good alignment but
limited healing of the fracture, which is
not unusual in open tibia fractures at
this location.

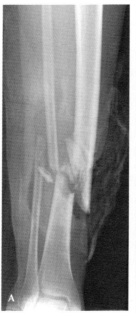
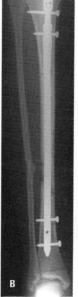
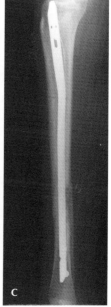

Figure 18-20: Dislocation of the Knee

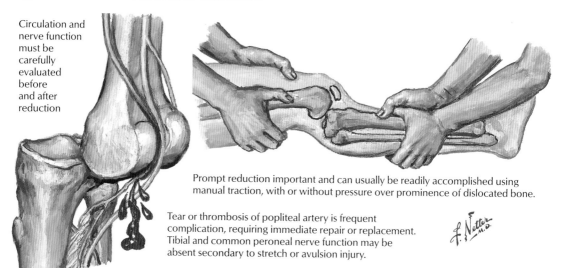

Circulation and nerve function must be carefully evaluated before and after reduction

Prompt reduction important and can usually be readily accomplished using manual traction, with or without pressure over prominence of dislocated bone.

Tear or thrombosis of popliteal artery is frequent complication, requiring immediate repair or replacement. Tibial and common peroneal nerve function may be absent secondary to stretch or avulsion injury.

motion, and tenderness medial to the patella. AP, lateral, and sunrise radiographs should be reviewed for possible avulsion fractures.

Patients who have sustained one dislocation of the patella are likely to experience additional episodes, particularly if they have predisposing factors. Recurrent episodes tend to occur with less trauma and milder symptoms than the initial episode.

The principles of treatment are to reduce pain and approximate the torn medial structures so that the vastus medialis heals in a normal instead of a lengthened position, which would enhance the possibility of recurrent instability. Initial treatment includes a compressive dressing and protective splint with the knee in extension. Aspiration of the hemarthrosis should be considered when there is a significant effusion. Isometric quadriceps exercises initially are done with the splint on. Reevaluate the patient every 2 weeks, and when medial tenderness resolves, institute motion and more vigorous strengthening exercises.

Associated osteochondral avulsion fractures that are intra-articular are uncommon but should be removed. Recurrent instability that does not respond to nonoperative treatment necessitates proximal and/or distal realignment of the extensor mechanism.

Dislocation of the Knee

Dislocation of the knee occurs secondary to multiple ligament injuries, usually of the ACL, the PCL, and one of the collaterals. Dislocation can occur in a high-energy trauma or it can occur as an isolated sports accident, that initially may be perceived as a relatively trivial injury. Dislocation of the knee can be a serious, limb-threatening injury because popliteal vessel tears occur in approximately one third. Anterior dislocations are the most common type.

The patient should be examined carefully for possible nerve or vascular injury. The dislocation should be reduced in an expedient manner (**Figure 18-20**). Any vascular injury requires emergency repair. Most studies recommend ACL and PCL reconstruction in 3 to 4 weeks.

Ligament Injuries

Collateral Ligament Injuries

An isolated MCL sprain results from an impact on the lateral aspect of the limb that causes a valgus force without rotation, such as occurs in football (see **Figure 5-6**). Isolated LCL sprains are less common and occur with a varus force.

Figure 18-21: Rupture of the Anterior Cruciate Ligament

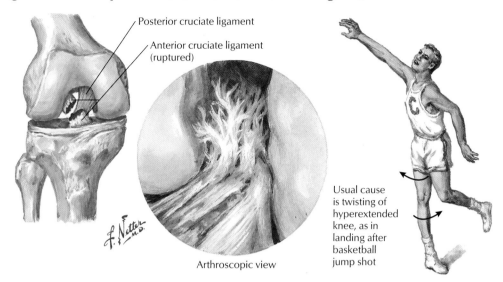

Posterior cruciate ligament

Anterior cruciate ligament (ruptured)

Arthroscopic view

Usual cause is twisting of hyperextended knee, as in landing after basketball jump shot

Most patients note tenderness on the involved side but are able to walk. The site of maximum tenderness varies, as the ligament may be partially or completely torn at any site. Isolated MCL or LCL sprains cause swelling of the adjacent tissues but do not create the significant joint effusion commonly observed in meniscal or cruciate ligament injuries.

Evaluate ligament stability in the following sequence. Assess collateral ligament stability by applying varus and valgus stress with the knee in full extension and 25° of flexion. In full extension, the posterior capsule and cruciate ligaments contribute to varus/valgus stability. Therefore, laxity in full extension indicates greater disruption of ligamentous structures. Laxity is based on joint opening: grade 1 (0 to 5 mm), grade 2 (5 to 10 mm), and grade 3 (>10 mm). Grade 3 valgus laxity in full extension indicates that the MCL and the posteromedial capsule are torn. Grade 3 varus laxity in full extension indicates tearing of the LCL and posterolateral capsular complex. Concomitant ACL or PCL tears also are more likely if grade 3 varus or valgus laxity is present at full extension. With the knee in flexion, the posterior capsule and cruciate ligaments are relaxed; therefore, instability that is observed only in this position indicates iso-lated collateral ligament injury. For example, pain on varus stress with less than 10 mm opening in full extension and more than 10 mm opening in 25° of flexion suggests an isolated complete LCL tear. Evaluate the knee for other injuries, particularly an associated meniscal or cruciate ligament tear.

Nonoperative treatment of isolated collateral ligament injury is satisfactory. Initial pain, swelling, and muscle spasm may mask the degree of injury. Management of MCL and LCL sprains requires ongoing evaluation for possible associated meniscal and cruciate injuries.

Anterior Cruciate Ligament Tears

The ACL is the primary restraint to anterior translation of the tibia; it also contributes to internal rotation and varus/valgus instability with the knee in extension. The anatomic configuration of its two bundles ensures functional tautness throughout the arc of motion, with the anteromedial bundle taut in flexion and the posterolateral component taut in extension. Although it may be torn by a contact injury, the ACL is most commonly injured without contact by a decelerating valgus angulation and external rotation force. In basketball, the ACL is commonly torn when a player lands from jumping with the knee in hyperextension and the tibia in internal rotation (**Figure 18-21**).

Examination shows a marked effusion, and most patients with an acute knee hemarthrosis have a torn ACL. The Lachman test is the most sensitive maneuver for detecting ACL tears. It is performed with the knee flexed to 20°. One hand placed laterally stabilizes the distal femur, and the other hand grasps the proximal tibia medially. The proximal tibia is pulled forward. With an intact ligament, minimal translation is felt and a firm end point is noted. With a torn ligament, more translation is noted, and the end point is soft. The hamstrings must be relaxed during the test to prevent false-negative findings.

Although not as sensitive as the Lachman maneuver, the anterior drawer test is easier to perform. It is performed with the patient supine, with the hamstrings relaxed, and the knee in 90° of flexion. The proximal tibia is grasped with both hands and pulled forward. Displacement >5 mm compared with the uninvolved side indicates an ACL tear.

Radiographs mostly rule out other injuries, but a lateral avulsion fracture (Segond fracture) indicating an associated lateral capsular tear may be present. If surgical reconstruction is planned, MRI is usually obtained to confirm diagnosis and to delineate associated injuries.

Cruciate ligaments do not heal with nonoperative treatment. With no treatment, the resultant recurrent instability makes return to previous level of sports participation unlikely and predisposes the patient to subsequent meniscal tears. Direct repair does not work. Intra-articular midpatellar bone-tendon-bone or hamstring tendon autograft reconstructive procedures provide the most consistent results, but allograft or extra-articular procedures are also used in selected cases. Possible complications include arthrofibrosis, repeat ACL tear, and patellar symptoms.

Posterior Cruciate Ligament Tears

The PCL provides primary restraint to posterior translation of the tibia. The PCL is the strongest knee ligament, and isolated PCL injuries are much less common than ACL tears.

Isolated PCL injuries usually occur with the knee in flexion, but may be secondary to a hyperextension injury (**Figure 18-22**). With severe extension/valgus/internal rotation contact injuries, the ACL is torn first, then the PCL is disrupted.

An effusion develops within 24 hours but is not as large as that observed in ACL tears. Assess PCL stability with the thumb sign and posterior drawer test. Place the leg in 90° of flexion. Usually, the tibial plateau is anterior to the femoral condyles, which permits the thumbs to rest on top of the tibial plateaus. With a disrupted PCL, the tibia falls back, and there is less space for the thumb. If the PCL is completely torn, the tibial plateaus are in line with the femoral condyles. Perform the posterior drawer test by applying a posteriorly directed force to the proximal tibia (see **Figure 18-22**). Increased posterior translation and a soft end point indicate PCL injury.

Isolated PCL injuries should be treated in a rehabilitation program that emphasizes increasing range of motion and quadriceps strengthening. Persistent or recurrent instability suggests concomitant meniscal tears. These patients may need reconstructive procedures.

Tendon Ruptures

A fall on a flexed knee can cause excessive eccentric loading of the extensor mechanism and rupture of the quadriceps or patellar tendon. A similar mechanism of injury can cause a patellar fracture. Quadriceps tendon ruptures generally occur in patients over 40 years old, while patellar tendon ruptures are more likely to occur in patients under 40 years of age. Predisposing factors to patellar tendon ruptures include diabetes mellitus, chronic renal failure, hyperthyroidism, gout, and multiple cortisone injections.

A large effusion and a palpable defect are usually present. The patient cannot actively extend the knee against gravity. With rupture of the patellar tendon, lateral radiographs show a patella that is higher than normal. Surgical repair is the treatment of choice for both quadriceps and patellar tendon rupture.

Figure 18-22: Rupture of Posterior Cruciate Ligament

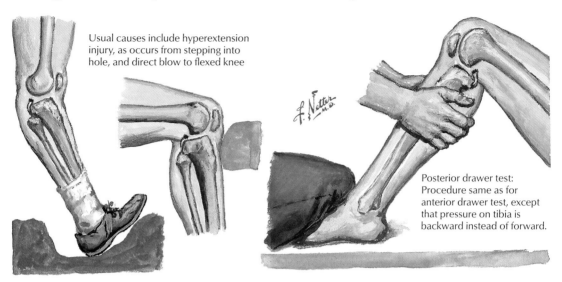

Usual causes include hyperextension injury, as occurs from stepping into hole, and direct blow to flexed knee

Posterior drawer test: Procedure same as for anterior drawer test, except that pressure on tibia is backward instead of forward.

PEDIATRIC CONDITIONS

Congenital Disorders of the Knee and Leg

Congenital dislocation of the knee causes striking hyperextension of the knee (**Figure 18-23**). The disorder ranges from a position-ing deformity that readily responds to short-term splinting to a resistant deformity that does not respond to serial casting and re-quires surgery. Associated hip dislocation and clubfoot commonly accompany true dislocation of the knee.

Congenital dislocation of the patella is often

Figure 18-23: Congenital Dislocation of the Knee

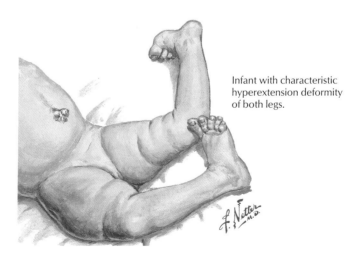

Infant with characteristic hyperextension deformity of both legs.

overlooked at birth because the infant's patella is small and often cannot be palpated in its lateral dislocated position. A persistent flexion contracture and external rotation of the tibia suggest the presence of this condition. Because the patella does not ossify until 3 to 5 years of age, ultrasonography is helpful in confirming the diagnosis. Operative treatment is necessary and requires an extensive lateral release and medial imbrication/realignment.

Posteromedial bowing of the tibia is usually obvious at birth; however, because the bowing causes the foot to be in apparent dorsiflexion and valgus, the disorder initially may be misdiagnosed as a calcaneovalgus foot (**Figure 18-24**). The condition is idiopathic, unilateral, and causes the affected limb to be short. The bowing gradually is corrected with growth, so realignment osteotomy is not necessary. Variable degrees of leg-length discrepancy persist and may require a shoe lift and possibly a contralateral epiphysiodesis.

Anterolateral bowing of the tibia may not be obvious at birth, is associated with neurofibromatosis, and frequently progresses to *congenital pseudarthrosis of the tibia,* a condition that results in an unstable extremity and requires complicated operations that have a high failure rate (**Figure 18-25**). In infants with anterolateral bowing of the tibia, bracing may prevent progression to pseudarthrosis.

Fibular hemimelia is a sporadic congenital deletion. Leg-length discrepancy is universal, is less severe if the fibula is partially present, and ranges from 2 to 16 cm at skeletal maturity. The deletion often includes the lateral aspect of the foot with the absence of one or more lateral rays and abnormalities of the tarsal bones causing valgus alignment of the hindfoot and equinus contracture of the ankle. The tibia may be bowed anteriorly. Mild shortening of the femur and mild hypoplasia of the lateral femoral condyle with subsequent genu valgum often are observed with complete absence of the fibula. Treatment depends on the severity of the condition. If the anticipated limb-length discrepancy is large (8 to 16 cm), if the foot is dysfunctional, or if both occur, the best treatment is disarticulation at the ankle and prosthetic fitting during the first 2 years of life. In a patient with a functional foot and anticipated shortening of less than 30% of the opposite side, other modalities to equalize leg lengths may be considered.

Tibia hemimelia is partial or complete absence of the fibula. Associated deletions of one or more of the medial rays and equinovarus foot deformity are common. Tibia hemimelia may be sporadic or be an autosomal dominant inherited disorder. Familial disorders are often bilateral and have upper extremity deletions. With unilateral involvement, the anticipated leg-length discrepancy

Figure 18-24: Posteromedial Bowing of the Tibia

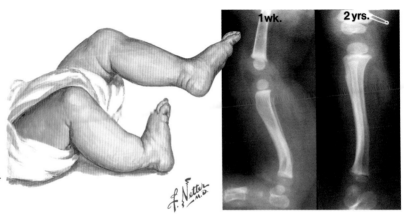

Posteromedial bowing. Convexity of bow in distal third of tibia and fibula directed posteriorly and medially. Spontaneous correction usually obviates need for realignment osteotomy, but leg-length discrepancy often persistent.

Figure 18-25: Anterolateral Bowing of Tibia and Congenital Pseudarthrosis of Tibia

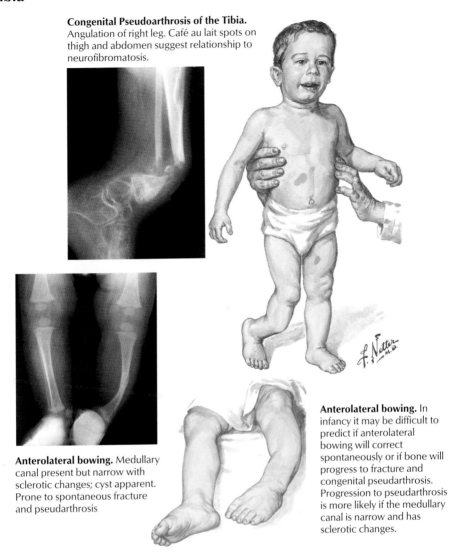

Congenital Pseudoarthrosis of the Tibia. Angulation of right leg. Café au lait spots on thigh and abdomen suggest relationship to neurofibromatosis.

Anterolateral bowing. Medullary canal present but narrow with sclerotic changes; cyst apparent. Prone to spontaneous fracture and pseudarthrosis

Anterolateral bowing. In infancy it may be difficult to predict if anterolateral bowing will correct spontaneously or if bone will progress to fracture and congenital pseudarthrosis. Progression to pseudarthrosis is more likely if the medullary canal is narrow and has sclerotic changes.

is large. If the proximal tibia is present and the quadriceps can actively extend the knee, disarticulation of the ankle and prosthetic fitting before age 2 years is the best treatment option. If the proximal tibia is absent or the quadriceps muscle is dysfunctional, a knee disarticulation and appropriate prosthetic fitting provide the best function.

Tibia Vara

Children with *infantile tibia vara* have persistent and progressive genu varum (see Chapter 3). Infantile tibia vara develops from excessive loading and subsequent deficient growth of the medial aspect of the proximal tibial physis. Associated factors are obesity and walking at an early age, when the knee is

Figure 18-26: Infantile Tibia Vara

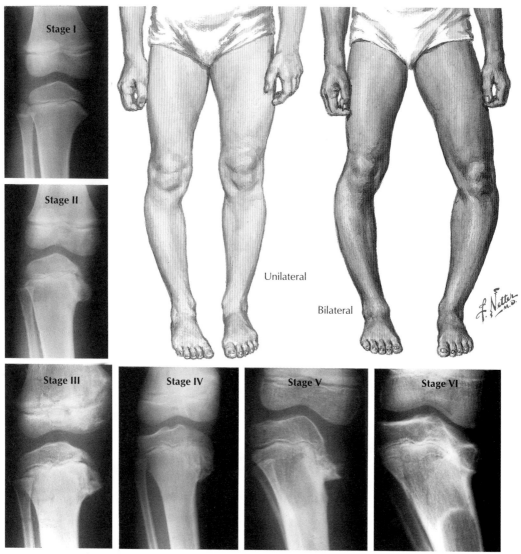

Radiographs demonstrate stages of Infantile Tibia Vara: progressive deformity of medial side of proximal tibial epiphysis and development of metaphyseal beak

in greater varus and walking may abnormally load the medial side of the physis.

Children with infantile tibia vara typically present for evaluation at between 18 and 36 months. In addition to genu varum, the disorder is associated with internal tibial torsion (**Figure 18-26**). Radiographs at this age usually do not demonstrate the diagnostic inferior sloping of the metaphysis that is present

at an older age, but measurement of the tibial metaphyseal-diaphyseal angle can help differentiate physiologic genu varum from infantile tibia vara. Bracing may correct the genu varum in children younger than 3 years. Realignment osteotomy is required for older children.

Adolescent tibia vara is progressive genu varum that insidiously develops, usually after

9 years of age. This disorder results from excessive compression and subsequent deficient growth of the medial aspect of the proximal tibial physis. Risk factors include morbid obesity, male sex, and African American race. If the physis is open, hemiepiphysiodesis should be performed on the lateral aspect of the physis. After skeletal maturity, realignment osteotomy should be performed to correct any residual deformity.

Osgood–Schlatter Disease

Osgood-Schlatter disease results from repetitive microtrauma at the insertion of the patellar tendon into the secondary ossification center of the tibial tuberosity. Onset of the condition is during early adolescence and coincides with the development of this ossification center, which is a weak link to repetitive quadriceps contraction. Overuse explains the 4 times greater incidence in athletic versus sedentary children. Patients present with a painful prominence of the anterior tibial tubercle.

Examination shows swelling and tenderness at the tibial tubercle but no restriction of motion (see **Figure 10-6**). Radiographs may be normal or may show heterotopic ossification and fragmentation of the tibial tubercle.

Treatment consists of activity modification to allow healing of microscopic avulsion fractures. Short-term immobilization for 4 to 8 weeks may benefit patients with severe or recalcitrant symptoms. If the patient is a highly competitive athlete, the parents and patient must understand that return to full sports activity often is not possible for 6 to 10 months.

ADDITIONAL READINGS

DeLee JC, Dres D Jr, Millder MD, eds. *DeLee and Drez's Orthopaedic Sports Medicine: Principles and Practice*, 2nd edition. Philadelphia, Pa: WB Saunders; 2003.

Harner CD, Vince KG, Fu FH. *Techniques in Knee Surgery*. Philadelphia, Pa: Lippincott, Williams and Wilkins; 2000.

Insall JN, Scott WN. *Surgery of the Knee*; 3rd edition. Philadelphia, Pa: Churchill Livingstone; 2001.

Sculco TP, Martucci EA, eds. *Knee Arthroplasty*. New York, NY: Springer; 2001.

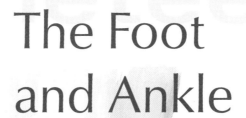

The Foot and Ankle

Judith F. Baumhauer, MD

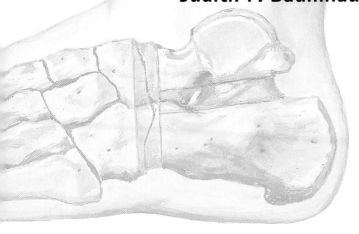

ANATOMY AND BIOMECHANICS

The foot is composed of 26 bones with multiple articulations held together by strong ligaments (**Figure 19-1**). It provides a stable mobile platform for standing, walking, and running through a complex balance of muscle contractions and sensory feedback. Power for motion comes from 10 extrinsic tendons crossing the ankle joint and many intrinsic muscles with origins in the foot (**Figure 19-2**).

The ankle is a hinge joint with articulations between the tibia, fibula, and talus. The weight-bearing surface of the tibia articulates with the spool-shaped surface of the talus. The ankle has a mortise and tenon configuration, with the talus being the tenon articulation and the medial malleolus and distal fibula (lateral malleolus) forming the articu-

lating sides of the mortise. As is typical with hinge joints, the capsule is thin in the plane of motion but supported by collateral ligaments. The thick *deltoid ligament* has four components that extend from the medial malleolus to the talus, calcaneus, and navicular (**Figure 19-3**). The *lateral ligament complex* includes the anterior and posterior talofibular ligaments and the calcaneofibular ligament.

The foot is commonly divided into the forefoot, midfoot, and hindfoot. The forefoot contains 5 metatarsals and 14 phalanges and is separated from the midfoot by the tarsometatarsal joint (of Lisfranc). The midfoot includes the 3 cuneiforms, the navicular, and the cuboid and is separated from the hindfoot by the transverse midtarsal joint (of Chopart).

Figure 19-1: Bones of Foot

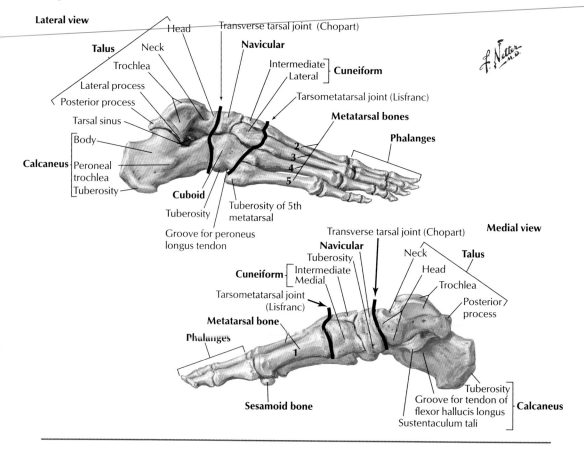

Figure 19-1: Bones of Foot *(continued)*

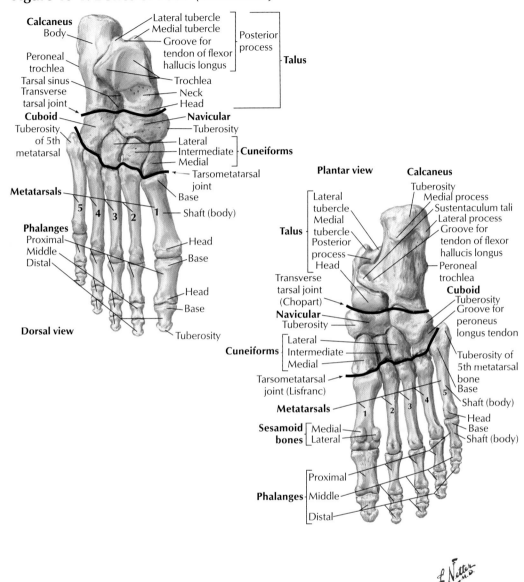

The hindfoot contains 2 bones—the talus and the calcaneus.

The *plantar fascia* originates from the calcaneal tubercle, inserts on the base of the proximal phalanges, and acts as a windlass to support the longitudinal arch of the foot during the midstance phase of gait (**Figure 19-4**). As the weight-bearing stresses are shifted to the foot and the toes are dorsiflexed, the plantar fascia is stiffened and pulled forward under the metatarsal heads. This elevates the longitudinal arch and plantarflexes the metatarsals.

The major plane of ankle motion is dorsiflexion and plantarflexion. Inversion and eversion of the foot, as well as the ability to

Figure 19-2: Bony Attachments of Muscles of Foot

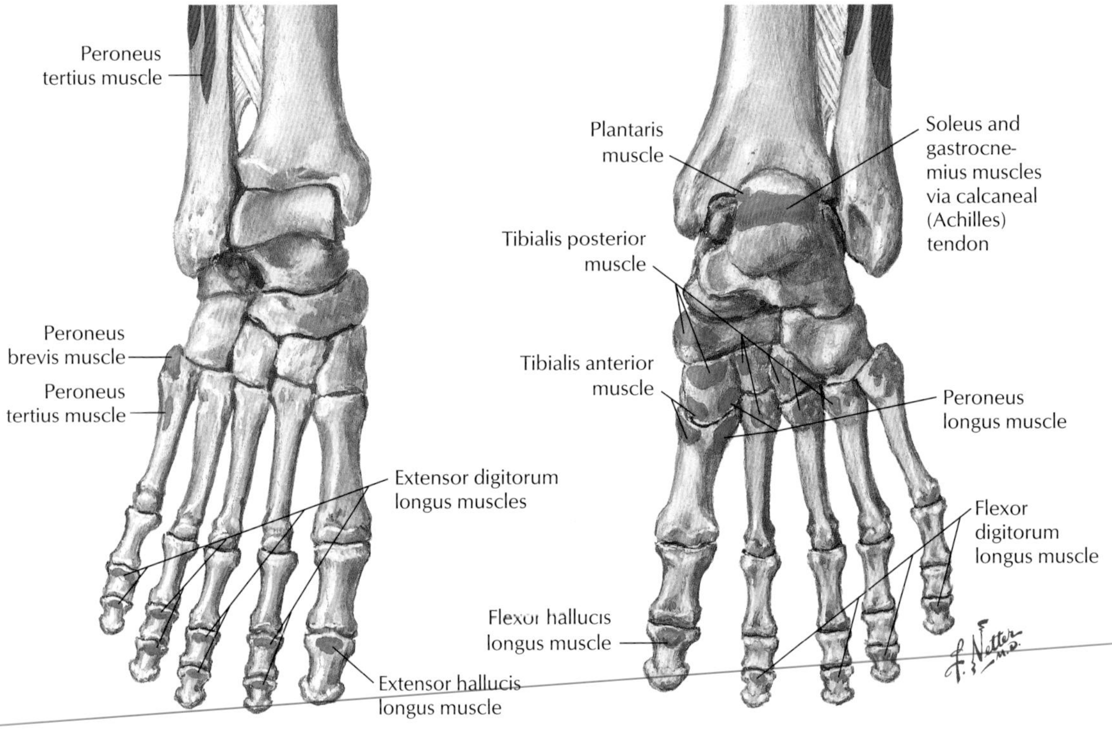

Peroneus tertius muscle

Peroneus brevis muscle

Peroneus tertius muscle

Extensor digitorum longus muscles

Extensor hallucis longus muscle

Plantaris muscle

Tibialis posterior muscle

Tibialis anterior muscle

Flexor hallucis longus muscle

Soleus and gastrocnemius muscles via calcaneal (Achilles) tendon

Peroneus longus muscle

Flexor digitorum longus muscle

accommodate to uneven ground, occur primarily at the subtalar (talocalcaneal) joint. Limited abduction and adduction of the forefoot occur at the transverse midtarsal joints (i.e., the ball-and-socket talonavicular joint and the calcaneocuboid joint). Very little motion occurs in the midfoot joints (the 3 cuneiform-navicular joints and the 5 tarsometatarsal joints). Flexibility in the fourth and fifth tarsometatarsal joints, however, does provide accommodation to uneven ground. The plane of motion at the toe joints is dorsiflexion and plantarflexion. Composite motions are supination, which includes forefoot adduction, hindfoot inversion, and ankle plantarflexion, and the opposite pronation, which includes forefoot abduction, hindfoot eversion, and ankle dorsiflexion.

Muscles posterior to the axis of the ankle joint—gastrocnemius-soleus, tibialis posterior, flexor hallucis longus, flexor digitorum longus, peroneus longus, and peroneus brevis—plantarflex the ankle joint (see **Figures 19-2** and **19-4**). Musculotendinous structures that pass anterior to the ankle axis—tibialis anterior, extensor hallucis longus, extensor digitorum longus, and peroneus tertius—dorsiflex the ankle (**Figure 19-5**). Muscles passing medial to the axis of the subtalar joint—tibialis posterior, flexor hallucis longus, flexor digitorum longus, and tibialis anterior—provide inversion motion. Structures lateral to this axis—extensor hallucis longus, extensor digitorum longus, peroneus longus, peroneus brevis, and peroneus tertius—produce eversion motion.

In all, 6 nerves and 3 vessels supply the foot.

Figure 19-3: Ligaments of the Ankle and Foot

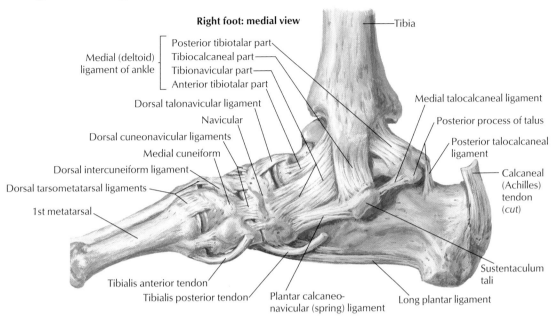

Right foot: medial view

Tibia

Medial (deltoid) ligament of ankle
- Posterior tibiotalar part
- Tibiocalcaneal part
- Tibionavicular part
- Anterior tibiotalar part

Dorsal talonavicular ligament

Navicular

Dorsal cuneonavicular ligaments

Medial cuneiform

Dorsal intercuneiform ligament

Dorsal tarsometatarsal ligaments

1st metatarsal

Medial talocalcaneal ligament

Posterior process of talus

Posterior talocalcaneal ligament

Calcaneal (Achilles) tendon (cut)

Sustentaculum tali

Tibialis anterior tendon

Tibialis posterior tendon

Plantar calcaneo-navicular (spring) ligament

Long plantar ligament

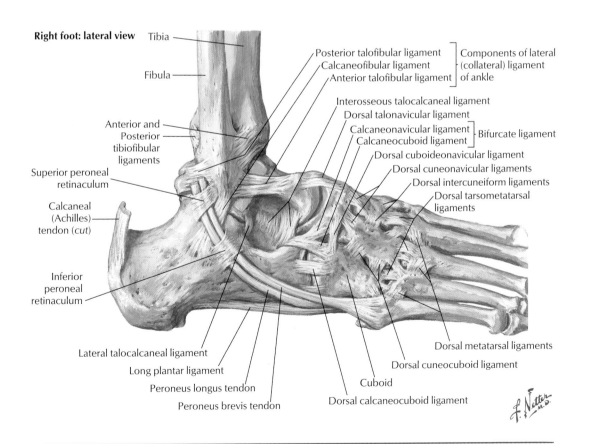

Right foot: lateral view

Tibia

Fibula

Anterior and Posterior tibiofibular ligaments

Superior peroneal retinaculum

Calcaneal (Achilles) tendon (cut)

Inferior peroneal retinaculum

Lateral talocalcaneal ligament

Long plantar ligament

Peroneus longus tendon

Peroneus brevis tendon

Posterior talofibular ligament
Calcaneofibular ligament
Anterior talofibular ligament
} Components of lateral (collateral) ligament of ankle

Interosseous talocalcaneal ligament

Dorsal talonavicular ligament

Calcaneonavicular ligament
Calcaneocuboid ligament
} Bifurcate ligament

Dorsal cuboideonavicular ligament

Dorsal cuneonavicular ligaments

Dorsal intercuneiform ligaments

Dorsal tarsometatarsal ligaments

Dorsal metatarsal ligaments

Dorsal cuneocuboid ligament

Cuboid

Dorsal calcaneocuboid ligament

Figure 19-4: Muscles, Arteries, and Nerves of Sole of Foot

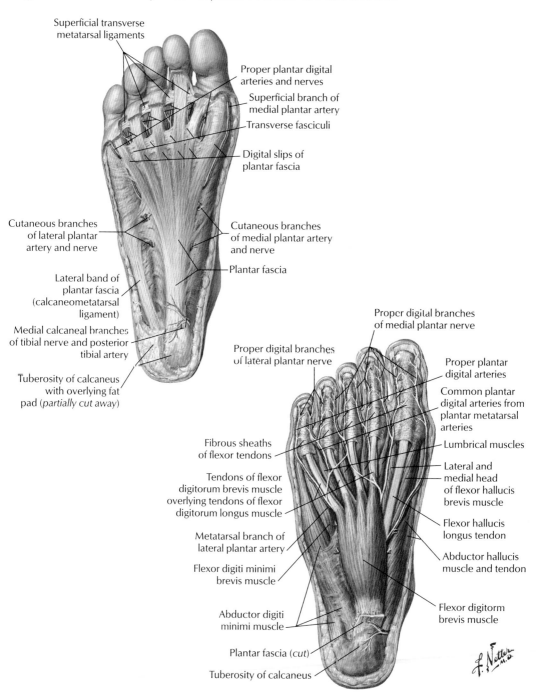

Superficial transverse metatarsal ligaments

Proper plantar digital arteries and nerves

Superficial branch of medial plantar artery

Transverse fasciculi

Digital slips of plantar fascia

Cutaneous branches of lateral plantar artery and nerve

Cutaneous branches of medial plantar artery and nerve

Plantar fascia

Lateral band of plantar fascia (calcaneometatarsal ligament)

Medial calcaneal branches of tibial nerve and posterior tibial artery

Tuberosity of calcaneus with overlying fat pad (*partially cut away*)

Proper digital branches of medial plantar nerve

Proper digital branches of lateral plantar nerve

Proper plantar digital arteries

Common plantar digital arteries from plantar metatarsal arteries

Lumbrical muscles

Lateral and medial head of flexor hallucis brevis muscle

Flexor hallucis longus tendon

Abductor hallucis muscle and tendon

Flexor digitorm brevis muscle

Fibrous sheaths of flexor tendons

Tendons of flexor digitorum brevis muscle overlying tendons of flexor digitorum longus muscle

Metatarsal branch of lateral plantar artery

Flexor digiti minimi brevis muscle

Abductor digiti minimi muscle

Plantar fascia (*cut*)

Tuberosity of calcaneus

Figure 19-5: Common Peroneal Nerve

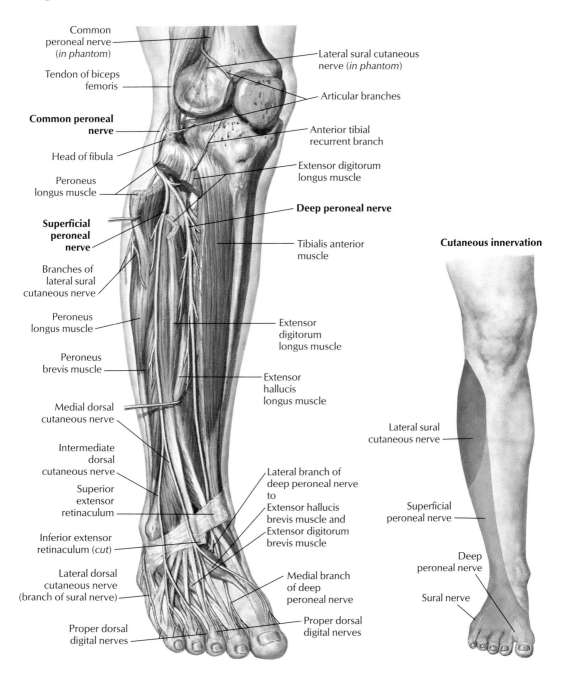

Common peroneal nerve (*in phantom*)

Tendon of biceps femoris

Common peroneal nerve

Head of fibula

Peroneus longus muscle

Superficial peroneal nerve

Branches of lateral sural cutaneous nerve

Peroneus longus muscle

Peroneus brevis muscle

Medial dorsal cutaneous nerve

Intermediate dorsal cutaneous nerve

Superior extensor retinaculum

Inferior extensor retinaculum (*cut*)

Lateral dorsal cutaneous nerve (branch of sural nerve)

Proper dorsal digital nerves

Lateral sural cutaneous nerve (*in phantom*)

Articular branches

Anterior tibial recurrent branch

Extensor digitorum longus muscle

Deep peroneal nerve

Tibialis anterior muscle

Extensor digitorum longus muscle

Extensor hallucis longus muscle

Lateral branch of deep peroneal nerve to Extensor hallucis brevis muscle and Extensor digitorum brevis muscle

Medial branch of deep peroneal nerve

Proper dorsal digital nerves

Cutaneous innervation

Lateral sural cutaneous nerve

Superficial peroneal nerve

Deep peroneal nerve

Sural nerve

Terminal branches of the *saphenous nerve* provide cutaneous sensation on the medial side of the foot, and the *sural nerve* innervates the lateral side. The *deep peroneal nerve* provides sensation to the dorsum of the first interspace, whereas the superficial peroneal nerve provides sensation to the remainder of the dorsum of the foot (**Figures 19-5** and **19-6**). The *tibial nerve* divides into *medial and lateral plantar nerves* that supply the numerous small plantar muscles and the bottom of the foot (see **Figure 19-4**). The *posterior tibial artery* accompanies the tibial nerve and likewise divides into medial and lateral plantar branches. The *anterior tibial artery* continues on the dorsal aspect of the foot as the *dorsalis pedis artery*, gives off medial and lateral tarsal branches, and ends by dividing into the arcuate artery and the deep plantar artery (see **Figure 19-6**). The perforating branch of the peroneal artery is typically small, but it may be the principal source of the blood supply to the dorsum of the foot when the dorsalis pedis is absent.

The gait cycle during walking and running consists of stance and swing phases (**Figure 19-7**). In normal walking, the *stance phase* goes from ipsilateral heel-strike to ipsilateral toe-off and occupies 62% of the gait cycle. *Swing* is from toe-off to ipsilateral heel-strike and is the remaining 38% of the gait cycle.

The stance phase includes an initial period of double-limb support, an intermediate phase of single-limb support, and a terminal stance phase of double-limb support. The initial period of double-limb support, also called the *loading response,* starts with *heel-strike,* ends with *opposite toe-off,* and occupies 12% of the gait cycle. Normal heel-strike occurs on the lateral aspect of the heel, with the ankle in the neutral position and the foot positioned into supination. As the foot progresses to foot flat, the ankle goes into plantarflexion, and the hindfoot progresses into valgus and pronation. This permits shock absorption and allows the foot to accommodate to uneven ground.

Single-limb support (midstance) corresponds to the swing phase of the contralateral limb and marks a reversal from stance limb absorption to stance limb propulsion. For momentum to advance the body over a stationary foot, the foot must move to a rigid lever. This is accomplished by inversion of the heel and locking of the subtalar and Chopart joints as the ankle goes into dorsiflexion. During the second phase of double support, the ipsilateral foot goes from heel-off to toe-off, with the ankle demonstrating progressive plantarflexion.

PHYSICAL EXAMINATION

Inspect the foot and ankle from all four sides with the patient standing, then supine. Assess heel alignment from the back. The normal finding is slight valgus with no lateral toes visualized. With pes planovalgus (flatfoot), the lateral toes are visible from the posterior view. From the anterior view, look at the alignment of the toes and the relationship of the forefoot to the hindfoot. Inspect the foot on the medial side for a high arch (cavus foot), flatfoot, or asymmetry of the foot. On the lateral side, look for prominence of the posterior calcaneus and abnormal swelling. Inspect the plantar aspect of the foot for callosities, prominence of the metatarsals, or ulceration. Assess the alignment of the foot during the different phases of gait. Palpate the foot and ankle for abnormal tenderness or swelling. This finding might indicate synovitis, tenosynovitis, plantar fasciitis, or degenerative arthritis.

To measure ankle motion, the *zero starting position* is with the foot perpendicular to the tibia. *Dorsiflexion* is movement of the foot toward the anterior surface of the tibia; *plantarflexion* is movement of the foot in the opposite direction (**Figure 19-8**). Normal ankle dorsiflexion is 10° to 20°, and plantarflexion is 35° to 50°. *Inversion* (inward turning of the heel) and *eversion* (outward turning of the heel) are estimated visually (**Figure 19-9**). The *zero starting position* is with the ankle in slight dorsiflexion, which limits side-to-side motion from the ankle and therefore allows better assessment of talocalcaneal mobility. Supination and pronation are difficult to quantify. Comparison with the unaffected

Figure 19-6: Muscles, Arteries, and Nerves of Front of Ankle and Dorsum of Foot

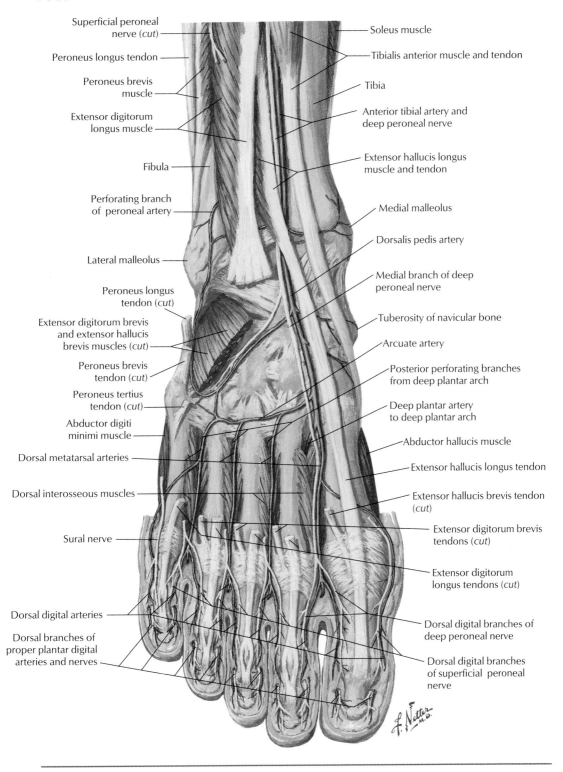

Superficial peroneal nerve (*cut*)

Peroneus longus tendon

Peroneus brevis muscle

Extensor digitorum longus muscle

Fibula

Perforating branch of peroneal artery

Lateral malleolus

Peroneus longus tendon (*cut*)

Extensor digitorum brevis and extensor hallucis brevis muscles (*cut*)

Peroneus brevis tendon (*cut*)

Peroneus tertius tendon (*cut*)

Abductor digiti minimi muscle

Dorsal metatarsal arteries

Dorsal interosseous muscles

Sural nerve

Dorsal digital arteries

Dorsal branches of proper plantar digital arteries and nerves

Soleus muscle

Tibialis anterior muscle and tendon

Tibia

Anterior tibial artery and deep peroneal nerve

Extensor hallucis longus muscle and tendon

Medial malleolus

Dorsalis pedis artery

Medial branch of deep peroneal nerve

Tuberosity of navicular bone

Arcuate artery

Posterior perforating branches from deep plantar arch

Deep plantar artery to deep plantar arch

Abductor hallucis muscle

Extensor hallucis longus tendon

Extensor hallucis brevis tendon (*cut*)

Extensor digitorum brevis tendons (*cut*)

Extensor digitorum longus tendons (*cut*)

Dorsal digital branches of deep peroneal nerve

Dorsal digital branches of superficial peroneal nerve

Figure 19-7: Phases of Gait

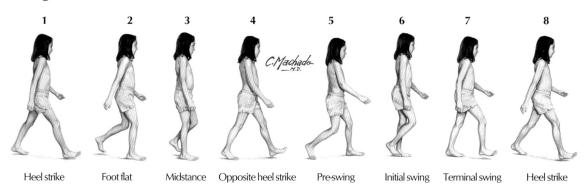

1	2	3	4	5	6	7	8
Heel strike	Foot flat	Midstance	Opposite heel strike	Pre-swing	Initial swing	Terminal swing	Heel strike

foot provides the best assessment of these composite motions.

Grading muscle strength starts by placement of the muscle in a contracted position and the other muscles that have similar function in positions that eliminate or lessen their activity during the test. Therefore, when testing the anterior tibialis muscle, place the foot in dorsiflexion and inversion and ask the patient to pull the foot into more dorsiflexion and at the same time flex the toes (which eliminates the activity of the toe extensors) while you provide resistance in the opposite direction (see section on muscle testing in Chapter 12).

Figure 19-8: Ankle Dorsiflexion/Plantarflexion

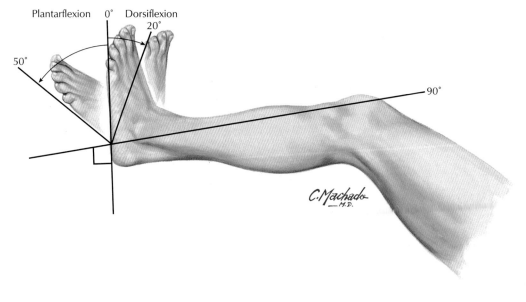

Figure 19-9: Inversion and Eversion

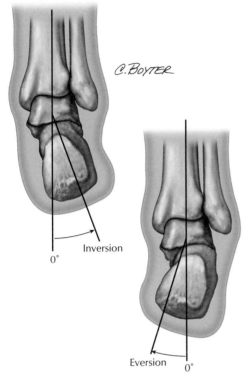

Most precise clinical measurement performed with patient prone and knee flexed. Place ankle in slight dorsiflexion to limit side-to-side motion at the ankle; therefore, providing better isolation of talocalcaneal mobility.

DEGENERATIVE DISORDERS

Arthritis of the Foot and Ankle

Osteoarthritis and traumatic arthropathy are the most common types of arthritis of the foot and ankle. Common sites include the first metatarsophalangeal (MTP) joint, midfoot (Lisfranc joints), talonavicular joint, talocalcaneal joint, and ankle joint (**Figure 19-10**). *Hallux rigidus* is the term for degenerative arthritis of the great toe MTP joint.

Patients report activity-related pain and swelling in the region of the affected joint. With ankle arthritis, pain frequently is localized to the anterior aspect of the joint. With talocalcaneal arthritis, pain typically is localized to the lateral aspect of the hindfoot. Swelling and osteophytes are obvious with arthropathy of superficial joints and motion is restricted in joints that have substantial movement.

Nonoperative treatment includes shoe modification or the use of supportive orthotics. For hallux rigidus or midfoot arthritis, a stiff-soled shoe may alleviate symptoms. For end-stage arthritis in the foot, arthrodesis is the most common surgical procedure (**Figure 19-11**). Dorsal cheilectomy or resection arthroplasty may be used to treat patients with hallux rigidus, and total joint arthroplasty may be indicated for patients with ankle arthritis.

Plantar Fasciitis

Plantar fasciitis, the most common cause of heel pain in adults, results from periostitis of the calcaneus at the origin of the plantar fascia. Plantar fasciitis is more common in females and in obese persons, but it is not associated with any particular foot type. Patients relate the insidious onset of pain that is particularly severe with first steps in the morning or when rising from a sitting position at the end of the day. Palpation with pressure demonstrates tenderness at the medial process of the calcaneal tuberosity. Radiographs show an osteophyte (heel spur) in 50% of patients; however, this spur is not the source of pain and is noted in 20% of asymptomatic adults.

Differential diagnosis includes tarsal tunnel syndrome (tibial nerve compression at the ankle with resultant plantar foot paresthesias), traumatic rupture of the plantar fascia (marked pain in the middle portion of the plantar fascia and swelling), seronegative spondyloarthropathy (enthesitis that is typically bilateral, and with other sites involved), and stress fracture of the calcaneus (medial and lateral heel pain that is activity related but not severe on awakening).

Most patients can be managed nonoperatively, but they should be counseled that it commonly takes 6 to 12 months for symptoms to resolve. Effective modalities include orthotics that unload the heel, exercises to

Chapter 19

Figure 19-10: Radiographs Depicting Arthritis in Various Sites of the Foot

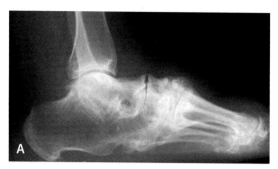
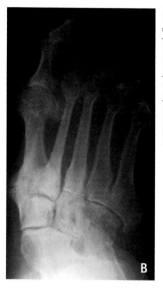
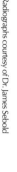

Radiographs courtesy of Dr. James Sebold

Arthritis of midfoot. Lateral radiograph (A) and standing AP radiograph (B) of the foot of a 61-year-old female with narrowing and degenerative changes in the tarsometatarsal and naviculocunieform joints. Arthritis secondary to transfer of stress following triple arthrodesis several years previously for foot deformity related to Charcot-Marie-Tooth disease. Obesity is a secondary factor. Toes demonstrate Charcot fragmentation secondary to the peripheral neuropathy.

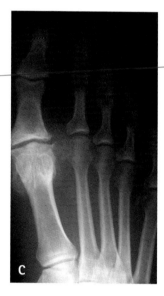
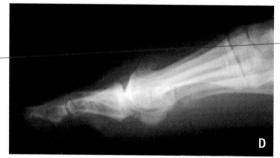

Hallux rigidus: arthritis of great toe metatarsophalangeal joint. Standing AP radiograph (C) and standing lateral radiograph (D) of a 42-year-old male with 10 year history of progressive pain in great toe and enlargement of dorsum of the toe. Pain increased with walking and especially aggravated with walking on inclines. No history of injury. Examination showed bony osteophytes and marked restriction of great toe metatarsophalangeal motion with only 10° of extension and 5° of flexion. Radiographs show narrowing of the joint and marked osteophyte formation, particularly on the lateral and dorsal aspects of the metatarsal.

stretch the Achilles tendon, night splints to keep the Achilles tendon on stretch, and steroid injections. Recalcitrant symptoms may require partial release of the plantar fascia.

Posterior Tibial Tendon Dysfunction

The posterior tibialis muscle is a major supporting structure of the midfoot during single-limb support. Not only does the posterior tibialis muscle actively contract during this phase of gait, but its tendon insertion extends beyond the navicular to all of the midfoot tarsal bones. Thus, this muscle provides an active supporting sling to counterbalance weight-bearing stresses.

Dysfunction of the posterior tibialis tendon (PTT) is the most common cause of acquired

Figure 19-11: Triple Arthrodesis

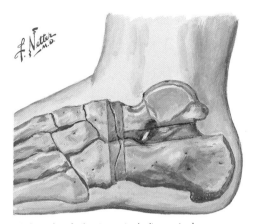

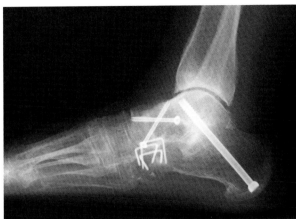

Triple arthrodesis. Bone, including articular surfaces, removed at talocalcaneal, talonavicular, and calcaneocuboid joint.

Lateral radiograph showing triple arthrodesis with internal fixation of talocalcaneal joint with 7.3 mm screw, cross 4.5 mm screw fixation of talonavicular joint, and staple fixation of calcaneocuboid joint.

flatfoot in adults (**Figure 19-12**). The cause is multifactorial. Associated factors include female gender; obesity; preexisting flatfoot or accessory navicular; rheumatoid arthritis, or other inflammatory arthropathy; steroid use; and, in younger patients, elevated levels of CW6 human leukocyte antigens. The site of dysfunction correlates with the blood supply to the PTT, which includes a 14-mm zone of hypovascularity beginning 40 mm proximal to the tendon insertion at the navicular tubercle. This hypovascular zone is further challenged by mechanical stress on the PTT as it makes a sharp turn behind the medial malleolus.

PTT dysfunction may result from tenosynovitis (inflammatory cell proliferation) or tendinosis (collagen degeneration with areas of focal necrosis). The latter is more common and in this situation the excursion and function of the tendon are lost. Increased stress is placed on surrounding ligamentous structures, which gradually elongate. As a result, pes planovalgus develops. Initially, the deformity is flexible, but over time, it becomes rigid and ultimately may cause a secondary valgus ankle arthropathy.

Early symptoms include pain on the medial aspect of the ankle and longitudinal arch. Swelling is noted over the PTT. In the standing position, increased heel valgus and "too many lateral toes" may be observed on the posterior view. Standing on the toes is difficult, painful, and abnormal. Normally, when a person stands on the toes, the heel is pulled into varus by action of the PTT, but in PTT dysfunction, the heel remains in valgus or has only limited inversion on this test. With the development of fixed deformity, passive inversion is limited, and the longitudinal arch remains flattened in a non–weight-bearing position.

If only tenosynovitis is present, casting or bracing to limit the excursion of PTT may eliminate the inflammatory response. If symptoms persist after 3 months, tenosynovectomy or tendon transfer—most commonly, flexor digitorum longus to the posterior tibial tendon, which is often combined with a medial displacement osteotomy of the calcaneus—is indicated.

In the patient who has tendinosis, nonoperative options include a medial heel wedge, foot orthotic, or an ankle-foot orthosis (AFO). Surgical treatment yields better results in earlier stages of PTT dysfunction. If the deformity is not fixed, options include a tendon transfer combined with Achilles tendon lengthening and realignment procedures such as medial displacement osteotomy and/or lateral col-

Figure 19-12: Posterior Tibial Dysfunction

Dysfunction of posterior tibial tendon may result from tenosynovitis of tendinosis. Symptoms include pain and swelling over course of tendon and loss of tendon function results in loss of longitudinal arch

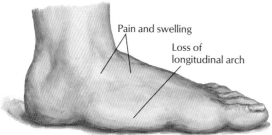

Pain and swelling

Loss of longitudinal arch

Medial view of pronated foot reveals flattened longitudinal arch

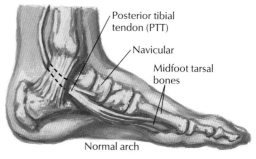

Posterior tibial tendon (PTT)

Navicular

Midfoot tarsal bones

Normal arch

Insertion of posterior tibial tendon extends beyond navicular to all midtarsal bones of foot and is the major supporting structure of midfoot

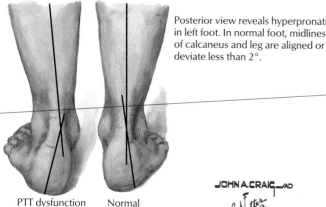

PTT dysfunction   Normal

Standing. In the standing position, increased heel valgus and "too many lateral toes" may be observed on posterior view

Posterior view reveals hyperpronation in left foot. In normal foot, midlines of calcaneus and leg are aligned or deviate less than 2°.

JOHN A. CRAIG—AD

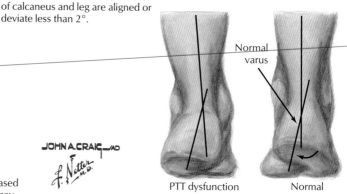

Normal varus

PTT dysfunction   Normal

Heel rise. On toe standing, normal PTT function pulls heel into varus. PTT dysfunction allows heel to remain in valgus poisition

---

umn lengthening of the calcaneus. With a fixed deformity, arthrodesis of the hindfoot joint is required.

DEFORMITIES OF THE FOOT

Hallux Valgus (Bunion Deformity)

Hallux valgus is lateral deviation of the great toe at the MTP joint. The medial aspect of the metatarsal head becomes prominent (bunion) and may be irritated and painful secondary to

shoe wear (**Figure 19-13**). Extreme angulation can cause lesser toe deformities, particularly the second toe overlapping the great toe with a subsequent hammertoe deformity.

The site of maximum tenderness is usually over the medial eminence and its hypertrophic bursa. Assess first MTP motion (which is usually normal), flexibility of the deformity, pronation of the hallux, and any lesser toe, first metatarsocuneiform joint, or hindfoot abnormalities.

Figure 19-13: Hallux Valgus

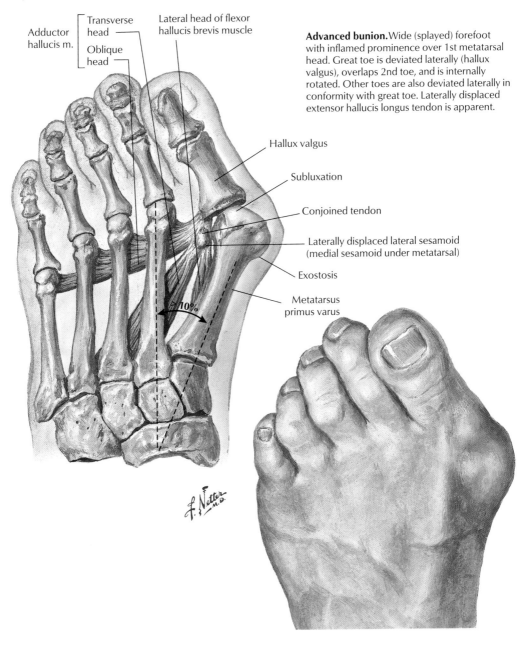

Adductor hallucis m.
— Transverse head
— Oblique head

Lateral head of flexor hallucis brevis muscle

Advanced bunion. Wide (splayed) forefoot with inflamed prominence over 1st metatarsal head. Great toe is deviated laterally (hallux valgus), overlaps 2nd toe, and is internally rotated. Other toes are also deviated laterally in conformity with great toe. Laterally displaced extensor hallucis longus tendon is apparent.

Hallux valgus

Subluxation

Conjoined tendon

Laterally displaced lateral sesamoid (medial sesamoid under metatarsal)

Exostosis

Metatarsus primus varus

10%

An anteroposterior (AP) radiograph is used to measure the hallux valgus angle and the intermetatarsal (IM) angle between the first and second metatarsals. Normal hallux valgus is less than 15°, and the normal IM angle is less than 11°. Radiographs are also assessed for sesamoid displacement, congruity and erosion of the MTP joint, shape of the metatarsal head, and any valgus deviation at the interphalangeal joint.

Nonoperative treatment includes shoes with adequate width at the forefoot, occasional stretching of the shoe at the deformity, and/or a longitudinal arch support to decrease pronation. High heels increase pressure on the great toe and should be avoided. The indication for surgery is persistent pain. Asymptomatic feet, no matter how severe the deformity, should be managed nonoperatively. The choice of numerous surgical options is based on the degree of deformity, the IM angle, and the degree of joint congruity and erosion.

Lesser Toe Deformities

Lesser toe deformities include claw toes, hammertoes, and mallet toes (**Figure 19-14**). A *claw toe* has hyperextension at the MTP joint and flexion at the proximal interphalangeal and distal interphalangeal joints. Claw toes are similar to claw finger deformities (see Chapter 16) and most commonly are secondary to a peripheral neuropathy that causes weakness of the intrinsic muscles or an inflammatory arthropathy such as rheumatoid arthritis or an idiopathic synovitis that causes laxity of the MTP joint and secondary mechanical dysfunction of the intrinsic muscles. Neurologic disorders that most often cause claw toes are diabetes mellitus and Charcot-Marie-Tooth disease. In patients with claw toes, all lesser toes are commonly involved. Pain and calluses develop on the dorsum of the proximal interphalangeal (PIP) joint, on the toe tips, and on the plantar surface of the foot beneath the depressed metatarsal head.

Hammertoe is a flexion deformity of the PIP without contracture of the MTP or distal interphalangeal (DIP) joint. The MTP joint may appear hyperextended when the patient is standing, but it is flexible with the foot at rest. Shoewear causes pain and callus formation on the dorsum of the PIP joint. A *mallet toe* has a flexion deformity at the DIP joint with or without hyperextension at the MTP joint. Pain and callus develop at the tip of the toe. Hammertoes and mallet toes are often secondary to improperly fitting shoes, particularly high-heeled and pointed-toe shoes. These deformities may be isolated to a single toe, with the second toe most commonly involved.

Nonoperative management includes wearing of shoes with adequate space in the toe-box and avoidance of high-heeled shoes. Metatarsal pads or orthotics, often combined with extra-depth shoes, may be helpful in alleviating abnormal pressure. Cushions for the corns may be helpful with hammertoes and mallet toes. Refractory cases may benefit from surgical intervention to correct the soft tissue and bony deformities.

Pes Cavus

A *cavus* foot has a high arch with the forefoot in plantarflexion relative to the hindfoot. The hindfoot is usually in varus (ie, a cavovarus foot) (**Figure 19-15**). Other components associated with a cavus foot include a plantarflexed first metatarsal and claw toes. The condition may be congenital or may develop during childhood or in the adult years. The cause is usually an underlying neuromuscular disorder, but the condition may be idiopathic or may occur secondary to incomplete correction of a clubfoot disorder (**Table 19-1**). Cavus foot secondary to neurologic conditions typically involves relative weakness of the intrinsic muscles of the foot and variable muscle imbalance of the extrinsic muscles.

Examination of a patient with no previous diagnosis includes evaluation for a possible neurologic or spinal disorder. Standing radiographs of the foot and lumbar spine should be obtained. Nerve conduction studies, electromyography, and magnetic resonance imaging (MRI) of the spine may be indicated. The *Coleman block test* is helpful in differentiating a

Figure 19-14: Lesser Toe Deformities (Claw Toe, Hammertoe, and Mallet Toe)

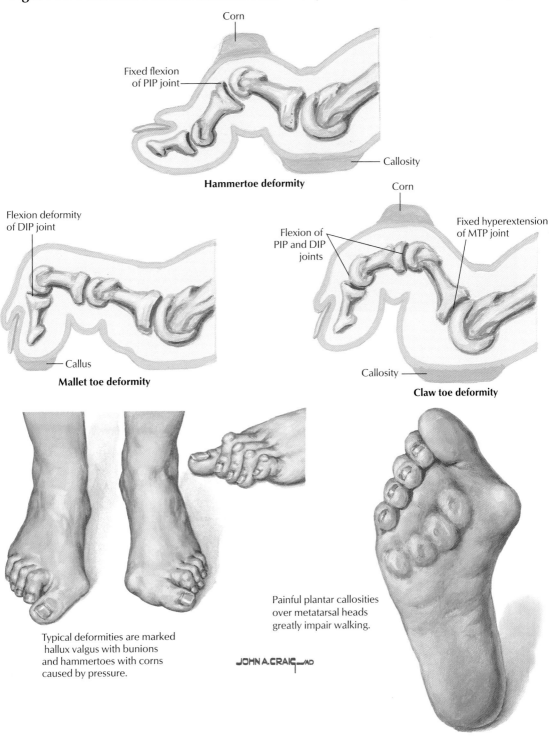

Corn

Fixed flexion of PIP joint

Callosity

Hammertoe deformity

Flexion deformity of DIP joint

Callus

Mallet toe deformity

Corn

Flexion of PIP and DIP joints

Fixed hyperextension of MTP joint

Callosity

Claw toe deformity

Typical deformities are marked hallux valgus with bunions and hammertoes with corns caused by pressure.

Painful plantar callosities over metatarsal heads greatly impair walking.

JOHN A. CRAIG—AD

Figure 19-15: Cavovarus Foot

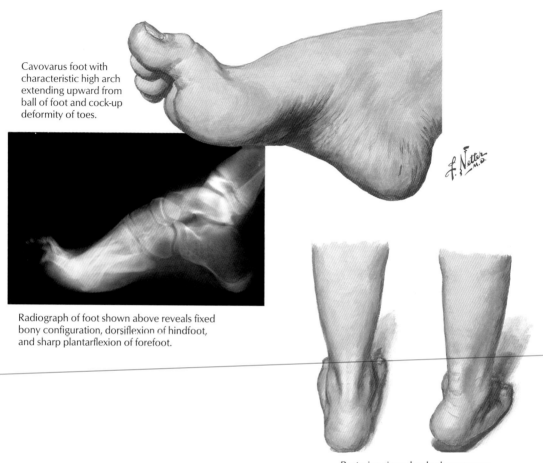

Cavovarus foot with characteristic high arch extending upward from ball of foot and cock-up deformity of toes.

Radiograph of foot shown above reveals fixed bony configuration, dorsiflexion of hindfoot, and sharp plantarflexion of forefoot.

Posterior view clearly shows varus deformity of affected right foot.

Coleman Block Test

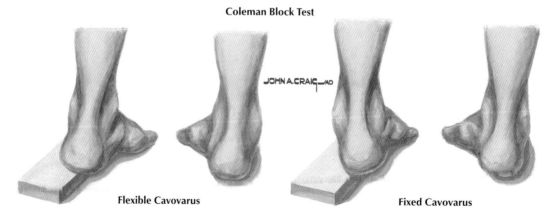

Flexible Cavovarus   **Fixed Cavovarus**

Table 19-1

Disorders Associated With Cavus Foot

Neurologic conditions
Spinocerebellar degenerative conditions
  Friedreich ataxia
Anterior horn cell deficiency
  Spinal muscular atrophy
  Poliomyelitis
  Arthrogryposis
Spinal cord abnormalities
  Diastematomyelia
  Lipomyelomeningocele
  Myelomeningocele
  Spinal cord tumors
Tethered spinal cord
Peripheral neuropathies
  Hereditary sensory motor neuropathies
  (Charcot-Marie-Tooth disease)
  Diabetic neuropathy
Clubfoot, incomplete correction
Idiopathic conditions
Trauma
  Compartment syndrome, foot/leg

flexible from a fixed hindfoot varus and in determining treatment. A 1-inch wooden block is placed under the patient's hindfoot and lateral forefoot, with the first metatarsal head off the block. With a *flexible deformity*, the hindfoot will evert into valgus when the plantarflexed first metatarsal is not bearing weight.

Nonoperative treatment includes shoe modifications, orthotics, and bracewear. Surgical treatment of any spinal pathology may stop, slow, or reverse the foot deformity. Cavus deformities are likely to progress in children, and surgical treatment is often needed in this age group. In adolescents and adults, secondary changes often require surgical reconstruction that addresses the multiple components of the deformity, including plantar fascia release, selected tendon transfers to improve muscle balance, Achilles tendon lengthening to treat equinus contracture, lateral closing wedge osteotomy of the calcaneus to correct heel varus, dorsal closing wedge osteotomy of the first metatarsal to correct a plantarflexed first metatarsal, and claw toe realignment. Arthrodesis is required for patients with hindfoot arthritis and a fixed cavus malalignment.

MISCELLANEOUS CONDITIONS

Morton Neuroma

Morton neuroma is not a true neuroma but entrapment of an interdigital plantar sensory nerve in the forefoot by the transverse metatarsal ligament and the underlying plantar fascia. Perineural fibrosis and thickening of the nerve develop. Morton neuroma most frequently occurs in the third web space, perhaps because this interdigital nerve is relatively tethered by its formation from both the medial and lateral plantar nerves. Morton neuroma occurs less frequently in the second web space and is very uncommon in the first and fourth web spaces. The condition is more frequently found in females, probably because high-heeled shoes keep the MTP joints in extension—a position that increases pressure from the transverse metatarsal ligament.

Patients note burning pain in the forefoot that radiates to the toes. This pain is activity related and is aggravated by shoes with high heels and a narrow toe box. Examination may demonstrate decreased sensation in the involved web space. The pain may be reproduced by application of upward pressure on the plantar surface of the foot with one hand (which puts the nerve between the metatarsal heads), followed by compression of the forefoot with the other hand. A palpable click during this maneuver is a positive *Mulder click*.

Nonoperative treatment involves wearing of shoes with wide toe boxes and low heels. A metatarsal pad may be helpful. An injection with lidocaine and steroid may be both diagnostic and therapeutic. Excision of the affected nerve is the usual treatment for persistent symptoms. The pain relief can be immediate and striking. The "physiologic neuroma" that develops at the cut end of the nerve can cause recurrent pain if the excision is not proximal enough.

Ingrown Toenail

An ingrown toenail occurs when the distal margin of a nail grows into the adjacent skin (nailfold), causing inflammation and sometimes secondary infection. The condition is most often limited to the great toe. Predisposing factors include improper trimming of the nail; a curved shape of the nail; and environmental factors such as tight shoes, humidity, and direct trauma.

An ingrown toenail is characterized initially by pain, inflammation, and swelling (**Figure 19-16**). Purulent drainage may develop, along with increased erythema and swelling. Treatment in the early phases of the condition includes warm soaks, placement of dental floss under the nail to direct its growth away from the skin, wearing of open-toe shoes, modification of activities, and education on proper nail trimming. Antibiotics and partial or complete excision of the nail are necessary if the pain is severe or the condition is persistent.

TRAUMATIC CONDITIONS

Ankle Fractures

Fractures of the ankle occur through a variety of mechanisms (**Figure 19-17**) and may injure the lateral malleolus (distal fibula), the medial malleolus, the posterior malleolus (posterior distal tibia), and the collateral ligaments. *Bimalleolar* injuries include fractures of the distal fibula and medial malleolus, fractures of the distal fibula combined with tearing of the deltoid ligament, and uncommon fractures of the medial malleolus combined with disruption of the lateral ankle ligaments. *Trimalleolar* fractures include fractures of the posterior malleolus. Posterior dislocation of the ankle may accompany an unstable injury, particularly a trimalleolar fracture.

Evaluation should include palpation for sites of increased tenderness. Radiographs should include AP, mortise (15° internally rotated AP), and lateral views of the ankle. A *stable fracture* is an isolated fracture without ligamentous disruption on the contralateral side of the ankle. Functional bimalleolar injuries (eg, fracture of the distal fibula and disruption of the deltoid ligament) usually show displacement of the talus in the ankle joint. However, an isolated fracture of the distal fibula or medial malleolus with significant tenderness over the contralateral ligaments but without radiographic displacement of the talus should be treated as an unstable injury unless stress radiographs show that the joint is stable.

Most stable ankle fractures can be treated symptomatically, with commencement of weight bearing in a short leg cast or clamshell walking boot as tolerated. The most common stable ankle fracture is a supination–external rotation injury limited to the lateral malleolus.

Most unstable ankle fractures are treated surgically because even 1 mm of lateral displacement of the talus reduces the contact

Figure 19-16: Ingrown Toenail

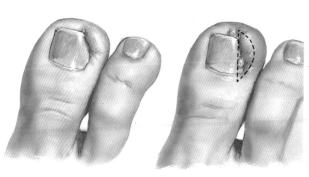

D. Mascaro

Broken lines show lines of incision for excision of lateral $1/4$ of toenail, nail bed, and matrix

Ingrowing skinfold

Inflamed and infected ingrown toenail

Table 19-2
Types of Ankle Fracture

Stable injuries
  Lateral malleolus
  Medial malleolus
  Posterior malleolus
Unstable injuries
  Bimalleolar fracture
  Trimalleolar fracture
  Trimalleolar fracture-dislocation

area of the talus by 42%, which may lead to traumatic arthropathy. Concomitant dislocation requires urgent reduction to reduce tension on compromised soft tissue.

Calcaneus Fractures

The calcaneus is the most commonly fractured tarsal bone. Most calcaneus fractures occur after a significant axial load, such as a fall from a height or a head-on motor vehicle accident. Pain and swelling of the hindfoot are usually obvious. Tenderness should be sought in other areas—particularly the back—

because concomitant fracture of the lumbar spine is relatively common. Other associated injuries include fracture of the femoral neck, tibial plateau, and ankle.

Calcaneus fractures are classified as extra-articular or intra-articular. Most commonly, the axial load is transmitted through the talus, which is wedged into the calcaneus, causing an intra-articular fracture of the posterior facet of the subtalar joint (**Figure 19-18**). The primary fracture line divides the posterior facet joint into anteromedial and posterolateral fragments. Secondary fracture lines are frequent, with resultant marked comminution and depression of the posterior facet.

Assess function of the superficial and deep peroneal, medial, and lateral plantar nerves and sural nerves distal to the fracture. Pulses, capillary refill, and temperature of the toes should be assessed. Distal paresthesias and increased swelling in the midfoot suggest a possible compartment syndrome of the foot. In addition to AP, lateral, and oblique radiographs of the foot, obtain radiographs of the spine or other areas (selected on the basis of tenderness). Special views of the hindfoot

Figure 19-17: Lauge-Hansen Classification of Ankle Fracture*

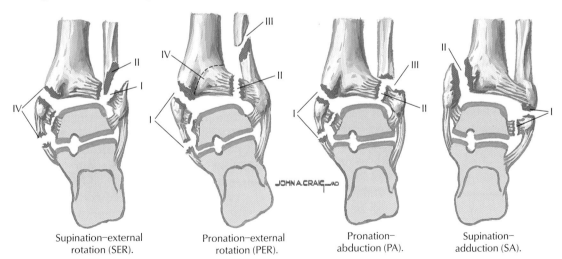

Supination–external rotation (SER).

Pronation–external rotation (PER).

Pronation–abduction (PA).

Supination–adduction (SA).

*Classification based on position of planted foot at time of injury (supinated or pronated) and direction of injuring force. Numbers are the order of fracture or ligament tear. For example, with a SER fracture, the anterior talofibular ligament is the first structure torn, followed by an oblique/spiral fracture of the distal fibula (stage II), followed by fracture of the posterior lip of the tibia (stage III), followed by either transverse fracture of the medial malleolus or tear of the deltoid ligament (stage IV). SER injury may only include stage I and II.

and computed tomographic (CT) scanning may be indicated.

Most extra-articular fractures are treated nonoperatively with casting or bracing for immobilization, avoidance of weight bearing, and early motion. Intra-articular fractures are usually treated operatively if the displacement is significant or joint depression makes the subtalar joint incongruent. Older adults and smokers may do better with nonoperative management, including avoidance of weight bearing and early motion. Operative intervention is delayed for up to 3 weeks to allow adequate reduction of swelling and reduced risk of wound necrosis. Because of frequent marked comminution, common sequelae of intra-articular calcaneus fractures include traumatic arthropathy and loss of subtalar motion.

Fracture of the Talus

Fracture of the talus is relatively uncommon (accounts for approximately 1% of all foot fractures). The neck of the talus is the most common site of injury (**Figure 19-19**). A talar neck fracture usually results from a motor vehicle accident or a fall from a height. The mechanism of injury is high-velocity axial load from the anterior cortical lip of the distal tibia with the ankle in dorsiflexion. With continued energy, the surrounding soft tissues are disrupted and the joints become incongruous; with extreme injury, the body of the talus is dislocated posteromedially.

Potential complications include delayed union, nonunion, osteonecrosis of the body of the talus, and secondary traumatic arthropathy of the ankle and/or subtalar joint, and avascular necrosis of the body of the talus with subsequent arthropathy of the ankle and/or subtalar joint. Greater displacement of the fracture is associated with increased risk of complications, but because of the vulnerability of the blood supply to the talus, even type I fractures may develop osteonecrosis.

Principles of examination, initial radiographs, and the need for special views and CT scanning are similar to calcaneus fractures. Type I talar neck fractures are initially treated

in a non–weight-bearing cast with the foot in slight plantarflexion. Displaced talar neck fractures require early reduction and internal fixation to minimize the risk of complications.

Tarsometatarsal (Lisfranc) Fracture–Dislocations

Injuries to the tarsometatarsal (Lisfranc) joint complex can range from isolated ligamentous injuries with minimal or no joint displacement to ligamentous injuries with severe displacement with or without associated fractures. Usually, a high-energy injury causes abduction or adduction of the forefoot, with some rotational component to the tarsometatarsal joints—for example, horseback riders who have a foot caught in a stirrup when they are thrown from their horses. However, the injury may result from a relatively trivial event, such as stepping into a hole with axial compression and abduction force at the Lisfranc joint.

Lisfranc fracture-dislocation has three typical patterns: (1) homolateral injury—all five rays displaced laterally; (2) isolated dislocation—the first medial ray is dislocated medially; and (3) divergent pattern—first ray deviated medially and the lateral 2 to 5 rays move laterally (**Figure 19-20**). A common associated injury is "nutcracker" fracture of the cuboid due to an abduction force of the lateral rays on the cuboid.

Examination reveals swelling and tenderness at the midfoot. A trivial foot sprain may be the initial impression, and the true extent of injury may be missed. Radiographs should be carefully examined for discontinuity of the following radiographic lines: (1) the medial cortex of the base of the second metatarsal base should line up with the medial cortex of the middle cuneiform on the AP view, and (2) the medial cortex of the fourth metatarsal should line up with the medial cortex of the cuboid on the oblique view. Other signs of injury include increased diastasis between the first and second metatarsals on the AP or oblique view, and dorsal displacement of the metatarsals in relation to their respective tarsal bones on the lateral view. When radiographic findings are

Figure 19-18: Intra-articular Fracture of the Calcaneus

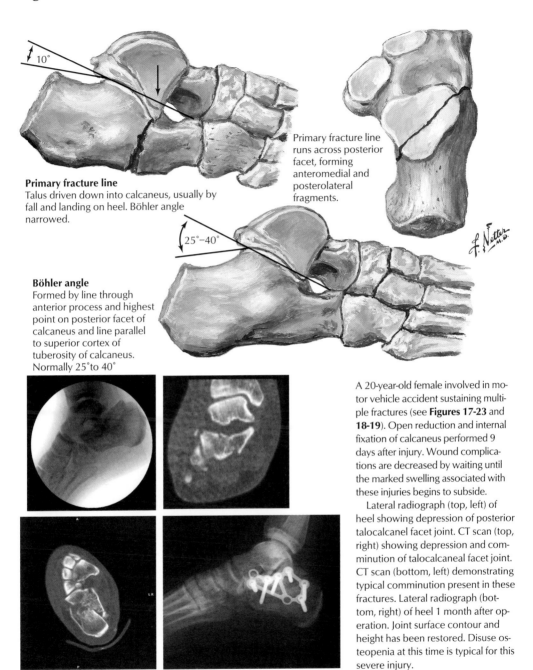

Primary fracture line
Talus driven down into calcaneus, usually by fall and landing on heel. Böhler angle narrowed.

Primary fracture line runs across posterior facet, forming anteromedial and posterolateral fragments.

Böhler angle
Formed by line through anterior process and highest point on posterior facet of calcaneus and line parallel to superior cortex of tuberosity of calcaneus. Normally 25° to 40°

A 20-year-old female involved in motor vehicle accident sustaining multiple fractures (see **Figures 17-23** and **18-19**). Open reduction and internal fixation of calcaneus performed 9 days after injury. Wound complications are decreased by waiting until the marked swelling associated with these injuries begins to subside.

Lateral radiograph (top, left) of heel showing depression of posterior talocalcanel facet joint. CT scan (top, right) showing depression and comminution of talocalcaneal facet joint. CT scan (bottom, left) demonstrating typical comminution present in these fractures. Lateral radiograph (bottom, right) of heel 1 month after operation. Joint surface contour and height has been restored. Disuse osteopenia at this time is typical for this severe injury.

Figure 19-19: Fracture of Talar Neck

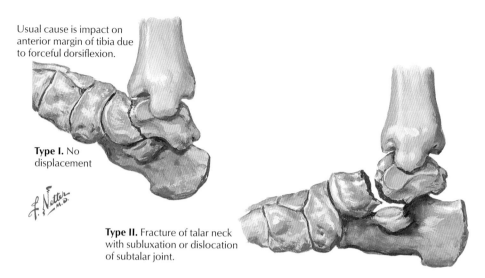

Usual cause is impact on anterior margin of tibia due to forceful dorsiflexion.

Type I. No displacement

f. Netter M.D.

Type II. Fracture of talar neck with subluxation or dislocation of subtalar joint.

normal but the examination indicates possible injury, a simulated weight-bearing view of the foot, CT scan, or MRI can denote the injury complex.

Nondisplaced fractures may be treated with cast immobilization and avoidance of weight bearing for 3 months. Fractures with any degree of displacement are treated with open reduction and internal fixation. Although the midtarsal joints have limited motion, their stability is critical for normal walking. Therefore, even 1 to 2 mm of residual displacement may cause traumatic arthropathy.

Fractures of the Metatarsals

Metatarsal fractures are common and occur secondary to trauma or repetitive stress (**Figure 19-21**). Most isolated metatarsal fractures can be treated nonoperatively by wearing of a stiff-soled, open-toed shoe. Displacement in the sagittal plane, intra-articular fracture, and multiple metatarsal fractures with shortening require surgical intervention to prevent altered pressure at the dorsum of the foot or abnormal MTP mechanics. A common problematic metatarsal fracture is a fracture of the fifth metatarsal that occurs at the

metaphyseal-diaphyseal junction (zone 3). This area has a tenuous blood supply, and bone healing is often delayed. Treatment options include non–weight-bearing immobilization for up to 3 months or screw fixation supplemented with a weight-bearing cast or brace.

Fractures of the Phalanges

Fractures of the phalanx result from either an axial load to the toe tip ("stub toe") or a crush injury from heavy objects that land on the toes. These fractures are acutely painful. Most are treated nonoperatively with a stiff-soled shoe, elevation, weight bearing as tolerated, and buddy-taping to the adjacent toe. Dislocations of the metacarpophalangeal (MP), PIP, or DIP joints require immediate reduction and subsequent buddy-taping. Displaced intra-articular fractures of the MTP joints of all toes and of the interphalangeal (IP) joint of the great toe may require reduction and pinning.

Fractures in Children

Fractures of the foot and ankle are relatively uncommon in children. Most injuries are min-

Figure 19-20: Injury to Tarsometatarsal (Lisfranc) Joint Complex

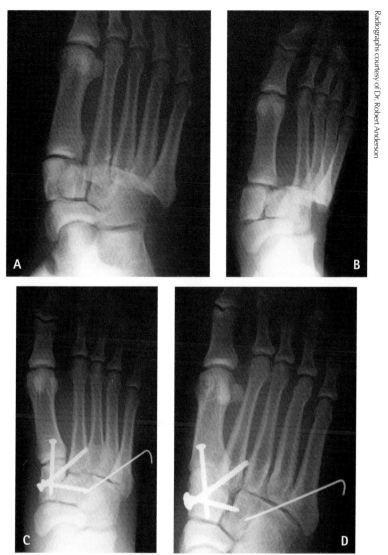

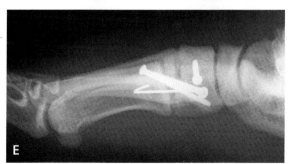

(A) AP radiograph of foot at injury; (B) radiograph of foot at injury. Postoperative AP (C), oblique (D), and lateral (E) radiographs of foot.

26-year-old male who fell while participating in sports sustaining an axial compression of the plantarflexed foot. Injury radiographs (A and B) demonstrate Lisfranc fracture-dislocation with disruption of the tarsometatarsal joints with associated fracture of base of 2nd metatarsal and subluxation of the medial cuneiform– navicular joint. Patient was treated with reduction and internal fixation (C to E). Medial column, which has no significant motion, was treated with screws to provide the rigid immobilization required for these joints. Lateral column has some flexibility and, therefore, was fixed with a smooth pin that was later removed. Patient returned to competitive sports activities.

Figure 19-20: Injury to Tarsometatarsal (Lisfranc) Joint Complex *(continued)*

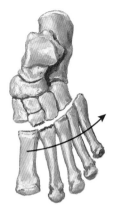

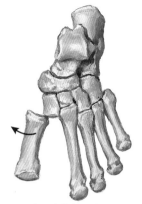

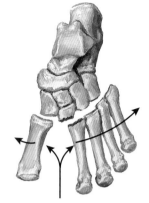

Homolateral dislocation. All five metatarsals displaced in same direction. Fracture of base of 2nd metatarsal

Isolated dislocation. One or two metatarsals displaced; others in normal position

Divergent dislocation. 1st metatarsal displaced medially, others superolaterally

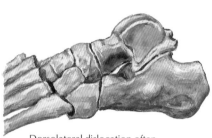

Dorsolateral dislocation often best seen in lateral view

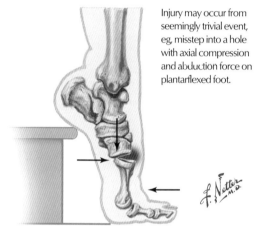

Injury may occur from seemingly trivial event, eg, misstep into a hole with axial compression and abduction force on plantarflexed foot.

imally displaced and can be treated by cast immobilization. Exceptions include intra-articular fractures of the distal tibia and open fractures (**Figure 19-22**). Lawnmower accidents are the most common cause of open foot and ankle injuries in children. These high-velocity, contaminated injuries require meticulous débridement and frequently necessitate partial amputation of the foot, as well as reconstructive skin coverage operations. Intra-articular fractures of the distal tibia are most often physeal fractures. These injuries require open reduction and internal fixation if the joint displacement is 2 mm or greater.

TENDON AND LIGAMENT INJURIES

Achilles Tendon Rupture

Rupture of the Achilles tendon typically occurs in middle-aged males who are participating in sports activities, especially basketball. The rupture typically occurs in a relatively avascular area 4 to 6 cm proximal to the tendon's insertion.

A typical patient reports, "I was starting to jump and felt a sudden onset of severe pain, like a gunshot went through my calf." However, the severe pain resolves, the patient can walk with a limp, and the injury may be mislabeled as a sprain. Examination shows

Figure 19-21: Injury to Metatarsals

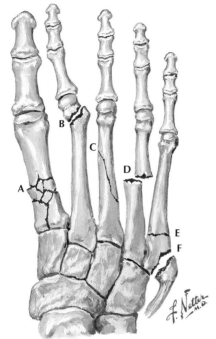

Types of fracture of metatarsal. A. Comminuted fracture. B. Displaced neck fracture. C. Oblique fracture. D. Displaced transverse fracture. E. Fracture of base of 5th metatarsal. F. Avulsion of tuberosity of 5th metatarsal.

tenderness in the area of the rupture. A palpable defect may be appreciated. The most sensitive and reliable sign is a positive *Thompson test* (**Figure 19-23**).

A delay in the diagnosis causes contraction of the muscle, difficulty in approximating the tendon, and compromised results. The advantages of nonoperative versus surgical repair are debatable. Nonoperative treatment starts with casting or bracing of the ankle in plantarflexion that is followed by gradual transition to the neutral position. The ruptured tendon is somewhat like a shredded mop, and operative repair does not achieve the tight approximation that is possible with a lacerated tendon. Decreased strength of the gastrocsoleus muscle and the possibility of re-rupture accompany each modality.

Ankle Sprain

Ankle sprains are usually inversion injuries that involve the anterior talofibular and/or lateral calcaneofibular ligaments. Although very common, ankle sprains are not always simple injuries, and they may include injury of the syndesmosis ("high" ankle sprain) and/or the deltoid ligament.

Patients typically report an inversion injury with a "pop" and the acute onset of swelling and difficulty walking. Examination should include palpation of different ankle ligaments for increased tenderness and elsewhere on the foot to exclude other possible inversion injuries, such as a fracture of the fifth metatarsal. Injury to the syndesmosis is suggested by pain on compression of the tibia and fibula 4 cm above the ankle (the squeeze test). The *anterior drawer* test is performed with the ankle in 10° to 20° of plantarflexion. Steady the tibia with one hand while pulling the heel anteriorly. Increased translation of the foot indicates injury of the anterior talofibular ligament.

To decrease the risk of chronic ankle instability, severe ankle sprains should be protected from reinjury, and functional rehabilitation then begins.

First Metatarsophalangeal Joint Sprain

First MTP joint sprain usually results from hyperextension. This injury is commonly called a "turf toe" because of its high incidence among persons playing sports on artificial turf. Grade III complete tears have marked swelling and tenderness. Radiographs are obtained to exclude other injuries. Nonoperative treatment includes compression wraps and a stiff-soled shoe worn for 1 to 3 weeks. Return to sports is possible in 4 to 8 weeks.

PEDIATRIC CONDITIONS

Clubfoot

Clubfoot (talipes equinovarus) is a common congenital deformity that includes ankle plantarflexion, hindfoot varus, midfoot cavus,

Figure 19-22: Fracture of Tibia in Children

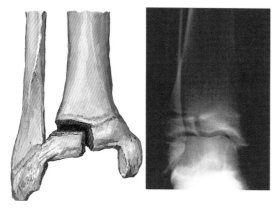

Tillaux (Salter-Harris type III) fracture of distal tibia. Fracture line extends partially across growth plate and vertically through epiphysis. Medial portion of growth plate and epiphysis remain intact.

and forefoot adduction (**Figure 19-24**). The deformity may be unilateral or bilateral, is twice as common in males, and varies in severity. Children with clubfoot typically are otherwise normal unless they have an underlying disorder such as arthrogryposis, myelomeningocele, congenital construction band syndrome, or chromosomal abnormality. Autosomal dominant inheritance with variable penetrance plays a role in some patients. The genetic association is more prevalent in the Polynesian population.

The goal of treatment is a plantigrade foot

that will function well in walking activities throughout the adult years. This goal is best achieved with corrective manipulation and serial casting implemented shortly after birth, as described by Ponsetti. An Achilles tenotomy may be necessary to facilitate cast correction. With incomplete correction, surgical release of tight structures to allow repositioning of the foot may be required. Complete medial, posterior, and lateral release should be delayed until the child is 8 to 10 months of age. Even with an excellent result, ankle and subtalar motion is less than

Figure 19-23: Thompson Test

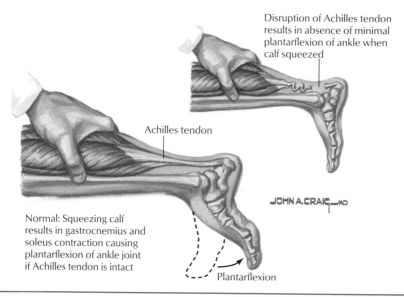

Disruption of Achilles tendon results in absence of minimal plantarflexion of ankle when calf squeezed

Achilles tendon

Normal: Squeezing calf results in gastrocnemius and soleus contraction causing plantarflexion of ankle joint if Achilles tendon is intact

Plantarflexion

JOHN A.CRAIG—AD

Figure 19-24: Congenital Clubfoot

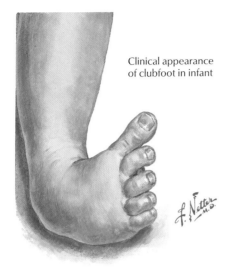

Clinical appearance of clubfoot in infant

normal, and the affected foot and calf are smaller than normal (obvious with unilateral involvement).

Calcaneovalgus

Calcaneovalgus, a postural anomaly secondary to intrauterine crowding, is very common in neonates. The ankle is markedly dorsiflexed (the foot may be pressed against the anterior surface of the tibia), and the heel is in valgus. The differential diagnosis includes *congenital vertical talus* and *lipomyelomeningocele*. Unless neuromuscular disorders are present, spontaneous correction occurs.

Metatarsus Adductus

Metatarsus adductus is a common congenital deformity characterized by medial deviation of the forefoot (**Figure 19-25**). Examination shows convexity at the lateral border of the midfoot-forefoot junction. The deformity may resolve spontaneously; this is more likely in patients with a flexible deformity (a foot that can be abducted beyond or to the line bisecting the heel). Serial casting is usually successful if persistent deformity is noted at 6 months of age.

Polydactyly

Polydactyly may be preaxial or postaxial (**Figure 19-26**). The accessory toe may be a partial toe or an entire toe, or it may include the metatarsal. Polydactyly causes problems with shoe wear. Amputation of the accessory digit with reconstruction of collateral ligaments and tendons is best performed around 8 to 10 months of age—a time when anesthetic problems are less likely but before the child begins to walk.

Syndactyly

Syndactyly in the toes occurs alone or in association with multiple other congenital abnormalities and syndromes (see **Figure 19-26**). Three types of syndactyly have been described that may be inherited as an autosomal dominant condition. Type I is most common and involves partial or complete webbing of the second and third toes. The fingers may similarly be involved. Type II is char-

Figure 19-25: Metatarsus Adductus

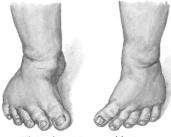

Bilateral metatarsus adductus

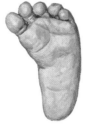

View of sole shows medial deviation of forefoot

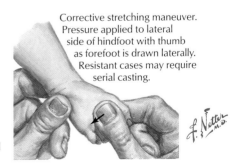

Corrective stretching maneuver. Pressure applied to lateral side of hindfoot with thumb as forefoot is drawn laterally. Resistant cases may require serial casting.

Figure 19-26: Polydactyly, Syndactyly, Congenital Curly Toe, and Overlapping Fifth Toe

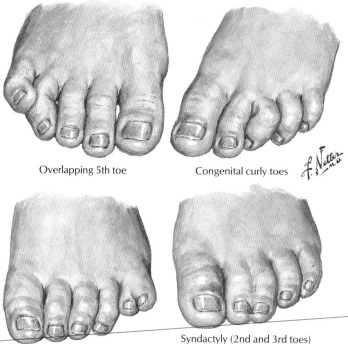

Overlapping 5th toe   Congenital curly toes

Polydactyly

Syndactyly (2nd and 3rd toes)

acterized by syndactylization of the fourth and fifth toes, and duplication of the fifth toe is common. Type III involves syndactylization of the toes with a metatarsal fusion. Syndactyly of the toes rarely causes functional problems, and surgical treatment is unnecessary unless growth causes angular malalignment.

Macrodactyly

Macrodactyly occurs when one or more digits are significantly larger than the adjacent toes. Common associated conditions are neurofibromatosis and hemangiomatosis. The static form of macrodactyly is evident when the infant is born, and subsequent growth of the enlarged digit occurs in proportion to the remaining digits. In the progressive type of macrodactyly, growth is more rapid in the affected area than in the rest of the foot. The second and third toes are more commonly in-volved. Overgrowth of forefoot soft tissues and metatarsals may be present.

Surgery is indicated when shoe fit and foot function are compromised. Procedures include reduction and syndactylization to maintain toe alignment, soft tissue debulking combined with ostectomies or epiphysiodesis, toe amputation, and ray amputation. Ray amputation often provides the best long-term results.

Congenital Curly Toe

Curly toe is characterized by flexion and medial rotation of the toe (see **Figure 19-26**). The lateral three toes are most often affected. The condition is usually idiopathic, but curly toe may be an inherited trait. Most children are asymptomatic. Strapping is ineffective. If problems develop with shoe wear, tenotomy of the toe flexors is usually successful in a young child.

Overlapping Fifth Toe

An overlapping fifth toe is a common familial condition that consists of contracture of the dorsal and medial capsules of the metatarsophalangeal joint and short extensor tendons (see **Figure 19-26**). The proximal phalanx is dorsally displaced, adducted, and rotated. The condition is commonly bilateral. When other toes are involved, congenital shortening of the associated metatarsal is common.

Approximately 50% of patients have shoe-fitting problems that warrant surgical treatment. Options include syndactylization of the fifth and fourth toes; proximal hemiphalangectomy; or a reconstructive procedure that involves a relaxing dorsal incision, lengthening of the extensor tendons, release of the contracted portion of the MTP joint capsule, and temporary pinning of the toe. Amputation of the toe is used to treat severe deformity or recurrent overlapping.

Flatfoot

Pes planus, more commonly called *flatfoot,* is a low or absent longitudinal arch that is commonly associated with increased heel valgus (pes planovalgus). It is useful to classify the disorder as a flexible or rigid deformity. *Flexible flatfoot* is more common and in many people, particularly young children, is a variation of normal foot posture (**Figure 19-27**). Patients with a flexible flatfoot have a visible arch when they are sitting and no restriction of subtalar motion (inversion and eversion). A *rigid flatfoot* is revealed by persistent flattening of the longitudinal arch in non–weight-bearing positions and restriction of subtalar motion. Flexible flatfoot is almost always bi-

Figure 19-27: Flexible Flatfeet

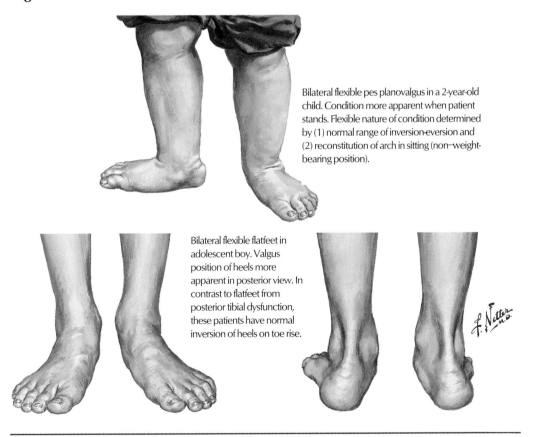

Bilateral flexible pes planovalgus in a 2-year-old child. Condition more apparent when patient stands. Flexible nature of condition determined by (1) normal range of inversion-eversion and (2) reconstitution of arch in sitting (non–weight-bearing position).

Bilateral flexible flatfeet in adolescent boy. Valgus position of heels more apparent in posterior view. In contrast to flatfeet from posterior tibial dysfunction, these patients have normal inversion of heels on toe rise.

lateral, but rigid flatfoot may be bilateral or unilateral.

Patients with flexible flatfeet are often asymptomatic. This is almost universal in early childhood. During the second decade, activity-related aching pain may be noted in the region of the longitudinal arch. Adolescents with symptomatic flatfeet often have an associated contracture of the Achilles tendon and limited ankle dorsiflexion.

Flatfoot that initially is flexible may progress to a rigid deformity. In children, this progression is more likely to occur with neuromuscular conditions that cause hypotonia or conditions associated with abnormal ligamentous laxity (eg, Marfan syndrome and Ehlers-Danlos syndrome). Severe idiopathic flatfeet may become rigid in obese adolescents or older adults.

Standing radiographs of the foot are indicated in patients with rigid flatfoot or symptomatic flexible flatfoot. Typical findings include medial deviation of the talus on the AP radiograph and plantarflexion of the talus on the lateral view.

Parents of young children with asymptomatic flexible flatfeet should be counseled that the degree of flattening of the longitudinal arch often improves, that orthotics or special shoes have not been shown to enhance the development of the arch, and that most adults with flatfeet are asymptomatic. Older patients with symptomatic flexible flatfeet can usually be managed nonoperatively with orthotics and heel cord–stretching exercises. For persistent and disabling symptoms, osteotomy to lengthen the lateral column, combined with lengthening of a contracted gastrocsoleus muscle, is indicated. Arthrodesis is necessary if joint deterioration has occurred.

In infancy, a rigid flatfoot most often occurs secondary to congenital vertical talus. This condition is uncommon and may be idiopathic or associated with myelomeningocele, arthrogryposis, or chromosomal abnormalities such as trisomy 18. Patients have a rigid, rocker-bottom foot secondary to a markedly plantarflexed (vertical) and medially deviated talus. Most patients require surgical realignment.

Tarsal Coalition

Tarsal coalition is an abnormal connection between two tarsal bones; it is the most common cause of a rigid flatfoot. The coalition may be fibrous or cartilaginous but often ossifies during adolescence—the time when symptoms typically develop. The two most common sites of tarsal coalition are between the calcaneus and the navicular and between the medial facet of the talus and the calcaneus. Patients with calcaneonavicular coalitions typically become symptomatic between the ages of 9 and 13 years, whereas patients with talocalcaneal coalitions generally develop symptoms later, between the ages of 12 and 16 years. Of note, some patients are asymptomatic, with their coalition discovered as an incidental radiographic finding.

Patients with tarsal coalition typically present with the insidious onset of activity-related hindfoot pain. In addition to pes planovalgus, the patient walks with the leg externally rotated (**Figure 19-28**). Peroneal spasticity is noted on attempted inversion. An oblique radiograph of the foot readily demonstrates a calcaneonavicular coalition; however, CT scanning is often required to confirm the presence of a talocalcaneal coalition.

Orthotics may control mild symptoms, and short-term cast immobilization can be helpful in treating patients with more severe pain. With persistent symptoms, excision of the coalition, along with interposition of fat or muscle tissue to minimize the risk of reossification, is indicated for a calcaneonavicular coalition and a talocalcaneal coalition that involves less than 50% of the facet. Arthrodesis is required for larger talocalcaneal coalitions or recurrent symptoms after excision.

Calcaneal Apophysitis

Calcaneal apophysitis, also called *Sever disease*, is most commonly seen in prepubertal active children. Affected children note activity-related posterior heel pain. The condition results from repetitive stress and microfracture of the calcaneal apophysis. This weak link is obliterated when the apophysis fuses to the main body of the calcaneus.

Figure 19-28: Tarsal Coalition

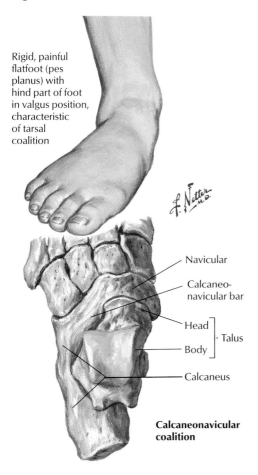

Rigid, painful flatfoot (pes planus) with hind part of foot in valgus position, characteristic of tarsal coalition

Navicular

Calcaneo-navicular bar

Head ⎤
Body ⎦ - Talus

Calcaneus

Calcaneonavicular coalition

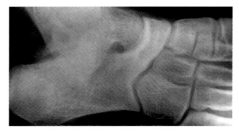

Solid, bony calcaneonavicular coalition evident on oblique radiograph

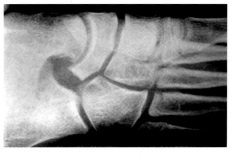

Postoperative radiograph

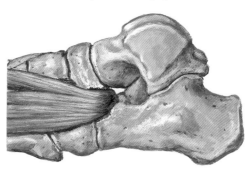

Extensor digitorum brevis muscle interposed after resection to minimize risk of recurrence

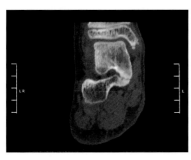

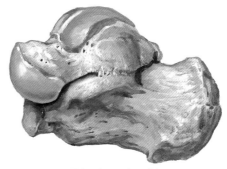

Talocalcaneal coalition

Medial facet talocalcaneal coalition. CT scan of foot in a 7-year-old male with several month history of activity-related, medial hindfoot pain. Examination demonstrated restricted inversion and eversion, peroneal spasticity on "quick" inversion, and a rigid pes planovalgus foot deformity. Radiographs, as is often the case with this site of coalition, did not demonstrate the bony abnormality. CT scan shows a narrowing of the medial talocalcaneal facet joint consistent with fibrocartilaginous coalition.

Positive examination findings are limited to tenderness at the posterior aspect of the heel. Furthermore, routine radiographs are not diagnostic because sclerosis of the calcaneal apophysis is normal. Nonoperative treatment modalities include activity modification, heel cushion inserts, and, for resistant cases, short-term cast immobilization. Operative treatment is not necessary.

Accessory Navicular

An accessory navicular is a secondary ossification center at the primary attachment site of the posterior tibialis tendon into the navicular that does not unite (**Figure 19-29**). It is often associated with flatfoot deformity. Patients may be asymptomatic or have varying degrees of discomfort and swelling that are activity related or caused by pressure from shoes on the bony prominence. The activity-related symptoms are probably caused by an inefficient

transfer of stress at the bone-tendon interface. Examination reveals prominence and focal tenderness over the medial aspect of the navicular. Pes planus may be present. An oblique radiograph of the foot confirms the diagnosis.

Treatment is directed toward relief of symptoms. Shoe modifications may alleviate pressure from the bony prominence, and casting for 4 to 6 weeks may relieve symptoms of repetitive microfracture at a synchondrosis. Resection of the accessory navicular, with reattachment of the posterior tibial tendon, is the treatment of choice for persistent symptoms. Alternatively, in some patients, fusion of the accessory bone to the navicular may be a better option.

Köhler Disease

Köhler disease is osteonecrosis of the navicular. This uncommon condition is usually seen in children between the ages of 2 and 9

Figure 19-29: Accessory Navicular

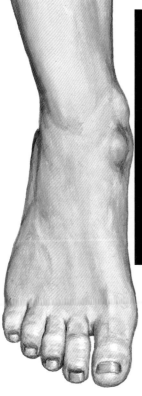

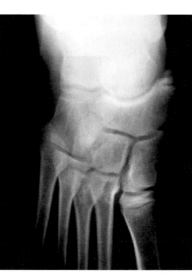

Radiograph reveals excessively large navicular with separate ossification center on medial aspect

Tender, inflamed bony prominence on medial aspect of foot over navicular

Figure 19-30: Köhler Disease

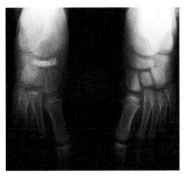 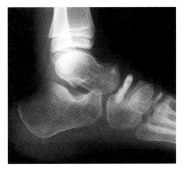

Anteroposterior radiograph shows sclerotic, wafer-shaped navicular in right foot.

Radiographs reveal characteristic changes in navicular of involved right foot.

years. An insidious onset of a limp and tenderness in the area of the navicular are the most common symptoms. Bilateral changes occur in 20% of cases. Radiographs demonstrate a thin, wafer-shaped navicular with patchy areas of sclerosis and rarefaction and loss of the normal trabecular pattern (**Figure 19-30**). Short-term casting followed by orthotic support enhances the healing process. Even without treatment, the osteonecrosis will resolve without sequelae.

Freiberg Infraction

Freiberg infraction is osteonecrosis of the metatarsal head. This disorder is most likely a result of axial loading trauma; therefore, the second metatarsal is almost always involved. Symptoms usually appear during the adolescent years with the insidious onset of forefoot pain that is activity related. The discomfort is aggravated by the wearing of high-heeled shoes. MTP motion may be limited, and pain is noted at extremes of MTP flexion and extension. Mild dorsal swelling may be observed at the MTP joint. Early in the disease process, radiographs may be normal. Subsequent findings include flattening of the metatarsal head, fragmentation, and progressive degeneration of the joint.

Treatment in the early phase of the disease process is designed to limit weight-bearing stress and includes activity modification, metatarsal pads, and a stiff-soled shoe. For patients with persistent symptoms, operative intervention to remove loose bodies and realign the metatarsal head may be necessary. With late arthritis, resection of the base of the proximal phalanx has produced good results.

ADDITIONAL READINGS

Coughlin MJ, Mann RA, eds. *Surgery of the Foot and Ankle*, 7th edition. Philadelphia, PA: Mosby; 1999.

Myerson MS. *Reconstructive Foot and Ankle Surgery*. Philadelphia, Pa: W.B. Saunders; 2005.

Thordarson DB, ed. *Foot and Ankle*. Philadelphia, Pa: Lippincott Williams and Wilkins; 2004.

Glossary of Common Orthopaedic Terms

Abduction: Movement of a body part away from the midline.

Adduction: Movement of a body part toward the midline.

Ankylosis: Marked stiffness of a joint secondary to bridging bone, cartilage, or connective tissue. Typically observed in a joint affected by end-stage arthritis.

Antalgic: Avoiding pain. "Antalgic gait" is a commonly used term that describes walking affected by lower extremity injury or arthritic condition. The affected side has a shortened stance phase.

Anteversion: Abnormal internal torsion of a bone (usually the femur).

Arthrodesis: Operative procedure to fuse a joint. The essence of the procedure is excision of remaining articular cartilage followed by positioning and fixing the bones so that bone growth is promoted across the joint. A successful arthrodesis eliminates motion, provides pain relief, and stabilizes the joint.

Arthroplasty: Operative procedure to mobilize a joint. Total joint arthroplasty is typically performed by removing the arthritic surfaces on both sides of the joint and replacing them with implants.

Cavus: Excessive height of the longitudinal arch of the foot.

Closed fracture: A fracture that does not disrupt the skin.

Closed reduction: Manipulation of a fracture or dislocation to restore acceptable alignment. No incision is made.

Comminuted: Fracture that has more than two fragments.

Condyle: A rounded process at the end of a long bone.

Contraction: Shortening of a muscle to provide joint motion (physiologic).

Contracture: Fixed shortening of a muscle, ligament, and/or joint capsule that results from injury, disease, or prolonged immobilization (pathologic).

Cox-, Coxa: Hip.

Cubitus: Elbow. Cubitus varus is adduction deformity of the elbow. Cubitus valgus is the opposite deformity.

Delayed union: A delay in normal fracture healing. A delayed union may progress to an established pseudarthrosis, or continued repair may produce a solid bony union.

Diaphysis: The shaft of a long bone.

Dislocation: Complete disruption in the normal relationship of two bones that form a joint (ie, no contact of the articular surfaces). The direction of the dislocation is described by the position of the distal bone. For example, with an anterior dislocation of the shoulder, the humerus is displaced anterior to the scapula.

Epiphysis: The end of a long bone in a child that develops from one or more secondary ossification centers.

Equinus: Plantarflexed position of the ankle.

Fracture: A traumatic break in the integrity of a bone.

Fracture-dislocation: Fracture of the bone associated with dislocation of its adjacent joint.

Genu: Knee.

Greenstick: An incomplete fracture that disrupts only one side of the bone. This type of fracture is seen more often in children because of the greater plasticity of their bones. The disrupted cortex is on the tension side of the injury.

Hallux: Great toe.

Impacted: A fracture in which one fragment is driven into the other, conferring a degree of stability.

Joint capsule: Fibrous tissue that encloses a joint.

Kyphosis: Posterior curvature of the spine.

Ligament: Specialized collagenous tissue that spans two bones. Ligaments function to stabilize joints.

Lordosis: Anterior curvature of the spine.

Malunion: Healing of a fracture in an unacceptable position.

Meniscus: A fibrocartilaginous structure interposed between articular cartilage to serve as a protective buffer. In the knee, the medial and lateral menisci are semicircular, wedge-shaped structures on the periphery of the joint that diminish walking and running stresses across the articular surface of the knee.

Metaphysis: The broad portion of a long bone. In adults, the metaphysis is adjacent to a joint. In children, the broad portion of the bone includes the epiphysis, the physis, and the metaphysis.

Myelopathy: A diseased state of the spinal cord caused by compression or a disease process.

Neuropathy: An abnormal condition involving a peripheral nerve.

Nonunion: Failure of a fracture or an osteotomy to unite.

Open fracture: A fracture that disrupts the skin.

Open reduction: An open surgical procedure in which normal relationships are restored to a fractured bone or dislocated joint.

Osteomyelitis: Infection of bone.

Osteotomy: Operative procedure in which a bone is cut and realigned.

Pes: Foot.

Pes planus: Flattening of the longitudinal arch of the foot. Pes planovalgus is a flat foot with associated heel valgus.

Physis: The growth plate. Specialized cartilaginous tissue between the metaphysis and the epiphysis in long bones of children. Provides growth in length of the bone.

Plantar: Pertaining to the sole of the foot.

Pseudarthrosis: A false joint produced when a fracture or arthrodesis fails to heal.

Retroversion: Abnormal external torsion in a bone (usually the femur or humerus).

Scoliosis: Lateral curvature of the spine.

Spondylolisthesis: A slippage or subluxation of one vertebral body in relationship to the one below. The slippage may be anterior, posterior, or lateral.

Spondylolysis: Unilateral or bilateral defect in the pars interarticularis. If bilateral, spondylolisthesis may develop.

Sprain: Partial or complete tear of a ligament.

Strain: Partial tear of a muscle, usually at the musculotendinous junction.

Subluxation: An incomplete disruption in the relationship of two bones that form a joint.

Synovium: The thin membrane of tissue that lines a joint capsule. It attaches to bone at the juncture of articular cartilage and bone.

Tendon: A cord of specialized collagenous tissue that connects muscle to bone.

Tenosynovium: Sheath around a tendon.

Tenotomy: Operative division of a tendon.

Torus: A fracture, seen most commonly in children, that buckles only one side of the cortex.

Tuberosity: A bony elevation or protuberance that is commonly the site of muscle or tendon attachment. The greater tuberosity of the femur is the insertion site for gluteus medius and minimus tendons.

Valgus: Angulation of a distal bone away from the midline in relation to its proximal partner. Genu valgum is a knock-knee deformity.

Varus: Angulation of a distal bone toward the midline in relation to its proximal partner. Genu varum is a bowleg deformity.

Frank H. Netter, MD

Frank H. Netter was born in 1906, in New York City. He studied art at the Art Student's League and the National Academy of Design before entering medical school at New York University, where he received his MD degree in 1931. During his student years, Dr. Netter's notebook sketches attracted the attention of the medical faculty and other physicians, allowing him to augment his income by illustrating articles and textbooks. He continued illustrating as a sideline after establishing a surgical practice in 1933, but he ultimately opted to give up his practice in favor of a full-time commitment to art. After service in the United States Army during World War II, Dr. Netter began his long collaboration with the CIBA Pharmaceutical Company (now Novartis Pharmaceuticals). This 45-year partnership resulted in the production of the extraordinary collection of medical art so familiar to physicians and other medical professionals worldwide.

Icon Learning Systems acquired the Netter Collection in July 2000 and continued to update Dr. Netter's original paintings and to add newly commissioned paintings by artists trained in the style of Dr. Netter. In 2005, Elsevier, Inc. purchased the Netter Collection and all publications from Icon Learning Systems. There are now over 50 publications featuring the art of Dr. Netter available through Elsevier, Inc.

Dr. Netter's works are among the finest examples of the use of illustration in the teaching of medical concepts. The 13-book *Netter Collection of Medical Illustrations*, which includes the greater part of the more than 20,000 paintings created by Dr. Netter, became and remains one of the most famous medical works ever published. The *Netter Atlas of Human Anatomy*, first published in 1989, presents the anatomical paintings from the Netter Collection. Now translated into 16 languages, it is the anatomy atlas of choice among medical and health professions students the world over.

The Netter illustrations are appreciated not only for their aesthetic qualities but, more importantly, for their intellectual content. As Dr. Netter wrote in 1949, ". . . clarification of a subject is the aim and goal of illustration. No matter how beautifully painted, how delicately and subtly rendered a subject may be, it is of little value as a *medical illustration* if it does not serve to make clear some medical point." Dr. Netter's planning, conception, point of view, and approach are what inform his paintings and what make them so intellectually valuable.

Frank H. Netter, MD, physician and artist, died in 1991.

Index

Note: Page numbers followed by f indicate figures; t indicates tables.